HYPNOSIS

Psychology Series
Series Editor: James E. Alcock, Ph.D.

Other titles in the series:

HYPNOSIS

The Cognitive-Behavioral Perspective

edited by
Nicholas P. Spanos
and
John F. Chaves

Prometheus Books
Buffalo, New York

To my mother, Pauline, who made it all possible.

——N. P. S.

To my mother, Mary, and my children: John, Christina, Eric, and Victor

——J. F. C.

Library of Congress Card Catalog number: 88-43037

ISBN 0-87975-469-9

Preface

The essays included in this collection present a coherent view toward the topic hypnosis, what we have called the cognitive-behavioral perspective. With this perspective we attempt to nest hypnotic phenomena within the larger fields of social-influence processes and cognitive behavior modification. Utilizing concepts derived from these fields, we underline deficiencies in some of the traditional approaches to the topic of hypnosis, but we also present an alternative conceputalization that has both clinical and theoretical significance.

Our views regarding hypnosis were most strongly shaped during our many years of association with Dr. Theodore X. Barber. While we were still graduate students at Northeastern University, Ted invited us to collaborate with him in his laboratory at the Medfield Foundation, where he encouraged and supported us. He became a kind of adopted mentor, though neither of us was ever formally his student. Ted defined scholarship for us, showed us what it was like to work hard, and shared with us the professional struggle endured by those who chose to swim against the tide. His energy, his dedication, and his generosity with his time will alwyas serve as a model for us. It will be obvious to readers familiar with Ted's pioneering work on hypnonsis that he has had an enormous influence on our views.

Professor Theodore Sarbin from the University of California at Santa Cruz has also had a profound influence on our views, both though personal contact and through his persuasive and eloquent writing. We are grateful for his friendship and honored by his including us in his annual "Role-Theorist" celebrations together with his many students, friends, and collegues.

All of the other contributors to this volume, students and colleagues alike, have influenced how we think about hypnosis. We thank them for their intellectual stimulation and for their friendship.

We owe a debt to our many colleagues and friends from the early days at Northeastern University and at the Medfield Foundation. In particular Drs. John McPeake and Martin Ham stimulated our thinking on many occasions and collaborated with us from time-to-time. We are grateful for their friendship. On a different note, Professor Harold S. Zamansky, from whom both of us took courses at Northeastern University, will no doubt find this book confirming his worst fear: that in rejecting the traditional perspective on hypnosis, we have thrown the baby out with the bath water.

iii

Last but not least we thank Joan Drummond and Marlene Hewitt for their unwavering secretarial support and Natalie Gabora and Lynn Jarrett for proofing many of the chapters.

Professor Spanos's work on this volume was supported in part by grants from the Social Sciences and Humanities Research Council of Canada, the Medical Research Council of Canada, and the Natural Sciences and Engineering Research Council of Canada. Professor Chaves's work on this volume was supported in part by a sabbatical leave from Southern Illinois University.

Nicholas P. Spanos
Ottawa, Ontario
Canada

John F. Chaves
St. Louis, Missouri
USA

Contents

PART THREE: HYPNOTIC PROCEDURES
IN APPLIED SETTINGS

PART FOUR: THEORETICAL OVERVIEWS
AND EMERGING PARADIGMS

PART FIVE: POLITICS AND PROSPECTS

Introduction

The Cognitive-Behavioral Alternative in Hypnosis Research

Nicholas P. Spanos and John F. Chaves

For most laypeople and many research workers and health care providers the term "hypnosis" connotes an altered or trance state of consciousness that is supposedly induced by certain repetitive verbal rituals known as hypnotic induction procedures. According to popular mythology, "hypnotized" subjects are transformed from active, planning, self-directed agents into passive automata whose experiences and behaviors come under the control of the hypnotist. At first blush, the behavior of responsive hypnotic subjects appears consistent with this popular myth. Thus, the hypnotized subject given a suggestion for arm rigidity appears to struggle in a vain attempt to bend his outstretched arm. The subject "regressed" to age five claims in a childlike voice that she is in the first grade; when asked to write her name, she prints it in large, poorly formed block letters. The "hypnotically amnesic" subject behaves as though she has lost control over her own memory functions and is unable to remember her own name. The "hypnotic hallucinator" opens his eyes and pets a nonexistent kitten that he has been told is in his lap. In short, the behavior of responsive hypnotic subjects very clearly appears to be out of the ordinary and therefore to require explanation in terms of unusual or out-of-the-ordinary causes.

SPECIAL PROCESS ACCOUNTS

Traditionally, the attempts made by psychologists and psychiatrists to provide scientific accounts for hypnotic behavior accepted at face value the idea that hypnotic procedures transform people from intentional agents to entranced automata. Since Mesmer's development of the theory of animal magnetism in

9

the late eighteenth century, theories in this area have usually begun with the presumption that hypnotic behavior differs in fundamental ways from normal, everyday social behavior. Hypnotic behavior is thought to result from mechanistic forces, agencies, or mental processes that, in some manner, displace the cognizing intending self and lead automatically to the generation of hypnotic responses (Sarbin, 1962). Theories that posit such unusual mental processes or states of consciousness to explain hypnotic responding may be labeled special process theories (Spanos, 1986b).

Contemporary special process theories do not deny that social psychological variables such as subjects' attitudes and expectations play some role in hypnotic responding. Nevertheless, these theories tend to downplay the importance of such factors and relegate them to a position of secondary importance. Also deemphasized in these perspectives is a view of the subject as actively involved in generating and achieving the effects called for by suggestions. Thus, from the perspective of special process theories, hypnotic responsiveness is accounted for in terms of mechanistic events that happen to subjects and that cause them to respond. For instance, hypnotic responsiveness is thought to reflect a capacity for passively experiencing "dissociations" among cognitive subsystems (Hilgard, 1977). Supposedly, hypnotic reductions in pain do *not* reflect subjects actively attempting to distract themselves from or to reinterpret noxious stimulation. Instead, "hypnotic analgesia" reflects the dissociation of pain behind an amnesia-like barrier (Hilgard, 1977a). The failure of subjects to recall a word list following an amnesia suggestion supposedly does *not* reflect their attempts to deflect attention away from the recall task. Instead, the memory of the list words is somehow dissociated from conscious control, and subjects are conceptualized as having lost control over their own memory processes (Kihlstrom, Evans, Orne & Orne, 1980). The reports by hypnotic hallucinators that they "see" a suggested object only vaguely, that the suggested object wanes in vividness and appears partially transparent, do not reflect the supposedly honest but incomplete attempts of cooperative subjects to generate visual imagery with eyes open. Instead, such reports are conceptualized as reflecting an unusual form of logic (i.e., "trance logic") that stems from the propensity of "hypnotized" people to experience a tolerance for logical incongruity (Orne, 1959; Orne & Hammer, 1974).

Throughout the nineteenth and early twentieth centuries special process views of hypnosis were sustained by the belief that hypnotic procedures produced highly unusual behaviors that transcended the capacities of nonhypnotized individuals. For example, hypnotic age regression was thought to actually reinstate the psychological organization of childhood. "Regressed" people were believed to have access to childhood memories and childlike patterns of cognitive activity and behavior that were indistinguishable from the memories, cognitive patterns, and behaviors of actual children (e.g., Gidro-Frank & Bowersbush, 1948; True, 1949). Relatedly, hypnotic suggestions for deafness and for color blindness were thought to give rise to experiences that were indistinguishable from organically produced deafness and colorblindness (Erickson, 1938, 1939). Hypnotic suggestions for blister formation were thought to give rise to actual blisters (Ullman,

1947), and hypnotic suggestions to engage in immoral or criminal activities were thought to cause the compulsive or automatic occurrence of the immoral or criminal behavior in question (Kline, 1958; Rowland, 1939; Young, 1948). In short, during the nineteenth and early twentieth centuries special processes theories benefited from the strongly held presumption that hypnotic procedures led to unusual cognitive changes (i.e., a trance state) that, in turn, greatly facilitated the automatic occurrence of responses to suggestions that called for highly unusual behavioral phenomena.

The special process view has also dominated the clinical application of hypnotic techniques. Within recent years, there has been a proliferation of clinical applications of hypnosis to problems in health psychology and behavioral medicine, as well as other psychotherapeutic applications. In general, there appears to have been a wide proliferation in the kinds of clinical problems to which hypnotic techniques have been applied. In the vast majority of these applications, the special process view of hypnosis has been the guiding force. Only occasionally have investigators attempted to bridge the apparent gap between hypnotic and nonhypnotic interventions.

The specialness of the hypnotic intervention has been reinforced further by the codification of special ethical standards by professional societies concerned with hypnosis. These standards pertain to such matters as the professional qualification and training thought necessary to use hypnosis. The Division of Psychological Hypnosis (Division 30) of the American Psychological Association (APA) undertook "Project Enlightenment" designed to educate other psychologists about hypnosis and help guide formulation of policy by the APA Council of Representatives. The resulting position paper began with the assertion that hypnosis is an altered state of consciousness.

CRITICISMS OF SPECIAL PROCESS VIEWS

Criticisms of special process views began with the report of the Royal Commission that investigated mesmerism in late eighteenth-century France. After a series of clever experiments the commissioners concluded that the effects attributed by Mesmer to an animal magnetism that flowed between the operator and the patient could be accounted for more parsimoniously in terms of imagination and expectant desire (Buranelli, 1975). However, the aim of the Royal Commission was not so much to account for the phenomena of mesmerism as to discredit Mesmer, his theoretical system, and his influence (Darnton, 1968). Mesmerism was not, of course, destroyed by the Royal Commission. Instead, it spread from France to the rest of Western Europe and America, became intertwined with a range of philosophical and occult ideas, and passed through complex phases of acceptance and rejection by the official science and medicine of the nineteenth and twentieth centuries (Ellenberger, 1970).

Throughout this period repeated criticisms were leveled against one or more aspects of mesmerism (and later hypnosis). However, the early critics of hypnosis—

to an even greater extent than many of its proponents—were caught up in the mechanistic/positivist heritage of the nineteenth century. Consequently, neither the proponents nor the critics possessed the conceptual tools that would enable hypnotic behavior to be understood as historically rooted, context generated, goal-directed action. Instead, early critics of hypnosis were restricted, by and large, to claiming either that hypnotic behaviors were faked, that hypnotists were the credulous dupes of wily and dishonest subjects, or that the subjects themselves were suffering from one form or another of "nervous" or "hysterical" disorder that accounted for their behavior without the necessity of positing mystical or occult explanations (Sarbin, 1962).

COGNITIVE-BEHAVIORAL PERSPECTIVES

The beginnings of the modern cognitive-behavioral perspectives toward hypnosis represented by the essays in this volume can be traced to the seminal work of Robert White (1942). Like many of his predecessors, White (1942) believed that hypnotic responding involved an altered state of consciousness and that hypnotic subjects were able to transcend normal capacities. Importantly (and somewhat inconsistently), White (1942) also conceptualized hypnotic responding as social behavior that was determined by subjects' implicit expectations and guided by their attempts to present themselves in terms of what they believed the hypnotist was looking for. Thus, for White (1942), hypnotic behavior was motivated, goal-directed, and interpersonal. Hypnotic subjects were conceptualized as sentient agents who used the information transmitted to them by the hypnotist to develop and continually refine their own image of what constituted "being hypnotized." Moreover, responsive hypnotic subjects were motivated to present themselves in terms of the conception that they and the hypnotist shared concerning what constituted hypnotic behavior. White's (1942) ideas had an important influence on the special process theories developed by Orne (1959) and Shor (1959) as well as on the more radical formulation developed by T. R. Sarbin (1950).

T. R. Sarbin and Role Theory

Sarbin was the first theorist to explicitly reject the notion that hypnotic responding required an explanation in terms of altered states of consciousness. Sarbin (1950) built on White's central insight that hypnotic responding was goal-directed action. Heavily influenced by the symbolic interactionist perspective in social psychology, Sarbin (1950) conceptualized hypnotic responding from a dramaturgical perspective. As the name implies, this perspective draws its explanatory metaphors from the theater. People are conceptualized as actors whose interactions are guided by the information they possess about one another's social roles. Roles are defined reciprocally, and interaction proceeds through mutually negotiated self-presentation and reciprocal role validation. Role enactment is rule governed and involves the tacit understandings of the actors concerning how the situation is defined, and the behaviors that are considered appropriate to that definition of the situation.

From this perspective hypnotic responding is viewed as role enactment. Hypnosis refers not to a "state" or condition of the person, but to the historically rooted conceptions of hypnotic responding that are held by the participants in the mini-drama that is labeled as the hypnotic situation. Thus, hypnotic responding is viewed as context dependent; determined by subjects' willingness to adopt the hypnotic role, by their understandings of what is expected of them in that role, by how their understandings of role requirements change as the situation unfolds, by how they interpret the ambiguous communications that constitute hypnotic test suggestions, and by how feedback from the hypnotist and from their own responding influences the definitions they hold of themselves as hypnotic subjects.

Central to Sarbin's (1950) role theoretic view is the notion that hypnotic role enactments are goal-directed actions. Contrary to the implications of special process theories, and contrary to the verbal reports that subjects themselves sometimes proffer, hypnotic responses are *not* automatic happenings. Instead, they are goal-directed doings, actions or achievements (Coe & Sarbin, 1977). The communications that constitute the unfolding hypnotic situation often convey to subjects the idea that hypnotic responses are involuntary occurrences (e.g., your arm is becoming stiff and rigid). From the role theoretic perspective communications of this kind act to tacitly inform subjects that their responses are to be defined as occurrences; as events that happen to them rather than as enactments that they carry out. Subjects who succeed in responding to these veiled communications succeed in imaginatively transforming their situation. They come to interpret their own goal-directed actions as automatic happenings.

Thus, from Sarbin's (1950) role theoretic perspective hypnotic behavior is seen as continuous with and a function of the same determinants as other complex social behaviors. Hypnotic behavior appears unusual and out of the ordinary not because it has unusual causes, but because the hypnotic role is defined as calling for unusual and nonordinary behavioral enactments.

Although his reformulation of hypnosis in terms of role enactment was ground-breaking, Sarbin conducted relatively little empirical work in the area of hypnosis. Throughout the 1960s, however, his ideas greatly influenced the voluminous experimental work conducted by T. X. Barber.

T. X. Barber and Experimental Hypnosis

Barber (1969), like Sarbin (1950), explicitly rejected the notion that hypnotic behavior required explanation in terms of an altered state of consciousness. Instead, his research was aimed at delineating the social psychological antecedents that gave rise to hypnotic responding. Much of Barber's (1969) empirical work involved the straightforward application of a relatively simple experimental design. Subjects were randomly assigned to three treatments. Those in one group were administered an hypnotic induction procedure, those in a second were administered brief instructions exhorting them to try their best to respond to the forthcoming suggestions (i.e., task-motivational instructions), and those in a third (control) group were simply asked to imagine whatever was suggested to them. Following these preliminaries subjects in all treatments were administered the same suggestions and their responses were compared quantitatively.

Using this design Barber and his associates examined a wide range of suggested behaviors including age regression, amnesia, hallucination, muscular strength and endurance, perceptual alterations (e.g., suggested deafness and color blindness), pain reduction, time distortion, memory enhancement, and others (for reviews see Barber, 1969; Barber, Spanos & Chaves, 1974). The results of these studies indicated the following: (a) The base rate of occurrence for response to even difficult suggestions like those for amnesia and hallucination was much higher than usually supposed. In other words, control subjects administered no special preliminaries of any kind frequently enacted the criterion responses called for by suggestions for age regression, hallucination, amnesia, pain reduction, and so on. (b) The administration of an hypnotic induction procedure produced only a small increment in responsiveness to suggestions above baseline levels. (c) Task-motivational instructions given to nonhypnotic subjects produced as large an increment in responsiveness to suggestion as did hypnotic induction procedures.

Barber's (1969) work, along with that of Sutcliffe (1960, 1961), Orne (1959), and others, also demonstrated that many of the more dramatic responses associated with hypnosis were, in fact, quite different from what they appeared to be. For example, Barber's (1969) careful reviews of the literature made it clear that self-injury could not be ruled out as the cause of the blisters in any of the published cases that purported to demonstrate hypnotically induced blister formation. Relatedly, upon close examination the behavior of hypnotically age-regressed subjects was found to differ from that of real children in a number of crucial respects. More specifically, Barber (1969) came to describe age-regressed subjects as adults who behave the way that they *believe* children behave. To the extent that their notions concerning childhood behavior are inaccurate (and this is frequently the case), their age-regressed performances are off the mark. Along similar lines, objective indexes of perceptual functioning indicated that hypnotically deaf subjects, despite their verbal reports to the contrary, continued to process auditory information, and hypnotically blind subjects continued to process the visual information that they claimed not to see (Barber, 1969). Work conducted in the laboratories of Orne (Orne & Evans, 1965) and Coe (Coe, Kobayashi & Howard, 1973) also made it clear that so called immoral, self-destructive, or criminal behavior induced by hypnotic suggestion was as likely to occur in nonhypnotic as in hypnotic subjects given the relevant suggestions. Furthermore, the occurrence of such responding was shown to be more closely tied to subjects' knowledge that they were participating within the protective confines of an experimental situation, than to any effects produced by hypnotic procedures per se.

Taken together Barber's (1969) repeated demonstrations that hypnotic responses were not extraordinary, and that such responses could be easily matched by the behavior of nonhypnotic subjects provided the empirical underpinnings that legitimated the view that hypnotic responding was goal-directed social-action. Special process views of hypnosis had long been sustained by the mystifying belief that hypnotic responding was extraordinary and, therefore, required the positing of extraordinary causes. Barber's (1969) extensive and systematic work was without a doubt the singlemost important factor in driving home the basic *ordinariness* of hypnotic responding, and therefore, its amenability to explanations that were framed in the terms used to account for other "ordinary" social behavior.

CONTEMPORARY COGNITIVE-BEHAVIORAL RESEARCH

In the 1970s and 1980s investigators who were heavily influenced by the frameworks of Sarbin and Barber applied these ideas to the in-depth study of discrete hypnotic phenomena. Sets of systematically conducted studies appeared on the contextual and cognitive underpinnings of suggested auditory and visual hallucinations (Spanos & Radtke, 1981), suggested amnesia (see chap. 5 by Coe), suggested pain reductions (see chaps. 9, 10, 11 by Spanos, Chaves, and D'Eon, respectively), the experience of involuntariness during suggested responding (see chap. 4 by Lynn, Rhue & Weekes), and suggested perceptual distortions (see chap. 6 by Jones & Flynn and chap. 7 by St. Jean). In each case, the phenomenon in question was reconceptualized as a doing or achievement of motivated, sentient agents who retained (rather than lost) control over their own actions, and who used contextual information to guide their responding in terms of the ends they wished to achieve.

Also appearing during this period were a series of studies that challenged the traditional view that individual differences in hypnotic responsiveness (called hyponotic susceptibility or hypnotizability) were best conceptualized as resulting from the operation of a relatively immutable trait or cognitive capacity (Diamond, 1977; Sachs, 1971; Spanos, 1986a). Instead of inferring stable traits, these investigators emphasized the stable nature of the hypnotizability test situation, and the relatively stable attitudes, interpretations, and preconceptions that people brought to that situation. Hypnotic responding was conceptualized as involving sets of modifiable attitudes, cognitive skills, and interpretations of task demands, and a number of "training packages" were developed to teach the role-relevant skills, attitudes, and interpretations in an attempt to enhance hypnotizability (see chap. 1 by Bertrand).

The present volume brings together literature reviews and theoretical statements written by investigators whose own research has been influenced by the cognitive-behavioral tradition associated with the formulations of White, Sarbin, and Barber. The book is divided into five major sections. The first provides critical overviews dealing with the conceptualization and assessment of hypnotizability and hypnotic depth reports, and with contemporary research dealing with the stability, modifiability, and correlates of hypnotizability. The second section provides comprehensive and critical reviews of the research literature associated with a number of discrete hypnotic phenomena as studied in laboratory contexts. Represented here are in-depth reviews of phenomena traditionally described as central to an understanding of hypnosis as a research area. Included here are chapters on the experienced involuntariness associated with hypnotic responding, hypnotic amnesia, hypnotic alterations of perceptual responding, hypnosis and time estimation, "trance logic" responding, and the hypnotic reduction of experimental pain.

Mesmerism and hypnosis began as applied disciplines and, until the middle of the twentieth century, most of the research associated with hypnosis had an applied focus. Most of the applications of hypnotic procedures have been in medical, dental, or psychotherapeutic settings, but particularly in recent years, there has been a growing interest in the use of hypnotic procedures in various forensic settings. The chapters in our third section review research on the varied applications of hypnotic procedures. These include several chapters on the use of hypnotic procedures for pain control in various medical and dental settings, as well as critical reviews of the literature dealing with the influence of hypnotic intervention on warts, blisters, and other dermatological changes, and the influence of such interventions in the treatment of cancer patients. This section closes with a critical examination of the literature relating to the forensic applications of hypnosis.

The fourth section provides three theoretical overviews. Each takes a somewhat different slant, and each attempts to provide a useful heuristic framework for organizing the available data concerning hypnosis and for guiding new research avenues.

Finally, the last section includes a chapter by Coe that delineates underlying economic and political factors that nurture the continued mystification of hypnotic phenomena and that reinforce the maintenance of special process accounts. This chapter takes issue with the "official" view of hyponosis researchers as objective, value-free "seekers-of-truth," and demonstrates how the divergent goals held by different interest groups within the field color the conceptualizations and definitions of hypnosis that they proffer. The chapter also provides argument and data to show that practitioners have a need to view hypnosis as a special phenomenon that causes unusual changes in the subject.

Part One

Hypnotic Susceptibility
Measurement, Correlates, and Modification

1

The Assessment and Modification of Hypnotic Susceptibility

Lorne D. Bertrand

Hypnotic susceptibility is traditionally defined as the degree of responsiveness to suggestions exhibited by subjects following a hypnotic induction procedure. During the past half century numerous scales have been developed in an attempt to enable assessment and quantification of susceptibility. This chapter discusses two issues that are central to the concept of hypnotic susceptibility: the first section will deal with selected issues in the assessment of susceptibility and will provide a brief overview of the scales that are currently available. This discussion is not exhaustive; rather, it deals with a representative sample of the available instruments. In the second section, the notion of modification of hypnotic susceptibility is discussed, and the available literature on this topic reviewed.

THE ASSESSMENT OF SUSCEPTIBILITY

Attempts to quantify subjects' level of responsiveness to hypnotic suggestions using standardized measurement instruments have had a long history. The development of these scales was intended to facilitate the prediction of subjects' performance during future hypnotic testing. The majority of these scales include two components: a hypnotic induction procedure, followed by a series of test suggestions that are representative of the behaviors assumed to fall within the domain of hypnosis. Following testing, subjects are assigned a susceptibility score that reflects their responses to the suggested effects.

A wealth of normative data was presented on the earliest scales, which are still widely used today. These scales were constructed by Weitzenhoffer and Hilgard (1959, 1962) and named the Stanford Hypnotic Susceptibility Scale: Forms A, B, and C (SHSS:A,B,C).[1] Hilgard (1965) noted that these scales were basically a revision and extension of an earlier instrument developed by Friedlander and

Sarbin (1938). Forms A and B of the SHSS (Weitzenhoffer & Hilgard, 1959) are parallel scales containing very similar items and were intended to be used when testing subjects on more than one occasion was desirable. Each of these scales contains twelve suggestions that represent three general types. The first type of suggestion informs subjects that some behavior is happening to them (e.g., hand lowering, moving hands apart, eye closure), and they are scored as passing each suggestion if the appropriate overt movement is observed. The second type of suggestion instructs subjects that they cannot perform some behavior and then challenges them to try to perform the response (e.g., hand lock, eye catalepsy, arm rigidity). Subjects are scored as passing these suggestions if the overt behavior that they are challenged to perform does not occur within a specified time. The final type of suggestion calls for some sort of cognitive or perceptual alteration (e.g., insect hallucination, posthypnotic response, amnesia) and a pass score is obtained if subjects make an overt response that is consistent with the suggestion (e.g., trying to shoo the insect away). Each suggestion is scored on a dichotomous pass/fail basis, yielding for each subject a single susceptibility score ranging from 0 (no suggestions passed) to 12 (all suggestions passed).

Normative data (Hilgard, 1965) indicated that the distribution of scores on the SHSS:A and B was roughly bell-shaped, albeit with a slight positive skew. When scores were collapsed into the categories of low, medium, and high susceptibility based on cut-off scores of 0–4, 5–7, and 8–12 respectively, the majority of the subjects in the normative sample scored in the low range (42 percent), with 28 percent scoring medium, and 30 percent scoring high. Factor analyses of the SHSS:A and B indicated the presence of three factors corresponding to the three types of suggestions discussed above (Hilgard, 1965). It was also found that differences in difficulty existed between these three groups of suggestions. Suggestions calling for simple motor responses were least difficult (i.e., passed by the greatest number of subjects), followed by the challenge suggestions, with the items calling for cognitive alterations proving to be the most difficult.

Coe and Sarbin (1971; Sarbin & Coe, 1972) have argued that the emergence of different factors in susceptibility scales reflects an artifact of difficulty level rather than the specific content of the suggestions themselves. According to this position suggestions of roughly equivalent difficulty levels (i.e., suggestions that have an equal probability of being passed) cluster together in factor analyses, which results in the generation of separate factors. According to Coe and Sarbin (1971), this artifact has led researchers to conclude that hypnotic susceptibility is multidimensional and that different cognitive abilities are employed in passing different types of suggestions, when in fact hypnotic susceptibility is best conceptualized as involving a single underlying cognitive dimension. In support of their hypothesis, Coe and Sarbin (1971) reanalyzed three studies (Ås & Lauer, 1962; Das, 1958; Hilgard, 1965) in which they demonstrated that the composition of susceptibility factors was related to item difficulty.

In response to the Coe and Sarbin (1971) findings, Tellegen and Atkinson (1976) noted that item difficulty and item content are confounded in standard scales. These investigators pointed out that, although the three factors that typically emerge during factor analysis of susceptibility scales differ in difficulty level, they also differ in terms of the the type of response that is required (i.e., simple motor movement, resisting a challenge, cognitive alteration), thus making it difficult to determine whether the factors are related to differing difficulty or differing content (cf. Balthazard & Woody, 1985 for a further discussion). In support of this notion Tellegen and Atkinson (1976) employed a multiple response choice scale rather than the typical dichotomous scale that controlled statistically for difficulty level. They reported that the usual motor and challenge factors neverthelsss emerged (these investigators did not employ any cognitive items in their study). On this basis, they argued that the multifactorial nature of susceptibility scales can best be conceptualized as reflecting different underlying psychological dimensions. However, one limitation of the Tellegen and Atkinson (1976) results was their use of a multiple response scale. Since previous research had employed a dichotomous, pass/fail criterion, the extent to which the Tellegen and Atkinson (1976) findings can be generalized to the typical susceptibility testing situation is unclear. As noted by Balthazard and Woody (1985), the use of a multiple response scale obscures the determination of easy versus difficult items because the issue of passing and failing individual items becomes arbitrary. Although the issue of the multidimensionality of susceptibility has not been definitively dealt with, a recent investigation by Spanos, Pawlak, et al. (1987) provided some support for the hypothesis that susceptibility can be accounted for by a single broad dimension.

Perceiving a need for an additional scale that included more difficult cognitive items, Weitzenhoffer and Hilgard (1962) produced Form C of the SHSS. An additional modification of this version was that the items were ordered from least to most difficult, allowing testing to be terminated for an individual subject following several failures. The distribution obtained with Form C is similar to that obtained with the earlier versions, the only difference being a somewhat more pronounced positive skew, owing to the greater number of difficult items (Hilgard, 1965).

The same year that the SHSS:C was published, Shor and Orne (1962) presented the Harvard Group Scale of Hypnotic Susceptibility: Form A (HGSHS:A). A revision of the SHSS:A, the HGSHS:A was designed with economy in mind: the entire procedure can be recorded on audiotape and administered to large groups. The advantage, of course, is that data from many individuals may be collected in the same period of time required to test an individual subject on any of the Stanford scales. An additional modification on the HGSHS:A is that the subject scores his or her own responses, thus eliminating the need for an experimenter/observer to monitor the subjects' responses. Numerous normative studies have been provided on this scale in addition to the original Shor and Orne (1963) norms (Coe, 1964; Laurence & Perry, 1982; Sheehan & McConkey, 1979), and the HGSHS:A has been found to correlate substantially with the SHSS:A and B, although its correlation with the SHSS:C has proved to be somewhat lower, once again due to the relatively large number of difficult items on the latter scale (Evans & Schmeidler, 1966).

The scales discussed thus far all have one important commonality: obtaining scores on these instruments involves assessing subjects' degree of overt response to each suggestion. In other words, the only criterion employed in determining whether a particular suggestion is passed is whether the subject made the appropriate overt response that was suggested. None of these scales assesses whether subjects who overtly passed a suggestion also experienced the corresponding subjective effects associated with that suggestion. For example, the overt behavior associated with an arm heaviness suggestion is simply the lowering of the arm; the corresponding subjective experience would be the perception of the arm as actually *feeling* heavy.

Recognizing the need for a scale that assessed both overt and subjective aspects of response, Barber and Calverley (1963) constructed the Barber Suggestibility Scale (BSS; see also Barber, 1969, for a discussion of a large number of studies that have employed this scale). The BSS contains eight suggestions similar to those employed on the earlier scales; an objective score is obtained by summing the number of suggestions to which the appropriate overt response is observed. Following testing, subjects are requested to complete a questionnaire that asks them to rate the degree (on a 0–3 scale) to which the suggested behaviors felt subjectively compelling. These scores are then summed to yield a subjective score. Another modification introduced in the BSS was that the scale could be administered with or without a prior hypnotic induction procedure. A great deal of Barber's research (reviewed in Barber, 1969) involved a comparison of responses to suggestions following a hypnotic induction with responses to the same suggestions following nonhypnotic "task-motivation" instructions—a set of brief instructions designed to enhance subjects' motivation to experience the subjective effects—that contains no mention of hypnosis. Thus the BSS can be employed under hypnotic or nonhypnotic conditions.

A study using the BSS (discussed in Barber, 1969) compared the responses of subjects given the scale preceded by (*a*) a hypnotic induction, (*b*) task-motivation instructions, or (*c*) no instructions (control). Results indicated that the hypnotic and task-motivation groups exhibited equivalent levels of overt and subjective response, and these groups scored higher on both aspects of the response than the control subjects. These findings indicate that brief, nonhypnotic preliminary instructions are as effective as a hypnotic induction procedure in enhancing the level of responsiveness to suggestions.

The most recent scale to emerge is the Carleton University Responsiveness to Suggestion Scale (CURSS; Spanos, Radtke, et al., 1983c). This instrument consists of seven test suggestions following a hypnotic induction procedure. In line with the HGSHS:A, the CURSS can be administered to individuals or groups and may be either experimenter- or subject-scored. The CURSS provides three susceptibility scores for each subject. Consistent with earlier scales, the CURSS provides an objective measure of response (CURSS:O) that reflects the number of suggestions to which the appropriate overt response was made. The CURSS:S (subjective) dimension provides an index of the degree to which the response to each suggestion was perceived as subjectively compelling. A significant addition to the CURSS is the OI (objective-involuntariness) dimension. This subscale assesses the degree to which each suggestion objectively passed was experienced as a primarily involuntary, as opposed to a voluntary, occurrence.

Normative data on the CURSS indicate that it exhibits test-retest correlations (Spanos, Radtke, et al., 1983a) of a magnitude similar to those reported for the Stanford scales (Hilgard, 1965), and that it correlates as highly with the SHSS:C and the HGSHS:A as these scales correlate with each other (Spanos, Radtke, et al., 1983b). However, the CURSS is a more reliable scale for selecting subjects who score in the high range of susceptibility than either the SHSS:C or the HGSHS:A (Spanos, Radtke et al., 1983b).

The Classic Suggestion Effect

Most hypnosis investigators assert that the experience of hypnotic behavior as an involuntary occurrence is a hallmark of hypnosis, and this pattern of responding has been referred to as the "classic suggestion effect" (K. Bowers, 1981; Spanos, Rivers & Ross, 1977; Weitzenhoffer, 1974, 1978, 1980). However, seldom has the experience of involuntariness been assessed; instead, the authors of the earlier scales simply assumed that if a suggestion is overtly passed, then it must also have been experienced as involuntary (Weitzenhoffer, 1980).

However, research has suggested that this assumption is invalid (e.g., Spanos, Rivers et al., 1977); in fact, the senior author of the Stanford scales has stated that the failure to assess experienced involuntariness is a major shortcoming of these instruments (Weitzenhoffer 1980). Normative data presented on the CURSS (Spanos, Radtke, et al., 1983a 1983b, 1983c; Spanos, Salas, et al., 1986) support these assertions and indicate that approximately half of the items that are overtly passed are experienced as primarily voluntary enactments rather than involuntary happenings.

In opposition to the findings of Spanos et al. (1977, 1986), Spanos, Radtke, et al. (1983a, 1983b, 1983c), and Weitzenhoffer (1980), some authors assert that the Stanford scales do adequately assess the classic suggestion effect (e.g., K. Bowers, 1981; Hilgard, 1981; Kihlstrom, 1985). K. Bowers (1981) presented the results of a study in which he assessed both overt responding and the experience of involuntariness on the SHSS:A and C. Results of this investigation indicated that a substantial portion of overtly passed items on the Stanford scales were rated as primarily voluntary. While Bowers's discussion focused on the objectively passed items that were rated as involuntary, the discrepancy between objective responding and the experience of involuntariness was still apparent in his data.

More recently, Kihlstrom (1985) has suggested that the hypnotic induction procedure used with the CURSS implicitly biases subjects toward overt behavioral compliance with the test suggestions, and that this bias is responsible for the discrepancy between O and OI scores. Kihlstrom further argued that this compliance effect does not present a problem with the Stanford scales, and that these scales do provide an adequate assessment of the classic suggestion effect.

Spanos, Lush, et al. (1986) provided a direct test of Kihlstrom's (1985) compliance hypothesis. Subjects in this study were administered both the CURSS and a group version of SHSS:C on separate days. Additional subscales were added to the SHSS:C to enable the assessment of subjective and involuntariness aspects of response. Half of the subjects received the CURSS induction prior to the test suggestions from the CURSS and the SHSS:C; the remaining subjects received the SHSS:C induction prior to receiving both scales. Results of this experiment indicated that, regardless of the type of induction employed, equivalent and significant O-OI discrepancies were observed on both scales. Thus, Kihlstrom's hypothesis that the CURSS induction biases subjects to overt compliance proved untenable.

We now turn to a discussion of the modification of hypnotic susceptibility, a topic that has generated much controversy and a great deal of research in the past two decades.

MODIFICATION OF HYPNOTIC SUSCEPTIBIITY

Hypnotic susceptibility has been found to be relatively stable over intervals as long as ten years (Hilgard, 1965). This stability has led some investigators to conclude that susceptibility represents a traitlike personality attribute. This attribute is held to be a preexisting capacity for dissociation (K. Bowers, 1976; Hilgar, 1977, 1979). Individual differences in this dissociative capacity are believed to account for both the range of susceptibility scores in any sample and the relatively high test-retest correlations on susceptibility scales. Although these investigators acknowledge a role for social psychological variables such as attitudes and expectations in determining susceptibility scores, these variables are presumed to operate *in addition* to the basic ability to experience dissociation (K. Bowers, 1976; Kihlstrom, 1985; Perry, 1977). From this perspective, large gains in susceptibility would not be obtained using any training procedure since training may enhance the relatively minor effects of social psychological variables but will have little if any effect on dissociative ability. This position is well delineated by the following quotation:

> There is no good evidence that a nonresistant low-scoring [subject] or patient can be made into a somnambulist by a course of training . . . . Once resistances have been overcome, and the individual is cooperative, the level of hypnotizability tends to remain quite constant and, what is interesting, that level is remarkably well predicted by initial testing, with only a few deviant cases. (Hilgard, 1982, 396)

On the other hand, social psychological accounts of hypnotic behavior do not hold that any sort of dissociative mechanism is necessary to achieve optimal response to hypnotic suggestions. From this perspective, variables such as subjects' interpretations of the demands contained within suggestions, the use of suggestion-appropriate imaginings, attitudes, and expectations interact to produce responsiveness to suggestions. At this point, an example will be useful. In a typical suggestion for arm levitation subjects are informed that their arm is beginning to feel lighter and lighter, and as it begins to feel lighter, it begins to rise in the air." Further, they are told to "imagine that your arm is like a balloon. Imagine that air is being pumped into it making it feel lighter and lighter" (Spanos, Radtke, et al., 1983d). From a social psychological position this suggestion can be viewed as including two requests. First, it tacitly asks subjects to raise their arms and, second, it asks them to disavow responsibility for their movement and experience it as an involuntary occurrence (Bertrand & Spanos, in press; Spanos, 1982). Subjects can respond to the first request in one of two ways: they can comply with the request and raise their arms, in which case they will objectively pass the suggestion. Alternatively, they may adopt a passive "wait and see" attitude whereby they will not make an overt movement; instead, they will wait passively to see if their arms will rise of their own accord. When they do not rise they fail the suggestion. In response to the second request, subjects who objectively pass the suggestion may engage in the cognitive imagining strategy contained within the suggestion (i.e., arm as balloon), in which case they can attribute their behavior to the balloon rather than to their own voluntary movement. In this case, subjects will exhibit the classic suggestion effect by overtly enacting the required behavior, but also by experiencing it as an involuntary occurrence.

From the social psychological position, then, the stability of hypnotic susceptibility over time reflects the fact that most subjects do not undergo any training designed to modify their interpretations of test suggestions or their utilization of suggestion-related imaginings between the two testings. A prediction of this position is that if subjects are administered a training procedure that is designed to modify these variables, substantial increments in susceptibility may be obtained. We now turn to a discussion of the research that has dealt with the modification of susceptibility.

Attempts to Enhance Dissociative Ability

A number of studies have employed modification procedures designed to produce alterations in consciousness, thereby increasing hypnotic susceptibility. These studies have used such varied procedures as meditation training (Heide, Wadlington & Lundy, 1980; Spanos, Gottlieb & Rivers, 1980; Spanos, Stam, et al., 1980), "personal growth" training (Tart, 1970), repeated hypnotic induction procedures tailored to individual subjects (Ås, Hilgard & Weitzenhoffer, 1963; Cooper et al., 1967), and electroencephalographic (EEG) biofeedback training (London, Cooper & Engstrom, 1974). Although most of these procedures produced significant enhancements in susceptibility, the actual magnitude of the increases was quite small (a detailed review of these studies may be found in Diamond, 1974, 1977, 1982; Perry, 1977).

Other studies have been premised on the assumption that increasing subjects' levels of relaxation during hypnosis will lead to enhancements in susceptibility. Three studies (Simon & Salzberg, 1981; Wickramasekera, 1972, 1973) reported that electromyographic (EMG) biofeedback training resulted in substantial increases in susceptibility. However, these investigators did not provide information regarding baseline EMG levels or changes in EMG levels across training sessions, thus making it unclear whether the reported changes in susceptibility levels were related to changes in EMG levels. Two recent studies (Radtke et al., 1983; Spanos & Bertrand, 1985) found that EMG training did not lead to enhancements in susceptibility, even though this training did lead to higher levels of relaxation. Other studies employing progressive relaxation training procedures rather than biofeedback also reported no or small enhancements in susceptibility (Leva, 1974; Springer, Sachs & Morrow, 1977; Simon & Salzberg, 1981; Radtke et al., 1983). A study reported by Sanders and Reyher (1969) suggested that sensory restriction procedures produced large increments in susceptibility; however, a number of failures to replicate this effect are available (Levitt et al., 1962; Shor & Cobb, 1968; Talone, Diamond & Steadman, 1975).

The data reported thus far are consistent with a dissociation hypothesis of hypnotic behavior. Since the capacity to experience dissociation is believed to be unmodifiable, none of these procedures could be expected to produce dramatic enhancements in susceptibility. However, these data are also consistent with a social psychological approach to hypnosis. According to this position, subjects' interpretational sets and utilization of cognitive strategies, as well as attitudes and expectations, are held to be the important variables leading to hypnotic responsiveness. None of the procedures discussed above attempted to manipulate these factors, thus the failure to observe substantial increments in susceptibility is not surprising.

Studies Based on Social Psychological Models

A large number of studies have attempted to modify the social psychological variables discussed above and, in general, have met with considerably greater success than the procedures discussed earlier. One early investigation (Sachs & Anderson, 1967) initially employed low- and medium-susceptible subjects and gave them several training sessions that included discussion of the subjective experiences associated with various suggestions; practice of various suggestions; and the presentation of reinforcement for appropriate responses. Following training, subjects were posttested using the same instrument on which they had been pretested. Results indicated a substantial increment in both objective responses (mean increment of 4.00 on the 12-point SHSS:C; Weitzenhoffer & Hilgard, 1962), and on the subjective experiences scale (mean increment of 3.5 on the 24-point scale). Unfortunately, this study did not incorporate a no treatment control group, so the increments in susceptibility could not be assumed with certainty to have resulted from the training sessions.

This problem was rectified in a study by Kinney and Sachs (1974); in addition, a second posttest was given one month after an initial posttest to ascertain the long-term effects of training. Results indicated that susceptibility significantly increased from pretest to initial posttest and remained at the higher level on the second posttest for the treatment group; control subjects exhibited no changes across testings. A further investigation by Springer, Sachs, and Morrow (1977) compared this training procedure with a progresssive-relaxation procedure and found that susceptibility was enhanced to a much greater degree with training than with relaxation.

Although these early studies provided support for the contention that hypnotic susceptibility can be modified by manipulating social psychological variables, three problems limit their generalizability. First, although the training procedures used in each study were similar, these procedures were not standardized, so it is impossible to determine what differences in methods individual subjects received. Second, only one study (Sachs & Anderson, 1967) assessed subjective experiences, and these subjective experiences did not measure perceived involuntariness of response, a defining characteristic of the "classic suggestion effect" as discussed above. Finally, subjects in these studies were posttested using only the same susceptibility scales on which they had been pretested, a method that did not allow for the generalization of the results to novel suggestions.

A number of studies have taken these criticisms into account and have reported positive results. For example, Diamond (1972) employed a standardized training procedure that included information designed to dispel negative attitudes of hypnosis, along with information that clarified the responses and subjective experiences that were expected of subjects. This information was presented by a videotaped model who was also shown responding to various suggestions. Results indicated that subjects who received this complete training package scored significantly higher than they had on the pretest on two different posttests of overt susceptibility. Moreover, this training package led to greater enhancements than training procedures that included only the motivational instructions and the behavioral modeling, only motivational instructions alone, or a no-treatment control group. In short, the Diamond study indicated that training procedures that include information designed to clarify subjects' interpretations of the types of responses expected of them during hypnosis are optimal for producing enhancements in susceptibility. A study by Commins, Fullam, and Barber (1975) used a similar training package and achieved comparable results, although the susceptibility increments were of smaller magnitude than those reported by Diamond (1972).

Other studies have exposed subjects to attempts to modify only a single social psychological variable such as attitudes or imagery strategies (e.g., Gur, 1974; Reilley et al., 1980; Crouse & Kurtz, 1984). In all cases, these single variable studies produced only small susceptibility enhancements. These findings suggest that modification attempts that employ procedures containing multiple components will be the most effective in enhancing susceptibility. A number of recent studies using the same training package have attempted to delineate the components that are necessary to produce large and reliable increments in susceptibility. The results of these studies will be summarized in the next section.

The Carleton Skill Training Package

A line of research initiated by Spanos and his colleagues has employed a standardized modification procedure (the Carleton Skill Training Package [CSTP]) and has obtained evidence that large and stable enhancements in susceptibility can be obtained following a single training session. This procedure is premised on the assumption that responding to hypnotic suggestions, and experiencing the corresponding subjective effects, can be most usefully conceptualized as a skill and, like most skills, can be learned and improved upon with appropriate training and practice.

The CSTP consists of three relatively distinct components, each of which is intended to address a social psychological variable believed to be related to hypnotic responsiveness. First, subjects are presented with tape-recorded introductory information that is designed to dispel myths about hypnosis, as well as any anxieties that subjects may have at the prospect of becoming hypnotized. The primary objective of presenting this information is to foster positive attitudes about hypnosis. The second component includes a discussion of the ambiguities contained in hypnotic suggestions and the importance of employing suggestion-consistent imaginings to produce the experience of involuntary responding. Subjects are informed that suggested behaviors do not just happen, but rather that they represent responses that subjects must actively cause to happen. To reinforce this information, subjects then view a two-part videotape in which a model is seen overtly responding to four different suggestions while concurrently verbalizing the imaginings and sensations she is experiencing while she performs the responses. The second part of the videotape consists of an interview with the model following each suggestion, in which she provides a more detailed description of her cognitive activity during her responses. The final component of the package involves a series of practice suggestions in which subjects are encouraged to make use of the strategies they have heard discussed in order to enact the suggestions and also to produce the corresponding subjective experience of involuntariness.

The first research to employ this training package was reported by Gorassini and Spanos (1986). These investigators tested subjects who had pretested as low or medium on the CURSS (Spanos, Radtke, et al., 1983c) in one of four groups. Subjects in one group received the complete training package described above, followed in separate sessions by posttests on both the CURSS and a version of the SHSS:C (Weitzenhoffer & Hilgard, 1962) modified for group administration. Overt and subjective response to suggestions was assessed during each susceptibility testing. A second group received the initial information designed to inculcate positive attitudes, as well as the opportunity to practice suggestions; however, this group did not view the videotape of the model responding to suggestions and discussing her strategies. A third group simply received practice with various suggestions without any interpretational information. A fourth group served as a no-treatment control and did not receive any information between the pretest and the two posttests.

Results of this study indicated that subjects in the complete package, the information plus practice, and the practice-alone groups scored significantly higher on the overt dimension of the CURSS on posttest than did the no-treatment control group. However, subjects who received the complete CSTP exhibited a substantially greater enhancement (mean change score of 2.97 on the 7-point overt scale) than did subjects in any of the other groups. Interestingly, on the objective-involuntariness dimension of the CURSS, only subjects given the complete package exhibited a significant increment from pre- to posttest. A similar pattern of results emerged on the SHSS:C posttest, with over 50 percent of the initial low-and medium susceptible subjects in the complete training group scoring in the high ranges on both the CURSS and the SHSS:C. These findings strongly suggest that substantial increments in both objective and involuntariness aspects of hypnotic responding can be obtained by employing a modification package that trains subjects in the appropriate interpretation of the ambiguous demands contained in most suggestions, as well as by training them in the appropriate use of cognitive strategies not only to enact the required overt response, but also to interpret this response as an involuntary occurrence.

Further research by Spanos and his colleagues has been aimed at delineating the critical variables in the CSTP that are responsible for the large increments in overt and subjective responding. A study by Spanos, Robertson, et al. (1986) compared the complete CSTP with a partial training package that included only information designed to clarify misconceptions about hypnosis and to inculcate positive attitudes along with information that encouraged subjects to engage in suggestion-related imaginings. However, no information was given regarding how suggestions were to be interpreted. Subjects were shown the videotape of the model responding to various suggestions, but the interview in which the model discusses her interpretation of each suggestion was omitted. A third group did not receive any training; instead, these subjects were instructed to simulate the behavior of an excellent hypnotic subject on both posttests (Orne, 1979). Once again, a fourth group served as a no-treatment control and simply received the pretest and two posttests with no intervening training. Results indicated that subjects given both the complete CSTP and partial training showed equivalent enhancements in positive attitudes toward hypnosis; however, subjects in the complete-package treatment exhibited much larger increments in both objective and subjective components of susceptibility than did subjects in either the partial training or no treatment groups. Interestingly, subjects instructed to simulate hypnosis showed higher overt and subjective susceptibility scores on the posttests than did subjects in any other group. We shall return to this finding in the next section.

In a further investigation, Spanos, Cross, et al. (1987) assessed subjects on measures of imagery vividness and absorption before exposure to the complete CSTP. In addition, after training but before their susceptibility posttest, attitudes toward hypnosis were assessed. Results indicated that the gains exhibited in susceptibility following exposure to the CSTP were predicted by both attitudes and imagery vividness. In short, subjects who continued to hold negative attitudes following training showed much smaller increments in susceptibility than did subjects whose attitudes were positive. Likewise, a high degree of imagery vividness prior to training was associated with larger gains in susceptibility than were lower scores on imagery.

The Spanos, Robertson, et al. (1986) and the Spanos, Cross, et al. (1987) studies indicated that the combination of positive attitudes, the presence of imaginal skills, and the presentation of a training procedure that provides subjects with an appropriate interpretational set are the necessary components for producing substantial enhancements in hypnotic susceptibility. The absence of one or more of these components will lead to small gains in susceptibility.

The Validity of Modification

One issue that must be dealt with in any research that relies on subjective reports is that of compliance. In any modification training procedure, a considerable amount of time is spent with individual subjects in attempting to increase their responsiveness. In addition, subjects are aware of the purpose of the research. These two aspects of the modification experiment raise the possibility that subjects may be simply complying with the experimental demands, engaging in the appropriate overt behavior, and then rating their responses as involuntary occurrences in the absence of the actual subjective effects called for by the suggestions. In short, these subjects may be simply faking throughout their posttest sessions. To answer this potential criticism, it is necessary to examine the data from a number of sources.

Some studies have posttested modified subjects on tasks that are quite different from those in which they received practice during training (e.g., Gfeller, et al., 1985; Spanos, de Groh & de Groot, 1987), and, in addition, in a number of studies the posttests have been conducted by an experimenter different from the person who conducted the training session (e.g., Gorassini & Spanos 1986; Spanos, de Groh & de Groot 1987). In fact, the experimenters who carried out the posttests typically were unaware of subjects' group assignments. In all of these studies subjects who had obtained higher scores following modification passed the novel suggestions, regardless of the identity of the experimenter. While these results do not rule out compliance as a possible account of the findings, they do suggest that if subjects are simply faking they are doing so with great consistency across both novel suggestions and different experimenters.

A study by Spanos et al. (1986) added further evidence against a compliance interpretation. These investigators tested subjects who had been modified nine to thirty months earlier on the SHSS:C. The experimenter who conducted this posttest was not the same person who had trained the subjects originally. Results indicated that these subjects maintained substantial gains in susceptibility even after this relatively long interval. These findings suggest not only that training-induced increments in susceptibility are stable over time, but also argue against a compliance interpretation. It is likely that any demands for compliance would be considerably lessened after this period of time.

The most striking evidence against a compliance interpretation comes from studies in which modified subjects have been compared with simulators and with natural high susceptibles who scored in the high range on various scales without undergoing a training procedure. For example, Gorassini and Spanos (1986) compared their modified high susceptibles with a group of natural highs that were matched according to their overt CURSS scores. These groups did not differ on either subjective experiences or ratings of nonvolition. Importantly, modified and natural highs showed equivalent discrepancies between their overt and involuntariness scores, a pattern discussed earlier. If modified subjects were simply complying with experimental demands, one might expect that they would rate all of their overt responses as involuntary happenings, rather than exhibiting the normal discrepancy. The studies by Gfeller et al. (1985) and Spanos, de Groh, and de Groot (1987) also found that the responses of modified subjects on novel suggestions were indistinguishable from those of natural highs.

The Spanos, Robertson, et al. (1986) study compared the responses of modified high susceptible subjects with those of subjects instructed to simulate high susceptibility. Most investigators recognize that simulating subjects tend to overplay the hypnotic role and respond to a great degree to most test suggestions (e.g., Orne, 1979; Spanos, 1986). When simulating and nonsimulating high susceptible subjects perform differently, it suggests that the nonsimulating subjects are not simply engaging in faked behavior. Spanos, Robertson, et al. (1986) found that simulating subjects obtained higher posttest scores on all dimensions of the CURSS than did modified high susceptibles. Importantly, while nine out of fifteen modified subjects exhibited the typical discrepancy between overt responding and ratings of nonvolition, all but one simulating subject obtained identical objective and involuntariness scores. This pattern of findings suggests that compliance is not a viable explanation for the performance of subjects who have been administered a modification training procedure.

OVERVIEW AND CONCLUSIONS

Numerous methods have been devised for assessing the capacity of individuals to experience suggested effects during hypnosis. Many of these scales have been carefully standardized, and a great deal of normative data have been presented on them. The relative stability of susceptibility over time has led to speculation about whether any procedures can be used to enhance scores on these scales. Thus, several attempts to modify hypnotic susceptibility have been reported, and the results of these attempts hold implications for the current theoretical controversy in hypnosis. On the one hand, investigators who view hypnosis as an altered state of consciousness have argued that the primary determinant of an individual's susceptibility is his or her ability to experience dissociation. Because this ability supposedly reflects a stable, traitlike characteristic, it is very difficult, if not impossible, to modify. Early modification studies appeared to support this conclusion because they typically obtained only small enhancements in susceptibility.

The alternative theoretical perspective, based on social psychological models, suggests that hypnotic behavior is strategic and does not reflect the operation of a dissociative mechanism. According to this position, subjects respond or do not respond to hypnotic suggestions in accordance with their attitudes, expectations, and interpretations of the often-ambiguous demands that constitute hyponotic situations. Susceptibility is viewed as a skill that can be substantially enhanced by providing subjects with training that attempts to clarify these ambiguities and inculcate positive attitudes and expectancies. Consistent with this view, a number of recent studies employing the Carleton Skill Training Package have obtained large increments in both overt and subjective aspects of susceptibility. These results argue strongly against views of susceptibility as a trait-like characteristic, and instead suggest that hypnotic responsiveness can be understood by examining the social psychological variables that operate in the hyponotic situation.

NOTES

Preparation of this chapter was supported by a Natural Sciences and Engineering Research Council of Canada Postdoctoral Fellowship. Address correspondence to Lorne D. Bertrand, Department of Psychology, The University of Calgary, 2500 University Drive N.W., Calgary, Alberta, Canada, T2N 1N4.

1. By necessity, only a few representative susceptibility scales can be discussed in this chapter. The interested reader is referred to a chapter in Edmonston (1986), which provides an exhaustive catalogue of methods for assessing susceptibility from the 1800s through the late 1970s.

2

Correlates of Hypnotic Susceptibility

Margaret de Groh

INTRODUCTION

Since the inception of hypnosis research, investigators have attempted to ascertain the "type" of individual that responds to hypnotic suggestions. For example, Charcot (1882) and many of his nineteenth-century contemporaries (e.g., Janet, Babinski) believed that only those constitutionally predisposed to hysteria could be hypnotized. This view was dispelled only after numerous studies clearly demonstrated that clinically diagnosed hysterics were no more hypnotizable than nonhysterics or even "normal" (i.e., college students) controls (for a review see Barber, 1964). Yet, even after college students became the most common experimental subjects, many investigators still expected "abnormal" personality characteristics to separate the hypnotically responsive from the unresponsive. Many studies investigated the relationship between hypnotic susceptibility and such variables as neuroticism and repression, as well as subscales of the Minnesota Multiphasic Personality Inventory (MMPI). Although some positive results were reported, the majority of studies failed to find a relationship between hypnotic responding and these indexes of psychopathology. Barber (1964) offers an extensive review of studies investigating the relationship between susceptibility and neuroticism as well as repression, and Hilgard (1965) and Deckert and West (1963) have reviewed the results of the MMPI and susceptibility.

In recent decades the search for a link between hypnotic responding and psychopathology has waned. Repeated demonstrations of intraindividual consistency in hypnotic susceptibility levels (as measured with standardized scales; see chap. 1), however, have maintained the search for enduring personality characteristics that may successfully predict responsiveness. Personality inventories such as the California Psychology Inventory (CPI), the Maudsley Personality Inventory (MPI), and the Myers-Briggs Inventory (MBI) have all been correlated with susceptibility.

Once again, extensive reviews of the largely negative results have been reported elsewhere (see Barber, 1964; Hilgard, 1965; Hilgard & Lauer, 1962).

The relationship of hypnotic susceptibility to a variety of other specific personality characteristics, such as extraversion (see Barber, 1964), locus of control (Austrin & Pereira, 1978; Diamond, Gregory, Lenney, Steadman & Talone, 1974; Klemp, 1969), persuadability/influenceability (Moore, 1964), and social desirability (Dermen & London, 1965), have also been investigated. Again, although some positive results have been reported, the correlations have been small, and even these positive results have often been followed by failures to replicate.

Given the largely negative results obtained with psychopathology measures, it is not surprising that some researchers turned their attention to the relationship of positive "adjustment" characteristics to susceptibility. The relationship of hypnotic susceptibility to sociability (Barber, 1956; Dermen & London, 1965; Lang & Lazovik, 1962), emotional stability (Barber, 1956; Levitt, Brady & Lubin, 1963; Weitzenhoffer & Weitzenhoffer, 1958), cooperativeness (see Barber, 1964), and trust (Barber, 1960; Barber & Glass, 1962; Roberts & Tellegen, 1973) have all been investigated. At first the results of positive adjustment variables were encouraging. Unfortunately, positive results were usually obtained in studies employing small sample sizes (e.g., Barber, 1956, 1960; Lang & Lazovik, 1962; Levitt, Brady & Lubin, 1963), and attempts to replicate with larger samples frequently failed (e.g., Barber & Glass, 1962; see Barber, 1964, for a review).

The disappointing results obtained with personality variables led to a shift in emphasis that produced more promising results. Both state and nonstate theorists have focused on the delineation of what might loosely be defined as the attitude and the aptitude components of hypnotic responsiveness. Specifically, the relationship between hypnosis-specific attitudes and expectations to hypnotic susceptibility has received extensive attention. With respect to the aptitude or skill component of hypnotic responsiveness, researchers have focused primarily on the relationship between hypnotic susceptibility and measures of imagery and imaginative involvement.

Studies of attitudinal and imaginal skill correlates of hypnotic susceptibility will be the primary focus of this review. More positive than negative results have been reported in studies that have correlated imaginal variables with susceptibility. As this statement implies, however, inconsistencies as well as disappointing results (e.g., low correlations with susceptibility) have also been common. This review will try to specify some of the reasons for inconsistent results.

It should be noted that a variety of scales have come into use since Weitzenhoffer and Hilgard (1959, 1962) popularized susceptibility testing with development of the Stanford Hypnotic Susceptibility Scales, Forms A through C (see chap. 1). Undoubtedly, differences among susceptibility scales have contributed to the variability in the results to be reviewed. Comparisons among the various scales, however, have usually demonstrated satisfactory convergent validity (e.g., Ruch, Morgan & Hilgard, 1974; Spanos, Radtke, Hodgins, Bertrand, Stam & Moretti, 1983; Tellegen, 1979). Despite similarities among scales, the results will be reported with reference to the specific susceptibility scales used.

As further consideration of susceptibility scales refines our understanding of the differences underlying test suggestions, such information may prove useful.

HYPNOSIS-SPECIFIC ATTITUDES/EXPECTATIONS AND SUSCEPTIBILITY

Most theoretical accounts of hypnotic responsiveness have acknowledged the influence of attitudes toward hypnosis (e.g., Spanos & Barber, 1974; Sheehan & Perry, 1977). However, controversy has concerned the degree and scope of influence associated with this component. Kihlstrom has suggested that the role of attitudinal variables represents one of the primary points of departure for state and nonstate theorists (Shor, Pistole, Easton & Kihlstrom, 1984).

At one extreme, attitudes and expectations have been allotted a relatively minor role. The "transient" nature of attitudes and expectations has led some to argue that more enduring characteristics will ultimately determine individual differences (Hilgard, 1965, 1975; Perry, 1977; Shor, Orne & O'Connell, 1966). At the other extreme, some researchers have considered subjects' attitudes and beliefs (i.e., expectations) of primary importance. For example, Barber (1964) suggested that the intraindividual consistency observed with repeated susceptibility testing may reflect the consistency of subjects' hypnosis-specific attitudes. Recently Kirsch (1985) has gone even further by suggesting that subjects' expectations for hypnotic responding are the unmediated cause of hypnotic behavior. An intermediate view maintains that positive attitudes and expectations are necessary but not sufficient for high levels of hypnotic responsiveness (Spanos, 1982; 1982; Spanos, Brett, Menary & Cross, 1987). Therefore, the dismissal of attitudes as somehow less important (than aptitude variables) because they may be modified is rejected. Recent evidence suggests that some subjects can be highly resistant to attempts to change their attitudes toward hypnosis (Spanos, Cross, Menary, Brett & de Groh, 1987).

Attitudes toward Hypnosis and Hypnotic Susceptibility

The relationship of attitudes toward hypnosis and hypnotic responsiveness has usually been assessed in terms of linear correlations. The methods for measuring attitudes, however, have varied considerably. Two studies have compared the hypnotic responsiveness of subjects with presumably "opposite" extreme (i.e., high/low) attitudes toward hypnosis (Diamond et al., 1974; Rosenhan & Tomkins, 1964). In both studies, subjects' reported "desire to participate" in hypnosis experiments constituted the hypnotic attitude measure. Rosenhan and Tomkins found that high-preference females were significantly more susceptible than low-preference females. The susceptibility level of high-and low-preference males did not differ. Diamond et al., however, found the preference scores of 110 males to significantly correlate r = .41 with their SHSS:A scores (males only tested). Diamond et al. also found a high degree of convergent validity (r = .73) between their "Preference for Hypnosis" measure and a more specific attitudes-toward-hypnosis scale (see Diamond et al., 1974). Diamond's more specific attitude measure also significantly correlated r = .47 with subjects' SHSS:A scores.

Unlike the approach outlined above, most researchers have investigated the relationship between hypnosis-specific attitudes and susceptibility using the full range of scores on both variables. Table 1 (p. 36) lists some of the reported correlations between hypnosis-specific attitudes scores and susceptibility scores. As one can see, a direct question assessing subjects' willingness to cooperate (i.e., one-item cooperative attitude scale) has exhibited low to moderate correlations with susceptibility. The Cooperative Attitude Scale has shown a slightly stronger relationship with the more difficult susceptibility scales (e.g., SHSS:C; CURSS). Correlations, however, are still of only moderate magnitudes at best.

Hypnotic Adjective Scales have produced some mixed results (see table 1). Melei and Hilgard's (1964) scale, and Barber & Calverley's (1966) revision, asks subjects to apply different adjectives to hypnosis. Both of these scales sum across items in the absence of statistical data supporting the unidimensional relationship of the adjectives.

Other scales have attempted to assess subjects' hypnosis-specific attitudes through direct questioning. London's Hypnosis Survey has yielded mixed results (see table 1). Inconsistencies may be due to the survey's low internal reliability (Dermen & London, 1965; London et al., 1962) and low test-retest reliability (London, Cooper & Johnson, 1962). It would appear that the beliefs and perceptions London and his associates investigated should not be treated as synonymous, either in their relationship to each other or in their relationship to susceptibility.

The Carleton Attitude Scale, however, has produced reliable results across two studies (see table 1). Further, total scores on this scale are normally distributed (de Groh et al., 1987, Spanos, Brett, et al., 1987), internally reliable (Spanos, Brett, et al., 1987), and demonstrate acceptable test-retest reliability (Spanos, Salas, Menary & Brett, 1986). As table 1 indicates, however, correlation magnitudes for large samples have been low.

Most researchers have recognized that hypnosis-specific attitudes play a role in hypnotic responsiveness. Given low correlation magnitudes, however, some have attempted to temper the importance of attitudes relative to other (e.g., "aptitude") variables (Bowers, 1976; Hilgard, 1975; Perry, 1977; Shor et al., 1984). Spanos, Brett, et al., however, suggested that low correlation magnitudes between these two variables may result from applying a linear assessment technique (i.e., correlation) to a nonlinear relationship. Specifically, Spanos and his associates found that the relationship between hypnosis-specific attitudes and susceptibility was fan-shaped. Subjects with low attitude scores almost always obtained low susceptibility scores, while those with at least moderate attitudes were represented at all susceptibility levels. This interpretation is consistent with suggestions that low hypnosis-specific attitudes suppress hypnotic susceptibility (see Hilgard, 1979; Perry, 1977; Spanos, Brett, et al., 1987).

TABLE 1.

CORRELATIONS FOR HYPNOSIS-SPECIFIC
"ATTITUDE" SCALES AND HYPNOTIC SUSCEPTIBILITY

Attitude Scales	Susceptibility Scales	r Values*	Sample Size
One-Item Cooperative Attitude Scale			
Spanos, Pawlak, D'Eon, Mah & Ritchie (1986)	HGSHS:A	r = .33	91(c)
	SHSS:C	r = .37	91
Spanos, Radtke, et al. (1983, Study 2)	CURSS	r = .40	102(c)
(Retest)	SHSS:C	r =.36	102
Spanos, McPeake & Churchill (1976)	BSS	r = .28, ns	36(f)
		r = .23, ns	55(m)
Hypnotic Adjective Scales			
Helei & Hilgard (1964)[1]			
Subjects with no previous hypnotic experience	SHSS:A	r = .37	125(f)
		r = .07,ns	161(m)
(Retest)	SHSS:C	r = .34	125(f)
		r = .06, ns	119(m)
Spanos, McPeake & Churchill (1976)	BSS	r = .24, ns	36(f)
		r = .15, ns	55(m)
Spanos & McPeake (1975a)	HGSHS:A	r = .23	83(f)
		r = .35	100(m)
Yanchar & Johnson (1981)	HGSHS:A	r = .35	99(c)
London's Hypnosis Survey			
London, Cooper & Johnson (1962)			
Experience/Interests	SHSS:A	r = .30	86(f)
Perceptions of Hypnosis		r = .40	86
Dermen & London (1965)			
Experience Interest	HGSHS:A	r = .49	97(f)
		r = .32	80(m)
Carleton Attitude Scale			
Spanos, Brett, Menary & Cross (1987)	CURSS	r = .31	315(f)
		r = .28	264(m)
de Groh, Cross & Spanos (1986)	CURSS	r = .27	180(f)
		r = .22	120(m)

All r values (unless otherwise specified) significant at p< .05, two-tailed.
*r values significant a[1] p< .05, one-tailed.
Key: f = females subjects only; m = male subjects only; c = females and males combined.
[1]Melei and Hilgard (1964) analyzed separately those males and females with previous hypnotic experience (n = 32 males; n = 22 females). For females, both SHSS:A and SHSS:C scores failed to correlate with initial attitude scores (r = .29, ns and r = .22, ns respectively). Males' initial attitude scores significantly correlated r = .40 with SHSS:C scores but failed to correlate with SHSS: A scores (r = .01).

More importantly, however, whether a relationship (fan-shaped or linear) is obtained between attitudes and susceptibility may be dependent on the characteristics of the populations that are sampled. For instance, college students (most samples have been taken from college populations) with strong negative attitudes toward hypnosis may simply fail to volunteer for hypnosis experiments. Brady, Levitt, and Lubin (1961) found that fear of hypnosis interfered with volunteering behavior in a subpopulation of student nurses. If volunteer status is partially dependent on a subject's hypnosis-specific attitudes, this may help to explain the inconsistent results reported in table 1. Significant linear correlations are unlikely to emerge in a sample that does not contain subjects with detrimental attitudes. If sampling procedures result in a sample generally high on attitudes, correlations performed on this truncated range will suggest no relationship between attitudes and susceptibility.

That the samples used in most hypnosis studies may be far from random also suggests care when generalizing to populations other than college students. There is some evidence to suggest that restricting sampling to college students may produce substantial distortion in the shape of hypnosis-specific attitude distributions. Hendler and Redd (1986) recently compared the hypnosis-specific attitudes of 277 undergraduates with the hypnosis-specific attitudes of 105 chemotherapy patients. The chemotherapy patients were significantly more likely than the undergraduates to perceive hypnosis as confusing and frightening (the undergraduates were more likely than the patients to perceive hypnosis as interesting). Chemotherapy patients were also more likely to perceive hypnosis as a powerful phenomenon involving involuntary responding, loss of control, and unconscious processes. The authors also cited numerous anecdotal accounts of patients who were unwilling (because of various fears) to participate in therapy involving hypnosis.

Whether the attitudes of chemotherapy patients, rather than college students, more accurately reflect the hypnosis-specific attitudes of the population in general requires further study. One notable limitation to Hendler and Redd's findings is that the mean age of their patient sample was sixty-one years (the mean age of their college population was not reported). Age as a possible contributing factor to attitude differences was not examined. Finding that college samples are biased (i.e., sophisticated) with respect to attitudes toward hypnosis could have an important impact on, among other things, our perceptions of the distribution of hypnotic susceptibility.

Attitudes: Concluding Remarks

Implicit in the remarks of some researchers is the notion that once subjects are provided with information designed to inculcate positive hypnosis-specific attitudes, hypnotic responsiveness becomes largely dependent on aptitude variables (see Bowers, 1976; Perry, 1977; Shor et al., 1984). Some preliminary results from studies designed to enhance hypnotic susceptibility in low-susceptible college students (i.e., modification research) suggest that attitudes should not be so easily dismissed. Spanos, Cross, et al. (1987) found that despite attempts to inculcate their male subjects with positive hypnosis-specific attitudes, attitudes scores still exhibited wide variability and significant, moderately high correlations with post-training susceptibility scores (females exhibited uniformly high-attitude change). Finally, researchers should not presume that the attitude measures developed thus far successfully tap all the perceptions and beliefs that may influence hypnotic responsiveness.

Expectations and Hypnotic Responsiveness

Most researchers in the area of hypnosis have operationally defined expectations either in terms of subjects' global ratings of their predicted degree of hypnotic responsiveness or in terms of subjects' summed predictions for passing a specific set of test suggestions, their beliefs about their own hypnotic responsiveness (e.g., whether they expect to be hypnotized; whether they expect to pass specific test suggestions). It is interesting to note that positive attitudes toward hypnosis are not necessarily accompanied by high expectations for hypnotic responding. In two separate studies, the proportion of subjects who were willing to be hypnotized was much higher than the proportion of subjects who expected hypnosis to be successful (London, 1962; Pistole, 1979, cited in Shor et al., 1984).

It appears that deterimental attitudes suppress hypnotic responsiveness and that positive attitudes may be necessary but not sufficient for high susceptibility. The relationship between subjects' expectations and actual performance, however, may be even less straightforward. Shor (1971) pointed out that expectations may interact with other factors, making the relationship between expectancies and actual performance highly complex (for an excellent illustration of this complexity, see Shor, 1971, 163).

Shor's ideas were probably based on his observation that the expectations of *naive* subjects produced, at best, low correlations with subsequent susceptibility level, as indicated in table 2. In fact, Barber and his associates suggested that the predictions of naive subjects are of little value because such subjects lack the experiences necessary to make accurate predictions (Barber, Spanos, & Chaves, 1974). Naive subjects, particularly those who are willing to respond, may simply be registering a "guess" as to their own susceptibility level. This reasoning predicts a substantially higher association between expectancies and susceptibility in hypnotically experienced subjects.

Two studies have produced contradictory results with respect to this issue. On the one hand, Melei and Hilgard found a much higher correlation between expectancies and susceptibility in their experienced females (n = 22; r = .65 with SHSS:A; r = .56 with SHSS:C) than in their naive females (see table 2). For experienced males, however, expectancies and susceptibility failed to significantly correlate. Dermen and London, on the other hand, found expectancies and susceptibility to correlate higher in their naive subjects than in their experienced subjects (r=.28 in experienced females and r = .33 in experienced males). The sample sizes for experienced subjects were small (n = 29 and n = 16 respectively), and these correlations were not significant.

TABLE 2.

CORRELATIONS FOR EXPECTATIONS AND HYPNOTIC SUSCEPTIBILITY,
NAIVE SUBJECTS ONLY

Expectancy Measure	Susceptibility Scales	r Values*	Sample Size
One-Item Expectancy Measures			
Melei & Hilgard (1964	SHSS:A	r = .26	125(f)
		r = .16	161(m)
Retest	SHSS:C	r = .29	121(f)
		r = .24	119(m)
Spanos, Pawlak, et al. (1986)	HGSHS:A	r = .45	91(c)
Retest	SHSS:C	r = .34	91
Dermen & London (1965)	HGSHS:A	r = .49	56(f)
		r = .35	52(m)
Expectancies for Passing Specific Hypnotic Suggestions			
Shor (1971)	HGSHS:A	r = .25	164(c)
Shor, Pistole, Easton, & Kihlstrom (1984)	HGSHS:A	r = .34	432(c)

Susceptibility retest scores correlated with subjects' initial expectancy scores.

One problem inherent to both of these studies is that subjects who simply stated that they had previously attempted hypnosis were the ones defined by the experimenters as "experienced." This criterion, of course, leaves the context within which subjects were exposed to hypnotic procedures uncontrolled (e.g., experimental setting; entertainment). In two separate studies Spanos and his associates adopted a within-subjects design that provided more control over the degree of exposure to hypnosis that subjects received. Spanos, Radtke, Hodgins, Bertrand, Stam, and Moretti (1983, Study 2) tested a mixed sample of subjects (n = 107) first on the CURSS, and several weeks later tested the same subjects on the SHSS:C Initial (i.e., naive) expectancy ratings significantly correlated r = .40 with CURSS scores while subsequent (i.e., experienced) expectancy ratings significantly correleated r = .50 with SHSS:C scores. In another study, Spanos, Radtke, Hodgins, Bertrand, Stam, and Dubreuil (1983) tested a large mixed sample of subjects (n = 152) twice on the CURSS. Initial (i.e., naive) expectancy ratings produced a low (r = .21) though statistically significant correlation with initial CURSS scores. Subsequent (i.e., experienced) expectancy ratings, however, produced a moderately high and significant correlation of r = .48 with CURSS retest scores.

That naive subjects may simply register an expectancy "guess" also finds impressive support from two other studies (Council & Kirsch, 1983; Council, Kirsch & Hafner, 1986). In these studies, subjects' expectancy ratings on ten different hypnotic suggestions were gathered at two critical points in the experimental procedure. The first set of expectancy ratings was gathered before the hypnotic induction was administered. The second set of expectancy ratings was gathered after the hypnotic induction but before the actual test suggestions were administered. The correlations between preinduction expectancy ratings and subsequent hypnotic responsiveness were similar to the results of Shor and his associates (see table 2). Preinduction expectancy ratings and SHSS:C scores failed to correlate above $r = .25$ in three separate samples (see Council & Kirsch, 1983; Council et al 1986). Correlations between postinduction expectancies and SHSS:C scores, however, were substantially higher. In two of the samples, postinduction expectancies and susceptibility correlated $r = .55$ and in the third sample these two variables correlated $r = .58$. The number of subjects in all three samples was greater than ($n = 50$, and all correlations were highly significant. Clearly, the expectancy ratings made by subjects after the hypnotic induction were more consistent with their subsequent hypnotic performance than the expectancy ratings made prior to a hypnotic induction.

Although the work of Spanos and his associates and Kirsch and his associates employed different measures of expectancies, their findings reveal one important similarity: "experienced" subjects are more accurate in their assessment of subsequent hypnotic responsiveness. The results of Kirsch and his associates are of particular interest for they suggest that the subject's experiences during the induction procedure provided sufficient information for the emergency of a more consistent relationship between subject's expectancy ratings and actual performance.

Expectancies: Concluding Remarks

The theoretical role of expectancies for hypnotic responsiveness remains controversial. For Kirsch, subjects' expectancies represent the primary determinant of hypnotic responsiveness (Kirsch, 1985; Council et al. 1986; Council & Kirsch, 1983). The superiority of postinduction expectancies arises because a subject's experiences during a hypnotic induction alter his expectancies. Furthermore, Kirsch argues that subsequent responding varies as a function of these altered expectancies; response expectancies are seen as the direct cause of a subject's response to hypnotic suggestions.

An alternative hypothesis holds that subjects' experiences during a hypnotic induction either support or fail to support preconceived notions of what a hypnotic experience "should" be like. For example, a subject who, prior to the actual induction, fully expects to respond to hypnosis may find her experiences during the induction procedure to be inconsistent with her expectations. This subject would conclude that she was not hypnotized. Another subject may find his experiences during the induction consistent with his preconceived notions of becoming deeply hypnotized. This subject would probably expect that once the actual suggestions started, he would be highly responsive. The new (postinduction) expectation for failure on the part of the first subject and success on the part of the second subject may well influence subsequent behaviors. For example, those who believe that the hypnosis is "working" may be more likely than those who do not to cooperate further, image the contents of the suggestions, and so on. The reason for positing a unmediated relationship between expectancy for success and actual performance, however, is not obvious. Postinduction expectancies fail to even account for half of the variance in susceptibility scores, which is much less than one would expect from a cause-and-effect relationship. Future research should focus on discerning which subjects are responsible for lowering correlation magnitudes. Subjects with high postinduction expectancies who fail to respond to test suggestions would be difficult to account for in terms of Kirsch's hypothesis.

IMAGERY

The relationship of imagery to hypnotic responsiveness has received extensive attention (see Sheehan, 1979). The concept of imagery is multifaceted and studies have examined the relationship of susceptibility to both performance measures (e.g., accuracy of imagery recall; preference for visual processing) and subjective aspects of imagery (e.g., imagery control; imagery vividness). The primary focus, however, has been on the predictive power of imagery vividness, and this review will be limited to that issue.

Imagery Vividness

The paper-and-pencil tests used in hypnosis research for assessing subjects' imagery vividness evolved out of the work of Betts (1909). Betts's developed a 190-item questionnaire that elicited imagery vividness responses across seven sensory modalities; Sheehan (1967a) shortened the original scale for practical use in experimental settings. This abridged version, which includes five items for each of the seven sensory modalities,[1] has demonstrated high correspondence with the original questionnaire (Sheehan, 1967a). Sheehan's Questionnaire on Mental Imagery (QMI) has been used extensively both within and outside the hypnosis area. An alternative 15-item variation of Betts's original questionnaire, developed by Shor et al. (1966), has also been used extensively in hypnosis research. This questionnaire also includes different sensory modality items but emphasizes visual imagery vividness. A third scale, Mark's Vividness of Visual Imagery Questionnaire (VVIQ; Marks, 1973), contains 16 items that are similar in many respects to the visual imagery section of the Betts scale.

Summary results for the relationship of these three scales to susceptibility are presented in table 3 (p. 42). As can be seen, inconsistent results have been obtained using all three scales. In addition to the results presented in table 3, Farthing, Venturino, and Brown (1983) cite three other studies (Crawford, 1978,

1979; McKinley & Gur, 1975) that have found significant positive correlations between the VVIQ and hypnotic susceptibility, and Perry (1973) cites two other studies finding no statistically significant correlation between imagery vividness (multimodal scales) and susceptibility (Jenness, 1965; Morgan & Lam 1969). The VVIQ, which assesses only visual imagery vividness, does appear to have produced more stable correlations with susceptibility than other vividness measures.[2]

TABLE 3.

CORRELATIONS FOR IMAGERY VIVIDNESS
AND HYPNOTIC SUSCEPTIBILITY

Attitude Scales	Susceptibility Scales	r Values*	Sample Size
Vividness of Visual Imagery Questionnaire (VVIQ)			
t'Hoen (1978)	SHSS:C	r = .28	108(c)
Crawford (1978)	SHSS:A	r = .41	31(f)
(composite scores)	SHSS:C	r = .36	25(m)
Bowers (1978; high and low susceptibles)	HGSHS:A	r = .32, ns	n=32(c)
Questionnaire on Mental Imagery (QMI)			
Hilgard, Sheehan, Monteiro & Macdonald (1981)	HGSHS:A	r = .15	237(c)
		r = .26	92(c)
Diamond & Taft (1975)	HGSHS:A	r = .15	237(c)
		r = .36, ns	23(m)
Hilgard (1979)	SHSS:C	r = .32	55(f)
		r = .17, ns	65(m)
Sutcliffe, Perry & Sheehan (1970)	SHSS:C	r = .20, ns	42(f)
		r = .58	53(m)
Perry (1973)	SHSS:C	r = .02, ns	26(f)
		r = .17, ns	36(m)
Vividness of Mental Imagery (VMI)			
Spanos, Pawlak, et al. (1986)	HGSHS:A	r = -.21	91(c)
	SHSS:C	r = .-29	91
de Groh, Cross & Spanos (1986)	CURSS	r = .19	180(f)
		r = .15, ns	120(m)
Spanos, McPeake & Churchill (1976)	BSS	r = .01, ns	36(f)
		r = .18, ns	55(m)

*Unless otherwise specified, all r values significant at p< .05, two-tailed.

Unlike the VVIQ, the QMI and VMI have been described as tests of primarily nonvisual imagery vividness (Palmer & Field, 1968). One possible explanation for the more variable results of multimodal scales with respect to susceptibility may be that scoring procedures sum across responses to different sensory modalities. Hiscock (1978) found the visual and auditory portions of the QMI to correlate around r = .4 in two separate mixed-gender samples. While these subsections of the QMI demonstrate some convergence, there is also a large proportion of unique variance. In addition, White, Ashton, and Brown (1977) found significant differences in QMI modality strengths for both males and females. Scale formats differing from the QMI have also produced significant modality-strength differences (e.g., Brower, 1947; Lindauer, 1969; see also McKeller, 1972).

Despite these results, some researchers have argued for the presence of a general imagery-vividness dimension underlying the modalities of multimodal scales. Factor analytic results are cited as primary support for this interpretation. Factor analyses have produced a general imagery factor (with moderate loadings) before rotation (Sheehan, 1967b; Wagman & Stewart, 1975; White, Ashton & Law, 1974), and a higher-order dimension among modality specific factors after rotation (White et al., 1974). Consistent with these results, both of the multimodal scales have been shown to be internally reliable (QMI; Sheehan, 1967a; VMI; Shor et al., 1966). In addition, White et al. reviewed reported test-retest reliabilities for the QMI. Although longer time intervals produced lower reliability coefficients, results after the longest period (twelve months) were still acceptable.

Nevertheless, the idea of looking at separate modalities does have some tradition within the area of hypnosis (e.g., Arnold, 1946). With a sample of forty male and female subjects, Arnold found that in response to a "body sway" suggestion (i.e., imagine falling . . .), subjects who reported kinesthetic imagery or a combination of visual and kinesthetic imagery showed more overt "sway" than subjects who reported visual imagery alone. Farthing et al. (1983) attempted to extend Arnold's findings. Their study employed two new scales, one to assess visual imagery vividness alone, and one to assess a combination of visual and kinesthetic imagery. Both scales correlated significantly (r = .25) with HGSHS:AA ideomotor items. The authors viewed their results as tentative since both of the scales were new. It should be noted also that their format did not necessarily assess whether some subjects expressed more kinesthetic imagery than others.

Hypnotic susceptibility has come to be operationally defined in terms of scores on standardized susceptibility scales, most of which include test suggestions emphasizing different modalities. For example, most scales include visual and auditory hallucination suggestions. Whether, for example, a "pure" measure of auditory imagery vividness would better predict responsiveness to an auditory suggestion awaits further investigation.

Imagery Vividness and Susceptibility: Deviations from Linearity

Despite the inconsistent results of both multimodal scales, most researchers have continued to stress the importance of imagery vividness for successful hypnotic responding (e.g., Sheehan, 1979). Inconsistencies have often been attributed to the inherent "imprecision" of trying to quantify subjective experiences (e.g., Perry, 1973; see also Sheehan, 1979, for an excellent review of other possible contributing factors). Another partial explanation for low and nonsignificant correlations, however, may be attributed to the "shape" of the relationship between imagery vividness and susceptibility.

Several independent laboratories have found the relationship between imagery vividness and susceptibility to deviate from linearity (de Groh et al., 1985; Hilgard, 1979; Barnard & Spanos, 1988; Sutcliffe, Perry & Sheehan, 1970). In conformance with some theoretical interpretations, subjects with lower imagery vividness scores fail to achieve high levels of susceptibility. However, as vividness scores increase, the degree of variability in susceptibility scores has been found to increase. Thus, unlike subjects with lower vividness scores, knowledge that a subject reports *vivid* imagery is of little predictive value. As depicted in figure 1, subjects with vivid imagery are represented at all levels of susceptibility.

The "fan-shaped" relationship depicted in figure 1 may help to explain the inconsistent correlations obtained between susceptibility and imagery vividness. If a particular sample lacks subjects with low vividness scores and/or lacks subjects with high susceptibility scores (random sampling error), as may be the case when smaller samples are used, the chances of finding a significant linear relationship is reduced (see fig. 1). With larger samples, deviations from linearity will inevitably lower linear correlation magnitudes.

The same reasoning may also account for the inconsistent gender-specific results reported in this area (see table 3). De Groh et al. found highly similar fan-shaped scatterplots for male and female subjects. In that study it would appear that imagery vividness significantly correlated with susceptibility for females only (see table 3) because more females than males were tested. Such findings suggest caution when interpreting gender-specific results.

Some researchers have emphasized the influence of detrimental attitudes toward hypnosis to explain why some vivid imagers fail to respond to test suggestions (e.g., Sheehan, 1979; Sutcliffe et al., 1970; Perry, 1973). If detrimental attitudes represent the primary moderating influence, one might expect that consideration of subjects with only positive attitudes toward hypnosis would produce a more linear relationship between susceptibility and imagery vividness. De Groh et al. found only partial support for this interpretation. When subjects with only positive attitudes toward hypnosis were considered (only those above the 75th percentile), the correlation between imagery vividness and susceptibility increased from $r = .17$ to $r = .33$. The fan-shaped relationship between the two variables, however, remained (see fig. 1). When males and females were analyzed separately, the same pattern was found: correlations increased, but the fan distribution remained.

Figure 1. Scatterplot for Imagery Vividness and Hypnotic Susceptibility
A Representation of Data from de Groh et al. (1985)

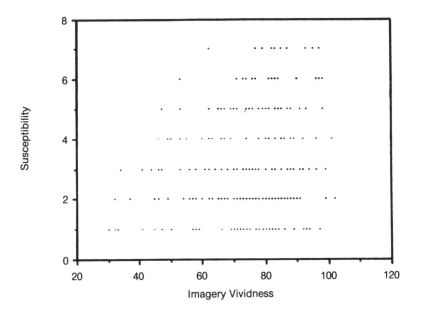

Scatterplot for Imagery Vividness and Hypnotic Susceptibility
(Lower Attitude Subjects Omitted)

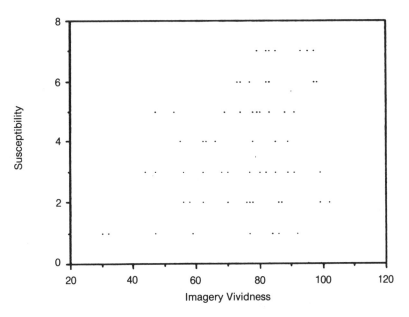

Imagery Vividness: Concluding Remarks

The critical point outlined above is that before and after controlling for attitudes, low-susceptible subjects appear to exhibit more variability in their vividness scores than high-susceptible subjects. Therefore, simply concluding that high susceptibles exhibit significantly higher vividness of imagery scores than low susceptibles can obscure the important fact that a large proportion of low susceptibles report vivid imagery. While the importance of statistical tests of significance cannot be denied, examination of scatterplots should aid in more accurate interpretations of results.

Although positive attitudes toward hypnosis appear to be a prerequisite for hypnotic responsiveness, and detrimental attitudes may inhibit vivid imagers' involvement in hypnosis, the picture is still incomplete. Some vivid imagers with positive attitudes still fail to respond to test suggestions. Accounting for these individuals may require a broader understanding of the role of imagery in hypnotic responding. For example, Coe, Allen, Krug, and Wurtzman (1974) pointed out that vividness questionnaires ask subjects to image, briefly while responding to test suggestions may require sustained imagery. Perhaps vivid imagers who pass hypnotic suggestions, as opposed to vivid imagers who don't, differ in their ability to sustain imagery.

Alternatively, how subjects interpret test suggestions is an important component of hypnotic responding (Gorassini & Spanos, 1986). Adopting the appropriate interpretation set involves the subject's tacit acknowledgment that successful hypnotic responding requires goal-directed behavior. When subjects adopt the appropriate interpretation, vivid imagery may aid their objective and subjective responding to test suggestions. However, subjects who fail to adopt the interpretation necessary to pass suggestions (e.g., those who simply wait for something to happen to them) will not make use of their imagery skill.

Along these lines, a number of studies have demonstrated that cultivating positive attitudes toward hypnosis, teaching imaginal strategies, as well as teaching the appropriate way to interpret the ambiguous aspects of test suggestions, result in substantial increases in hypnotic susceptibility levels (Cross & Spanos, in press; Gfeller, Lynn, Pribble & Kvinge, 1985; Gorassini & Spanos, 1986; Spanos, Cross, Menary, Brett & de Groh, 1987; Spanos, de Groh & de Groot, 1987). Spanos, Cross, et al. also found that imagery vividness may play an important role in the successful enhancement of subjects' susceptibility level. In that study imagery vividness (VMI) was significantly correlated with susceptibility gains (i.e., posttraining susceptibility scores) for thirty female subjects ($r = .32$). The correlation between these two variables for thirty males was near zero. The importance of imagery vividness for males, however, surfaced when several attitude measures and the VMI were included as potential predictors of susceptibility in a stepwise multiple-regression analysis. Two attitude measures and the VMI were entered and accounted for approximately 50 percent of the variance in males' posttest susceptibility scores. The VMI was entered last, suggesting that once attitudes were statistically controlled, imagery vividness scores were associated with successful gains in hypnotic susceptibility.

These results suggest that exposure to skill-training packages designed to enhance the use of imaginal strategies and to adopt the appropriate interpretation set may not be enough. Successful execution of test suggestions may require the ability to image vividly. This conclusion, however, is tentative. As Spanos et al. pointed out, skill-training procedures emphasized the use of imaginal strategies to pass test suggestions. The skill-training procedure may have contributed to an expectation of success in vivid imagers and an expectation of failure for those with poor imagery. Consequently, the relationship of posttraining susceptibility scores to imagery vividness levels may have been an artifact of the experimental procedure.

IMAGINATIVE INVOLVEMENT

In 1974 Spanos and Barber suggested that the role of imaginative involvement in hypnotic responding appeared to be an area of convergence for state and nonstate theorists. The concept of imaginative involvement (often treated as synonymous with absorption) refers to the process of elaborating upon "make believe" situations, while reinterpreting or failing to reflect upon information that contradicts the reality status of the make-believe situation (O'Grady, 1980; Shor, 1970; Spanos & Barber, 1974). Josephine Hilgard (1979) saw an important distinction between the role of imaginative involvement and imagery vividness in hypnotic responding. According to Hilgard, no matter how vivid subjects' imagery, the absence of imaginative involvement during hypnosis will leave subjects unresponsive.

Much research in this area has focused on the development of measurement scales that attempt to capture those experiences predictive of hypnotic responsiveness. Hilgard (1979), however, relied primarily on extensive interviews with subjects in an attempt to delineate experiences (i.e., interests/involvements) that predicted susceptibility. As will be shown, many of the experiences that became the focus of involvement questionnaires (e.g., absorption-ABS scale; Tellegen & Atkinson, 1974) were also of central importance in Hilgard's interviews.

Development of Involvement Scales

Attempts to identify the types of involvements outside the hypnotic context that might predict hypnotic susceptibility began with the work of Shor (1960). Shor was primarily interested in the frequency of "hypnotic-like" experiences: those experiences outside of the hypnotic context that he felt might reflect the components necessary for hypnotic responsiveness. Shor's work demonstrated that many of the items included in his Personal Experience Questionnaire (PEQ; Shor, 1960) were not uncommon in normal college students. This realization initiated quantitative attempts to relate the reported frequency of "hypnotic-like" experiences to levels of hypnotic susceptibility.

Shor, Orne, and O'Connell (1962) expanded the original PEQ to 149 experience items covering a wide range of experiences.[3] In an attempt to identify those items positively associated with susceptibility, Shor et al. calculated phi coefficients between the susceptibility scores of twenty-nine subjects and their frequency and intensity scores for each item. The intensity measure identified 45 items that correlated with susceptibility scores at or above a set criterion level. Cross-validation using twenty-five specially selected subjects yielded a correlation around r = .45 between summed intensity scores and SHSS:C scores.

Subsequent attempts to demonstrate a relationship between susceptibility and various renditions of the PEQ have not been very successful (Barber & Calverley, 1965; Dermen & London, 1965; London, Cooper & Johnson, 1962). Although Nowlis (1969) did find a significant correlation between PEQ and HGSHS:A scores (r = .36; n = 34), he failed to replicate this result in a second sample (r = -.03; n = 40). Bowers (1971) reported a significant relationship between these two variables for females only (r = .39; males, r = .09, ns). Unfortunately, all of these studies differed not only in the items used to represent the PEQ, but also in the "response-type" elicited from subjects (i.e., intensity, frequency, or simple occurrence). None of the response types have proven superior and all three have produced contradictory results (see also Hilgard, 1965; Shor et al., 1966).

The Experience Inventory of As (1963) represents another attempt to identify those experiences related to susceptibility. Using a variety of items (n = 60)[4] similar in many respects to those of Shor et al., As (1963) found total EI scores to correlate significantly with susceptibility (consolidated scale; see As 1963) r = .36 and r = .31 in two separate samples of females (n = 50 and n = 52, respectively). Similar correlation magnitudes were reported for a sample (n = 50) of males (r = .35 with SHSS:A scores and r = .47 with SHSS:C scores; As, 1962, cited in Hilgard, 1965). Van Nuys (1973) also found the EI to correlate significantly with HGSHS:A scores r = .53 in a sample of forty-seven males (females were not tested).

As (1963) also attempted to "purify" his inventory (as Shor and his associates had attempted to do) by selecting out those individual items that significantly correlated with susceptibility. As (1963) hoped to find a subset of items that produced a stronger relationship with susceptibility than the overall scale. The best subset of individual items were ascertained for each of his two female samples. Of the 60 EI items, only 16 in the first sample and 17 in the second sample were positively correlated with susceptibility beyond the 10 percent level of significance. The correlation between susceptibility and summed subset items was significantly enhanced within the sample from which they were selected. When subsets of items were applied to their respective "replication" samples, however, correlation magnitudes dropped and faired no better than total EI scores.

Given these results, As (1963) suggested that to produce a significant relationship between susceptibility and subjective experience items from sample to sample would require an inventory covering a broad range of experiences. The instability of As's smaller subset, however, may have had more to do with his use of by-item correlations as the criterion for item inclusion. Dichotomous responses to specific items are often unreliable, thus increasing the probability of sample-specific results. As one might expect, therefore, As's experiences items appeared "unstable" by significantly correlating in one sample, but failing to correlate significantly in another sample.

The reliability of a smaller subset of items may have been enhanced by summing together conceptually related "experience" items. Many of the experience items that correlated in at least one of As's (1963) samples could be classified under one of two theoretical dimensions that As, O'Hara & Munger (1962) deduced from factor analyzing a subset of EI items. Moreover, the factor analytic results suggested that the two dimensions, labeled Role Absorption and Tolerance for Unusual Experiences (see note 4), were conceptually distinct (i.e., orthogonal). As's (1963) objective of a reliable subset of experience items might have been achieved if he had, for example, summed together Role Absorption items. This approach, the logical step after his factor analytic results, was not pursued.

Lee-Teng (1965) was the first to assess the degree of association between susceptibility and a group of supposedly conceptually similar "experience" items summed together as a unit or subscale. Lee-Teng's Hypnotic Characteristic Inventory (HCI) included five 12-item subscales.[5] It should be noted that Lee-Teng restricted the types of experiences she investigated. Specifically, her HCI did not include experiences reflected in the second factor of As et al. (e.g., perceptual distortion and mystical experience items).

Lee-Teng's *rationally constructed* subscales produced some positive results. In a sample of 105 males and females, only three of the five subscales (trancelike experiences, role playing, and impulsivity vs. rationality) correlated significantly with SHSS:C scores. Only the role-playing subscale correlated higher with susceptibility (r = .38) than the total HCI (r = .33), and this difference may easily be attributed to chance. Further, all three of the subscales that produced positive results also demonstrated the highest degree of convergence with the total HCI. Since Lee-Teng's rationally constructed subscales may have demonstrated convergence among themselves, it is difficult to discern whether particular subscales would have shared unique or only common variance with susceptibility.

The Absorption Scale

The most widely used "experience" scale within the hypnosis area has been Tellegen and Atkinson's (1974) Absorption (ABS) scale. Scale construction followed the same conceptual format as previous research in this area. The majority of Tellegen and Atkinson's original items were chosen either because a statistically significant relationship with susceptibility had been demonstrated previously (e.g., As, 1963; Roberts & Tellegen, 1973), or because items were part of subscales Lee-Teng Lee-Teng (1965) found to be related to susceptibility. Unlike previous scale construction methods, however, these authors focused primarily on empirically demonstrated similarities among experience items.

The development of the original absorption scale involved two important stages. First, the responses of 481 female subjects to the original 71 items were factor analyzed. Eleven factors were interpreted. Factors with at least two items were considered, and many of the items exhibited nontrivial loadings on more than one factor. Items were included within a particular factor based on their highest loading. Tellegen and Atkinson's primary objective was to demonstrate a higher-order structure among these eleven factors. The authors reasoned that if particular sets of items exhibited systematic loadings across factors, further analysis would allow a higher-order structure to emerge.

A second factor analysis included thirteen scores for each subject, the eleven factors mentioned above, plus two other scales, Block's Ego Resiliency and Block's Ego Control (see Tellegen & Atkinson, 1974). The results for two separate samples of female subjects (sample 1, n = 142; sample 2, n = 171) were almost identical. Of the original eleven factor scores, the same six showed moderate to high loadings on only one factor.

In their original article Tellegen and Atkinson (1974) argued that this factor comprised examples of absorbed experiences and episodes of "total" attention during which the individual devotes "full commitment of available perceptual, motoric, imaginative and ideational resources to a unified representation of the attentional object (p. 274)." For Shor (1970), this underlying component was termed a fading of one's "Generalized Reality Orientation." Tellegen and Atkinson's conceptual definition of an absorbed experience appears to place no restriction on the properties of the object toward which the individual may attend. Items included on the ABS scale, however, appear to be tapping a restricted constellation of experiences, both in content and with respect to the selection procedure (i.e., for the most part, items demonstrating a relationship with susceptibility were considered).

After Tellegen and Atkinson's original publication, Tellegen (1976) expanded the Absorption (ABS) scale in conjunction with a larger personality inventory, the Differential Personality Questionnaire (DPQ). This questionnaire contains 300 items, and sixteen subscales of which the ABS scale is just one. Tellegen, in his description of the ABS scale contained in the DPQ, outlines the particular contexts tapped by many of the items on the scale. Individuals high on the Absorption scale were described as responsive to music, art, and nature. Tellegen also suggested that these individuals were more likely to become involved in imaginative experiences and fantasy.

Consistent with this description, the ABS scale[6] has demonstrated a moderate association with scales measuring daydreaming (Crawford, 1978, 1982) and fantasy-proneness (Lynn & Rhue, 1986). The ABS scale has also demonstrated divergent validity by failing to correlate significantly with traditional personality variables as well as measures of psychopathology (e.g., O'Grady, 1980; Tellegen & Atkinson, 1974; Spanos & Moretti, 1988; Spanos, Stam, et al., 1976).

The ABS scale, however, has also demonstrated a moderate association with such variables as mysticism (Spanos & Moretti, 1988) and imagery vividness (Crawford, 1982; Hilgard et al., 1981; Spanos et al., 1976), as well as attitudes and expectancies toward hypnosis (Council & Kirsch, 1983; Council, Kirsch & Hafner, 1986; Spanos, Brett, et al., 1987; Spanos et al., 1976). Moreover, the ABS has been shown to load with imagery vividness and hypnosis-specific attitude variables in factor analytic studies (Spanos, D'Eon, Pawlak, et al., 1988; Spanos, Rivers & Gottlieb, 1978). These studies are not devoid of methodological problems, the most serious being small mixed-gender sample sizes. Despite problems, however, this finding was effectively replicated.

The wide range of different variables with which the ABS scale significantly correlates provides indirect evidence that the scale may contain divergent subcategories. Consider, for example, that there appears to be no shared variability between imagery vividness and hypnosis-specific attitude variables (see de Groh et al., 1985; Spanos, McPeake, et al., 1976), yet both correlate with the absorption scale. It would appear that the variability absorption and imagery vividness share is different from the pattern that variability absorption and attitudes have in common.

That the ABS scale may contain subcategories is by no means inconsistent with Tellegan and Atkinson's (1974) original findings. In fact, their objective of demonstrating a higher-order structure among their primary factor scales leaves open this possibility. Consequently, although Tellegen and Atkinson (1974) may have achieved their objective of demonstrating a higher-order structure (or dimension), the primary (or second-order) factors (or subscales) may also be of interest. While the potential ABS subscales would probably be correlated, they may also demonstrate unique variance that oculd be of interest both within and outside the area of hypnosis.

Tentative support for the existence of divergent subscales within the ABS scale comes from the work of Ronnestad (1985) who first content analyzed and then factor analyzed the 34-item absorption scale. Ronnnestad's content analysis resulted in four subscales.[7] Ronnestad tested his hypothesis of four subscales by factor analyzing 176 males' and females' responses on ABS items, with the restriction of four factors. Each of the theoretically derived subscales correlated r = .70 or above with only one of the empirically derived subscales. All the theoretical subscales produced moderate to low correlations with the other three empirically derived subscales.

Unfortunately, intercorrelations among the factor analytic subscales were not reported. Further, while the degree of convergence between a particular rational and empirical subscale was respectably high (r < .70) they were obviously not perfect. Ronnestad did not address these discrepancies. Finally, the generalizability of these results is open to question. The most obvious concern is that Ronnestad first hypothesized four subscales and then carried this restriction over into his empirical analysis. The possibility of a more parsimonious factor structure was not investigated.

The results of prior research, however, suggest that Ronnestad's subscales may have some validity. Descriptive examples from Ronnestad's Cognitive Perceptual subscale (see note 7) suggest that a portion of the ABS scale may be tapping an imagery vividness component. According to Ronnestad, almost one-third of the ABS items fell into this category. Although some researchers have suggested that vivid imagery is necessary for deep "affective" involvement (e.g., Sheehan, 1979), this hypothesis has not been systematically tested. In addition, in the factor analysis reported by As et al. (1962), two factors (labeled

Role-Absorption and Tolerance for Unusual Experiences) show similarities to two of Ronnestad's subscales. The Role-Absorption factor showed some similarities to Ronnestad's Affective/Regressive subscale and the Tolerance for Unusual Experiences showed some overlap with Ronnestad's Mystical subscale (see notes). Recall that As et al. reported their two factors to be orthogonal. These results combined suggest a degree of independence may exist among prospective subscales that is not trivial.

Absorption and Hypnosis

Most researchers have considered, the ABS scale to be a stable, unidimensional index of subjects' imaginative involvement outside of the hypnotic context (Finke & MacDonald, 1978; Kihlstrom et al., 1980; O'Grady, 1980; Spanos et al., 1983). The ABS scale and susceptibility scales have demonstrated low to moderate correlations, with some nonsignificant results. Table 4 presents most of the studies that have correlated these two variables. The findings obtained by Kihlstrom et al. are representative of the trends in this area. These authors found the average correlation between ABS scores and HGSHS:A scores across six mixed-gender samples to be $r = .27$ (the range of the correlations was not reported). Sample sizes ranged from 110 to 426, and all correlations between the ABS and HGSHS:A scores were signficant. For the most part, studies with larger sample sizes ($N < 50$) have reported correlation magnitudes of less than $r = .35$. The exceptions have been studies using more difficult susceptibility scales (see table 4).

Kihlstrom's use of mixed-gender samples is also consistent with research in this area. Studies that have analyzed males and females separately have found slightly higher correlation magnitudes for females, and in some male samples correlations between absorption and susceptibility have failed to achieve statistical significance. Given these findings, some researchers have suggested (e.g., Bowers, 1971) that the relationship of "experience" items and susceptibility may be moderated by gender. Whether this is true remains to be tested. When interpreting these results, however, one should keep in mind that Tellegen and Atkinson's original scale construction involved all female samples. Furthermore, numerous studies have found females to score significantly higher than males on absorption (Crawford, 1982; Farthing et al., 1983; Spanos, Brett et al., 1987; Spanos & McPeake, 1975a; Yanchar & Johnson, 1981), with one exception (Finke & MacDonald, 1978). While magnitude differences have often been small, this may help to explain the slightly higher correlation between absorption and susceptibility for female subjects.

Whether women are more likely than men to engage in the experiences included on the ABS or are simply more willing to acknowledge such experiences also requires further study. Unfortunately, little work has been done beyond simply demonstrating that gender differences exist. Moreover, the picture is further complicated by tentative findings suggesting that the relationship between absorption and susceptibility is not linear.

TABLE 4.

CORRELATIONS FOR ABSORPTION
AND HYPNOTIC SUSCEPTIBILITY

Susceptibility Scales	r Values*	Sample Size
Barber Suggestibility Scale (BSS)		
Spanos, McPeake & Churchill (1976)	r = -.13, ns	36 (f)
	r = .23, ns	55(m)
Harvard Group Scale of Hypnotic Susceptibility (HGSHS:A)		
Hilgard et al. (1981)	r = .13	237 (c)
	r = .33	92 (c)
Spanos, Stam, Rivers & Radtke (1980)	r = .32, ns	34 (c)
Farthing, Venturino & Brown (1983)	r = .35	122 (c)
Spanos & McPeake (1975a)	r = .43	83 (f)
	r = .37	100(m)
Spanos & McPeake (1975b)		
Hypnotic Context (favorable)	r = .41	44 (c)
Hypnotic Context (unfavorable)	r = .17, ns	42 (c)
Spanos, D'Eon, Pawlak, Mah & Ritchie (1988)	r = .19, ns	91 (c)
Yanchar & Johnson (1981)	r = .29	99 (c)
Tellegen & Atkinson (1973)	r = .27	142 (f)
(GSHS, variation of HGSHS:A)	r = .43	171 (f)
Carleton University Responsiveness to Suggestion Scale (CURSS:O)		
Spanos, Radtke, Hodgins, et al. (1983a)		
Study 2	r = .30	102 (c)
Spanos, Brett, Menary & Cross (1987)	r = .41	250 (f)
	r = .18	213(m)
Stanford Hypnotic Susceptibility Scale (SHSS:C)		
Spanos, Pawlak, et al. (1986)	r = .28	91 (c)
Finke & MacDonald (1978)	r = .39	160 (f)
	r = .32, ns	28(m)
Crawford (1982)	r = .57	31 (f)
Composite scores SHSS:A and SHSS:C	r = .36, ns	25(m)
Spanos, Radtke, Hodgins, et al. (1983a) study 2	r = .24, ns	102 (c)

*Unless otherwise indicated, all r values significant at p< .05, two-tailed.

Absorption and Susceptibility: Deviations from Linearity

Some evidence suggests that the relationship between ABS scores and susceptibility scores is fan shaped (Crawford, 1982; Spanos, Brett, et al., 1987). It has been suggested that individuals scoring low on the ABS scale, for the most part, also achieve low susceptibility scores. As ABS scores increase into the upper range on the scale, however, susceptibility scores vary considerably (see Spanos, Brett, et al., 1987). That the relationship between absorption and susceptibility may violate the assumption of homoscedasticity has not been as systematically investigated as the relationship between imagery vividness and susceptibility. Shor et al.'s (1966) discussion of their results for "experience" items (PEQ) and susceptibility scores, however, also hints at this relationship.

Partial explanation for this fan shape may be that subjects' attitudes toward hypnosis and the hypnotic context mediates the relationship between absorption and susceptibility. Specifically, subjects high on the ABS scale may fail to achieve high levels of susceptibility due to detrimental attitudes. This was confirmed by Spanos, Brett, et al. who found that when only subjects with positive attitudes toward hypnosis were considered (i.e., above the median), the magnitude of the correlation between ABS and susceptibility scores increased. Unfortunately, Spanos, Brett et al. did not report on whether "weeding out" those with low attitudes substantially reduced the degree of heteroscedasticity. The mediating effects of hypnosis-specific attitudes on the relationship of other variables to hypnotic susceptibility (e.g., imagery vividness) suggests that the fan shape may remain (see imagery section).

The ABS scale appears to be another measurement tool in which the range fails to discriminate high- and low-susceptible subjects. Subscales, however, may prove useful in making this discrimination. It may be that moderate- to high-absorption subjects who respond to test suggestions are systematically endorsing different types of absorption items in comparison with higher-absorption subjects who fail to respond. As it stands, summing across the ABS experience items makes this hypothesis untestable.

Experience Questionnaire: Summary

Refinement of a scale reflecting experiences and involvements apparently related to susceptibility culminated with the development of the ABS scale. As mentioned previously, researchers have considered the ABS to be a stable index of subjects' degree of imaginative involvement outside of the hypnotic context. Unfortunately, researchers have often ignored the fact that no published data have addressed either the internal consistency or test-retest reliability of the ABS scale. Furthermore, theorists should keep in mind that interpretation of the underlying construct of the ABS scale is confounded by the contextually specific nature of many of its items, an observation underscored by the work of J. Hilgard ([1970]/1979). Since, for the most part, item inclusion was based on observed correlations with susceptibility, whether the ABS scale indexes imaginative involvement or the situationally specific interests (or lack of interest) of high- versus low-susceptible subjects is still unclear.

Situationally Specific Interests

Josephene Hilgard ([1970]/1979) launched an in-depth study of subjects' involvement in a variety of situationally specific activities. These activities included subjects' degree of involvement in literature, drama, religion, music, and "aesthetic" involvement in nature. Hilgard also investigated subjects' degree of physical space travel (or adventuresomeness) and mental space travel (interest in mind-altering drugs, science fiction, and Eastern philosophy). Interviewers' ratings for these different areas were categorized (high, medium, low or high, low depending on the variable), as were subjects' SHSS:C scores (high, medium, low or high, low, again depending on the variable). Significant chi-squares were found for level of reading involvement, drama, aesthetic involvement in nature, and physical and mental space travel. There was a tendency for subjects involved in drama, nature, or mental space travel to be relatively high in susceptibility, and subjects rated as low on these interests to be relatively low in susceptibility. For reading and physical space travel, however, significant chi-squares resulted because subjects rated lower on these interests tended to be lower in susceptibility. Subjects rated as "involved" in reading or physical space travel were represented in comparable proportions at all susceptibility levels.

Several criticisms leveled against Hilgard's approach have questioned the reliability of her results.[8] Nevertheless, some support has been obtained for Hilgard's findings. Davis, Dawson, and Seay (1978) had fifty-six subjects rate 16 items representing seven different areas of involvement investigated by Hilgard. Sixteen "high" and "low" involvement scorers were chosen and administered the SHSS:A. The mean SHSS:A score for the high-involvement group (m = 8.1) was significantly higher than the mean for the low-involvement group (m = 5.7). Given the possible fan-shaped relationship between "experience" items and susceptibility, one would expect low-involvement scores to be accompanied by correspondingly low-susceptibility scores. One would also predict more variability in the level of hypnotic responsiveness among those with high-involvement scores. Since Davis et al. failed to provide standard deviations for their data, this hypothesis could not be investigated.

Two studies (Baum & Lynn, 1981; Fellows & Armstrong, 1977) have spe- cifically investigated the relationship between reading involvement and susceptibility. High- and low-susceptible subjects (on the HGSHS:A) were asked to rate their *own* level of reading involvement in passages ascertained by the authors to exhibit high fantasy content. Although sample sizes were small (approximately ten subjects per group), both studies found the level of involvement in fantasy material to be higher for high susceptibles than for low susceptibles. As predicted by Hilgard (1979), Baum and Lynn found this relationship to hold only for high fantasy material.

Other findings of Fellows and Armstrong, however, signal caution regarding conclusions drawn about the relationship between susceptibility and imaginative reading involvement. Low susceptibles in that study perceived their involvement in the experimental test as an *underestimation* of their normal level of involvement in imaginative literature of their own choosing. Further, given Hilgard's results for reading involvement and susceptibility (i.e., those high in reading involvement were represented at all susceptibility levels), it is possible that differences between high- and low-susceptible subjects may be due to a comparatively small number of lows who fail to become involved in imaginative material. Again, these studies failed to report standard deviations for their data. As it stands, further research is necessary to clarify whether levels of imaginative reading involvement clearly discriminate high- and low-susceptible subjects.

Childhood Experiences and Susceptibility

Hilgard also investigated subjects' retrospective reports for different types of childhood experiences. Two particular areas of childhood experiences—reports of imaginary companions during childhood and reports of parental punishment levels—have also received attention from other researchers.

Subjects' recollection of imaginary playmates is an "experience" item that has been tested both within (As, 1963; As, O'Hara & Mungar, 1962; Shor, 1960) and outside (Barber & Calverley, 1965; Barber & Glass, 1962) the context of "experience" questionnaire development. No consistent relationship between susceptibility and reports of imaginary companion(s) was found. Inconsistent results may be due, in part, to the low frequency rate of reported imaginary companions among college students. In a mixed sample of 391 students, Hilgard found that only 17 percent reported imaginary companions, a frequency rate comparable to previous findings (As et al., 1962; Shor, 1960). It is possible that failures to find a relationship between reports of imaginary companion(s) and susceptibility may simply stem from testing samples that contain too few subjects who reported imaginary companions. If this is the case, then involvement with an imaginary companion during childhood is clearly not necessary for high susceptibility, a conclusion Hilgard herself acknowledges. More importantly, however, the mean susceptibiity level of subjects who reported imaginary companions in Hilgard's study failed to differ from the mean susceptibility level of subjects who did not report imaginary companions. In essence, Hilgard's results indicated that having an imaginary playmate during childhood did *not* increase the probability of being a high susceptible.

The relationship of childhood punishment levels and adult susceptibility levels, however, has produced a different pattern of results. The results do suggest that severe levels of punishment during childhood may be one avenue resulting in high fantasy involvement during adulthood (and by extension high levels of susceptibility). For example, Hilgard (1979) found that reported childhood punishment levels correlated r = .30 with SHSS:C scores in a mixed sample of 187 students. In addition, Nash, Lynn, and Givens (1984; Study 2)[9] compared the susceptibility level of 16 subjects self-defined as physically abused during childhood, with the susceptibility level of 300 subjects self-defined as not physically abused. Thirteen (approximately 81 percent) of those physically abused during childhood achieved high scores on the HGSHS:A. Of the 300 nonabused subjects, only 40 percent achieved high HGSHS:A scores. A chi-square analysis yielded a significant difference in the distribution of susceptibility scores for abused and nonabused subjects.

Several researchers have suggested that severe (i.e., abusive) environments may serve as a catalyst for increased imaginative activity during childhood (Fraiberg, 1968; Overstad, 1981; Tower, 1982; Wilson & Barber, 1981). For example, some of Wilson and Barber's "fantasy addicts" reported using fantasy during childhood as a means of escaping a bad environment. All of Wilson and Barber's subjects were also excellent hypnotic subjects. Rhue and Lynn's (1988) comparison of high, medium, and low fantasy-prone subjects quantified Wilson and Barber's anecdotal findings. All six of the subjects in their total sample (n = 59) who were defined as physically abused during childhood fell into their high fantasy-prone group. In another study (Lynn & Rhue, 1986), high fantasy-prone subjects exhibited significantly higher HGSHS:A scores than both medium and low fantasy-prone subjects. Consequently, physical abuse during childhood may bear an indirect relationship to hypnotic responsiveness.

One should keep in mind that aversive childhood environments are best thought of as only one possible pathway to high levels of fantasy involvement (and susceptibility) in adulthood. Researchers have not always been clear on this point. For example, Rhue and Lynn stated that high fantasy-prone subjects reported *significantly more* frequent and severe physical abuse during childhood than either medium or low fantasy-prone subjects. Six of the twenty-one high fantasy-prone subjects in their study were physically abused during childhood. It is quite likely that these subjects were primarily responsible for group differences on punishment measures. In fact, high fantasy-prone subjects exhibited significantly more variability than lows on both of the "frequency of punishment" measures used. Granted, for this sample it would appear that those physically abused as children became "fantasizers" during adulthood. One should not lose sight of the fact, however, that most of Rhue and Lynn's high fantasy-prone subjects (approximately 71 percent) were *not* abused during childhood.

APTITUDE AND ATTITUDE COMPONENTS AS COMBINED PREDICTORS

This review has examined the role of hypnosis-specific attitudes, expectations, imagery vividness, and imaginative involvement in hypnotic responding and the types of measurement scales that have been developed to assess these "aptitude" and "attitude" components of susceptibility. Although the possible moderating effect of hypnosis-specific attitudes has been touched on briefly, the combined predictive power of these variables has not yet been addressed.

A number of studies have looked at the proportion of variance in susceptibility scores explained by a linear combination of absorption and various attitude and expectancy measures (Spanos, Brett, Menary & Cross, 1987; Spanos & McPeake, 1975a; Spanos, Radtke, Hodgins, Bertrand, Stam & Moretti, 1983; Yanchar & Johnson, 1981). All but one of these studies used multiple regression with either forward or stepwise selection techniques to determine the predictive power of the predictor variables. The results of most studies suggested that despite intercorrelations among predictors, linear combinations of these predictors accounted for more variance in susceptibility scores than the predictors in isolation. The proportion of variance predictors shared with susceptibility ranged from $R^2 = .18$ to $R^2 = .30$. As one can see, much of the variance in susceptibility scores remained "unexplained." Consequently, some researchers also investigated specific models in an attempt to enhance the predictability of hypnotic responsiveness.

A Moderating Variable: Hypnosis-Specific Attitudes

The importance of positive attitudes toward hypnosis as a prerequisite for successfully passing test suggestions has been recognized by both state and nonstate theorists (see Spanos & Barber, 1974, for a review). Therefore, one might expect that subjects with strong negative attitudes toward hypnosis would evidence low levels of hypnotic responding regardless of their level on another (e.g., aptitude) variable. This reasoning has led some researchers to argue that attitudes may moderate the relationship of susceptibility and predictors, such as absorption.

One way of investigating this issue involves introducing into the multiple-regression model an "interaction" term (Wiggins, 1973) represented by the cross product of predictor variables. Attempts to enhance significantly the prediction of subjects' susceptibility scores using product terms, however, were unsuccessful (Spanos et al., 1983; Yanchar & Johnson, 1981).

An alternative method of investigating the moderating effects of attitudes has involved dichotomizing subjects into two groups, those with higher attitudes and those with lower attitudes, and observing the "differential predictability" of susceptibility scores on a specific variable (e.g., absorption). Normally this type of approach would be rejected as less sensitive than the introduction of product terms. Results in the hypothesized direction, however, were reported. For example, Spanos, Brett, et al. (1987) used this method to test whether hypnosis-specific attitudes moderate the linear relationship between absorption and susceptibility. The correlation magnitude of absorption and susceptibility was higher for subjects with positive attitudes than for subjects with more negative attitudes toward hypnosis. Yet, even among subjects selected for high hypnosis-specific attitudes, the variance ABS scores and susceptibility scores shared was modest.

De Groh et al. (1985) applied the same technique to investigate the moderating effects of hypnosis-specific attitudes on the relationship between imagery vividness and susceptibility. Using the same criterion as Spanos et al., correlation magnitudes for VMI scores and susceptibility scores within high-and low-attitude groups failed to exhibit any appreciable difference (below the 25th percentile on attitude measure r = .31; above the 25th percentile r = .18). However, when a more stringent criterion for *positive* attitudes was used (above the 75th percentile), the correlation between imagery vividness and susceptibility increased to r = .33, p< .05.

While these results are not compelling, they are in the predicted direction. Recall, however, that de Groh et al. found the fan-shaped relationship between susceptibility and imagery vividness still remained (see imagery vividness section). For subjects with only high attitudes, low susceptibles were equally likely to exhibit low vividness scores as high vividness scores (de Groh et al., 1985).

It would appear that the models investigated to date are still far from complete. Viewing attitudes as a moderator variable, while making some conceptual sense, has not substantially increased the predictability of hypnotic responsiveness. A more far-reaching concern, however, is the validity of the predictors themselves with respect to hypnotic responding. Recently, the necessity of absorption for a model of hypnotic responsiveness has been seriously challenged. In fact, recent findings may profoundly alter the way we interpret many of the results presented thus far.

Absorption and Susceptibility: Context Dependent?

Council, Kirsch et al. (1986) suggested that prior findings of a significant correlation between absorption and susceptibility are the consequence of administering the ABS scale within the context of hypnotic-susceptibility testing. Council et al. found their review of the literature to be consistent with this argument. In studies reporting a significant linear relationship between these two variables, absorption was assessed in a context explicitly associated with subjects' hypnotic-susceptibility testing. These authors also noted that all items on the ABS scale are positively keyed and face obvious, allowing easy self-assessment by subjects. It is this self-assessment that is viewed as influencing subjects' subsequent hypnotic respon-siveness. Since this influence can occur only if subjects perceive a connection between their responses on the ABS scale and susceptibility testing, Council et al. predicted no relationship between ABS scores and susceptibility scores when the ABS scale was administered to subjects outside of the hypnotic context.

To test this hypnothesis, Council et al. compared the correlation between ABS and SGSS (Stanford Group Scale; see Council et al., 1986) scores for subjects who rated the ABS scale outside of the hypnotic context (n = 64) with the correlation between these two variables for subjects (n = 64) who rated the ABS scale just prior to being administered a hypnotic induction. When absorption was measured within the hypnotic context, a subjective measure of subjects' responsiveness correlated significantly with ABS scores (r = .31), while objective susceptibility scores failed to correlate significantly (r = .22, ns). When absorption was measured outside of the hypnotic context, ABS scores failed to correlate with either subjective (r = -.14, ns) or objective (r = -.03, ns) susceptibility scores.

De Groot, Gwynn, and Spanos (1988) recently replicated the contextually dependent relationship between absorption and susceptibility for females only.

The relationship between these variables was assessed in three different groups. For two groups, the subjects were aware of a subsequent session that would assess their hypnotic susceptibility. One group of subjects was informed prior to completion of a questionnaire package that the researcher was interested in how their responses during the session would predict susceptibility. The second group was informed of the researcher's interest and of the subsequent susceptibility testing after the questionnaire package had been completed. For the third group, the experimenter made no mention of hypnosis or susceptibility testing. Subjects in this third group were later contacted by another experimenter for an apparently unrelated experiment assessing hypnotic susceptibility. The sample size for each condition was greater than n = 100 (approximately equal numbers of females and males were tested).

De Groot et al. analyzed the responses of males and females separately. For males, ABS scores failed to correlate significantly with CURSS:0 scores in all three groups. The results for females, however, were consistent with the findings of Council et al. Female subjects' ABS scores significantly correlated with CURSS:0 scores when hypnosis was mentioned before (r = .27) and after (r = .32) the questionnaires were filed out. When no connection between ABS responses and susceptibility testing was maintained, these two variables failed to correlate significantly (r = -.16, ns).

These studies do provide strong evidence for a context-dependent relationship between absorption and susceptibility. It would appear that when subjects are aware of subsequent susceptibility testing, they derive inferences from their ABS responses that influence their subsequent susceptibility level. These results, combined with previous findings on the shape of the relationship between absorption and susceptibility (when measured within the hypnotic context), suggest that any "influence" absorption scores have may be selective. Recall that some researchers reported that the relationship between ABS scores and susceptibility scores was fanshaped. De Groot (personal communication, 1986) also found the relationship between these variables to deviate systematically from linearity for his female subjects informed of susceptibility testing. In essence it would appear that the only reason researchers have found a relationship between absorption and susceptibility is because subjects with low ABS scores fail to achieve high levels of hypnotic responsiveness. Scoring high on absorption, however, may not contribute to a corresponding systematic enhancement of responsiveness.

Obviously variables must first demonstrate a consistent relationship with susceptibility within the hypnotic context in order for a context-dependent relationship to be proposed. As de Groot et al. noted, a variety of personality variables have been measured within the hypnotic context without a significant relationship with susceptibility emerging. One focus for further research, therefore, should examine why a context-dependent relationship with susceptibility emerges for absorption. What is special about the experiences described within this questionnaire that somehow influences subjects' subsequent level of responsiveness?

That a widely accepted variable, such as absorption, may be related to susceptibility only when tested within the hypnotic context may have important implications for other traditionally accepted variables, such as imagery vividness. Perhaps the relationship of imagery vividness and susceptibility is also dependent on vividness being assessed within the hypnotic context. My review of the literature suggested that, like absorption, imagery vividness has also been routinely measured within contexts associated with hypnosis. Moreover, two studies (Perry, 1973; Spanos, D'Eon, et al., 1988) measured imagery vividness after susceptibility testing and found no relationship between these two variables. Sutcliffe et al. (1970) also measured imagery vividness after susceptibility testing and found a significant correlation for males only. This suggests another avenue for further research.

SUMMARY

An extensive number of variables have been investigated in relation to hypnotic susceptibility. As theoretical perspectives concerning hypnosis have changed, so have the variables of primary interest. Yet even in recent investigations, researchers have exhibited little concern for either the reliability of their measures or the generalizability of their results. Unanswered questions still remain, even with respect to imagery vividness (a construct whose measurement has received systematic attention). A more accurate understanding of the psychometric properties of our measurement scales can only help to generate a clearer picture of the relationship of these variables to hypnotic responding.

In attempting to delineate those variables related to susceptibility, researchers have relied primarily on linear correlation results. With respect to all of the variables reviewed, such a statistical technique alone may be misleading. Visual analyses of the relationship of susceptibility to attitudes (Spanos, Brett, et al., 1987) imagery vividness (de Groh et al., 1986; Hilgard, 1979; Sutcliffe et al. 1970), and absorption (Crawford 1982; Spanos, Brett et al. 1987) have all suggested a systematic deviation from linearity. Low scores on all of these predictors appeared to be associated only with low-susceptibility scores, while higher scores on all of these predictors were associated with all levels of hypnotic susceptibility. Descriptive measurement techniques should aid in discriminating among linear relationships, systematic deviations from linearity, and situations where no relationship is present.

A hypnosis session is a highly specific contextual event. Perceiving subjects as active participants in the hypnotic session has been central to nonstate theories of hypnotic responding. Nevertheless, many state and nonstate theorists have paid insufficient attention to the fact that subjects are not only aware that they are being tested, but they are also aware that the questionnaires they complete are related to the researcher's hypotheses concerning their performance. Consequently, researchers have taken at face value quantitative assessments of the relationship between predictors and susceptibility. Recently, however, the reactive effect of the ABS scale on subsequent hypnotic responding has called into question previous interpretations. Whether the context dependency observed between absorption and susceptibility will generalize to other "aptitude" variables remains to be seen. The utility of the scales, however, should not be dismissed prematurely. While ABS experience items may not signify an important "aptitude" for hypnotic responding, it may offer insights into subjects' perceptions of hypnosis.

NOTES

1. Sensory modalities: visual, auditory, kinesthetic, cutaneous, gustatory, olfactory, and organic.

2. Researchers have reported the VVIQ to be internally reliable (Gur & Hilgard, 1975; Marks, 1973; McKelvie & Gingras, 1974). Acceptable test-retest reliabilities have also been reported (Gur & Hilgard 1975; Marks, 1963), with one exception (McKelvie & Gingras, 1974).

3. Some illustrative examples from Shor et al. (1962, p. 58). Have you ever had the experience of walking in your sleep? Have you ever become so absorbed in listening to music that you almost forgot where you were? Have you ever been able to ignore pain? Has everything in your line of vision become blurry or strange, as if you were dreaming? Do you find yourself unwittingly adopting the mannerisms of other people?

4. Some illustrative examples from As, O'Hara, and Mungar (1962, pp. 24–25): *Tolerance for Unusual Experiences Factor*—Have you ever carried on real conversations with another person while you were asleep? Do you think there are events and things that cannot ultimately be explained logically? *Role Absorption Factor*— Have you ever had the experience of being caught up by music or dancing so that you became enraptured by it and had it live and express itself through you so that you as yourself seemed to cease to be during it? Have you ever participated (been caught up) in a crowd action (mass demonstrations, mass audiences, dormitory raids, riots, rallies, etc.) and found yourself doing and feeling things that you would not normally do or feel?

5. Subscales and illustrative examples from Lee-Teng (1965, p. 384). Those subscales significantly correlated with susceptibility are indicated by an asterisk. *Conformity versus Autonomy:* In general, do you prefer to follow rather than to direct? *Trancelike Experiences*:* When you dance, do you often feel that the music and mood are being expressed through your movements, while you yourself fade into the background? *Role-Playing*:* While watching a movie or show do you sometimes become so involved that you feel yourself participating in the action? *Impulsivity versus Rationality*:* When faced with a decision, do you usually ponder and weigh all aspects carefully (reverse scoring)? *Concentration and Absorption:* Do you often have trouble keeping you mind on what you should do (reverse scoring)?

6. Some researchers in the hypnosis area have retained the original 20-item ABS scale (from Tellegen & Atkinson, 1974), while others have adopted the 34-item ABS subscale from the DPQ. Consistent with the approach of researchers in this area, results (and interpretation) of the two scales will be treated as synonymous. One should keep in mind, however, that future research may uncover meaningful differences between the two versions.

7. Categories (subscales) and illustrative examples from Ronnestad (1985). *Affective/Regressive (13 items):* I can be greatly moved by eloquent or poetic language. *Congitive/Perceptual Engagement (10 items):* My thoughts often don't occur as words but as visual images. *Dissociative (6 items):* If I wish I can imagine that my body is so heavy that I could not move it if I wanted to. *Mystical Inclination (5 items):* I often know what someone is going to say before he or she says it.

8. The reliability of Hilgard's results is weakened by her method of apparently categorizing her variables in a way that produced the best results. In addition, Drake and Nash (1986) have noted that interviewers' ratings may have been biased since they were often aware of subjects' susceptibility level and research hypotheses. Further, for the activities reported here, preliminary results indicated that interrater reliabilities were quite low. Finally, the phenomenological experiences of subjects were estimated by the interviewers rather than the subjects without first demonstrating some correspondence between the two.

9. In Study 1 (Nash et al. 1984) parental disciplinary practices were gathered directly from the parents of sixteen high- and fourteen low-susceptible subjects. Based on parental accounts, high

and low susceptibles failed to differ on the severity of punishment measure. There are several possible explanations for these apparently inconsistent results. For example, it would appear that a distinction between physical punishment (i.e., discipline) and physical abuse may be important. It is possible that only severe physical abuse during childhood is associated with later hypnotic responsiveness. Hilgard's in-depth interviews with students (and subjects' self-ratings; Nash et al., Study 2) may have proved more sensitive at detecting severe abuse than Nash's telephone interviews with parents. Alternatively, both studies suggest that severe physical punishment during childhood is not a necessary condition for high susceptibility. With this in mind, it is not surprising that Study I found no difference among high and low susceptibles and the severity of punishment measure.

3

Hypnotic Depth as Social Artifact

H. Lorraine Radtke

Hypnotic depth refers to a person's belief regarding the degree to which they were hypnotized, and current measures of "depth" reflect the idea that hypnotized persons are experiencing an altered state of consciousness (for recent reviews, see Laurence & Nadon, 1986; Radtke & Spanos, 1981; Tart, 1979b). Historically, the concept of "depth" was not distinguished from the concept of "susceptibility," and in fact, depth was inferred from subjects' response to suggestions (Edmonston, 1986; Sheehan & Perry, 1976; Weitzenhoffer, 1957). More recent formulations (e.g., Hilgard, 1965) distinguish between the behavioral response to hypnotic procedures (i.e., hypnotic susceptibility) and the subjective response (i.e., hypnotic depth). Nonetheless, the intent remains to assess the quantitative change in a person's state of consciousness.

Obviously, then, the concept of "depth" fits within a theoretical framework where hypnosis is conceptualized as involving some alteration in consciousness (e.g., Bowers, 1976; Evans, 1968; Hilgard, 1977; Kihlstrom, 1984; Orne, 1959). In fact, within this framework, depth ratings have been viewed as validating evidence for the existence of a hypnotic state (Conn & Conn, 1967; Hilgard, 1965, 1979; Hilgard & Tart, 1966; Sheehan & Perry, 1980; Tart & Hilgard, 1966). These investigators have argued that hypnotic procedures result in an identifiable qualitative shift in consciousness and that depth reports reflect the extent of this shift. Most importantly, depth reports are regarded as at least partly independent of the hypnotized person's actions and contextual variables. Hypnotic depth takes on a very different meaning however within the alternative social-psychological framework where hypnosis is construed as involving goal-directed behavior in response to the demands of a particular social context (Barber, 1969; Sarbin & Coe, 1972; Spanos, 1982, 1986; Wagstaff, 1981). Within this latter framework, depth ratings can be viewed not as objective self-observations of experience, but as contextually embedded interpretations of experience. In other words, depth ratings reflect a person's understanding of hypnosis that has emerged within a particular historical and cultural context.

Adopting a social-psychological orientation involves two important assumptions. First, it is assumed that knowledge does not arise directly from experience. Second, it is assumed that how we understand our world is a social artifact, and therefore, by implication, attributing one's experiences to being hypnotized is also a social artifact. Applying the first assumption to hypnotic depth, it is assumed that depth reports do not reflect a natural change in the state of a person's consciousness. In other words, there is no hypnotic trance that exists apart from the meaning hypnosis has come to acquire within our culture.[1] Indeed, careful examination of its research literature reveals that, aside from participants' overt responses to suggestion and their introspective reports, there are no objective criteria, such as physiological indicators, for the presence of a trance or dissociated state (Edmonston, 1979; Spanos, 1982; Sarbin & Slagle, 1972). Moreover, the experiences reported by research participants following hypnotic procedures are highly similar to those associated with other procedures involving minor sensory restriction, relaxation, EMG (electromyographic) and EEG (electroencephalographic) biofeedback, and mediation techniques requiring concentration (Aaronson, 1973, As & Ostvold, 1968; Barber & Calverley, 1969; Deikman, 1963; Edmonston, 1977, 1979; Field, 1965; Field & Palmer, 1969; Hilgard, 1965; Hunt & Chefurka, 1976; Morse, Martin, Furst & Dubin, 1977; Plotkin, 1979).

The second assumption draws our attention to the historical and cultural underpinnings of our understanding of hypnosis. The language used to describe the hypnotic experience has been adopted by convention and has emerged within a certain social relationship (hypnotist and research participant) that only makes sense within a specific socio-historic-cultural time period. This assumption then alerts us to the need to acknowledge explicitly how the understandings of both the hypnotist and the research participant impact on the participant's responses. The social situation becomes of primary importance, and we are led to examine how the actions of both hypnotist and participant reflect certain cultural values and beliefs.

The purpose of this paper is to review the literature on hypnotic depth and to evaluate it critically from a social-psychological perspective. It will be seen that hypnotic depth is a social phenomenon and as such must be studied within its social context.

MEASUREMENT OF HYPNOTIC DEPTH

Most of the measuring instruments developed to assess hypnotic depth require the research participants to indicate how hypnotized they felt at a particular point in time. Depth then is defined for research participants as a continuum ranging from "not hypnotized" through being hypnotized to varying degrees (e.g., "light, medium, deep"), and generally the research participants select a number to represent their experiences. These scales differ in a number of ways, however, including (a) the degree to which the scale values are concretely defined, (b) whether the research participants are asked to estimate their depth deliberately or automatically (e.g., "a number representing your depth will come to mind automatically"), and (c) the number of scale alternatives provided. In addition, there is wide variation across studies in the number of depth reports obtained within a single testing session. One example is a scale used by Tart (1963). The research participants were instructed to use the analogy of a yardstick when measuring their depth, and behavioral criteria were provided for different levels of depth. At a depth of 1 to 12, the research participants were to feel very relaxed and detached and to pass an arm levitation or arm rotation suggestion. At a depth of 30 and above, they were to be amnesic for the events taking place during the hypnotic condition. Another example, used by O'Connell (1964), was a simple 1 (awake) to 10 (hypnotized as deeply as possible) scale. Other researchers have used similar scales with variations in the number of scale alternatives (e.g., Barber & Calverley, 1966; Bowers, 1981; Cheek, 1959; Field, 1966; Hilgard & tart, 1966; Israeli, 1953; LeCron, 1953; Perry & Laurence, 1980; Sheehan & Dolby, 1974; Tart, 1966, 1970; Tart & Hilgard, 1966; Wedemeyer & Coe, 1981).

Researchers seldom provide a rationale for their use of a particular depth scale, and in general, there has been little systematic study of these scales other than to correlate them with a criterion such as hypnotic susceptibility. Moreover, two studies have shown that the wording of hypnotic depth scales significantly affects participants' reports (Barber, Dalal & Calverley, 1968; Radtke & Spanos, 1982). These studies suggest a need for greater attention to the meaning of the reports and will be discussed in greater detail below.

GROUP DIFFERENCES IN HYPNOTIC DEPTH

Many studies of hypnosis compare the responses of research participants exposed to a standard hypnotic-induction procedure with those of a control group exposed to some other instructions such as task-motivating instructions (Barber, 1969). A large number of these indicate that when given short nonhypnotic instructions aimed at motivating performance, research participants respond to test suggestions in the same way as participants who are given a standard hypnotic-induction procedure (for a review, see Barber, 1969). When comparisons of hypnotic depth are included, however, most studies have found that research participants given a standard hypnotic-induction procedure rated themselves as more deeply hypnotized than those given such nonhypnotic control procedures as task-motivating or imagination-control instructions (Connors & Sheehan, 1978; Gilbert & Barber, 1972; Ham & Spanos, 1974; Radtke-Bodorik, Spanos & Haddad, 1979; Spanos & Barber, 1968; Spanos, Ham & Barber, 1973; Spanos, Stam, D'Eon, Pawlak & Radtke-Bodorik, 1980), and only two studies have failed to find such differences (Connors & Sheehan, 1976; Sheehan & Dolby, 1974).

Two factors may be responsible for the observed group differences: defining the context as hypnosis or not hypnosis is one; the other is the different instructions administered to research participants in the hypnotic and nonhypnotic conditions.

A study by Spanos, Radtke-Bodorik, and Stam (1980) provided data relevant to this issue. They gave hypnotic and control groups identical instructions, but in the first case labeled them as hypnotic instructions and in the second case as nonhypnotic instructions. Although the study focused on the research participants' responses to an amnesia suggestion, depth ratings were also obtained. Consistent with earlier studies, research participants in the hypnotic group rated themselves as more deeply hypnotized than those in the nonhypnotic group. As the two groups received identical instructions, the factor likely responsible for this difference was the way in which the context was defined.

RELATIONSHIP BETWEEN HYPNOTIC DEPTH RATINGS AND OVERT RESPONSES

A number of studies have correlated hypnotic susceptibility, as measured by a standardized hypnotic-susceptibility scale, with hypnotic depth ratings. When the situation was explicitly defined as hypnosis, researchers obtained significant correlations, ranging from .23 to .88 between ratings of hypnotic depth and hypnotic susceptibility assessed by Forms A, B, and C of the Stanford Hypnotic Susceptibility Scale (SHSS:A, SHSS:B, Weitzenhoffer & Hilgard, 1959; SHSS:C, Weitzenhoffer & Hilgard, 1962), the Harvard Group Scale of Hypnotic Susceptibility Scale, Form A (HGSHS:A, Shor & Orne, 1962), and the Barber Suggestibility Scale (BSS, Barber, 1969; Barber & Calverley, 1966, 1969; Bowers, 1981; Council, Kirsh & Hafner, 1986; Hatfield, 1961; Hilgard & Tart, 1966; Kihlstrom, 1982; O'Connell, 1964; Perry & Laurence, 1980; Spanos, Ham & Barber, 1973; Tart, 1970; Wedemeyer & Coe, 1981).

When the testing situation was not explicitly defined as hypnosis, results were mixed. Hilgard and Tart (1966) reported significant correlations between scores on the SHSS:C and hypnotic depth for two of their four control groups. On the other hand, in studies correlating hypnotic depth and response to individual test suggestions no statistically significant relationship between these two variables has been found (Ham & Spanos, 1974; Spanos, Ham & Barber, 1973; Spanos & Barber, 1968). This discrepancy may be accounted for by the wording of the suggestions on the SHSS:C, which tends to define the situation as hypnosis even when a formal induction procedure is omitted.

It has been argued that research participants make inferences about their hypnotic depth based on their response to suggestions when they have prior reason to believe that hypnosis is relevant to their responding (e.g., when the situation has been implicitly or explicitly defined as one in which they will be hypnotized; Radtke & Spanos, 1981). The alternative position is that depth ratings reflect degree of hypnosis and that depth of hypnosis determines the level of hypnotic responding (Hilgard & Tart, 1966; Tart, 1970). For example, Tart (1970) asked research participants to report their hypnotic depth before responding to each test suggestion on the SHSS:C and found higher depth reports before suggestions that were subsequently passed than before suggestions that were subsequently failed. More recently, Wedemeyer and Coe (1981) replicated Tart's (1970) findings on eight of the nine SHSS:A test suggestions. When they compared the responses to each suggestion with depth reports obtained following the suggestion, however, on all nine suggestions they found higher depth reports following suggestions that were passed compared to those that were failed. Because the test suggestions are presented more or less in order of difficulty, both patterns may simply reflect participants' inferences that they are not as hypnotized once they begin to fail suggestions. As a consequence, they lower their depth ratings.

This hypothesis is further strengthened by the findings of Perry and Laurence (1980). They obtained retrospective depth reports on a 10-point scale for each of the items on the HGSHS:A. The Spearman rank order correlation between the test suggestions, ordered according to difficulty, and mean depth reports, ordered from smallest to largest, was .94, indicating that higher depth ratings were associated with easier items (i.e., those items with a higher percentage of "pass" responses). When the mean depth reports were plotted by test suggestion for the high (10–12), high-medium (7–9), low-medium (3–6), and low (0–2) susceptibles, the lines for the four groups did not overlap, reflecting the strong relationship between hypnotic susceptibility and hypnotic depth. Perry and Laurence (1980) suggested that the lines were actually parallel; however, no statistical test was performed. Assuming the lines were parallel, Perry and Laurence argued that the research participants did not base their depth reports simply on their objective responses to suggestions because the low and high susceptibles showed the same decreases and increases in hypnotic depth with increases and decreases in item difficulty. For example, although many low susceptibles did not pass item 7 (moving hands together), they nonetheless reported a higher mean depth on this item than on other items. Such a finding is consistent with a social-psychological interpretation of hypnotic depth. Research participants may experience some subjective changes in response to a suggestion (e.g., they were able to imagine their hands moving together to a slight degree) that are not reflected in an overt response. If they then base their depth ratings on both overt (i.e., behavioral) information and subjective information, then pass/fail information alone will not predict hypnotic depth.

RELATIONSHIP BETWEEN HYPNOTIC DEPTH RATINGS AND SUBJECTIVE EXPERIENCE

The studies already discussed focused on the relationship between hypnotic depth ratings and research participants' overt responses to suggestion, i.e., their behavioral responses. Depth also correlates with scores on an inventory developed by Field (1965) to assess components of subjective response to the hypnotic situation (Council et al., 1986; Kihlstrom, 1981, 1982; Spanos, Rivers & Gottlieb, 1978; Tart, 1970). In addition, both Kihlstrom (1982) and Council et al. (1986) assessed the relationship between hypnotic depth and subjective responses to each test suggestion. Following administration of the HGSHS:A, Kihlstrom (1982) obtained self ratings of (*a*) behavioral responses to each item (pass/fail), (*b*) subjective success on each item (pass/fail), and (*c*) hypnotic depth (10-point scale). Council et al. (1986) used the Stanford Group Scale (Finke & MacDonald, 1978) to assess susceptibility and also obtained self-ratings of (*a*) behavioral response (pass/fail), (*b*) subjective success (5-point Likert scale), and (*c*) hypnotic depth (Long Stanford Scale; Tart 1979a). In both studies, there was a stronger relationship between the research participants' subjective success or perceived success on the test suggestions and their hypnotic depth ratings (r's = .70 and .42, respectively) compared to the relationship between the participants' behavioral responses and their depth ratings (r's = .65 and .35, respectively). Nonetheless, in an earlier study (Barber & Calverley, 1969) depth reports correlated .75 with response to the test suggestions and .67 with "reports of unusual experiences," the reverse of the pattern reported by Kihlstrom (1982) and Council et al. (1986). Thus, the method of assessing subjective experiences may influence the strength of the correlation with depth reports.

These findings can be interpreted from a social-psychological perspective. This view does not deny that research participants have experiences such as "my arm feels lighter" or "it felt as though I could *not* open my eyes." Rather, the meaning that participants attribute to their actions is taken from the social context. In another context, these experiences would have a very different meaning. Attributing them to hypnosis is likely only when the context suggests that such an interpretation is appropriate.

RELATIONSHIP BETWEEN HYPNOTIC DEPTH RATINGS
AND EXPECTANCIES

The impact of expectancies on the hypnotic experience has yet to be investigated thoroughly; however, it has been suggested that research participants will define themselves as hypnotized if their experiences match their expectations (Barber, 1969; Sarbin & Coe, 1972). An early study by McCord (1961) found that what research participants expected to experience during hypnosis was very similar to the reported experiences that correlate with hypnotic depth, for example, relaxation, effortless responding to suggestion, and so on (Barber & Calverley, 1969; Tart, 1970; Spanos, Rivers, & Gottlieb 1978). In addition, when Barber and Calverley (1969) compared research participants who were equally responsive to suggestion but differed on their hypnotic depth ratings, they found that the participants who rated themselves as "medium" or "lightly" hypnotized rather than "deeply" hypnotized did so because they were (*a*) aware of what they were doing, (*b*) aware of their surroundings, (*c*) able to think of extraneous things, (*d*) able to hear extraneous sounds, and (*e*) not completely amnesic. This suggests that the otherwise responsive research participants rated themselves as "medium" or "lightly" hypnotized because their experiences conflicted with their expectations regarding hypnosis.

In a recent study examining the impact of expectancies or hypnotic responding, Stam and Fraser (1986) on two occasions assessed susceptibility using the SHSS:C. They compared a condition in which the research participants were asked to do whatever they could to "place themselves in hypnosis" with a condition in which the participants received the standard induction accompanying the SHSS:C. Three groups of participants were tested: (a) Group 1 received the standard induction during the first session and placed themselves in hypnosis during the second session, (b) Group 2 received the reverse order of testing, and (c) Group 3 received the standard induction during both sessions. There were no group or session differences in hypnotic susceptibility measured via the SHSS:C. An interesting interaction involving hypnotic depth emerged however. The research participants in Groups 2 and 3 showed no change in depth ratings (reported on a 10 cm visual analogue scale), but Group 1 reported significantly lower levels of hypnotic depth when they placed themsleves in hypnosis on Session 2 compared to Session 1 when they received the standard hypnotic-induction procedure. This order effect suggests that the research participants' expectancies affected their judgments of the subjective experiences accompanying hypnotic procedures. Presumably, the participants in Group 1 did not expect to experience the hypnotic suggestions as deeply when placing themselves in hypnosis as they did when hypnotic induction was provided. Those in Group 2, on the other hand, had no previous hypnotic experiences with which to compare their self-hypnotic experiences. Thus, their self-hypnotic experiences were judged to be as deep as those following a standard hypnotic-induction procedure. These results then provide at least indirect evidence of the impact of expectancies on reported hypnotic depth.

A few studies have directly examined the relationship between expectancies and hypnotic depth reports. Two obtained a moderate correlation between expected hypnotic depth and actual reported depth (Barber & Calverley, 1966, 1969), but a third found no relationship between the two variables (Council et al., 1986). The Council et al. (1986) study will be discussed in some detail, as it involved a complex and sophisticated approach to examining the relationships between subjective experience and overt response.

Using a path analysis, Council et al. (1986) examined the relationships among predicted hypnotic depth (preinduction depth), predicted response to suggestion (preinduction expectancies), actual hypnotic depth reported after the hypnotic induction procedure (postinduction depth), predicted response to suggestion obtained after the induction (postinduction response expectancies), behavioral and subjective response to suggestion, and ratings of subjective experience on the Field (1965) inventory. Postinduction hypnotic depth had an indirect effect on the behavioral and subjective responses to suggestion, which was mediated by the research participants' postinduction expectancies. On the basis of these findings, Council et al. (1986) argued that the experiences reflected in the depth reports affected the participants' response expectancies, which in turn affected their behavioral and subjective response to suggestion. There were, however, no direct effects of pre-induction depth ratings or response expectancies on postinduction depth.

At a superficial level these findings appear to contradict the view that research participants' preconceived notions about hypnosis impact on their depth reports. When examined more closely, one discovers reasons to exercise caution about this interpretation. An examination of the measures and procedures adopted by Council et al. (1986) suggests one possible problem. Pre-induction depth was assessed via 10 items taken from the Field (1965) inventory and included items such as "I will not be able to resist the experimenter's suggestion." Thus, it may be better thought of as a preinduction measure of expected subjective response to hypnosis. Postinduction depth was assessed via the Long Stanford Scale (Tart, 1979b) and consisted of a single rating on a 5-point scale. Thus, the measure of postinduction depth was consistent with the definition of "hypnotic depth" used throughout this paper. Although the pre-induction and postinduction depth ratings were not significantly correlated, both variables were correlated with the Field (1965) inventory (r's = .29 and .39, respectively). Moreover, the path analysis revealed a direct effect of preinduction depth on the subjective experiences assessed by the Field (1965) inventory. As the preinduction depth reports and the Field (1965) contained similar items, it is not surprising to find a relationship between the two measures. However, use of items from the Field (1965) inventory to measure preinduction depth confounded expected hypnotic depth and expected subjective response to suggestion. The anomalous findings clearly involve the postinduction depth rating, but since it involved a single rating, unreliability may have attenuated its correlation with the preinduction depth rating. Finally, given the assortment of factors that may affect the size of correlation coefficients and the converging evidence supporting the importance of expectancies, it would be premature to overemphasize the Council et al. findings until replication has been reported.

Two other studies have examined the impact of the hypnotist's opinion regarding a research participant's level of hypnotic depth (Barber, Dalal & Calverley, 1968; Wedemeyer & Coe, 1981). Barber, Dalal, and Calverley (1968) administered a hypnotic-induction procedure followed by a standardized hypnotic-susceptibility scale (BSS) to three groups. Following the hypnotic induction procedure, the hypnotist told one group that he thought they were hypnotized, told the second that he thought them not hypnotized, and gave the third no such information. The three groups did not differ significantly on hypnotic susceptibility, but the group told that they were hypnotized rated themselves as more deeply hypnotized than did the participants in the other two groups. In addition, participants told nothing scored higher on hypnotic depth than participants told they were not hypnotized. Thus, the research participants based their evaluations of their experiences on the hypnotist's expert opinion.

Using a different approach, Wedemeyer and Coe (1981) provided their research participants with the hypnotist's expectations prior to susceptibility testing and administration of the hypnotic-induction procedure. They were told that the hypnotist was interested (*a*) only in data from participants who gave deep state reports, (*b*) only in data from participants who gave low state reports, or (*c*) only in data from participants who gave either deep or low state reports. Depth reports were highest for the deep-expectation group, followed by the deep- or low-expectation group, and finally the low-expectation group. Deep-expectation participants also scored significantly higher on hypnotic susceptibility than the other two groups. It is apparent, then, that hypnotic depth reports are sensitive to contextual manipulations such as the hypnotist's opinion.

REPEATED ASSESSMENT OF HYPNOTIC DEPTH

When hypnotic depth is assessed on more than one occasion within an hypnotic session, the ratings tend to be relatively stable and, in particular, do not differ dramatically from depth reports given prior to the administration of the test suggestions (Hilgard & Tart, 1966; Tart, 1970). For example, Tart (1970) reported that 50 percent of the time depth reports did not change from one report to another and 35 percent of the time they changed by 1 point on a 10-point scale. Moreover, 86 percent of the research participants showed a change of 2 or fewer points as their maximum absolute change from one report to another. The Council et al. (1986) study notwithstanding, this may reflect the impact of expectancies that influence both hypnotic responsiveness and hypnotic depth ratings. In other words, expectancies may influence level of hypnotic responding and initial depth reports; when exposed to test suggestions the research participants may then make further decisions about their hypnotic depth based on the level of hypnotic responding. As a consequence, depth ratings obtained following the test suggestions will be consistent with depth ratings obtained prior to administration of the test suggestions and depth ratings will be consistent with level of hypnotic responding.

Wedemeyer and Coe (1981) reported findings that differ somewhat from those of Hilgard and Tart but that are nonetheless consistent with a social constructionist view. Susceptibility scores were more strongly correlated with the research participants' average depth reports (r = .61) than with their first depth report obtained immediately following the hypnotic induction procedure (r = .31). These results suggest that once the test suggestions are administered, research participants begin to base their depth reports on their responses to suggestions.

Although the data just discussed are open to alternative interpretations, other studies provide some support for the contention that research participants' knowledge of their performance on hypnotic test suggestions influences their hypnotic depth ratings. In three studies the research participants were asked to report the criteria they used to judge that they were hypnotized (Barber & Calverley, 1969; Tart, 1970; Wedemeyer & Coe, 1981). Barber and Calverley (1969) reported that participants who rated themselves as "deeply" hypnotized indicated that they did so because they responded successfully to the suggestions. In the other two studies, 21 percent (Tart, 1970) and 53 percent (Wedemeyer & Coe, 1981) of the subjects indicated that they based their depth reports on the intensity of their responses to the test item administered prior to the depth rating. The remaining participants reported other criteria that are consistent with the relaxation instructions and focus on bodily sensations that are contained in hypnotic-induction procedures, for example, body feelings and awareness or lack of awareness of the environment. Perceived involuntariness of responses was also reported as a criterion, and again, it must be noted that the standard wording of hypnotic suggestions generally implies involuntariness of response. In addition, involuntary responding is part of the common understanding regarding hypnosis (e.g., McCord, 1961). Thus, it seems likely that depth ratings reflect a combination of factors: expectancies generated by the participant's understanding of hypnosis, the context created by the researcher's actions and the instructions provided, and the participant's own response to these instructions.

Furthermore, in an interesting participant-observation study, Kidder (1972) reported that participants in a hypnosis workshop initially described their responses to hypnotic procedures with nonhypnotic terms (e.g., "I felt normal," "I was only imagining"). Through the guidance of the workshop leader participants learned to relabel their experiences in terms of hypnosis, for example, the leader directed their attention to the fact that they made certain responses in the absence of any external cause. By the end of the workshop, many of the participants came to define their experiences as due to hypnosis; in Kidder's words "the skeptics became convinced." Given that participants in hypnosis research are typically aware that hypnosis is involved, it is reasonable to expect that they will define their responses in terms of hypnosis and will base their hypnotic depth estimates at least partly on their level of responding.

WORDING OF HYPNOTIC DEPTH SCALES

A final contextual factor that has received some attention is the wording of hypnotic depth scales. Barber et al. (1968) asked research participants to compare experiences in the hypnotic state with experiences in the waking state. When asked whether the hypnotic state was *similar* to the waking state, only 17 percent of the participants responded that it was *not* the same (i.e., 17 percent indicated that hypnotic and waking experiences differ). When asked whether the hypnotic state was *different* from the waking state, however, 72 percent indicated that they differed. The wording of the question put to the participants, then, had a dramatic impact on the evaluation of their experiences, leading them to think either in terms of similarity or difference.

More recently, Radtke and Spanos (1982) hypothesized that regardless of their level of hypnotic susceptibility, research participants would be less inclined to report having been hypnotized when provided with a rating scale that offered alternative descriptors for their experiences. In other words, we allowed for the possibility that participants would have experiences during hypnotic susceptibility testing that they would *not* label as hypnotic experiences. The research participants were administered the HGSHS:A and then retrospectively responded to one of three depth scales. Scale 1 was a standard 4-point scale used in previous research (e.g., Spanos et al. 1978) with the alternatives (*a*) not hypnotized, (*b*) slightly hypnotized, (*c*) moderately hypnotized, and (*d*) highly hypnotized. Scale 2 also had four alternatives, but ratings were made on a continuum with varying degrees of hypnosis *and* absorption: (*a*) *neither* hypnotized *nor* absorbed, (*b*) absorbed *and* hypnotized to a slight degree, (*c*) absorbed *and* hypnotized to a moderate degree, and (*d*) absorbed *and* hypnotized to a high degree. Finally, Scale 3 provided seven alternatives: experiences were classified as (*a*) *neither* hypnotized *nor* absorbed; (*b*) absorbed *and* hypnotized to a slight, moderate, or high degree; and (*c*) absorbed to a slight, moderate, or high degree *but not* hypnotized.

For all three scales, the participants were classified as indicating that they were hypnotized to at least some degree or not hypnotized. On Scale 1 (hypnotized *or* not), 100 percent of the high susceptibles, 94 percent of the medium susceptibles, and 55 percent of the low susceptibles reported that they had been hypnotized to some degree. The results for Scale 2 (hypnotized and absorbed *or* not) were very similar with 96 percent of the highs, 89 percent of the mediums, and 61 percent of the low susceptibles reporting that they had been hypnotized to some degree. On Scale 3 (hypnotized and absorbed *or* absorbed but not hypnotized), however, only 64 percent of the high susceptibles, 18 percent of the mediums, and 11 percent of the lows indicated that they had been hypnotized to some degree. Thus, as predicted, at all susceptibility levels there were substantial drops in the proportion of participants reporting that they had been hypnotized when they were given the option of classifying their experiences along a continuum other than degree of hypnosis.

Although the effects of varied wording in this study were large and statistically significant, some participants (in particular, high susceptibles) continued to classify their experiences as being hypnotized to some degree. This is not surprising from a social-psychological perspective. After all, the situation was defined as involving hypnosis, the procedures employed were consistent with what one might expect of hypnotic procedures, and the high susceptibles were successful in imagining and experiencing what was suggested. Thus, a majority of high susceptibles would be expected to label their experiences as involving some degree of hypnosis. Their interpretation of their experiences as such, however, cannot be viewed as evidence for the existence of an hypnotic state. Rather, their intepretation is based on a desire to make sense of their experiences, and in the absence of conflicting information, it will reflect the context defined by the researcher.

CONCLUSION

The literature reviewed indicates that when asked to judge the extent to which they were hypnotized, research participants were influenced by a variety of factors: (*a*) whether the social context is implicitly or explicitly defined as involving hypnosis, (*b*) their overt and subjective responses to the suggestions, (*c*) their expectations and those of the hypnotist, and (*d*) the frame of reference provided by the assessment instrument. It has been argued that a social-psychological perspective can usefully guide our understanding of these effects. In particular, a social-psychological perspective emphasizes the social nature of the hypnotic interaction and the importance of historical, social, and cultural factors in determining our (that is, the hypnotist and the research participant) understanding of hypnosis. Hypnosis then is not seen as some natural psychological state that can be measured at least partly via hypnotic depth reports. It, and hypnotic depth reports, are seen as social artifacts. What remains to be done is an analysis of how popular conceptions of hypnosis fit within the broader framework of cultural values and beliefs about persons and social interaction and of the social institutions supported by those beliefs.

NOTE

1. This is similar to the analyses of anger and schizophrenia provided by Averill (1982) and Sarbin and Mancuso (1980), respectively.

Part Two

Specific Hypnotic Phenomena

4

Hypnosis and Experienced Nonvolition
A Social-Cognitive Integrative Model

Steven J. Lynn, Judith W. Rhue, and John R. Weekes

"I felt like I could not control my actions. . . . my hands felt like they were moving toward each other, and I could not prevent their touching." This hypnotized subject's account of her suggestion-related movements is not atypical. Descriptors such as "loss of control," "compelled," "passive," "automatic," and "effortless" color many hypnotized subjects' portrayals of their hypnotic responses. Not only is the hypnotized subject's feeling of involuntariness a compelling personal experience, but observers have long been intrigued and fascinated by such dramatic testimony. Indeed, the experience of involuntariness is one of the hallmarks of hypnosis, around which has coalesced an abundance of theoretical and research interest in hypnotic phenomena.

Hypnosis theorists of diverse stripe have attempted to account for what Weitzenhoffer (1974) has termed the "classical suggestion effect": the subject's "transformation of the essential, manifest, ideational content of a communication" into behavior that is considered involuntary. More than thirty years before Weitzenhoffer provided this characterization, White (1941) maintained that suggestion-related involuntariness was so central to the experience of hypnosis that it was incumbent upon theorists to address this domain of experience. In this chapter we will describe how hypnosis theorists have risen to the challenge of explaining the well-documented finding that hypnotizable subjects who pass test suggestions characterize their responses as more automatic or nonvolitional than subjects who fail suggestions (e.g., K. Bowers, 1981; P. Bowers, 1982; P. Bowers, Laurence, & Hart, 1988; Farthing, Brown & Venturino, 1983; Spanos, Bertrand, Rivers & Ross, 1977; Spanos, Radtke, Hodgins, Stam & Bertrand, 1983). The particular focus of our chapter will be on delineating a framework for understanding the experience of nonvolition. We will draw upon broadly defined social psychological

We would like to thank Wendi Cross, Joseph P. Green, and G. Daniel Lassiter for their helpful comments on an earlier version of this chapter.

and cognitive perspectives on hypnotic responding to advance an integrative perspective on hypnotic involuntariness. We will begin with a historical overview of conceptualizations of the experience of nonvolition.

HISTORICAL OVERVIEW

Since the dawn of thinking about hypnotic phenomena, the involuntary, compulsive aspect of hypnotic responding has been associated with special forces such as animal magnetism or fluids in the universe working through a powerful, active operator on a passive subject. Mesmer and Pursegur claimed that hypnotic phenomena depended upon the special prowess or supernatural skills of the hypnotist (Sheehan & Perry, 1976), under whose agency the "magnetized" person behaved as a virtual automaton. Spanos and Gottleib (1979) noted that despite technical differences among magnetists, by the early nineteenth century, the unique identity of mesmerism was largely shaped by the dominance-submissive aspects of the interaction and the view of the magnetized subject as an automaton. The correlated notions of automaticity and the passive subject survived the transition from magnetic doctrine to a more psychologically oriented view of hypnosis. Wells (1940) noted that the viewpoint that hypnotic behavior is involuntary dominated "the golden age of hypnotism"—the 1880s and 1890s—and united antagonists such as Janet and Charcot (Spanos, 1982; Spanos & Gottleib, 1979; Weitzenhoffer, 1978).

During this period it was common practice to question whether a subject was hypnotized if signs of initiative or "willpower" were exhibited. Only when the subject's normal or characteristic ways of behaving were superseded by "involuntary" behaviors associated with hypnosis, would the hypnotist be satisfied that the subject was duly hypnotized. Wells states (1940) that an inspection of influential writings from the latter half of the nineteenth century compels the conclusion that helplessness on the part of the subject was seen as an essential feature of successful hypnosis. The idea that a loss of volition constituted ultimate proof that the subject was hypnotized emanated from the influential hypnosis theories of the day.

THEORIES OF HYPNOTIC NONVOLITION

Braid

Conceptualizations of hypnotic involuntaries were influenced in various ways by Braid's theorizing. Braid (1843) soundly rejected the magnetic doctrine. He believed that the heightened responsiveness, passivity, and behaviors that resembled sleep following the hypnotist's ministrations were the result of a reflexlike process associated with staring fixedly at an object. Although Braid (1843) did not fully equate the hypnotic sleep with natural sleep, the analogy was perhaps inescapable given the physical parallels between the hypnotized and the sleeping person (e.g., eye closure, alterations in respiration and muscular tension). Braid acknowledged the importance of psychological variables such as suggestion effects, beliefs, and expectancies, particularly in his later writings (1846). And yet he did not abandon the belief that control processes and volition were distinct. This conclusion was based on his observation that subjects responded as predicted or directed by the hypnotist despite being "asleep." According to Braid's reasoning, if asleep, subjects were incapable of exercising choice and initiating actions (Gorassini, 1983).

The mechanism responsible for the involuntary quality of hypnotic behavior was monoideism: a state of enhanced concerted attention upon a single idea suggested by the hypnotist (Bramwell, 1903). In this state, imagination, belief, and expectancy are presumed to be heightened (see Sheehan & Perry, 1976). An inward focus of attention on a particular body part, especially when accompanied by the expectation that something would happen, was sufficient to cause a physical action via the mechanism of ideomotor action (Braid, 1846).

Berheim

Bernheim (1880), too, was impressed with the nonvolitional nature of hypnotic responding. In his now famous quote he stated, "The most striking feature of a hypnotized subject is his automatism" (p. 125). Bernheim (1886) defined suggestion broadly to encompass any idea that elicited responses that circumvented higher, volitional cortical processes and was mediated by a cortical reflex process termed "ideodynamic action" (Weitzenhoffer, 1986). Like Braid, Bernheim (1880) argued that motoric responses during hypnosis ensued following an "exaltation of the ideomotor reflex excitability, which effects the unconscious transformation of the thought into movement, unknown to the will" (p. 137). Relatedly, sensory or hallucinatory experiences could be accounted for by an ". . . exaltation of the ideo-sensorial excitability, which effects the unconscious transformation of thought into sensation, or into sensory image" (p. 137). This emphasis on physiological reflexive activity notwithstanding, Bernheim was aware that hypnotic behavior was an admixture of automatism and conscious, volitional activities and exhibited many features of intelligent, conscious behavior (Weitzenhoffer, 1978). Yet, when clients offered resistance, Bernheim would state, "Your nervous system is quiet; you have no will" (Bernheim, 1884, 1964, p. 3)

Hull

One thread of Braid's theorizing—the concept of ideodynamic action—weaves through the cloth of both Bernheim's thinking and other hypnosis theorists' accounts of involuntariness. As Gorassini (1983) has noted, although Hull (1933) couched his views in the vernacular of behaviorism, he echoed Braid's and Bernheim's view that ideodynamic action triggered an automatic behavioral response. Hull was in essential agreement with Bernheim's (1880) notion that "a peculiar aptitude for transforming the idea received into an act exists in a hypnotized subject" (p. 137). According to Hull (1930), this occurred when the hypnotized subject's muscles were particularly responsive to the hypnotist's suggestions following the reduction in active thought and symbolic activity produced by hypnosis. Hull also distinguished suggested and nonsuggested actions. He noted that, "One of the most characteristic differences between actions performed through the influence of suggestion and ordinary acts is that the latter are usually felt to be somehow willed, whereas the former are acts felt not to be willed" (p. 395).

Arnold

A more contemporary account of hypnosis, which traces its lineage to Braid's concept of monoideism, is Arnold's (1946) conceptualization of involuntariness. Arnold believed that imaginative processes are crucial determinants of the experience of nonvolition. According to Arnold, suggestions are invitations to imagine specific behaviors. In imagining what the hypnotist describes, the focus of attention narrows and the subject "relinquishes the control of his imaginative process." Sustained, uncontradicted imagining of a specific behavior leads automatically to the occurence of that behavior: The more vivid the imaginative process, the more pronounced will be the overt movements. According to Arnold, executing a movement as the result of imagining it represents a gradual intensification of the minimal motor nerve excitation accompanying imagination of the movement. Arnold wrote, "the experience of 'intention', of 'willing', is . . . absent from these imagined movements (p. 111)." The subjects' reports of nonvolition are viewed as accurate reflections of the supposed automatic nature of ideomotor action. Since the choice to imagine or not is under the subjects' control, however, they are capable of resisting suggested behavior by interrupting their imagining. Thus, subjects' reports of involuntariness do not imply an actual inability to resist the suggested behavior.

Dissociation Theory

Janet's dissociation theory of hypnosis represents an extension of Braid's views in the sense that ideomotor action results in automatized actions even though the ideas are dissociated or "split off" from normal consciousness and no longer subject to conscious control mechanisms (Gorassini, 1983; Spanos, Rivers & Ross, 1977). Weitzenhoffer (1986) has contended that the idea that essentially two psyches reside in every person evolved from an attempt to resolve the paradox of seemingly conscious behavior produced by a relatively passive or unconscious individual: One psyche was involved with consciousness and will; the other without will and consciousness but otherwise capable of carrying out the same activities.

Contemporary dissociation accounts (e.g., Hilgard, 1977, 1979; Kihlstrom, 1984; Kihlstrom, Evans, E. Orne & M. Orne, 1980; Miller & Bowers, 1986) also contend that divisions exist in the personality and that reports of nonvolition during hypnosis accurately reflect subjects' diminished control over behavior that is normally subject to conscious control. Kihlstrom (1984) has argued that perceived involuntariness is an essential property of the concept of dissociation. Hilgard (1977) captured the essence of the dissociation position by noting that "one of the most striking features of hypnosis is the loss of control over actions normally voluntary" (p. 115). He viewed these alterations in control as dissociations that occur at the level of the executive function of the personality that is responsible for volitional activity. Relevant subsystems of control are temporarily dissociated from conscious excecutive control and are instead directly activated by suggestion (Miller & Bowers, 1986). Hilgard argued that the operation of *dissociated cognitive subsystems* during hypnosis underlies 'subjects' diminshed control over muscular movements relative to more conscious, voluntary processes that mediate non-hypnotic, goal-directed experiences.

According to dissociation theory, nonmotoric responses such as analgesia and amnesia are potentially mediated by dissociative processes. For example, in the case of analgesia, the activation of a subsystem of pain control during hypnosis is temporarily less guided by plans and intentions than would ordinarily be the case. According to Miller and Bowers (1986), hypnosis is particularly conducive to the emergence of dissociative processes. This occurs because hypnosis attenuates subjects' generalized reality orientation (Shor, 1962), thereby affecting information processessing. Ideas processed in this fashion activate subsystems of cognitive control more or less directly, unencumbered by the mediation of higher executive processes (Miller & Bowers, 1986). Furthermore, although an activating idea and its subsequent enactment may be represented in consciousness, the psychological connection between them is not. This results in a state of affairs experientially quite different from purposeful, goal-directed behavior.

In the perspectives we have reviewed, subjects' reports of involuntariness are taken at face value. The experience of nonvolition is variously assumed to reflect reflexive, imaginative, or dissociative processes. Whatever the process, it is purported to derive from hypnosis or a special state of consciousness. Furthermore, the perspectives generally agree that the ability to focus attention and become absorbed in the events or imaginative activities called for by suggestion, to the exclusion of more reality-based perceptions, are fundamental to successful responding (see Orne, 1977; Sheehan & McConkey, 1982). Whether the theoretical account emphasizes the reflexive or the automatic, unconscious nature of hypnotic responding, hypnotic behavior is conceptualized as something that "happens" to subjects rather than something subjects are "doing" (Coe, 1987, 1978; Sarbin & Coe, 1979; Sarbin, 1984; Spanos, 1982, 1986c).

Social Psychological Theories

Not all theorists have endorsed the view that the hypnotized person is a passive participant who is transformed by hypnosis into an observer of his involuntary actions (Spanos, 1986c). Contemporary social psychological theorists (e.g., Barber, Spanos & Chaves, 1974; Sarbin & Coe, 1972; Spanos, 1986c) argue that hypnotic behavior is similar to other forms of behavior, and that despite subjects' feelings of involuntariness, they in fact retain control of their hypnotic behavior.

Perhaps the theorist who most influenced contemporary social psychological theories of nonvolition was White (1941) who conceived of hypnosis as an altered state. Yet his conception of hypnosis is more akin to contemporary social psychological theories than to so-called special process theories. The following quote represents his position and captures the essence of the contemporary social psychological viewpoint: "Hypnotic behavior is meaningful, goal-directed striving, its most general goal being to behave like a hypnotized person as this is continuously defined by the operator and understood by the subject" (p. 483).

White argues that there are several cogent reasons for adopting the concept of striving and rejecting the concept of automatism. First, many hypnotized subjects can successfully resist responding to suggestions that "are repugnant to their own deeper tendencies." Second, hypnotized subjects often improvise and elaborate on suggestions and suggested behaviors. Therefore, the initial suggestion does not constitute a sufficient cause or explanation. That subjects make substantial spontaneous additions to what is stated in the suggestion, marks the difference between automatism and a goal-directed striving to act as if hypnotized.

White's (1941) observations anticipate certain themes evident in modern social psychological formulations of hypnotic involuntariness. For instance, Coe (1987) virtually paraphrases White's (1941) comments in stating that social psychological approaches contend that hypnotic behavior is "purposeful, goal-directed strivings on the subjects' part to present themselves as hypnotized." Social psychological models conceptualize hypnotic responding as "scripted role enactment" in which subjects modify their responses strategically in terms of shifting role demands (Sarbin & Coe, 1972; Spanos, 1986a; Spanos, Salas, Bertrand & Johnson, 1988). Hypnotizable subjects are seen as active cognizers who are invested in meeting the requirements of hypnotic role behavior and are sensitively attuned to the broad demands of the testing context. Whereas social psychological accounts (Sarbin & Coe, 1972; Spanos, 1982, 1986c) underline the importance of understanding hypnosis in terms of how subjects present themselves to others through their actions, they also contend that subjects' hypnotic behavior is consistent with their role-related experiences and their self-perceptions (Spanos, 1986c).

Fundamental to the social psychological viewpoint (e.g., Barber, Spanos & Chaves, 1974; Coe, 1987; Sarbin & Coe, 1972, 1979; Spanos, 1981, 1982, 1986c; Spanos, Rivers & Ross, 1977) is the premise that hypnotizable subjects retain control over suggested responses. Hypnotic responses are regarded as goal-directed actions, and reports of involuntariness reflect context-generated interpretations of these goal-directed actions. A "central demand" of hypnosis is that subjects come to appraise their goal-directed responses to suggestions as involuntary "happenings." Sarbin and Coe (Sarbin, 1984; Sarbin & Coe, 1979) have observed that subjects' interpretations of their experiences reflect an implicit distinction between "doings" (seeing themselves as agents of goal-directed, purposeful actions) and "happenings" (viewing themselves as passive respondents). Spanos (Spanos, 1982; Spanos & Gorassini, 1984) has noted that "Interpreting behavior as an action involves attributing causality to the self (e.g., I did it), while interpreting it as a happening requires that causality be attributed to sources other than the self (e.g., It happened to me)."

According to the social psychological perspective, subjects' interpretations or attributions of involuntariness are evoked by multiple factors including preconceptions concerning hypnosis (e.g., Lynn, Nash, Rhue, Frauman & Sweeney, 1984; Spanos, Cobb & Gorassini, 1985; Spanos et al., 1987), the structure and wording of test suggestions (e.g., Spanos & Gorassini, 1984), patterns of imaginative activity that accompany response to many test suggestions (e.g., Spanos & Barber, 1972), context-generated expectancies (e.g., Kirsch, 1985; Lynn et al., 1984), and self-observation of hypnotic responses (e.g., Wedemeyer & Coe, 1981). In contrast to Arnold's (1946) viewpoint, social psychological accounts do not ascribe a causal role to subjects' imaginings. However, imaginings may legitimize and reinforce the interpretation that the actions occurred involuntarily. Thus, despite the subjectively compelling nature of subjects' reports of nonvolition, social psychological theorists have argued that it is incorrect to assume that such reports reflect an actual loss of control over responding by the subject.

A SOCIAL-COGNITIVE INTEGRATIVE MODEL OF INVOLUNTARINESS

In the discussion that follows, we will attempt to show that the automatic, robot-like appearance of certain hypnotized subjects is explicable in terms of constructs derived from social and cognitive psychology. In so doing, we reject the hypothesis that hypnotic responding is outside the realm of subjects' control, or is in any sense automatic or involuntary. We will argue that subjects' hypnotic performances and subjective experiences are shaped by the same needs that affect subjects' responses outside the hypnotic context: to maintain a sense of personal control, self-esteem, and the regard of others. We view subjects' expectancies, self-perceptions, and needs to be seen by others in a particular light as important response determinants, along with the need to optimize affect and minimize conflict. At the focal point of these sundry influences are the broad demands that emanate from the hypnotic context (Orne, 1959). These demands define the parameters of hypnotic conduct and role-related perceptions. In short, the hypnotized subject acts in terms of her aims, according to her point of view, and in relation to her interpretation of appropriate behavior and feelings.

We will adopt and embellish upon many of the explanatory constructs and determinants of involuntariness advanced by social and cognitive theorists. These include subjects' prehypnotic expectancies, situational and self-schemas/representations, interpretations and imaginative activities related to the wording and structure of hypnotic communications, and subjects' observations and attributions regarding their stream of awareness during hypnosis.

Situational Representations

Any behavior, action sequence, or feeling state can be identified or understood in diverse ways (e.g., Ryle, 1949; Wittgenstein, 1953). Which of the manifold possibilities for understanding a given action or feeling we adopt depends largely on the cues inherent in the situation and the way we interpret those cues.

Like other more mundane actions, our perceptions of hypnotic actions are structured in terms of situational and self-representations. We not only see ourselves as distinct personalities, but we also understand and interpret our actions in the context of specific situations (Trzebinski, 1985). Cantor, Mischel, and Schwartz (1982) have shown that situational representations consist of knowledge of the situation, details about the persons likely to be involved, and what is appropriate to them in these situations. Situational representations encompass scripts or schemas—knowledge structures about the nature and appropriate sequence of events or tasks in situations. These representations play a guiding role in social interactions (Abelson, 1981; Schank & Abelson, 1979; Tomkins, 1979, 1981a, 1981b), and correspond roughly to roles and role perceptions as discussed by role theorists (e.g., Coe, 1987; Sarbin & Coe, 1972).

Hypnotic subjects' expectancies, beliefs, and perceptions may be organized in a prototypic (Cantor & Kihlstrom, 1981; Hastie & Kumar, 1979; Turk & Salovey, 1985) fashion that includes representations of the attributes of hypnotizable individuals and characteristic behaviors performed by such individuals. Subjects' representations of hypnosis typically include not only the idea that hypnosis is an altered state of consciousness, but also the perception of the hypnotist as a Svengali-like figure, the belief that hypnotizable subjects are passive and receptive, and the idea that hypnotic suggestions are carried out automatically or effortlessly (McConkey, 1986; McCord, 1961; Wilson, Greene, and Loftus, 1986). For many subjects, then, merely defining the situation as hypnosis activates socio-cultural schema or prototypes that involve classifying everyday behaviors (e.g., raising of the arm) as involuntary.

It is useful to remember that even in nonhypnotic contexts we often attribute involuntariness to physiological or mental states. Kaufman (1970) gives the following example: "I am listening to a lecture, it is boring. My eyes begin to close. I try as hard as possible to keep them open; but they irresistibly close. I am unable to keep my eyes open. Someone notices and asks, 'Why did you close your eyes during the lecture?' I reply, 'I was unable to keep them open.'"

We typically dichotomize our own and others' experiences into the attributional categories or schemas of "actions" and "occurrences" (Kruglanski, 1975): Actions are voluntary, whereas occurrences are not. According to Kruglanski (1975), an action is commonly assumed to be determined by the actor's will, whereas an occurrence is largely independent of the will and is caused by factors other than the self. As social psychological theorists (Coe, 1978; Sarbin & Coe, 1979; Spanos, Salas, et al., 1988) have pointed out, people do not accept direct responsibility for "occurrences" or "happenings." The tactic of disclaiming of responsibility is expressed in statements about everyday actions like "It happened to me," "I was overcome," and "I was carried away." Hypnotic conduct, then, is not so far removed from other spheres of life, where linguistic artifice and the disclaiming of agency buttress perceptions of involuntariness by transforming "actions" into the category of "occurrences." Like many cognitive operations and activities, the identification or categorization of actions and the disclaiming of responsibility for thoughts and actions may or may not be conscious and well articulated (Wachtel, 1984). Nonetheless, the hypnotic context primes, that is, makes more accessible the attributional category of "occurrences," and thereby increases subjects' readiness to attribute suggestion-related hypnotic actions to automatic, will-less "happenings" (Spanos, Salas, et al., 1988; Spanos & Katsanis, 1988).

In summary, many subjects hold situation-specific beliefs about causal connections in the hypnotic context. The familiar event sequence of the hypnotized subject responding in close temporal contiguity to the hypnotist's suggestions, along with cultural stereotypes about hypnosis, promote the inference that dramatic hypnotic phenomena arise from the hypnotist's control over a passive subject. In general, the activation of hypnosis-specific schema requires little attentional processing, and like other examples of causal processing is well-automatized (White, 1988). However, in certain instances, to be described later in our discussion, when subjects have particular reason to contemplate the relation between hypnosis and suggestion-related involuntariness, automaticity is compromised.

Whereas Spanos and his associates contend that wide differences exist in the extent to which subjects wish to be hypnotized and believe that they can be hypnotized (e.g., Barber, 1969; Spanos, Brett, Menary & Cross, 1987), considerable agreement exists that individuals who *are* hypnotized respond to suggestions automatically. Spanos and his colleagues (Spanos, Salas, et al., 1988) have tested the contention that observers rate hypnotic behaviors as involuntary occurrences or happenings—that is, they invoke an occurrence schema to interpret hypnotic events. The authors conducted an interesting experiment in which subjects viewed a videotaped model who acted in one of three scenarios. In the first scenario, the model sat with eyes closed and head down listening to a voice that defined the situation as hypnosis (e.g., "Now that you are deeply hypnotized . . .") and then administered a passively worded suggestion for arm levitation (e.g., "Your arm is lighter and lighter, rising higher and higher"). The model responded to this suggestion by slowly raising her arm. The second scenario also involved the model responding to the arm levitation suggestion. However, the situation was not defined as hypnosis. In the third scenario the model was seen reading a book. When disturbed by a fly, she slowly raised her hand, tracked the fly, and swatted it with her hand.

In both open-ended testimony and on questionnaires, observers consistently described the fly-tracking behavior as a goal-directed action and the hypnotic response as an involuntary occurrence. Observers showed more variability when describing the behavior of the model who received the nonhypnotic suggestion: 70 percent of the subjects described the model as being in an altered state of consciousness and described her behavior as an involuntary occurrence. Observers consistently categorized the suggestion-related responses they viewed as involuntary. These findings provide strong support for the notion that prevailing cultural beliefs or occurrence schemas influence attributions of hypnotic responses.

We (Lynn, Snodgrass, Hardaway & Lenz, 1984) recently examined the relation between subjects' prehypnotic response expectancies and attributions of involuntariness. Before hypnosis, subjects rated the extent to which they believed their hypnotic responses would be a function of the hypnotist's ability and effort and their own ability and effort. We hypothesized that subjects' ratings of involuntariness after hypnosis would be associated with their prehypnotic attributions of response causality to external factors. Our research confirmed this prediction. Ratings of hypnotist ability and effort attributions made *before* hypnosis correlated positively with involuntariness ratings made *after* hypnosis at .44 and .34 respectively. These findings suggest that prehypnotic expectancies, along lines consistent with the evocation of an occurrence schema, have an influence on feelings of involuntariness during hypnosis.

In a second study, we (Lynn, Jacquith, Jothirathnam & Rhue, 1987) tested the hypothesis that dominant Western cultural beliefs about hypnosis (e.g., occurrence schemas) prime subjects to label their suggestion-related sensations and movements as involuntary. We administered the Harvard Group Scale of Hypnotic Susceptibility and measures of imagination, waking suggestion, and involuntariness to English speaking students at the University of Malaysia. We compared their performance with Malaysian students at Ohio University who had been resident in the United States for at least 6 months (average stay 2.5 years), and with native U.S. citizens who were students at Ohio University. Our findings were quite interesting. The mean scores on the measures of hypnosis, imagination, and waking suggestion were vitually identical across all three samples. However, in the sample of Malaysian students tested in Malaysia, where subjects were unfamiliar with Western ideas about hypnosis, none of the correlations among the measures were statistically significant. Whereas a measure of involuntariness failed to correlate with hypnotizability in the sample of Malaysian students tested in Malaysia, a significant correlation between involuntariness and hypnotizability was obtained in the sample of Malaysian students tested at Ohio University. Furthermore, in the sample of Malaysian students tested at Ohio University, all of the measures intercorrelated in a manner comparable to that of the native U.S. sample. Our findings provide support for the hypothesis that culturally bound expectancies mediate the relation between hypnotizability and involuntariness ratings.

Self-Representations

Perceptions of involuntariness are influenced not only by situational representations, but also by self-representations. Self-schemas (Epstein, 1973; Greenwald & Pratkanis, 1984; Markus, 1986; Kihlstrom & Cantor, 1983; Meichenbaum and Cameron, 1984) are generally described as affective-cognitive structures or theories about the self that lend coherence to one's experiences. Markus (1986) has advanced the concept of "possible selves" to account for motivation in the self-concept. Possible selves are not only the selves we could become or would like to become; but they also are the selves we are afraid of becoming.

Self-schemas structure interpretations of the self in relation to specific situations (Markus, 1986). Because hypnotic behavior occurs in an interpersonal context, with performance concerns tinged with personal and interpersonal themes, our self-schema, the impressions we attempt to convey, and the way we relate to others are intertwined. As a general rule, we desire to present ourselves to others in a favorable light (see Baumeister, 1982) in a manner congruent with our ideal self-image. The hypnosis context is no exception.

Self-schemas are often subjected to minimal personal reflection and often become automatic (Marcel, 1983). The connection between specific representations of the self and hypnotic behavior is therefore not necessarily obvious to the subject. Yet, whether fully articulated or not, hypnotic responsiveness undoubtedly has positive connotations for some subjects and negative connotations for other subjects. Hypnosis has positive connotations for subjects' whose beliefs about the attributes of a "good" hypnotic subject are consistent with valued, prized, or sought after attributes (e.g., cooperativeness, imaginativeness, flexibility, creativity). For such subjects "letting go," "being hypnotized," and experiencing suggestion-related involuntariness are consistent with personal goals and self-perceptions. Feelings of involuntariness, in turn, enhance hypnotic involvement and legitimize perceptions of being "hypnotized" in a recursive fashion.

Other subjects report considerable apprehension and fear about experiencing hypnosis. When McCord (1961) asked subjects who had never been hypnotized to describe how they thought they would feel if "in a hypnotic trance," the overtones of many of his subjects' responses were negative, threatening, and implied concerns about "being led." As McCord (1961) noted, such preconceptions could act as a deterrent to full involvement in hypnosis.

Some subjects are torn by a tug-of-war of conflicting forces that augment involvement and the adoption of role-relevant behaviors and feelings versus forces that constrain involvement. Curiosity, the demands for cooperation inherent in the situation, and the desire to please the hypnotist and to cooperate in a treatment or scientific endeavor, incline subjects to have hypnosis-related experiences (e.g., "invountariness"). However, countervailing fears and negative preconceptions can produce an internal dialogue marked by fears of losing control of one's mental processes and bodily functions, along with concerns about appearing passive, weak, and gullible. An aversion to experiencing an "altered state" of consciousness, as well as feelings of competitiveness and resentments against authority (i.e., the hypnotist) may also enter into the arena of conflict.

The term "psychological reactance" was introduced by Brehm (1966) to describe the feeling that is experienced whenever important freedoms are eliminated or threatened. The clinical literature (Baker, 1986; Levitan and Jevne, 1986; Murray-Jobsis, 1986) is replete with examples of "reactant" clients who are fearful of relinquishing control of feelings and actions and are resistant to fully experiencing hypnosis. The well-known hypnotist Milton Erickson recognized the necessity of allowing people the opportunity to maintain their sense of freedom and to resist control (Sherman, 1988).

Supplementing clinical lore, a body of research has shown that some subjects resist or oppose hypnotic suggestions in order to maintain their sense of freedom, appear nongullible, and "in control." Barber and Calverley (1964) found that hypnotic responding was virtually nullified in a group of subjects who were informed that hypnosis was a test of gullibility. More recently, how hypnotizable subjects who received suggestions for increased auditory sensitivity were shown to oppose suggested demands by exhibiting a heightened bias toward reporting the signal as absent rather than as present (Jones & Spanos, 1982). Spanos and Bodorik (1977) found that some low susceptibles tried not to appear hypnotized by actively attempting to remember rather than to forget following hypnotic amnesia suggestions. Studies have shown that low susceptibles are as capable as high susceptibles of reducing pain when encouraged to do so in a context that is not implicitly defined as related to hypnosis or as being controlled (D'Eon & Perry, 1983; Farthing, Brown & Venturino, 1984; Spanos, Kennedy & Gwynn, 1984; Spanos, McNeil, Gwynn & Stam, 1984; Spanos, Voorneveld & Gwynn, 1987).

We (Lynn, Weekes, Snodgrass, Abrams, Weiss & Rhue, 1984) recently examined high and low hypnotizable subjects' ability to move in opposition to motoric suggestions. For purposes of description, the experiment can be thought of as consisting of three phases. In phase one, an experimental assistant either administered prehypnotic instructions that informed subjects that control in hypnosis could be demonstrated by moving in the direction opposite that called for by a particular suggestion or he provided no prehypnotic information. In phase two the hypnotist administered two motoric suggestions, and in phase three, the hypnotist told the subjects not to respond to the two motoric suggestions that would follow, but only to think and imagine along with the suggestions. Paradoxically, the prehypnotic instructions administered in phase one had also informed subjects that, under these circumstances, "opposing" the hypnotist— demonstrating control—could be exhibited by moving in the direction called for by the suggestion.

As we predicted, relative to low hypnotizables, hypnotizable subjects in phase two reported greater involuntariness and exhibited fewer movements in opposition to suggestions when opposing the hypnotist was presented as a way of demonstrating control. In phase three—after the hypnotist told subjects not to respond to suggestions—the low hypnotizables, informed that moving in the direction of the suggestion was an indicator of being in control, moved in the direction of more suggestions than did uninstructed unhypnotizable subjects.

What was perhaps even more interesting was the finding that nearly a quarter of the low hypnotizables in phase three who were instructed that control could be demonstrated by moving in response to suggestion, demonstrated their control by moving in the direction opposite that called for by the suggestion. This type of response circumvented both the hypnotist's explicit directive (i.e., do not move) and the assistant's prehypnotic instructions (i.e., to move in the direction of the suggestion to exhibit control). No hypnotizable subject responded in this manner. Even when unhypnotizable subjects were uninstructed, several moved in opposition to the hypnotist's suggestions. Subjects' reports were most enlightening: The majority of unhypnotizables appeared to relish the idea that they were confounding or opposing the hypnotist. In contrast, hypnotizable subjects reported being highly conflicted about opposing the hypnotist. Our findings suggest that unhypnotizable subjects are not simply passive, uninvolved responders; rather they are motivated to actively and purposefully assert their independence from the hypnotist's influence.

In a recent study (Lynn, Weekes,, Neufeld, Weiss, Brentar & Zivney, 1987), we examined the effects of increasing hypnotic rapport and minimizing reactance on hypnotic responding and involuntariness reports in high and low hypnotizable subjects. In a contractual condition adapted from Sheehan and McConkey's (1976) research, subjects received audiotaped instructions about the experiment and interacted with a formal, aloof hypnotist who disclosed minimally and nonreciprocally in a prehypnosis self-disclosure task. In the collaborative condition, hypnosis was presented as a collaborative venture and the instructions were personally delivered by the hypnotist who was warm, friendly, and reciprocally disclosing in the self-disclosure task. After the manipulation, subjects' hypnotizability was tested on the Stanford hypnotizability scale (SHSS:C, Weitzenhoffer & Hilgard, 1962) and measures of liking, rapport, and involuntariness were obtained.

Although the manipulation affected subjects' liking and rapport with the hypnotist as intended, whether hypnotizable subjects interacted with a friendly or an aloof hypnotist, the majority scored as high hypnotizables, and rated their experiences as involuntary. In contrast, unhypnotizable subjects in the collaborative condition scored nearly three points higher on the hypnotizability scale and experienced their responses as more involuntary than their low susceptible counterparts in the contractual condition. Despite achieving this increment in responding, unhypnotizable subjects did not score as high as hypnotizable subjects in either condition. Nonetheless, our findings suggest that when reactance is reduced by encouraging unhypnotizable subjects to establish a collaborative relationship with the hypnotist, not only is responsivity to suggestion enhanced but the experience of involuntariness is also facilitated.

The class of reactions that we have described as reactance represents a complex of affective and behavioral responses. Reactant subjects critically and analytically monitor the self and the environment while assuming a defensive and resistant stance. Their instrumental cognitive set (Klinger, 1971) primes effortful, planned, voluntary behavior directed toward maintaining control and regulating affect in the hypnotic situation. Suggestion-related sensations and responses are matched and evaluated against a standard of performance based on the exhibition of control and resistance. In short, unhypnotizable subjects' behaviors and sensations reflect two regnant motives (Snyder & Higgins, 1988): to maintain feelings of personal control and to maintain self-esteem. For hypnotizable subjects, self-esteem maintenance and enhancement is oriented more toward experiencing than resisting hypnotic effects. Hypnotizable subjects adopt an experiential set based on a readiness to undergo experiential events that are suggested, a set in which experiences have a "quality of effortlessness, as if they happened by themselves, and in that sense, of involuntariness" (Tellegen, 1981, p. 222).

THE HYPNOTIC INDUCTION

Our discussion suggests that individual differences exist in terms of readiness or preparedness to respond to hypnotic suggestions (McConkey, 1979) and to adopt an experiential set to respond to hypnotic events (Tellegen & Atkinson, 1974; Tellegen, 1981). However, elements of the hypnotic induction, and the hypnotic situation more broadly cast, facilitate the development of an experiential set and perceptions of involuntariness. Typical hypnotic inductions orient the subject to relax physically and mentally, to focus attention directly on the hypnotist's communications and away from the environment and current concerns, and to engage in fantasy and give free rein to the imagination in accord with suggested experiences. Hypnotic inductions contain words or phrases that are commonly associated with passive or receptive mental states (e.g., sleep; you are becoming relaxed; your eyes are closing); the focus on sensations of relaxation, drowsiness, and sleepiness discourages the subject from adopting an analytical attitude and the search for causes of responding outside the framework of hypnosis. Furthermore, such words and phrases reinforce subjects' prehypnotic beliefs that events occur involuntarily. By exposing subjects to occurrence schemata-related cues, they make the schema more accessible (Herr, Sherman & Fazio, 1983; Higgins, King & Mavin, 1982; Wyer & Srull, 1981) and increase the likelihood that the schema will be adopted to categorize hypnotic experience as involuntary.

The wording of the induction also implicitly informs subjects that various effects are happening to them rather than being self-generated (Spanos, 1982). The hypnotist's soothing and relaxed tone of voice and altered speech patterns reinforce more explicit suggestions and role relationships (e.g., the passive subject) and help to define the experience of hypnosis as an "altered state" of consciousness marked by receptivity to suggested events. The belief that one is experiencing a receptive altered state that is the product of the hypnotist's suggestions, rather than one's purposeful efforts, is conducive to defining self-generated responses as involuntary.

Our perceptions and attributions are intimately associated with the words and linguistic forms that we adopt in order to understand and communicate our behaviors. Field (1979) performed a linguistic content analysis of hypnotic inductions that he contrasted with parallel analyses of formal and informal speech in nonhypnotic situations. He found that the hypnotic induction wording serves to direct attention inward, to reduce vigilance, and to diminish the importance of action on the environment. Whereas the induction absorbs subjects' attention and focuses awareness on concrete images, sensations and behavior, it diminishes abstract, logical, and critical thought processes.

If anything has the potential to vitiate the experience of nonvolition, it is critical or analytical thought. Langer (1978) has shown that thinking about or assessing behaviors as they are being enacted often destroys the spontaneous continuity of the action sequence. Furthermore, Atkinson and Allen (1979) found that subjects' who performed a fine-grained analysis of behavior tended to view it as deliberate and lacking in spontaneity (Atkinson & Allen, 1979). Hypnotic subjects who focus on breathing, or slight movements of their arms, for example, while failing to identify their actions as part of a smooth-flowing sequence of behaviors "caused" by suggestions, are unlikely to label their actions as involuntary. On the other hand, subjects who engage in mimimal critical thinking, yet perceive their movements and the hypnotists' suggestions to move as a single unit of analysis, are likely to label their suggestion-related actions as involuntary.

As Field noted, the hypnotist's language encourages nonspecific action or behavior without a clear-cut and understandable objective: The subject of action as well as the object of action are blurred—hypnotic behavior happens by itself, spontaneously, not with a deliberate decision. There is another sense in which the hypnotist-subject boundary is indistinct. It is the hypnotist who administers the suggestions and is, in this sense, "responsible" for hypnotic actions. Subjects' attributions of their responsiveness to the hypnotist carry a certain weight of legitimacy. The fact that responses follow suggestions to engage in a particular thought and behavior, probably contributes to the perceptions that hypnotic actions are in direct response to the suggestion and are not self-initiated. Indeed, if subjects uniquely or consistently associate hypnotic effects with the hypnotist or his suggestions, rather than with their efforts or to aspects of the hypnotic context, they are likely to identify their suggestion-related responses as involuntary.

In a related vein, subjects who exhibit rapport with the hypnotist may come to think of themselves and the hypnotist as a unit and therefore not distinguish their actions from the actions suggested by the hypnotist. Certain subjects perceive the hypnotist as a powerful figure through which their hypnotic behavior and performance are manifested. Sheehan and his colleagues (Dolby & Sheehan, 1977; McConkey, 1979; Sheehan, 1971, 1977, 1980; Sheehan & McConkey, 1982; Sheehan & Perry, 1976) have emphasized transference and rapport factors and stressed hypnotizable subjects' motivated involvement with the hypnotist and sensitivity to her perceived intent as critical factors in enhancing the compelling nature of hypnotic sugestions. A number of studies have shown that involuntariness reports are associated with ratings of rapport with the hypnotist (Lynn et al., 1984; Lynn et al., 1987; Lynn et al, 1988). In summary, elements of the hypnotic induction, rapport with the hypnotist, and the structure of the hypnotic relationship combine to decrease analytical thought and to promote attributions of involuntariness.

Hypnotic Experience

Our discussion suggests that alterations in information processing, such as a tendency toward the concrete rather than the abstract and the imagistic rather than the conceptual, which Miller and Bowers (1986) attribute to dissociative processes, may instead be attributable to induction wording. Suggested imagery also may encourage a receptive mode of experiencing (Deikman, 1973) versus analytic attending (Spanos, Gottlieb, & Rivers, 1976). Yet the tendency to dichotomize hypnotic experiences or information processing as either holistic or analytic, dissociative or nondissociative, for example, represents a simplification of subjects' cognitive processes and experiences during hypnosis, and detracts from a full understanding of involuntariness reports.

Hypnotic experience is not static or immutable. It can be thought of as a flow of interacting images, feelings, personal associations, and self-evaluations. These may be represented verbally and pictorially, and in tandem with suggestion-related sensations. In this "experiential stream," concrete and abstract thinking, and reality-based and fantasy-based thinking coexist (Sheehan and McConkey, 1982) and can operate together to foster responding in alignment with subjects' needs, goals, and expectancies. Imaginings, goal-directed strivings, and expectancies are viewed as integral, and perhaps inseparable facets of subjects' hypnotic experience. Responses to suggestions are rarely aptly described as purely cognitive or purely affective; more typically, they reflect a variegated and individualized blend of cognitive and affective responses. Involuntariness is only one aspect of subjects' response to hypnotic suggestion (Bowers, Laurence, & Hart, 1988), intermingled with other cognitive and affective events.

Individual differences and variability within a particular subject over the course of a hypnotic session are often evident with respect to the following foci of attention: suggestion-related absorption versus the experience of being an analytical observer of one's own actions; task-relevant versus task-irrelevant thoughts, and attention to suggestion-related imaginings versus objective aspects of the situation (McConkey, 1979). Like critical thought, assuming the role of spectator, attending to the objective reality of the situation, and task-irrelevant cognitions are hypothesized to short-circuit the feeling of involuntariness.

Because hypnotic experience is fluid and generally not construed in mundane or prosaic terms, it may tax subjects' attempts to understand and interpret their sensations and behaviors. Furthermore, hypnotic behavior is shaped by subtle contextual cues, such as the wording of suggestions, which subjects may fail to recognize as the determinants of their feelings and actions. To add to the complexities of understanding the causes and nature of actions, subjects' cognitive processes are often unavailable or relatively unavailable to conscious scrutiny (e.g., Nisbett & Wilson, 1977). Moreover, our vocabulary for bodily feelings and sensations is meager, and somatic feelings often are nebulous and defy adequate description (Sarbin & Coe, 1979). Thus, subjects not only have imperfect access to their mental states (Wilson, 1984), but they also have imperfect access to their bodily states.

We believe that hypnotic subjects resort to a verbal explanatory system in order to understand ambiguous or poorly understood internal states. Explanations based on a priori theories of hypnotic events (e.g., responses happen involuntarily) provide an interpretative framework, increasing subjects' readiness to adopt the language of the hypnotist and her suggestions to describe their experiences. Hypnotic language reinforces perceptions of involuntariness that have their seeds in prehypnotic conceptions. Combined, these influences increase the accessibility (Fazio, 1986; Salancik & Conway, 1975; Sherman, Zehner, Johnson & Hirt, 1983; Strack, Schwarz & Gschneidinger, 1985) of occurrence schemas. This position is consonant with the views of a number of investigators (e.g., Coe, 1978, Coe & Wedemeyer, 1981; Sarbin & Coe, 1979; Spanos & de Groh, 1983) who have maintained that involuntariness reports reflect, in part, retrospective evaluations or interpretations of ambiguous suggestion-related behaviors and experiences.

Hypnotists use a variety of strategems to promote the view, or to convey the illusion, that the hypnotist is powerful and that hypnosis is effective. Edmonston (1986) has observed that methods of handling resistant patients involve convincing the patient that natural physical events are the result of the hypnotist's manipulations and that the patient is capable of being hypnotized (Edmonston, 1986). A number of authors (Barber, Spanos, & Chaves, 1974; Edmonston, 1986; Spanos & Gorassini, 1984; Wickless & Kirsch, 1987) have noted that hypnotists often use techniques that involve suggesting naturally occurring responses (arm lowering of an outstretched arm), interpreting observed behavior as evidence of successful hypnotic responding, and preventing or reinterpreting failures to respond to suggestions. These devices can be quite successful in facilitating not only hypnotic responding (Barber et al., 1974; Edmonston, 1986; Wickless & Kirsch, 1987) but also involuntariness reports (Spanos and Gorassini, 1984). The wisdom of this approach is acknowledged in standardized hypnotizability scales that begin with so-called "warm up" items, such as eye closure or arm lowering, that capitalize on the coupling of suggestions with naturally occurring events.

Spanos and Gorassini (1984) found that a direct relationship existed between the degree of involuntariness and the congruence between the aim of suggestion and naturally occurring feedback. Suggestions that expose subjects to contradictory sensory information, such as levitation of an outstretched arm, would be difficult to interpret as involuntary. The authors found that subjects who were asked to imagine a force acting on their outstretched arm to make it feel lighter (arm rising) rated their experience as more voluntary than subjects asked to imagine a force acting on their arm to make it feel heavier (arm lowering).

In order to experience involuntariness in relation to an arm levitation suggestion, the subject must ignore or reinterpret contradictory proprioceptive feedback. Angelini and Stanford (1987) found that subjects who received suggestions for arm levitation rated their responses as more involuntary when the suggestions contained vivid suggestion-relevant imagery. They argued that the imagery served to divert subjects' attention from suggestion-incongruent proprioceptive information that interferes with a sense of perceived involuntariness.

These studies are consistent with the hypothesis that subjects identify their actions as involuntary to the degree that their experiences and sensations match or do not contradict their expectancies about involuntariness (e.g., Barber, 1969; Barber & Calverley, 1969; Sarbin & Coe, 1972; Spanos & Radtke, 1981). Expectancies about involuntariness are shaped not only by a priori theories about hypnosis, by hypnotic language, and by naturally occurring proprioceptive feedback, but also by the cues inherent in suggestions themselves. In order to highlight the importance and diversity of subjects' interpretations of the meaning of suggestions, we now turn our attention to the structure of suggestions.

THE STRUCTURE OF SUGGESTIONS

Even cooperative subjects do not universally experience hypnotic responses as involuntary: Some subjects respond to suggestions yet identify their reponses as voluntary. For example, Spanos and his colleagues found that between 45 percent (Spanos et al., 1977) and 55 percent (Spanos et al., 1983) of the subjects studied could be so described, whereas K. Bowers (1981) and P. Bowers (1982) found that about 20 percent of subjects who passed items perceived them as being volitionally performed. A somewhat lower percentage (15 percent) was reported by Weitzenhoffer (1974). P. Bowers and her colleagues (Bowers et al., 1988) used a "choice" scale that provided the discrete options of mostly voluntary, and an "intertwining of nonvolitional and volitional experiences"; 12 percent and 22 percent respectively, of subjects who passed suggestions endorsed these options. Whereas variability is evident across studies, perhaps because different scales were used to assess involuntary experiences, and because different scales were used to assess hypnotizability (P. Bowers et al., 1988), agreement exists that mismatches between behavioral criteria for passing suggestions and measures of nonvolition are far from rare.

Spanos (1981) has grappled with the problem of explaining mismatches by showing that subjects' interpretations of suggestions have important consequences for defining responses as involuntary. Involuntariness reports depend upon correctly discerning the intent and subtle implications of hypnotic suggestions, while ignoring contradictory information or interpretations.

Suggestions are more than simple descriptions of events or situations. They also convey the implication that the experiences suggested are to occur involuntarily. Hilgard (1963) noted that the typical suggestion indicates that something is going to take place "automatically" or "involuntarily." Spanos (1981) uses the following suggestion, taken from the "moving hands" suggestion from the Stanford HSS:A, to illustrate this point: "Now I want you to imagine a force attracting your hands toward each other, pulling them together. As you think of this force pulling your hands together, they will move together . . . closer and closer together as though a force were acting on them . . ." (pp. 21-22). The suggestion has two components: (1) a tacit request to move the arms and (2) a request to perceive the movement as a result of an imagined force, that is, as an involuntary movement outside the subject's agency.

Spanos (1981) outlines three ways in which subjects could respond to the suggestion. First, they may respond to neither of the requests and thereby fail the suggestion. This may occur either because they choose not to cooperate with the suggestion, or because they miss the import of the tacit request. Recent research

(Bowers et al., 1987) has shown that more than a quarter of subjects sampled believe that their responses started out voluntary but became involuntary. However, if subjects are unaware that they must initiate the movements that are to be self-defined as involuntary, and simply wait passively for their arms to "move together themselves," they will fail the suggestion. Furthermore, if subjects believe that they should remain passive, to "let things just happen," they are less likely to initiate the goal-directed cognitive activities necessary to respond to the suggestion (see Lynn, Snodgras, Rhue, & Hardaway, 1987; Spanos & de Groh, 1983). These subjects may, however, experience their *failure* to respond as an involuntary occurrence. Indeed, a number of studies (K. Bowers, 1981; P. Bowers, 1982; P. Bowers et al., 1988) have shown that a sizable minority of subjects—between 15 percent and 25 percent—experience their response to failed items as involuntary. Because of the relatively high frequency of mismatches—experiencing passed items as voluntary and failed items as involuntary—it appears to be important to include assessments of involuntariness along with behavioral responding in scales that purport to measure hypnotizability (Spanos et al., 1977; Spanos & Gorassini, 1984; Spanos et al., 1983; Weitzenhoffer, 1974, 1978).

The second pattern identified by Spanos (1981) addresses the problem of mismatches that we discussed at the outset of this section: The subject responds to the suggestion's implicit request while deemphasizing the request for involuntariness. That is, she responds overtly in terms of the suggestion while defining her response as occurring voluntarily. This might occur for a number of reasons. First, subjects might simply miss the import of the request for involuntariness. Second, subjects might be aware of the connotation of involuntariness but choose to ignore it. These subjects do not simply fake or merely comply with the suggestion; rather, they exhibit involvement in the suggested events and feel related sensations. However, they attribute their responses to their own efforts or to their willingness to "let it happen." Finally, subjects "fake" their hypnotic performance; that is, they fail to experience suggestion-related effects yet, for some reason, wish to convey the impression that they are hypnotized.

A third pattern involves responding to both requests implicit in hypnotic suggestions. That is, subjects both act in keeping with the suggestion and come to believe that their response is an involuntary occurrence. Research (K. Bowers, 1981; P. Bowers, 1982; Spanos et al., 1977; Weitzenhoffer, 1974) has shown that unselected subjects rate the majority of passed suggestions as involuntary, ranging as high as 67 percent of the items passed (Bowers, 1981).

Studies have demonstrated that suggestion structure is an important determinant of involuntariness reports. Investigations have compared subjects' involuntariness ratings following suggestions (e.g., "experience a force acting on your hands to move them apart") and following instructions (e.g., "move your hands apart from one another). If suggestions convey the tacit implication that control is relinquished to the hypnotist (Hilgard, 1965), and instructions convey no such implication, then subjects ought to rate their suggestion-related responses as more involuntary. Research with motoric (Spanos & Barber, 1972; Spanos & Gorassini, 1984; Spanos & de Groh, 1983; Spanos & McPeake, 1977; Spanos,

Spillane, & McPeake, 1976) and analgesia suggestions (Spanos & Katsanis, 1988) has shown this to be the case. That subjects generally report equivalent involuntariness in hypnotic and nonhypnotic conditions underlines the important role of suggestion structure.

Permissive versus Authoritative Suggestions

Hypnotic suggestions that differ in wording style convey divergent implications that affect involuntariness reports. Traditional suggestions involve an unambiguous tacit request for a specific response that is couched in authoritative language yet conveys the expectation that suggested effects will occur involuntarily. These suggestions are characterized by statements that are specific and command-like. We may contrast suggestions delivered in a direct, authoritative style with the following communication: "Sooner or later you might begin to wonder about going into a deep trance, and you may do that suddenly or rapidly, responding in your own unique way to all sorts of experiences I will suggest." These suggestions are delivered in a permissive style, provide the subject with a range of appropriate responses, and convey the implication that the subject is central to hypnotic events. Two recent studies found that despite responding equivalently in terms of overt response, subjects who received permissive suggestions rated their responses as feeling more voluntary than did subjects who received authoritatively worded suggestions (Lynn et al., 1987; Lynn et al., 1988).

Goal-directed Fantasies

Whether responsing to permissive or authoritative suggestions, hypnotizable subjects shift their thinking and modify their behavior in accordance with the changing demands of suggestions. As we have indicated, responding to suggestion is not aimless, without purpose, or lacking in direction; instead, it is goal-directed and strategic. Raising one's hand during a hand levitation suggestion occurs in alignment with imagining along with suggestions worded to imply that the hand will lift involuntarily (e.g., "Your hand is getting lighter and lighter, it will rise by itself"). Spanos (1971) hypothesized that subjects tend to define their overt response to suggestion as involuntary when they become absorbed in a pattern of imaginings termed goal-directed fantasy (GDF). GDF's are defined as "imagined situations which, if they were to occur, would be expected to lead to the involuntary occurrence of the motor response called for by the suggestion" (Spanos, Rivers, & Ross, 1977, p. 211). For instance, subjects administered a hand levitation suggestion would exhibit a goal-directed fantasy report (GDFr), if they report such events as imagining a helium balloon lifting their hand, or a basketball being inflated under their hand. Subjects involved in GDFs attend fully to their imaginings while ignoring or reinterpreting information that contradicts the "reality" of the imagined events (Spanos et al., 1977).

    Suggestions worded to stimulate GDFs provide subjects with a cognitive strategy for generating and intensifying feelings of involuntariness. Because the imaginative strategies are implicit in the wording of the suggestion, subjects are unlikely to attribute the feelings that ensue, from adopting the strategy, to their own agency. Studies have indicated that GDFrs are related to subjects' tendencies to define their overt responses to suggestion as involuntary occurrences (e.g., Lynn et al., 1987b; Spanos, 1971; Spanos, Spillane, & McPeake, 1976; Spanos & Barber, 1972; Spanos & Gorassini, 1984; Spanos & McPeake, 1976; Spanos, Rivers, & Ross, 1977), though not necessarily to their overt responding to suggestion (Buckner & Coe, 1977; Coe, Allan, Krug, & Wurzman, 1974; Spanos 1971, 1973; Spanos & Barber, 1972; Spanos & McPeake, 1974; Spanos, Spillane, & McPeake, 1976). These findings support the social psychological position that imaginings legitimize and reinforce the interpretation that the actions occurred involuntarily (e.g., Spanos et al., 1977). However, they do not provide support for Arnold's (1946) view that sustained and vivid imagining is intimately associated with hypnotic behavior.

Amnesia Suggestions

Different suggestions require different suggestion-related cognitions or strategies to enhance the perception of involuntariness. For example, amnesia suggestions initially instruct subjects to take an active role in the process of forgetting (e.g., "I want you to forget . . ."). The wording of .the suggestion is then subtly transformed to imply that the target material disappears effortlessly and involuntarily (e.g., "The words are disappearing . . . you will be unable to remember the words . . . they are disappearing from your mind . . .") (Spanos & Radtke, 1982). Some subjects interpret the tacit message of the suggestion as signifying that they should become distracted by focusing their attention on physical (e.g., sensations such as relaxation) or imagined events other than the target material (Spanos & Radtke-Bodorik, 1980; Spanos & Radtke, 1982). Simply saying to oneself, "I am unable to remember" could prove sufficiently distracting to interfere with access to the target material until the subject receives the hypnotist's "permission" to recall (e.g., "Now you can remember everything"). These "effortless forgetters" (Spanos & Radtke, 1982) are likely to identify their forgetting as occurring involuntarily (e.g., "The words disappeared by themselves"). In sum, subjects' interpretations of the requirements of hypnotic suggestions, and their active attempts to fulfill these requirements, mediate the identification of action as involuntary with respect to both amnesia and motoric suggestions.

We have noted that subjects generally respond in a manner consistent with demands inherent in the structure of communications. However, this is not invariably true. For example, Weitzenhoffer (1974) has argued that, in some instances, responses to intended instructions are rated as involuntary. Studies have shown that between a fifth (Spanos & Gorassini, 1984) and a third (Weitzenhoffer, 1974) of subjects rate their responses to instructions as mostly involuntary.

What can account for these findings? Whereas the wording of instructions themselves do not contain cues for responding involuntarily, subtle pressures to acquiesce to simple requests or instructions, engendered by the socialization process, create demands of their own. Furthermore, simple motoric actions are, through practice, highly automatized and require little conscious thought, deliberation, or effort for their execution. These two factors, when considered together, render subjects' involuntariness ratings of responses to simple instructions understandable. Indeed, instructed actions often have an involuntary quality outside of the context of the psychology experiment. This is nicely illustrated in subjects' responses to the childhood game of "Simon Says." To win this game, a person must resist responding unless an instruction such as, "lift your hand" is prefaced by the phrase "Simon says." The person playing the role of "Simon" typically delivers the instructions forcefully, authoritatively, and rapidly. Anyone who has played this game knows how difficult it is to inhibit response to the instruction when it is not preceded by "Simon says."

Our lexicon provides us with rich opportunities for construing hypnotic experience along a voluntary-involuntary dimension. However, terms such as "voluntary" and "involuntary" have multiple and varied connotations (Kimble & Perlmutter, 1970). Involuntary might be thought to mean spontaneous; effortless; not involving deliberation, choice, purpose, or unconscious for example. Because subjects do not share a uniform understanding or interpretation of what constitutes a voluntary or an involuntary response, and because rating scales used in hypnosis research have not provided clear definitions of what is or is not an "involuntary" response, it is not surprising that some subjects rate their responses to instructions as involuntary.

Spanos and de Groh (1983) tested the idea that subjects who received a suggestion that implicitly informed them that the response should be construed along a voluntary-involuntary dimension would show a close correspondence between open-ended reports of involuntariness and scale ratings indicating involuntariness. However, because instructions do not imply involuntary responding, subjects who respond to them might not reflect upon their suggestion-related experiences in terms of the involuntary-voluntary dimension until it is made salient by a rating scale assessing involuntariness after an open-ended question. Thus, Spanos and de Groh (1983) hypothesized that some subjects who received instructions would retrospectively rate their responses as involuntary on the rating scale but not describe them as such on the preceding open-ended questions.

The authors' predictions were confirmed. Almost all of the subjects who received suggestions and who rated their responses as involuntary had previously described them as involuntary in the open-ended question. In contrast, 13 percent of the subjects who responded to an instruction rated their response as "mostly" or "completely" involuntary, but only one of these subjects reported an involuntary experience in the open-ended questioning before they rated their response.

The Ability to Resist Suggestions

Cultural conceptions of the hypnotist as a Svengali-like figure hinge on the subject's purported inability to resist the hypnotist's commands. As we noted earlier, even early hypnosis luminaries such as Bernheim were impressed with the subjects' apparent loss of will and initiative. Perhaps the acid test of whether hypnotic behavior is involuntary is whether subjects are truly unable to resist suggestions.

A number of studies have examined subjects' ability to resist suggestions when specifically instructed to do so. Young (1927, 1928) found that all four subjects who gave themselves autosuggestions in advance of hypnosis to resist one of the items chosen from a list of suggestions were able to resist. In a second series, the subject and an experimenter decided in advance which suggestion the subject was to resist. Even though the suggestions were administered by another hypnotist, subjects were able to resist.

Wells (1940) repeated the second series of Young's experiment. Although Wells did not frame the suggestions in terms of "autosuggestions," as in the Young study, suggestions were not standardized, and the procedure was free to vary and adapted to each individual case. In advance of hypnosis, Wells's (1940) sixteen subjects were assigned an item to resist that was chosen by lot from an item pool. By contrast with Young's subjects, Wells's subjects, with minor exceptions, failed to resist.

Although the hypnotist did not know on which item resistance was being attempted, he was not blind to the hypotheses. Indeed, Wells was strongly committed to a particular outcome of the study. He concluded that complete helplessness is an essential feature of hypnosis, and that the subject who is not helpless is not a satisfactory subject. It is possible that Wells conveyed the impression to the subject that inability to resist was a sign of deep hypnosis. Indeed, when the experimenter was not successful in getting the subject to comply, he tried another method. Hilgard (1963) also criticized Wells's methodology, noting that when subjects were selected for participation, Wells emphasized helplessness, and urged them to try to resist while he hypnotized them. Thus, Wells chose subjects who had been unsuccessful in resisting hypnosis in their early experiences with it.

Hilgard (1963) examined the ability of twelve moderately high hypnotizable subjects to resist suggestions on an item that had been passed successfully on two previous days of testing. Hilgard's instructions emphasized that the experiment was designed to examine the degree of initiative and control retained by subjects during hypnosis. Although it was not communicated to subjects whether the expectation was that they would succeed or fail, they were asked to try to resist on two of the six trails. Hilgard found that one subject failed to resist either suggestion, five subjects resisted one of two, and six subjects resisted both suggestions. Subjects generally retained control during hypnosis, but many felt conflicted about responding. Furthermore, Hilgard (1963) noted that certain subjects' motivations and needs entered into the situation, claiming that "they didn't want to resist, it spoiled all the fun of hypnosis, it was like insisting that a child do something he doesn't want to do" (p. 12). These sorts of comments indicate that subjects retained control over their responding during hypnosis.

Levitt and Henderson (1980) pointed out that a number of factors, including subjects' perceptions of the purpose of the experiment and allowing subjects to choose their own points of resistance might have influenced the results. Using subjects unselected for hypnotizability, Levitt and Henderson tested ten subjects with the Stanford Scale Form A on two occasions. At the conclusion of the first session, subjects were told that the experiment was concerned with the degree of initiative and control that a person retains during hypnosis. They were informed that they should become deeply hypnotized but try to resist all of the suggestions that would be administered by a second hypnotist. The results were quite comparable to those obtained by Hilgard (1963): Of possible points of resistance, subjects successfully resisted on 36 percent, compared to 30 percent in Hilgard's study. The mean following the first induction was 5.1 versus 2.9 on the second induction, representing a reduction of a little more than 40 percent.

In a series of studies, Levitt and Baker (Baker & Levitt, 1988; Levitt, 1986; Levitt & Baker, 1983) examined subjects' ability to resist a hypnotist's suggestions when bribed with various monetary denominations (ranging from $5 to $100) by a "resistance instructor." Across four studies, the percentages of nonresisters varied from 33 to 53 percent of the subjects tested, and the correlation between resistance and hypnotic responsiveness varied from .37 to .54. A relation was also found between subjects' feelings about the resistance instructor and their resistance to hypnotic suggestions. However, the researchers' most interesting finding was that a substantial number (6 out of 12) of highly hypnotizable subjects who scored 11 or 12 on the Harvard Group Scale did not resist the hypnotist's suggestions despite being offered a bribe of as much as $100 to do so.

Although Levitt (1986) concluded that hypnotic influence is truly coercive for a small number of subjects and that their hypnotic performance is, in fact, truly involuntary, across all studies more than half of the subjects successfully resisted suggestions. Additionally, nonhypnotizable simulating subjects were not included in the experiments. It is therefore impossible to determine whether the experimental demand characteristics were responsible for subjects' purported "inability" to resist suggestions. Arguably, subjects who failed to resist despite being bribed could simply have been more invested in presenting themselves as deeply hypnotized than they were in collecting a sum of money for resisting the hypnotist. Failing to resist a hypnotic suggestion, despite being offered a large bribe to resist, would constitute powerful validation that one is an "excellent" hypnotic subject. Finally, whether the "bribe" was perceived by subjects as credible was apparently not evaluated.

It is very difficult to draw firm conclusions about the studies on resistance given the failure to include measures of subjects' perceptions of the experiment and the absence of appropriate control groups of imagining and simulating subjects. It does appear, however, that many hypnotizable subjects retain an ability to resist suggestions.

A number of studies have been designed to redress some of the problems of earlier research and to address contrasting predictions derived from hypnosis theories. In a series of studies conducted in our laboratory, hypnotic subjects were first hypnotized and then instructed to vividly imagine and experience motoric suggestions that were to follow, but to resist engaging in movements. We found that high hypnotizable subjects, when asked to resist suggested responses, often failed to do so, and afterward stated that their movements occurred despite their best efforts to counter or prevent them. In this context, movements may be thought of as a behavioral index of nonvolition. Hypnotized as opposed to imagining (Lynn, Nash, Rhue, Frauman & Stanley, 1983) and simulating subjects (Lynn et al., 1985) moved in response to countersuggestion and defined their suggestion-related responses as involuntary. Contrary to Arnold's ideomotor-action hypothesis, hypnotizable imagining subjects reported feeling as absorbed and involved in imaginings as did hypnotic subjects but resisted responding to suggestions.

Although the real-simulating differences obtained in our earlier research could be interpreted as supporting a neodissociation account of involuntariness, other findings (Lynn et al., 1985) suggested that the responses of both real and simulating subjects may be expectancy based. Simulating subjects relative to susceptible subjects, not only moved less but tended to report that other good subjects were less likely to move in response to countersuggestion. Several other studies (Sheehan, 1971; Spanos, Bridgeman, Stam, Gwynn & Saad, 1983) indicate that real-simulator differences may reflect between-group differences in expectancies arising from divergent experiences and experimental demands associated with the task of simulation.

In order to test the hypothesis that hypnotizable subjects are responsive to the broad expectational context in which the experiment is conducted and that involuntariness is mediated by active cognitive processes and expectancies, subjects' expectancies regarding the experience of nonvolition during hypnosis were manipulated prior to their being hypnotized and receiving countersuggestions. To be more specific, prior to hypnosis, subjects were informed either that other good hypnotic subjects could successfully resist suggestions and retain control over their movements or that other "good" subjects fail to resist suggestions and experience loss of voluntary control over their actions during hypnosis.

Our findings provided strong support for our hypothesis. Prehypnotic normative information had a strong effect on subjects' ability to resist the hypnotist and tended to affect subjects' report of suggestion-related involuntariness in line with induced expectancies about appropriate responding. Furthermore, hypnotizable subjects' reports of how other good subjects behave in the experimental context were found to closely parallel their own actions, which provided additional evidence that their experience of involuntariness is associated with expectancies regarding appropriate response. We also found that subjects' experience of involuntariness is not necessarily associated with reports of being hypnotized. When hypnosis is defined as involving voluntary control over actions, subjects report that they are both good hypnotic subjects and that they retain control over their actions. Finally, both simulators and hypnotizable subjects behaved in conformance with their expectancies rather than counterexpectationally.

This study also demonstrated that rapport plays a role in subjects' experience of involuntariness. When hypnotizable subjects were preset to move yet the hypnotist instructed them not to, subjects with highly positive rapport were more likely to respond to the hypnotist by fully resisting at least one suggestion than were subjects with less positive rapport. Thus, susceptible subjects with highly positive rapport resolved hypnotic conflict by achieving a compromise between meeting normative expectations (e.g., to respond) and complying with the hypnotist's counterdemand (i.e., to resist). Susceptible subjects with less positive rapport respond primarily in accordance with the normative expectations. These findings are supportive of the view, propounded by Sheehan and his colleagues (e.g., Dolby & Sheehan, 1977; McConkey, 1979; Sheehan, 1971; Sheehan, 1980) that some hypnotizable subjects may be specially motivated to be highly responsive to the hypnotist.

Research 'by Spanos, Cobb, and Gorassini (1985) provided support for the hypothesis that subjects' propensity to successfully resist suggestions depended on their construal of such behavior as congruent with presenting themselves as deeply hypnotized. To test this notion they placed high susceptible subjects in four different instructional conditions. Control subjects received no preparatory instructions. Subjects in the "ability to resist" condition were told that deeply hypnotized individuals were capable of both becoming very involved in test suggestions and simultaneously resisting them (i.e., try and prevent the overt response called for by the suggestion). Subjects in the "inability to resist" condition were told that deeply hypnotized individuals were incapable of resisting suggestions. Finally, subjects in an ambivalent information group were told that deeply hypnotized individuals' capacity to resist suggestions was unknown. All subjects were then hypnotized and administered four motoric suggestions. Subjects in the ability to resist treatment successfully resisted 95 percent of the suggestions and rated themselves as maintaining voluntary control over their behavior. Subjects in the remaining conditions passed (i.e., failed to resist) most suggestions, rated themselves as losing control of their behavior, and reported an inability to resist the suggestions. Subjects in all four groups were generally equivalent in their ratings of imaginal involvement and degree of experiencing suggested effects.

When examined together, these studies provide strong support for the position that hypnotic behavior is goal-directed and purposeful, and that subjects' reports of involuntariness are expectancy-based and mediated by contextual and relationship factors. Furthermore, when compared with Levitt and Baker's (Baker & Levitt, 1988; Levitt, 1986; Levitt & Baker, 1983) findings, the studies conducted in our laboratory and Spanos's, indicate that simply providing subjects with information about what constitutes responding like a "good" hypnotic subject is more effective than a monetary bribe as a means of influencing the ability to resist suggestions. Finally, several of the studies cited (Lynn et al., 1984; Spanos et al., 1985) failed to generate support for Arnold's (1946) position: Hypnotizable subjects were actively involved in imaginings, yet resisted suggestions when such behavior was perceived as appropriate in the experimental situation. A number of other studies have shown that the ideo-motor hypothesis does not provide a viable account of hypnotic behavior or involuntariness reports. Zamansky (Zamansky, 1977; Zamansky & Clar, 1986) found that hypnotizable subjects were able to respond to suggestions despite imagining inconsistent events. Kirsch, Council, & Mobayed (1987) showed that subjects who imagined incompatible events nonetheless responded to suggestions when lead to believe that imagining events incompatible with suggestions enhanced responding. Unfortunately, the studies by Zamansky and Kirsch and his colleagues did not include involuntariness measures.

Spanos, Weekes, and de Groh (1984) recently demonstrated that subjects could respond overtly opposite to suggestions while defining their responses as involuntary. The authors informed subjects that deeply hypnotized individuals could imagine an arm movement in one direction while their unconscious caused their arm to move in the opposite direction. Even though subjects so informed moved in the opposite direction, they imagined suggested effects and described their countersuggestion behavior as involuntary.

In a recent study, we (Lynn, Snodgrass, Rhue, & Hardaway, 1987) found that with instructions designed to increase the use of GDFs, low and high hypnotizable subjects reported equivalent GDF absorption and frequency of GDFs. However, hypnotizable subjects responded more and reported greater involuntariness than low susceptibles, even when their GDFs were equivalent. We therefore found no support for the hypothesis that sustained, elaborated suggestion-related imagery mediates response to suggestion (Arnold, 1946). We also failed to find support for Zamansky and Clark's (1986) hypothesis that low hypnotizable subjects, lacking the capacity to dissociate incompatible cognitions from relevant ones, are able to pass suggestions only when it is possible to become absorbed in them. Even when low and high hypnotizables were absorbed in GDFs to a comparable extent, low hypnotizables were not as responsive to suggestions as high hypnotizables.

Although correlational analyses revealed that subjects used GDF as a strategy to promote the experience of involuntariness, a finding consistent with other studies (e.g., Spanos & Barber, 1972; Spanos & Ham, 1975; Spanos & McPeake, 1977), GDF's were not associated with responding to suggestion. In contrast, subjects' beliefs about how imaginative subjects respond, and subjects' ratings of the degree to which imagining is associated with responding, predicted responding and involuntary experience. Thus, expectancies appear to be of greater import than imaginings as determinants of involuntariness reports.

The finding that hypnotizable and nonhypnotizable subjects construe the relation between imagining and the occurrence of suggested responses in very different ways suggests the following interpretation of the relation between hypnotizability and involuntariness: When instructed to do so, low hypnotizable subjects respond to suggestion by engrossing themselves in suggestion-related imagery. However, they fail, for the most part, to perceive a connection between their suggestion-related imaginings and moving in response to suggestion. This suggests that despite being absorbed in imagery, low hypnotizable subjects wait passively for suggested events to occur. Not surprisingly, nothing happens. In contrast, hypnotizable subjects take a much more active and constructive approach to the situation. They are successful in creating role-related experiences and behaving as suggested while simultaneously generating imagery of a kind that qualifies their responding as an involuntary happening.

The demonstrated relations among hypnotizability, cognitive construal, and involuntariness reports are compatible with the integrative model and with social psychological accounts of hypnotizability, which emphasize role-related beliefs and context-based expectancies rather than capacities for experiencing unusual cognitive changes (e.g., dissociations of cognitive controls, alterations in conscious state).

Posthypnotic Responding

Posthypnotic suggestions inform subjects to respond to a cue and perform certain acts after they are "awakened" from hypnosis. Traditionally, posthypnotic responding has been identified by two characteristics: The subject both experiences a compulsion to perform the act and a lack of awareness that the act was performed (Erickson & Erickson, 1941). Because the posthypnotic response is purportedly automatically triggered by a predetermined cue, some investigators have contended that it can persist outside the confines of the hypnosis experiment (e.g., Erickson & Erickson, 1941; Orne et al., 1968; Weitzenhoffer, 1953). However, evidence suggests (Fisher, 1954; Spanos, Menary, Brett, Cross & Ahmed, 1987; St. Jean, 1978) that posthypnotic responding is, in fact, not automatic but is instead mediated by situational cues and expectancies and can be thought of as goal-directed action (Spanos, Menary et al., 1987).

Fisher (1954) gave thirteen subjects the suggestion to scratch their ear each time they heard the word "psychology." After the posthypnotic response was elicited the hypnotist created the impression that the experiment was over by conversing with a colleague. During this time the cue word was used informally. The hypnotist then restructured the situation to intimate that the experiment was still in progress. Although all thirteen subjects responded to the formal testing of the cue word, nine failed to respond when the cue word was mentioned informally. Seven of the nine subjects who had stopped responding, responded again when they thought the experiment was again in progress. St. Jean (1978) found that when the experimenter left the room to attend to an emergency, almost all subjects stopped responding posthypnotically to a prerecorded auditory stimulus.

In a study conducted by Orne and his colleagues (Orne, Sheehan & Evans, 1968), seventeen hypnotizable and fourteen simulating subjects were given a posthypnotic suggestion to touch their foreheads each time they heard the word "experiment" for the next forty-eight hours. The hypnotist tested the suggestion in the experimental setting, and a secretary tested the suggestion as subjects left the building and returned the next day. Whereas five out of the seven highly hypnotizable subjects responded consistently away from the experimenter, no simulators did so.

Although designed to challenge Fisher's (1954) finding that expectations play a role in determining the performance of posthypnotic behavior, the study did not constitute a strong challenge. The five subjects who responded outside of the experimental setting all stopped responding when the hypnotist used the cue word with the clear intent of removing the original suggestion. Postexperimental inquiry revealed that these subjects stopped responding because they anticipated the suggestion's removal. Furthermore, posthypnotic responders could have guessed that the experiment was still in progress when tested by the secretary who was associated with the experiment and was not blind to all of the subjects' real-simulating status.

Spanos and his associates (Spanos, Menary et al., 1987) recently found that hypnotizable subjects' posthypnotic responding (e.g., cough out loud when you hear the word "psychology") was nill when tested in a context that subjects did not associate with their experimental situation. When the cue was embedded in a meaning context that was associated with the hypnotic role—tested formally by the hypnotist—subjects exhibited posthypnotic responding. However, when tested informally by a confederate who posed as a lost student and asked for directions to the *psychology* department, none of the hypnotizable and none of the simulating subjects responded to the cue word. Only one of the simulating subjects and none of the hypnotizable subjects responded to a second informal test by a second confederate who asked subjects, at the laboratory, if they were there for a *psychology* experiment. Spanos and his colleagues contend that these results indicate that posthypnotic responding is expectancy-mediated, goal-directed action.

Hoyt and Kihlstrom (1987) conducted two experiments that contrasted posthypnotic suggestion and waking instruction. In the first experiment, hypnotized subjects were given a posthypnotic suggestion to mail predated postcards to the experimenter for three weeks. Subjects were told to underline the date each time they mailed the postcard. Unhypnotizable subjects were given the same task as a waking instruction. The two groups were equally compliant in sending the postcards and in underlining the date. Furthermore, compliance to the posthypnotic suggestion did not last longer than to the waking instruction.

In a second experiment, the authors found that subjects who were presented with both a waking and a posthypnotic suggestion to respond to two different digit cues presented on a computer screen did not automatically favor the posthypnotic cue. Subjects who favored the posthypnotic cue when it appeared alone on trials when it did not conflict with the posthypnotic cue, also favored that cue when it conflicted with the waking cue, and vice-versa. Subjects responded significantly more accurately and faster to their favored cue than to their nonfavored cue. Subjects did not, therefore, behave like automatons who were compelled to respond to the posthypnotic suggestion. Subjects appeared to allocate resources to one task at the expense of the other task. Hoyt and Kihlstrom (1986) concluded that posthypnotic information processing is no different than nonhypnotic information processing.

Breaching Amnesia

Early attempts to pressure initially amnesic subjects to "breach" their hypnotic amnesia (e.g., Bowers, 1966; Kihlstrom, Evans, Orne & Orne, 1980) generally found that whereas approximately half of the initially amnesic subjects reversed their reports and indicated that they could remember, the remaining subjects continued to report amnesia. These findings have been viewed as reflecting a genuine inability of some amnesic subjects to recall due to their loss of conscious control over memory. Coe and his associates (Coe & Yashinski, 1985; Howard & Coe, 1980; Schuyler & Coe, 1981) have found that subjects can be classified on the basis of whether they rate their forgetting as under their control (i.e., voluntary) or beyond their control (i.e., involuntary) in hypnosis pretesting (session one). These researchers found that about half of amnesic subjects breached when exposed to procedures designed to accomplish this (e.g., attachment to a lie detector). However, subjects who had previously rated themselves as having voluntary control over memory were more likely to breach than those subjects who rated their forgetting as being beyond their control.

Coe (1983) maintains that subjects use their response to suggestion as a primary criterion for judging their reports of control. While trying to remember during the second "breaching" session, subjects rated their degree of perceived control. Subjects who changed their reports from being in control of remembering at pretesting, to not being in control of remembering during the second session did not exhibit recall at session two. Coe believes that the second experience of not recalling was sufficiently convincing to lead their subjects to decrease the amount of control they reported. Relatedly, subjects who changed their reports from having little control in session one to having more control in session two typically recalled more in the second session.

Although Coe and his colleagues did not succeed in completely breaching amnesia, other investigators have succeeded in doing so by defining breaching as compatible with successfully fulfilling hypnotic role demands. For example, in two experiments, Spanos, Radtke, and Bertrand (1985) used the so-called "hidden observer" to create expectancies that recalling forgotten material was appropriate. In their first study, subjects were informed that, while hypnotized, they possessed a hidden part of their mind that retained an awareness of information the conscious hypnotized part no longer remembered. In a second experiment, amnesic subjects were informed that they possessed two hidden observers—one in each cerebral hemisphere, and that in addition, abstract words were stored in one hemisphere and concrete words were stored in the other. In both studies, subjects initially showed complete amnesia. In the first study, when the hypnotist contacted their hidden observer all of the subjects recalled the target words; in the second study, subjects recalled abstract and concrete words when their respective hidden observers were contacted by the hypnotist. These studies, plus a recent investigation by Silva and Kirsch (1987) which showed that subjects breached amnesia who received prehypnotic information that instilled expectancies that hypnosis could enhance memory, indicate that amnesic subjects' inability to recall must be called into question. Indeed, like motoric and posthypnotic responding, amnesia does not qualify as an automatic or involuntary response that operates independently of the determinants of hypnotic responding that we have outlined in this chapter.

CONCLUDING COMMENTS

In this chapter we have presented an integrative model of the experience of nonvolition. We have attempted to show that the automatic, robot-like appearance of certain hypnotized subjects is explicable in terms of constructs derived from social and cognitive psychology. We believe that there are at least four reasons to reject the hypothesis that hypnotic responding is outside the realm of subjects' control, or is in any sense automatic or involuntary: (1) We have seen that hypnotic responses have all of the properties of behavior that is typically defined as voluntary. That is, they are purposeful, goal-directed, regulated in terms of subjects' intentions, and can be progressively changed to better achieve subjects' goals. Indeed, hypnotic behaviors occur because of subjects' over-arching goals rather than despite them. Like other voluntary behaviors, hypnotic behaviors and perceptions of involuntariness are shaped by psychological processes and situational factors that vary in their degree of accessibility to consciousness (e.g., Nisbett & Wilson, 1977). (2) It is well documented that hypnotizable subjects can resist suggestions when resistance is defined as consistent with the role of a "good" hypnotized subject (Lynn et al., 1984; Spanos, Cobb & Gorassini, 1985). (3) Hypnotic behaviors are neither reflexive/automatic (see Bargh, 1984) nor manifestations of innate stimulus-response connections (Kihlstrom, 1987). (4) Hypnotic performances consume attentional resources (Hoyt & Kihlstrom, 1987; Kihlstrom, 1987) in a manner comparable to nonhypnotic performances.

We have argued that hypnotizable subjects act in conformance with their perceptions of the hypnotized subject who, given the dominant cultural vision, is seen as responding automatically to suggestions. Subjects' identification of their actions as involuntary is in keeping with their understandings of appropriate hypnotic behavior, and their desire to fulfill hypnotic role demands. These understandings are shaped and defined by multiple and interacting factors including prehypnotic expectancies, self and situational representations, the structure of the hypnotic situation, rapport with the hypnotist, the wording of the suggestions, subjects' observations of their own behavior, and an array of subtle and not-so-subtle contextual influences.

Hypnotic subjects' cognitive activities clearly demonstrate their active attempts to fulfill the requirements of hypnotic suggestions (Sheehan & McConkey, 1982), which include experiencing suggestion-related effects as involuntary. The act of imagining, and other cognitive strategies we discussed, are not passive happenings; instead, they are goal-directed, purposeful, and attuned to personal strivings and changing contextual demands. We have contended that such "doings," particularly the act of understanding the self and one's behavior in the terms implied by the hypnotic context, the language of the induction, and the structure of the suggestion (e.g., as one being acted upon rather than as an actor), contribute to the perception of actions as involuntary reactions. That subjects often have a mental representation of hypnotic events (e.g., imaginings, sensations), suggests that a formidable degree of mental control exists (Vallacher & Wegner, 1987). At the same time, many of the cognitive operations and affective reactions that accompany hypnotic responding are not readily accessible to consciousness.

We discussed certain features of the hypnotic context that discourage awareness and analysis of the personal and situational factors that influence hypnotic behavior. To the extent that interests and intentions lack articulation, self-consciousness, and the perception of inner directedness, the sense of deliberate control of action is compromised (Fingarette, 1969; Sarbin, 1984). Even though the subject does not recognize that his feelings of involuntariness are a product of his own goals and understandings, even though he might not be aware of contingencies that affect his feelings, even though his sense of volitional direction and control may consist only of a peripheral awareness of directed activity, his behavior is, in fact, goal-directed, purposeful, and ultimately explicable in the same terms that account for nonhypnotic behavior.

5

Posthypnotic Amnesia
Theory and Research[1]

William C. Coe

The usual operational definition of posthypnotic amnesia is the nonreporting of certain events that the hypnotist suggested the subject could not remember. This definition, however, avoids the knotty problem of the credibility of the subject's not reporting. Nonreporting may be coterminous with "inability to report," "unwillingness to report," "being unable to remember," "confusion about instructions," "resistance," etc. The first section of this chapter raises the question "Is posthypnotic amnesia credible?"

Several laboratory examples will help to establish the boundaries of our discussion.

In the usual case subjects are administered a standard scale of hypnotic responsiveness that includes a suggestion for posthypnotic amnesia. Such a suggestion informs subjects that after they awaken they will not be able to remember anything that happened since they entered hypnosis. It is also suggested that they will be able to remember after the hypnotist provides an agreed-upon cue, e.g., "Now you can remember everything!" Subjects are awakened and asked to tell everything that has happened since they were hypnotized. Some subjects report very little of what happened. However, when the cue to remember is presented, they recall a good deal. Such subjects are judged to have been amnesic because (1) they did not report the specific happenings, and (2) they reported many of them when presented the remember cue ("reversibility"). Is their amnesia credible?

In another example, galvanic skin resistances (GSR) are monitored during the test for posthypnotic amnesia. Subjects are given a posthypnotic suggestion not to remember certain key words. During recognition testing, the key words are interspersed with other "neutral" words. Subjects demonstrating posthypnotic amnesia do not report recognizing the key words until they are given the reversibility cue. However, their GSR responses to the key words differ from their

110

GSR responses to the neutral words (Bitterman and Marcuse, 1945). While subjects said that they did not remember, their GSR responses suggested that they did. Is their amnesia credible?

In a third example, subjects learn two lists of words, one before they are hypnotized and one while they are hypnotized (for example, Coe, Basden, Basden & Graham, 1976). The list they learn while hypnotized has been constructed to create retroactive inhibition for the first list, that is, learning the second list increases the difficulty of recalling the first list. Some subjects are given a posthypnotic amnesia suggestion to forget the second list; others are given no suggestion. If posthypnotic amnesia has rendered the second list unavailable, then subjects who are amnesic for it should recall the first list at a higher level than subjects who are not amnesic for it. Recall of both lists is tested before posthypnotic amnesia is lifted. The results show that subjects who demonstrated posthypnotic amnesia for the second list, recalled the first list at the same level as subjects who were not amnesic for the second list. Thus, even though some subjects do not report the second list, it interferes with their recall just as much as it does for subjects who do report it. Again, their reports indicated they were amnesic, but their performance indicated they were not. Is their amnesia credible?

CRITERIA FOR CREDIBILITY

The above examples provide us with measures of posthypnotic amnesia that may be classified into two broad categories: (1) those that are presumably difficult to modify purposely, like physiological responses and subtle methods of testing memory (Coe, Basden and Basden & Graham, 1976; Coe, Taul, Basden & Basden, 1973; Cooper, 1972; Graham & Patton, 1968; Williamson, Johnson & Ericksen, 1965), and (2) those that can easily be modified, namely, verbal reports and some nonverbal communications.

Difficult-to-modify measures are employed for two reasons: (1) to reduce the possibility that subjects are merely withholding information, and (2) to evaluate the extent to which presumably forgotten material is available during recall. In general, such measures have demonstrated that the material that is supposedly forgotten is still as available to amnesics as it is to nonamnesics. If we choose difficult-to-modify measures as our criteria for the credibility of posthypnotic amnesia, the data force us to conclude that posthypnotic amnesia is not credible. This aspect of posthypnotic amnesia raises the so-called "paradox" of posthypnotic amnesia. Subjects claim *to not* remember, but at the same time they seem *to* remember.

That many initially amnesic subjects remember a good deal after the reversal cue speaks against the possibility that posthypnotic amnesia is the same as normal forgetting, or as never having learned the material in the first place (Bowers, 1975, 1976; Cooper, 1972). Thus, if we select as our criterion the similarity of posthypnotic amnesia to never having learned the material in the first place, or to normal forgetting, we are again forced to conclude that posthypnotic amnesia is not credible.

As we reject one criterion after another we are perforce led to another, namely, the extent to which the subject's phenomenological report of the experience is convincing. To be sure, we are entering a shadowy area of investigation. The validity of the self-report, an indirect measure of the experience, is difficult to evaluate. Nevertheless, it appears that the phenomenal experience is the only remaining viable criterion supporting the credibility of posthypnotic amnesia. We are therefore left with the task of evaluating self-reports as valid mirrors of phenomenal experience.

Simply saying "I can't remember" or "I don't remember," or showing reversibility is not an adequate indicator of phenomenal experience. Many subjects who are instructed to simulate hypnosis will produce these responses. Even so-called genuine hypnotic subjects may at times purposely falsify their reports for one reason or another. Failure to recall, and reversibility, are more convincing if subjects have responded positively to other hypnotic suggestions. However, because passing another suggestion can also result from volitional compliance, it cannot be accepted as a valid criterion for self-reports.

However, some self-reports are rather easily accepted as valid reflections of private experience. For example, reports implying that the experience of amnesia was not complete, or that it was not experienced at all, are generally easier to accept. We are likely to believe simulating subjects who say that they recalled almost everything when they were asked, but that they did not report it because they were trying to deceive the hypnotist. Likewise, we are likely to accept reports of subjects who say that they probably could have remembered if they had not purposely redirected their attention to other things. Such reports are not unusual or exciting; therefore, they are rather easy to accept, but these reports do not support the credibility of posthypnotic amnesia.

What about reports of unusual and counterexpectational experiences? Some of these may also be accepted as valid reflections of experience. Therefore, counterexpectational reports of not being able to remember, expressed with a high degree of conviction, remain the sole criterion in support of the crediblity of posthypnotic amnesia.

THEORIES

The major theoretical differences surrounding posthypnotic amnesia revolve around the issue of whether posthypnotic amnesia should be viewed as a "happening" or a "doing." Special-process theorists prefer "happenings." In opposition, social psychological theorists prefer "doings."

Special-process theorists postulate that subjects *cannot* remember. Posthypnotic amnesia is viewed like other everyday disruptions of memory, e.g., forgetting where one left one's car keys, or blocking out someone's name at a cocktail party (Kihlstrom, 1978). Cooper (1972), for example, states that "amnesia . . . has been traditionally viewed as being outside of the subjects volitional control and carried out automatically" (p. 248).

Social psychological theories postulate that subjects are best viewed as "doing" something not to recall, even to the extent that their failure to recall may be interpreted by them as out of their control, i.e., involuntary. Variables in the setting are believed to interact with subject variables in important ways, interactions are therefore emphasized (Coe, 1978; Spanos, 1986b).

Kihlstrom (1978), a special process theorist, stated that "we have analyzed the wider social context and determined the relative importance of contextual variables in amnesia. . . . Thus, we are led to shift our emphasis from the social context 'in which' amnesia occurs to the cognitive processes 'by which' it occurs" (p. 252). Unusual, special processes, like dissociations of materials and amnesic barriers, are postulated as accounting for subjects' inability to recall. It is postulated that memories are dissociated from conscious control so that they cannot be accessed voluntarily (Hilgard, 1974, 1977a, 1977b; Kihlstrom, 1978, 1983; Kihlstrom et al., 1980; Kihlstrom & Shor, 1978). Special process theorists also imply that hypnosis is best viewed as a special state of consciousness (e.g., Kihlstrom, 1978, p. 248; Hilgard, 1977b, p. 58). However, they are also careful to spell out that "special state" or "hypnosis" represents a "category of phenomena, not a causal agent" (Kihlstrom, 1978, p. 250).

The paradox of subjects seeming to know, but at the same time not to know is explained by special process proponents by comparing it to other memory findings. Posthypnotic amnesia should not be considered unusual, because other findings in memory research have shown that material can be available in memory storage but cannot be retrieved for recall. "A failure to remember simply means that the person cannot 'now' gain access to the target memory" (Tulving & Perlstone, 1966) or that he cannot construct a complete account based on what he has accessed (Brown & McNeil, 1966) (Kihlstrom, 1978, p. 251). The posthypnotic cue lifting amnesia presumably operates like other cues that help increase recall, e.g., recognition cues.

Subjects' verbal reports present a problem to theorists who focus on memory mechanisms. Kihlstrom (1978) recognizes that we are "ultimately thrown back on subjects' verbal reports of memory . . . because it is the only evidence that is admissible" (p. 251).

However, there is no way to investigate subjects' reports from a memory model, but we can explain them as the result of postulated changes in memory mechanisms. Take the example of someone who reports little or no remembering at testing and also reports little or no control over remembering (involuntariness). The special process theorist is left explaining the reports as the result of a dissociative barrier that prevents the retrieval of the forbidden material. However, the dissociative barrier, which bans the material from awareness, also accounts for the experience of involuntariness. The possibility of circular explanation is obvious. The barrier is postulated because of subjects' reports, and the reports are explained by the presence of the barrier.

What about those who do not report the forbidden material and say that their not reporting was voluntary? Or, what if they say their not reporting was involuntary because their jaws were stuck shut and they could not report? The hypothetical dissociative barrier must now take on quite different characteristics. In the first instance, the barrier must have created a dissociation from the retrieval mechanism but not from consciousness. In the second instance, the barrier allowed the material to be retrieved into awareness but also created an hysterical paralysis of the jaw to prevent its report.

In short, the special process theorist must accept verbal reports as either mirrors of private experience or not. Concepts are not available for evaluating the reports. Nevertheless, Kihlstrom (1978) defends the position: "It is worth remembering that whole subdisciplines of psychology—such as psychophysics—are predicated on the scientific acceptance of self-reports" (p. 251).

The social psychological view argues that the hypnosis setting and subject characteristics interact in important ways to determine both self-reports *and* personal experiences (Coe, 1978; Coe & Sarbin, 1977; Sarbin & Coe, 1972, 1979; Spanos, 1981, 1982, 1986b). Rather than trying to hold the setting constant in order to obtain one sort of self-report, interactions among setting and subject variables may be studied systematically. Predictions may be made as to what and how subjects report; post-hoc explanations are not necessary. Subject variables are clearly recognized as important, but the emphasis is on their interactions with setting variables. However, the subject variables are not those of memory, they are concepts like "expectations," "response-expectations," or "cognitive skills." Thus, subjects who respond to the suggestion for posthypnotic amnesia are viewed as actively employing their skills or abilities to fulfill their expectations for the role of "good" subject. Subjects of interest are those who objectively demonstrate posthypnotic amnesia by (1) reporting very little or none of the critical material, (2) reporting the experience as involuntary, and (3) recovering the materials on cue. Some of these follow the path of *deception*. They report their failure to recall as involuntary when they know it was not. Others follow the path of *self-deception*. They attribute their failure to recall to a personal inability to remember (an involuntary experience), *and* they believe their reports, even though the material was available for recall as evidenced by their recall after the reversibility cue.

Secrets and Believing

Another earlier article detailed an analysis of secrets and tried to show how such an analysis leads to a more complex texture of events than those considered by a special process approach (Coe, 1978). Conditions were pointed out under which subjects' reports of involuntariness are more likely to be believed, or not to be believed. Reports that are ambiguous, or given without conviction, are not likely to be accepted as evidence for a credible, posthypnotic amnesia. We are also less likely to believe reports that suggest a subject was purposely doing something to avoid recalling. The reports that are most likely to be accepted as valid are those that suggest a subject has expended effort to remember but was unable to do so, e.g., "No matter how hard I tried, something just blocked my memory" or "My mind was simply blank, I had no control, it was just blank."

It is also important to note that the listener's own belief system can take on importance in accepting counterexpectational statements as accurate reflections of private experience (Sarbin & Juhasz, 1970, 1975). The special process theorist is placed in the position of having to accept the involuntary quality of such reports as "happenings," and therefore as similar to other more common lapses of memory (e.g., forgetting where one left the keys). For the commonday experience of forgetting where one left one's keys, a rule-following explanation is more readily sought (Peters, 1958), e.g., the person was involved in other matters and not attending when he or she put the keys down. However, in the context of hypnosis, with its benign verbal suggestions that subjects will be unable to remember, reports of not remembering take on added importance, and more powerful inner explanations, like "dissociated subsystems" and "amnesic barriers," may be postulated. However, rather than focus on subject memory systems, the social psychological position postulates that a clearer understanding will follow from an examination of the interactions among the setting, participant characteristics, and interpersonal exchanges.

Self-Persuasion and Self-Deception

Even when we believe that subjects are convinced of their helplessness in recalling, different conclusions and different questions arise from a social psychological position than from a special-process one. The special process theorist asks "What force(s) is (are) operating to cause this experience?" The social psychological theorist asks "What leads people to believe in their counterfactual statements?" "What leads them to believe in their imaginings?" We are led to a social psychological analysis of self-persuasion and self-deception.[2,3]

To begin with, imagining is viewed as an active process, one of persons pretending, of persons covertly engaging in "as if" behavior, of persons performing at various levels of hypotheticalness (Sarbin, 1984; Sarbin & Coe, 1972; Sarbin & Juhasz, 1970). Even though people differ in their capacity for taking a hypothetical attitude, contextual characteristics will modify how they report about their hypothetical activity.

Hypnotic subjects may entertain the notion that it is "as if" they cannot remember (bend their arm, say their name, etc.). Yet, there are times when they drop the metaphorical connotations and state that they simply could not remember. If they are not withholding secrets, we are faced with explaining what leads them to believe in their hypothetical (fictive) activity.[4]

We have discussed in some detail elsewhere how the *degree of involvement in imaginings* encourages believability (Sarbin & Coe, 1972). The more involved in our hypothetical conduct (imagining), the more likely we are to accept it as literal, or "real." Spanos and McPeake (1974) provided empirical support for this notion. In brief, they requested hypnotized subjects to rate (1) the degree to which they were involved in their imaginings, (2) the extent to which they experienced their response as involuntary, and (3) the degree of credibility they assigned to their imaginings. Involvement was positively related to involuntariness, to credibility, and to hypnotic performance.

Contexts like hypnosis, which arouse expectations of unusual occurrences, also encourage participant involvement. Subjects are more likely to attend to their internal sensations than they normally would, and they may not have conventional code words for fully describing these experiences. Sarbin (1968) has outlined the general process. Many personal experiences, especially those whose sources derive from inner, somatic events, have no ready verbal referents. Yet, noticing them and communicating their occurrence becomes important in some contexts. We search for words that refer to known events that are similar (metaphors) in hopes of communicating about interesting, but ambiguous, experiences. For example, a person suffering stomach discomfort may say "It's as if my belly is on fire." Metaphors are commonly used to describe and relate experiences of personal interest.

Hypnotic subjects who become involved in what they are doing are likely to be surprised, interested, and perplexed by the sensations they experience. In the interest of communicating the unusualness of their experiences, they may drop the metaphorical characteristics of their words. In so doing, they transform the metaphor to myth, and causal properties may be assigned to it. Hypnotic subjects who report "It was as if I could not focus on what had happened," leaves the investigation open. The use of metaphorical description remains recognizable. But when subjects shift to mythic forms, such as "My mind was blank"—perhaps for the purpose of communicating the strangeness of their experience—ambiguity is reduced and causality is implied. Presumably, their experience can now be attributed to the workings of an inner force that prevents them from remembering. In sum, the *expectations of unusual occurrences,* which are stimulated by the setting, the *need to understand* unusual experiences, and the *need to communicate them,* all combine to encourage hypnotic subjects, who are involved in their imaginings, to employ mythic rather than metaphorical descriptions.

Other parameters of involvement also seem worth investigating. One is the possibility that under conditions of high involvement *more organismic systems* are involved than usual. Subjects are therefore faced with the added task of making sense of them, a task that further encourages literal statements rather than hypothetical ones. For example, highly involved worshipers are more likely to say that they "heard" God's voice than to say it was "as if" they heard God's voice.

The *degree of ambiguity* in the context can also be important and can interact with self-persuasion. The option of believing what one has reported, as opposed to not believing it, is more likely to be chosen as ambiguity increases. An example we have presented elsewhere is that of the sentry at night who hears a twig crack in the darkness (Sarbin & Coe, 1972). A choice must be made. "Is it an enemy? Is it something else?" The sentry's *expectations of reinforcement* enter into his decision. Challenging may be silly, but failing to challenge may be fatal. He chooses challenge, and a startled rabbit runs off through the brush. Never seeing the rabbit, he fires at the sounds. In telling the incident to his aroused comrades, he is likely to lose his doubts and state that he had in fact rousted an enemy. Although the circumstances are less critical, ambiguity in hypnotic settings may have similar effects. For example, hypnotic subjects may not report a few things that they fleetingly remember during the testing of posthypnotic amnesia. However, they may later become convinced that in fact they had not remembered anything. How much they were expected to forget may not have been very clear in the first place. So once committed to not remembering, it is easier to ignore the importance of their fleeting thoughts than to admit that they did not report some of the things they remembered.

A final variable that appears to influence believing one's self are the *expectations the setting holds for telling the truth*. Bem (1965, 1967) found that people were more likely to believe their own false statements when given under experimentally manipulated "honesty" conditions than under "dishonesty" conditions. He even suggested that the effect may be strong enough to lead people to believe false confessions. The relevance to hypnotic settings seems obvious. In both clinical and experimental hypnosis, implict and/or explicit expectations for honesty and truth-telling are likely to be given. Thus, it is likely that some posthypnotically amnesic subjects who report that they could not remember, come to believe their reports even though they initially had some doubts.

Furthermore, Bem hypothesized that people learn about their own beliefs by observing their own behavior. If so, hypnotic subjects who perceive the circumstances as ones for telling the truth will then begin to believe their own reports of not remembering from observing their own behavior. In turn, they may behave in ways that further enhance the credibility of their statements, convincing themselves, and the hypnotist, even more.

So far my analysis has purposely emphasized the effects of the setting, not because the setting is of primary importance, but rather because setting variables are at times considered "artifacts" of hypnosis (for example, Orne, 1969). Consequently, attempts are made to control setting variables rather than to investigate them. Viewing setting variables as not very important is a basic difference between social psychological theories and special process theories, the latter taking a more limited view of human conduct.[5] There is nothing inherently incorrect in Kihlstrom's (1978) cognitive position for example. However, memory is only a limited part of the larger context. A complete understanding of human conduct will only be found through study of the interrelatedness of all aspects of the context.

Doing As Not Remembering

Cognitive skills are important to most human endeavors, and experiencing posthypnotic amnesia is no exception. We take the position that subjects who produce posthypnotic amnesia employ skills—they *do* something—in order *not* to remember (Coe, 1973; Sarbin & Coe, 1972). I do not mean that subjects purposely set out to deceive or fake, although some apparently do, but rather that they are involved in their experiences and bring certain cognitive abilities to bear to assist them. I agree with Kihlstrom (1978) that a failure in retrieval, defined as not reporting, accounts in part for posthypnotic amnesia. Is the failure best viewed as a happening or a doing?

In a majority of an unselected population a failure in retrieval *does not* occur following a posthypnotic amnesia suggestion. About 67 percent do not respond to the suggestion; they report as many memories as do nonhypnotized persons. About one-third of the population, depending on the particular criteria employed, respond to suggested amnesia. Of this number, recent evidence suggests that many may simply not report what they remember. Spanos and Bodorik (1977) and Spanos and Radtke (1981, 1982) found that 40 percent to 63 percent of their "amnesic" subjects (total nonrecall) admitted postexperimentally that they had suppressed their reports. (Perhaps we should wonder how many did not confess?) If this finding is valid, it appears reliable, and if it is not restricted to their particular amnesic task (nine free recall words learned to criterion), at least half of our amnesic subjects are not very mysterious. The "skill" they employ is *not reporting*. It would be of interest, however, to discover what factors led them to keep their secrets.

There are, of course, still other amnesic subjects. It seems that about half, according to their own reports, do not try to forget and about half try to forget, but these groups do not differ in hypnotic susceptibility (Coe & Yashinski, 1985; Howard & Coe, 1980; Schuyler & Coe, 1981, 1987; Spanos & Bodorik, 1977; Spanos & Radtke, 1982; Sluis & Coe, 1987). The particular cognitive strategies or skills that these subjects use appear to vary. For subjects who try to forget, suppression appears to be a common strategy—they try not to think of the items. A good portion remember but choose not to report, and some try to distract themselves by focusing on other things. Subjects who report that they did not try to forget seem to use somewhat different strategies. Some report not being able to say the material even though they remembered it. For example, their throat or jaw is stuck. Others report a lack of motivation. They say, for example, they were too relaxed to make the effort, though they believe they might have recalled had they tried. A few subjects report feeling that they "have no role in causing the words to leave awareness or in keeping them out of awareness" (Spanos and Bodorik, 1977, p. 301). They feel relaxed and the material is just gone.

Earlier work by Spanos and Ham (1973) indicated that goal-directed fantasy (GDF) was important in posthypnotically forgetting the number "4." For example, subjects reported that they imagined a string of numbers with the "4" missing, or they saw it falling apart so that it was not there. When asked to count from 1 to 5 upon awakening, the number 4 would not be reported. Even so, when they rated themselves on whether or not they had thought of the number 4 while counting, only 10 percent claimed that they had experienced complete amnesia.

The foregoing discussion suggests that when subjects respond to suggested amnesia, the vast majority of them are doing something. They are either employing a cognitive strategy that assists them in not remembering or, with the same effect, they are doing nothing to help themselves remember. Apparently it is very rare for individuals to claim that they tried hard to remember, that they expended great effort to search for the proper tags—if you will—and felt that they were a victim of some inner change. To be sure, the evidence indicates a disruption in memory, but the disruption appears to be mostly self-imposed by the subjects' actions.

I will now turn to an evaluation of the research that is often quoted as evidence that posthypnotic amnesia (and hypnosis) is a special phenomenon.

RESEARCH PHENOMENON

It is important to explain data on posthypnotic amnesia; however, it is also important to evaluate the research *critically* before jumping to conclusions. In 1978, I evaluated the data on source amnesia, disrupted retrieval, and breaching posthypnotic amnesia (Coe, 1978). I will summarize those analyses then present more recent research.

Source Amnesia

Claims have been made that "source amnesia" represents a phenomenon unique to hypnosis. In turn, hypnosis becomes special and deserves special concepts for understanding it. Operationally, source amnesia refers to posthypnotically amnesic subjects who remember information they learned while hypnotized but claim that they do not remember where or when it was learned. Five studies provide the primary data (Cooper, 1966; Evans, 1979a, 1979b; Evans and Thorn, 1966; Gheorgin, 1967).

Claims were made that source amnesia was (1) a hypnosis, or state-dependent, phenomenon, (2) a process different from the usual recall amnesia, and (3) not related to experimental demands (social psychological factors).

Is source amnesia hypnosis specific? Evans and Thorn (1966) compared the frequency of spontaneous (not suggested) source amnesia in three hypnotized samples to one waking sample. Because 10 percent of the combined hypnotized samples showed source amnesia, compared to 2 percent of the waking sample, they concluded that source amnesia was the result of hypnosis. However, their method of scoring the presence or absence of source amnesia was critical to their conclusion. They chose a cut-off point on the 6-point scale below at item 4, or higher, as passing source amnesia. (The scale had no reported reliability.)

1. Questions recalled during test of recall amnesia.

2. Source of information correctly given when asked questions.

3. Probably knows source of information, confusion evident.

4. States source, but *S* appears to be guessing or deducing this.

5. Apparently *S* has no idea of source of information.

6. *S* invents or rationalizes source.

Choosing to include item 4 is problematic since subjects scored as "4" accurately recalled the source of the information, i.e., they correctly stated that they had learned the material during hypnosis. Thus, according to their report they did *not* demonstrate source amnesia. However, the authors apparently chose not to believe them. Kihlstrom (1978) defended Evans and Thorn's choice of a cut-off at "4." He stated, "Evans and Thorn did not arbitrarily choose to disbelieve their *Ss*: the criterion was chosen in recognition of the fact that many *Ss* will (correctly) attribute some unusual self-observation to hypnosis without having any direct awareness that this is the fact. . . . We must distinguish between memory and inference: and when we do, the incidence of posthypnotic source amnesia is found to be approximately 10 percent in the unselected sample" (p. 254).

Nevertheless, neither Kihlstrom nor Evans and Thorn describe how they could tell the difference between those subjects who were "inferring" the source from subjects who actually remembered the source. The lack of operational definitions and reported reliabilities certainly make the scale suspect as a valid measure of source amnesia.

If only items 5 and 6 are considered as source amnesia, the data change rather dramatically as shown below. With rescoring, only two of the hypnotic samples demonstrate higher source amnesia than the waking sample, and they were probably not statistically higher.

	Hypnotic 1	Hypnotic 2	Hypnotic 3	Waking	Comb. Hyp. Samples
Score of 4, 5, or 6	13%	11%	7%	2%	10%
Score of 5 or 6	2%	5%	5%	2%	4%

Cooper's (1966) study showed a similar pattern. Only 2 percent of his unselected *hypnotic* subjects showed spontaneous source amnesia when a strict criterion for passing was employed (he had no waking controls). But when the criterion was easier, 9 percent showed it. I suggested that caution be heeded before heralding source amnesia as a hypnotic-specific phenomenon.

Is source amnesia a different process from recall amnesia? I also challenged Evans and Thorn's (1966) conclusion that recall and source amnesia were probably independent phenomenon and that they arose from different underlying mechanisms. They reported correlations between source amnesia and recall amnesia in all four samples (including the waking sample) that were significant at the .01 level (.37, .38, .39, and .42). Cooper (1966) reported a correlation of .48 (p< .001) between the two "phenomena." Yet, Evans and Thorn chose to view the significant positive relationships as demonstrating independence!

Since my 1978 article there has been no argument or research supporting source amnesia as independent from recall amnesia. Thus, I still conclude that they are *not* independent.

Source amnesia is not related to social psychological factors. Evans (1979a) compared highly susceptible subjects (completely amnesic) with simulating subjects for spontaneous source amnesia (see Orne, 1969, for more details of design).

Subjects who showed complete recall amnesia were then asked questions, the answers to which they had learned while hypnotized, e.g., the color of an amethyst when it is exposed to heat. Because no simulating subjects gave correct answers, and about one-third of the real subjects showed source amnesia, Evans interpreted the results as evidence that the social psychological demands of the experiment could not account for source amnesia.

In 1978, I criticized Evans's conclusion on the basis that the demands on simulators compared to those on real subjects are not necessarily the same. Simulators are usually more alert to instructions and more careful in how they respond. Further, in Evans's case there was no chance to test the demands for *not reporting the source* because none of the simulators gave a correct answer to the questions in the first place.

I also argued that Cooper's (1966) study offered some support for the effects of social psychological variables in source amnesia. Because he found a significant order effect in a counterbalanced, repeated measures design where source amnesia was suggested in one session but not in the other, the possibility that changes in the experimental context affected the level of source amnesia was strong. Kihlstrom (1978) seemed to agree, but he argued that the results suggested that the "explicit demands contained in the suggestion" (p. 255) were not the important factors. I would not disagree. The important point is made: source amnesia is significantly effected by social psychological variables of the setting.

Since my 1978 paper, I know of only three empirical studies on posthypnotic source amnesia.[6] These were reported by Spanos, Gwynn, et al. (1988). The results *did not* support source amnesia as special but *did* support my 1978 criticisms and a social psychological view. The findings supported the notion that source amnesia represents one of several possible strategies for dealing with an ambiguous test situation (Coe, 1978; Spanos, 1986b; Wagstaff, 1981). Amnesic subjects find themselves in an ambiguous situation after they have answered a question learned under hypnosis and are then asked "How do you know that?" Because the appropriate response is not clear, some subjects choose the path of denying they know where the learning took place. Most others readily admit they learned it during hypnosis.

Three samples were compared in Spanos, Gwynn et al.'s (1988) first study: (1) high-susceptible subjects who were hypnotized before and during learning the critical material, (2) high-susceptible subjects who were given "task-motivational" (TM) instructions (Barber, 1969) before and during learning, and (3) low-susceptible subjects were instructed to simulate as in Orne's (1969) instructions. However, simulators were also told that excellent subjects, given an amnesia suggestion, rarely forget everything; instead, they tend to show partial forgetting. The purpose of the added instructions was to produce simulators who would answer the critical question later and then have a chance to act under the demands associated with being asked how they knew the answer. Source amnesia was scored dichotomously, i.e., did or did not show any source amnesia, using only criteria numbers 5 and 6 above as I suggested in 1978 (100 percent interjudge reliability reported). The percentage of source amnesia out of the total number of times it was possible was also scored on a continuous index.

One result showed that hypnotized subjects and TM subjects answered critical questions equally, but both were more likely to answer the questions than were simulating subjects. This finding demonstrates the well-known fact that simulators overestimate the responsiveness of highly susceptible subjects, even when they have been instructed that reals are likely to show only partial amnesia. However, of the simulators who had the opportunity to show source amnesia at least once, a higher percentage of them showed it than either the hypnotized or the TM subjects. The rate of continuous source amnesia was also higher for simulators than for those in the other two samples. Thus simulators, given the opportunity, show a level of source amnesia at least equal to reals. The obvious conclusion is that social psychological demands for the source amnesia response appear to be clearly present.

Further, the similarity of response between hypnotized subjects and TM subjects supports the notion that hypnotic source amnesia is not hypnosis specific, consistent with other studies showing that hypnotic and TM subjects respond similarly to many suggestions (see Barber, 1969; Barber, Spanos & Chaves, 1974).

Recall that the simulators in study 1 were informed that deeply hypnotized subjects tend to exhibit partial rather than complete amnesia. Experiment 2 tested the hypothesis that these explicit instructions for partial amnesia may have somehow cued simulators to exhibit source amnesia. This hypothesis suggests that simulators exhibited source amnesia in response to tacit demands conveyed by their instructions to show partial amnesia, while in nonsimulators (who did not receive instructions for partial amnesia) the occurrence of source amnesia reflected intrinsic characteristics of partial amnesia.

Study 2 examined this hypothesis by comparing low susceptible simulators, who were again told that deeply hypnotized subjects tend to show partial amnesia, with high susceptible nonsimulating subjects who were also told that deeply hypnotized subjects show partial amnesia. A third group consisted of high susceptible nonsimulating subjects given no information concerning partial amnesia.

If information about partial amnesia provides cues for source amnesia responding, it should do so for informed hypnotic subjects as well as for simulators. Consequently, informed hypnotic subjects (who presumably have both an intrinsic tendency toward source amnesia and demands for source amnesia) should exhibit more source amnesia than either uninformed hypnotic amnesics (intrinsic tendency but no demands) or simulators (demands but no intrinsic tendency). Contrary to this hypothesis, the results of study 2 indicated that the three groups of subjects showed equivalent rates of source amnesia. In other words, the occurrence of source amnesia among the simulators could not be explained away by suggesting that their instructions for partial amnesia had also inadvertently cued them to exhibit source amnesia.

The third study (Spanos, Gwynn et al. [1988]) examined the effects of subtly manipulating the demands for the occurrence of source amnesia. Three hypnotized samples were compared; they differed on their pre-experimental instructions. One sample (control) was told nothing about the experiment. A second sample (information only) was told that the study involved posthypnotic amnesia and that subjects could respond to PHA in one of three ways, and that no one response was better than another: (a) not show amnesia, (b) show partial or complete amnesia, or (c) remember material without being aware it was learned during the session. The third sample (information plus demand) was told the same as the second sample with the addition that the experimenter was particularly interested in source amnesia (the "c" option).

The results showed: (1) The three samples did not differ on the number of chances they.had for showing source amnesia. (2) Both dichotomous and continuous scoring showed a greater amount of source amnesia in the "information plus demand" group than in the other two, which were equal. Thus, source amnesia appeared to be simply one of several response strategies in that situation. When the experimenter legitimized it as role appropriate, its frequency increased substantially.

In conclusion, the research on source amnesia since 1978 supports the view that when it exists it is largely the result of social psychological variables operating in the hypnotic setting. It is not hypnosis specific, nor does it need to be accounted for by special processes. Source amnesia can be most parsimoniously viewed as one of several possible strategies for dealing with an ambiguous test situation.

Disrupted Retrieval and Organization of Recall

In 1978 I also reviewed studies said to demonstrate that posthypnotically amnesic subjects showed patterns of recall indicative of a temporary disruption in memory retrieval. Temporal sequencing, or seriation (recalling in the order of administration), and clustering in free recall had been examined.

The effects of recalling in temporal order had been investigated primarily by Evans and Kihlstrom (1973) and Kihlstrom (1977) (see also Kihlstrom & Evans, 1979). They recognized that the effects they reported were "subtle." Nevertheless, they suggested that the effects made a strong case for the presence of disrupted retrieval in amnesic subjects compared to nonamnesic subjects.

My examination of the studies suggested on the other hand (1) that their hypothesis may not have been tested after all, and (2) that the data could be interpreted as *not* supporting differences between amnesic and nonamnesic subjects as easily as it could be interpreted as in support of differences.

To begin with, I questioned whether or not "amnesic" subjects had actually been examined. The method for computing recall order precluded the inclusion of subjects who recalled fewer than three items on a standard hypnotic scale, the usual criterion for passing posthypnotic amnesia. Thus, most subjects who would have normally been scored as passing the amnesia item were eliminated. Further, the mean susceptibility level for subjects who showed disrupted retrieval was only slightly more than 6.0 on the SHSS:C (Weitzenhoffer & Hilgard, 1962), a level most investigators (including them) consider medium susceptibility. From the outset, then, the meaning of the studies for posthypnotic amnesia was at best difficult to evaluate and, at worst, irrelevant to posthypnotic amnesia.

Another problem also made Evans and Kihlstrom's conclusions questionable *even* if they had studied "partially" amnesic subjects. Table 2 (Evans & Kihlstrom, 1973) showed that more highly hypnotic scorers than low scorers showed disrupted order of recall. However, 36 percent to 49 percent of their *low* scorers also showed it. Such a high frequency in low susceptibles certainly did not seem to limit disrupted retrieval to highly susceptible, posthypnotically amnesic subjects.

Further, if we accepted the usual levels of probability, i.e., $< .05$, the differences in rho (the measure of disrupted recall) between susceptibility levels *were not* statistically supported on two out of three hypnotic scales (Table 3, Evans & Kihlstrom, 1973). Further, the same subjects were administered the HGSHS (Shor & Orne, 1962), the SHSS:B (Weitzenhoffer & Hilgard, 1959) and the SHSS:C (Weitzenhoffer & Hilgard, 1962) in that order, but there was no mention of the possible effects that repeated measures might have had on the results.

In Kihlstrom's 1977 study, differences in temporal order were reported between highs and lows in a new sample. Even so, the magnitude of the differences were quite small, though significant, except on the SHSS:C.

Since in both studies it is difficult to know how subjects' previous experiences may have affected their recall of SHSS:C items, I recommended a very tentative and cautious interpretation of the results. Since then, my misgivings about temporal sequencing (seriation) in recall have been largely confirmed. Two studies have been unable to replicate the effects, which questions the validity of its existence (Radtke & Spanos, 1981; St. Jean & Coe, 1981). In another study, unhypnotized, role playing subjects when given instructions to "pretend to remember on a few items," recalled in a "random and disorganized manner similar to Evans and Kihlstrom's "hypnotized subjects" (Wagstaff, 1977, p. 499). When not given the instruction, they recalled sequentially like Evans and Kihlstrom's insusceptible subjects. Thus, the effect may simply reveal what subjects do in order to comply with instructions.

Another important, methodological flaw has also been pointed out since then (Spanos, 1986b). The earlier studies had interpreted the negative relationship between *susceptibility level* and the degree of seriation at recall as support for a relationship between the degree of *amnesia* and seriation. The problem with that approach was that no measures of seriation were taken before amnesia or after amnesia. Thus, it could not be known whether seriation changed during amnesia or whether it was a characteristic of high and low subjects at other times as well (Spanos, 1986b, p. 456). In fact, three studies have supported the latter interpretation. Negative correlations for susceptibility and seriation have been found even *before* the amnesia suggestion is given (Radtke, et al., 1986; Schwartz, 1978, 1980). That is, higher susceptible subjects tend to show lower seriation even without amnesia.

More recent investigations have taken the direction of (1) using word lists rather than hypnosis items, (2) measuring amnesia unambiguously, and (3) assessing seriation, or subjective organization (SO), idiosyncratic strategies individual subjects develop for remembering a list of unrelated words) on recall trials before, during and after the amnesia suggestion.

Subjective organization (SO). Several studies have compared changes in SO before, during, and after cancelling the amnesia suggestion in subjects who showed partial amnesia and in subjects who showed no amnesia. Spanos, Radtke-Bodorik, and Shabinsky (1980); and Radtke, Spanos, and Bertrand (1983) found no evidence for an amnesia-specific breakdown in SO. Tkachyk, Spanos and Bertrand (1985) suggested that these studies may have failed to obtain a significant breakdown effect because of floor effects; subjects in these studies exhibited fairly low levels of SO even before they were administered the amnesia suggestion. In support of this hypothesis, Tkachyk et al. (1985) demonstrated that subjects who received a learning procedure that created high, initial levels of SO (i.e., presuggestion) later showed an amnesia-specific breakdown. In contrast, subjects who received a learning procedure that did not produce high, initial levels of SO failed to show an amnesia-specific breakdown.

Unlike Tkachyk et al. (1985), Wilson and Kihlstrom (1986) reported that subjects failed to exhibit an amnesia-specific breakdown in SO even when they attained high, initial levels of SO. However, the Wilson and Kihlstrom (1986) study is difficult to interpret because of a methodological shortcoming. To assess accurately an amnesia-specific breakdown, the SO performance of amnesic subjects must be compared to that of *nonamnesic* subjects (Spanos, Bertrand & Perlini, 1988). Unfortunately, Wilson and Kihlstrom (1986) did not conduct these comparisons. They lumped together amnesic and nonamnesic subjects and compared the SO performance of high, medium, and low susceptibles across the three trials. Finding no significant interaction between *susceptibility* level and trials, they inappropriately concluded that there was no interaction between level of *amnesia* and trials. The relationship between degree of amnesia and hypnotic susceptibility is at best moderate, and sometimes quite low. Therefore, inferences about the differences between the performance of amnesics and nonamnesics cannot be validly drawn from comparisons across susceptibility levels. In short, Wilson and Kihlstrom's (1986) failure to divide their sample into amnesics and nonamnesics makes the results of their study uninterpretable.

Seriation. Radtke, et al., (1983) failed to find an amnesia-specific breakdown in seriation in three separate experiments. However, as in the case of the SO experiments, not finding breakdown may have been related to subjects' low initial levels of seriation. Two studies (Kihlstrom & Wilson, 1984; Spanos, McLean & Bertrand, 1987) used a word list procedure that created very high levels of initial (presuggestion) seriation. Both studies reported an amnesia-specific breakdown in seriation. In addition, Spanos, McLean et al. (1987) found that amnesic subjects who had attained very high, initial levels of seriation exhibited a significantly larger seriation breakdown than amnesic subjects who had attained relatively low, initial levels of seriation. In summary, studies of SO and seriation suggest (1) that an amnesia-specific breakdown in organization is not an invariant (or even usual) accompaniment of hypnotic amnesia, and (2) a breakdown is only likely to occur when subjects show high levels of organization before the amnesia suggestion is administered.

Clustering. Clustering in free recall refers to the number of times two words from the same category (e.g., metals, birds, flowers, etc.) are recalled together. The subject's task is to learn a list of words composed of several categories while hypnotized. Posthypnotic amnesia is suggested for the list then recall is tested under posthypnotic amnesia. In 1978, I pointed out that this paradigm also faces the problem of completely eliminating amnesic subjects from inspection because subjects who report nothing, or few words, cannot be included in the computations. Even so, the findings of the studies that had evaluated clustering were inconsistent. Spanos and Bodorik (1977) found less clustering, i.e., disrupted retrieval, under posthypnotic amnesia. But Coe, Taul, and Basden and Basden (1973) did not. Kihlstrom (1978) suggested that the Coe, et al. subjects may not have learned the words well enough to begin with (35 word list, 3 trials), therefore, floor effects may have prevented them from showing disruption.

Given the apparent design problems and contradictory findings, I concluded in 1978 that disorganization in clustering need not be considered a characteristic of posthypnotic amnesia until it was well documented.

A series of studies since then have consistently found an amnesia-specific, disorganization effect. That is, amnesic subjects have shown significantly less clustering on the amnesia suggestion trial than on the trials before or after the suggestion, while nonamnesics have shown the same high levels of clustering across the three recalls (Perlini, Bertrand, and Spanos, 1988; Ham, Radtke & Spanos, 1981; Radtke-Bodorik, Planas & Spanos, 1979; Spanos & D'Eon, 1980; Spanos, Radtke-Bodorik & Stam, 1980; Spanos, Stam, D'Eon, Pawlak & Radtke-Bodorik, 1980).

However, most of the above studies used short, categorized word lists (9 items). Wilson and Kihlstrom (1986) used a 16-item list (4 words in each of 4 categories) and did not find an amnesia-specific, disorganization breakdown. Wilson and Kihlstrom (1986) concluded that the disorganization effect may only occur when the word lists are short.

In response, Perlini, Bertrand and Spanos (1988) claim that Wilson and Kihlstrom (1986) again failed to test appropriately for amnesia-specific, disorganization. As in their SO study, they compared high-, medium-, and low-susceptible subjects rather than amnesic and nonamnesic subjects. To clarify the Wilson and Kihlstrom (1986) findings, Spanos, Perlini et al. (1988) replicated the study's procedure of administering an amnesia suggestion to high- and medium-susceptible subjects who had learned a 16-item categorized list. However, before analyzing their data, they divided subjects into amnesics and nonamnesics. Contrary to Wilson and Kihlstrom's (1986) conclusions, by testing across amnesic categories rather than susceptibility levels, a significant disorganization effect was found for the amnesics, but not for the nonamnesics.

Two other studies have also found amnesia-specific disorganization effects on categorized lists of more than 9 items. Ham et al. (1981) used a 12-word, categorized list and Wagstaff and Carroll (1987) used a 20-word, categorized list. A disorganization in clustering therefore appears to be reliably associated with hypnotic amnesia for both short and longer word lists. Nevertheless, it is important to point out that wide individual differences have been found on amnesia and disorganized clustering. Several studies (Spanos & D'Eon, 1980; Spanos, Radtke-Bodorik, & Shabinsky, 1980; Spanos, Stam et al., 1980) have found that only about *half* of the amnesic subjects show disorganized clustering, the remaining amnesics cluster to a high degree. The meaning of such observations are not clear. One hypothesis would be that subjects employ individuated methods for achieving the same goals.

Processes in Disrupted Retrieval? Spanos (1986b) concluded that disrupted retrieval can best be viewed as the result of response strategies. Spanos and D'Eon (1980) showed that when both high- and low- susceptible subjects were instructed to write backward by threes instead of given an amnesia suggestion, both showed reduced recall and equal levels of disorganization in clustering. The same finding occurred when both high and low susceptibles were instructed to distract themselves during recall. Similarly, in Tkachyk, et al. (1985) and in Spanos, McLean, and Bertrand (1987) the same pattern was found for both SO and seriation; i.e., distracted subjects, who exhibited partial recall, behaved in the same way as partial amnesics. Spanos (1986b) concluded that the results did not support "the notion that disorganized recall is hypnosis-specific, a defining characteristic of hypnotic amnesia, or a reflection of dissociative capacities possessed only by high suggestibles" (p. 456). He favored an "inattention hypothesis" in explaining disorganized recall.

Wagstaff (1981a, 1981b, 1981c, 1982) also favors a social psychological interpretation of disorganized recall, but one that emphasizes "compliance" rather than "inattention." His arguments are based on the behavior of simulating subjects who are given instructions to pretend to forget some of the words. Wagstaff (1982) criticized the Spanos, Radtke-Bodorik and Stam study (1980) where simulators so instructed failed to show disorganization. He pointed out that only nine subjects had been tested, but even though nonsignificant, the results were clearly in the direction of disorganization. Wagstaff (1981c) found a significant disorganization effect when he examined 22 subjects, and concluded that "compliance as an artifact in the disorganization effect is not so easily dismissed" (Wagstaff, 1982, p. 42).

Wilson and Kihlstrom (1986) continue to interpret disorganized retrieval in terms of memory concepts. They claimed that "when words are organized by category clustering, posthypnotic amnesia tends to be an all-or-none affair" (p. 271). Combined with their conclusion that category clustering is at most only weakly disrupted when long lists are used, they conclude that the findings "are consistent with current models of category clustering in free recall" (references cited, p. 271). They treat subjective organization (SO) (also, according to them, not disrupted in posthypnotic amnesia) as analogous to clustering, even though they admit that there are no formal models available for SO.

Based on their 1984 study, Wilson and Kihlstrom also view serial organization as being "clearly disrupted in posthypnotic amnesia" (p. 372). Such a conclusion, however, clearly appears to be an overstatement. It is accurate that serial organization showed disruption in their 1984 study, but the results of the other studies reported above have not been at all clear. However, to buttress their position, they again offer speculative theories of memory that take the position that serial organization can be separated qualitatively from SO and category clustering. In conclusion: "If these speculations are correct, it would seem that the process underlying posthypnotic amnesia appears to affect selectively the temporal organization of events in memory" (Wilson & Kihlstrom, 1986, p. 272).

In my opinion, Wilson and Kihlstrom's (1986) position is an attempt to force the observations into a form that might make sense from the limited view of memory theory. However, because they choose not to consider concepts for dealing with situational factors, they are at a loss to explain events that do not conform with the "laws of memory."

Wilson and Kihlstrom (1986) also ignored Bertrand and Spanos's (1985) study where three samples of subjects were given different suggestions for selective amnesia on a three-category, three-words-per-category list: (1) forget the entire list (nine words), (2) forget the words in one category, and (3) forget one word from each category. The second two instructions encourage recall by clusters strategies, while the first instruction, the usual posthypnotic suggestion, encourages a disorganization recall strategy. The results supported the expectations. Of the partially amnesics, the first sample showed disorganization whereas the other two did not. What sort of "memory process" explains those results? What might be found if the same instructions were given for a thirty-five word list, seven categories, five words per category? The subject's task becomes a much more difficult one, with more to weed out and more to recall. A broader perspective than memory processes is needed to evaluate such a study meaningfully.

Finally, a major problem remains in that subjects who are characteristically judged to be amnesic cannot be included in studies of recall organization. By studying only partial recallers, we may have learned nothing about the most amnesic subjects, and they are really the ones of interest for studying the processes of posthypnotic amnesia.

Breaching Posthypnotic Amnesia

Breaching amnesia addresses the question whether subjects who initially respond to posthypnotic amnesia will report more before the reversal cue, when external pressures to recall are placed on them. If amnesia cannot be breached, subjects presumably have no control over remembering, which would support the view of posthypnotic amnesia as a "happening" (or a special process).

In 1978, I evaluated two studies that had claimed to demonstrate that posthypnotic amnesia cannot be breached (Bowers, 1966; Kihlstrom, Evans, Orne & Orne, 1980). They will be reviewed briefly along with my earlier conclusions.

Bowers (1966) designed a rather elaborate study to deceive subjects into believing that the experiment had ended before amnesia was removed. All subjects were high susceptibles. Half were hypnotized when given the posthypnotic amnesia suggestion. Half were read the same suggestion while awake, then asked to pretend that they had been hypnotized when they heard it. All showed high responsiveness to the suggestion with a second experimenter. Bowers then asked them to see a third person who needed subjects for pilot data, but he did not give the cue removing amnesia. He said, "And listen, since we're all finished here, *I want you to be completely honest with him, regardless of what I've said before.*" (p. 45, italics his). The responses to the third experimenter's questions showed that all of the simulators and 43 percent of the reals were aware of the amnesia suggestion. Also, all simulators, but only 14 percent of the reals, rated amnesia as voluntary.

Bowers interpreted the results as support for posthypnotic amnesia as a happening, i.e., a demand for honesty did not breach amnesia. I qualified his interpretation by pointing out that almost half of the real subjects reported being aware of their "amnesic" response (even though only a small percentage claimed that it was voluntary). I further criticized his procedures on the ground that the demands on simulators to "confess" were much stronger than the demands on the reals.

My evaluation of the Kihlstrom et al. (1980) study raised the issue of the differential strengths that various situational circumstances hold for breaching amnesia. Their design tested four groups. Following the administration of the Harvard Group Scale of Hypnotic Susceptiblity (HGS) (Shor & Orne, 1962), all subjects were tested for posthypnotic amnesia (three minutes to write down everything that they remembered), then different instructions were given to each group: (1) *retest*, asked to recall again, (2) *cue*, list the items in chronological order, (3) *challenge*, overcome amnesia by exerting more effort to recall, and (4) *honesty*, cautioned not to fail to report voluntarily what they actually remembered. Amnesia was tested a second time, was then lifted on cue, and then followed by a final recall.

The initially amnesic subjects in all four samples did not differ from each other on recalls 2 or 3. Because the three "breaching" groups did not recall more than the "retest" group at recall 2, the results were interpreted as evidence that posthypnotic amnesia was not breached. However, my examination of the data made it clear that about 50 percent of the subjects in *all four* samples breached. That is, each of the instructions led about half of the initially amnesic subjects to recall significantly more. Thus, the results could have as easily been interpreted as showing that *all four* instructions had a considerable effect on breaching amnesia. Kihlstrom (1978) did not agree. He offered the alternative hypothesis that posthypnotic amnesia, "at least in inexperienced subjects, remits with time regardless of demands" (p. 258). His hypothesis is evaluated later.

I concluded that the potency of the situational demands for breaching was an important variable. Kihlstrom (1978) agreed, but also argued that until someone obtained positive evidence with stronger demands, posthypnotic amnesia remained robust in the face of demands for extra effort to recall and for honesty in reporting.

Since my review, a number of studies have addressed the question of breaching.

Strength of Demands. We have evaluated the effects of stronger breaching demands and also the interaction of breaching with subjects' ratings of their control over remembering (Coe & Yashinski, 1985; Howard & Coe, 1980; Schuyler & Coe, 1981, 1987; Sluis & Coe, 1987). In the first four studies, we introduced "honesty demands" and "lie detector demands" after the initial testing for amnesia. In the "honesty" condition subjects were told that they should be completely honest and report *everything* that they could remember. In the "lie detector" condition they were told that the physiological apparatus to which they were attached acted like a lie detector; in some cases they were told nothing more, and in some cases they were told that it indicated they were *not* telling all they knew. Controls who were only asked to recall again were also included. In general, each breaching condition, compared to the control condition, created significantly more breaching. No one breaching manipulation was especially more effective than the others. However, breaching was not complete in the breaching samples, and it interacted with subjects' ratings of their control over remembering. That is, those who rated themselves as being in control of remembering (voluntaries) were more likely to breach, even in the control condition, than were those who rated themselves as not in control of remembering (involuntaries). Compared to the Kihlstrom et al. (1980) results, our breaching subjects recalled more at the second recall than our controls. Thus, we supported the hypothesis that stronger demands created more breaching, but there was still a considerable number of the initially amnesic who did not breach—about 50 percent, mostly "involuntaries."

Our most recent study considerably increased the demands for breaching (Sluis & Coe, 1987). As in the earlier studies, we preselected only highly susceptible subjects who had demonstrated amnesia on the HGS (Shor & Orne, 1962). Approximately half were categorized as "voluntaries" and half as "involuntaries" on the basis of their control ratings from the HGS amnesia response. They were then administered the individual Stanford Hypnotic Susceptibility Scale, Form C (SHSS:C Weitzenhoffer & Hilgard, 1962) with the usual posthypnotic amnesia item. After testing amnesia and obtaining another control rating, subjects were assigned to a breaching condition or a control condition (half voluntaries and half involuntaries, based on their HGS ratings). Breaching consisted of three manipulations over approximately fifty minutes. First, "honesty" instructions were administered, followed by second recall and control rating. Next, subjects were told that the physiological equipment indicated they were not telling all they knew ("lie"), followed by a third recall and control rating. They were next shown a videotape replay of their hypnosis session, then asked if they could really recall anything else (see, McConkey et al., 1981, next topic). A fourth recall and control rating followed. Finally, the reversal cue for amnesia was given followed by a fifth recall.

The control sample sat quietly for the same amount of time. At the times matching the breaching subjects' critical recalls, they were only asked if they recalled anything else then, followed by the recall and control ratings. Amnesia was lifted in the same way as for the breaching sample.

All but one of nineteen breaching subjects breached *completely* before amnesia was lifted. About fifty percent, on the HGS, nearly all voluntaries breached completely in the control condition. The involuntaries in the control condition recalled significantly more items at reversibility than they did over the three preceding recalls. Thus, for subjects who had initially claimed control over remembering (voluntaries), amnesia appeared to dissipate over time, whether or not they were under pressure to breach. However, involuntaries not under pressure to breach remained amnesic, while their counterparts who were under pressure breached.

We (Coe & Tucibat, 1988) recently selected twenty-one subjects (half voluntaries, half involuntaries) who had scored 9 or higher and passed posthypnotic amnesia on the HGS and tested them following the individual SHSS:C under the first two breaching conditions of the Sluis and Coe study ("honesty" and "lie"). Sixteen of the twenty-one breached almost completely. Three of the five remaining subjects were "pseudoamnesics," recalling only one or two items over all four recalls. Only two subjects remained amnesic until the reversal cue. The HGS voluntary/involuntary designation was not related to breaching. In fact, all but three subjects rated their first recall on the SHSS:C as *involuntary*. As they recalled more items at breaching trials, their ratings changed in the voluntary direction.

Our results in general support the hypothesis that most amnesic subjects will breach under adequate pressure. They *do not* appear to be passive persons who experience some sort of special process that interferes with their memory abilities. As pressure is added for them to remember more, they do so, to the extent that they have nothing left to remember when amnesia is lifted. Our results represent the "positive evidence" Kihlstrom (1978) requested that demonstrates that posthypnotic amnesia *does not* remain robust in the face of strong demands.

Recognition Testing. McConkey, Sheehan, and Cross (1980) and McConkey and Sheehan (1981) used a video replay of the hypnosis session to evaluate the extent to which subjects breach amnesia. They call their approach the "Experiential Analysis Technique" (EAT) (Sheehan, McConkey & Cross, 1978). Subjects are instructed to stop the tape at any time should they wish to comment on their experiences. It was believed that the playback acted as a "variant of recognition testing" for amnesic subjects and that showing the playback of the hypnosis session before amnesia was lifted would place on subjects the "most stringent demands" to breach.

The 1981 study was designed to replicate and extend the findings of the 1980 study where almost half of the subjects maintained amnesia (over half breached). Both simulators (low susceptibles) and reals (high susceptibles) were tested (Orne, 1969). The simulator were "assumed to provide an index of whether the differentiation of behavioral and experiential memories may be explained on the basis of cue demands" (p. 47). Subjects were first seen by an experimenter who gave them instructions, a second experimenter (hypnotist) administered the hypnosis session including posthypnotic amnesia for it, and a third experimenter administered the EAT, telling subjects that the video would help them to remember. They were instructed to stop the tape and describe their experience whenever they remembered anything. After the viewing, the hypnotist returned, administered a second recall test, then cancelled amnesia.

The results were reported separately for the subjects' recall of behaviors and for their subjective reports about their recall. Real subjects were classified as amnesic or not based upon the number of items they recalled before viewing the tape (two or fewer items versus more than two items). Viewing the tape did not erase the differences between the initially amnesic and initially nonamnesic. However, objective data for breaching were evident. Of the initially amnesic, 62.5 percent recalled more than two items after viewing (breached?)? The initially amnesic (1) gained a mean of 2.94 items after the viewing; (2) showed a similar mean recall level after viewing (5.40 items) as the initially nonamnesics had before the viewing (5.25 items); and (3) did not differ from the nonamnesics on the number of times they stopped the tape—the measure of recognition memory. The last finding could be interpreted as showing that the initially amnesic subjects breached completely on recognition memory.

The subjective reports during viewing suggested that the three types of subjects differed somewhat. Amnesics generally expressed an inability, or difficulty, in recalling the events being viewed. The nonamnesics commented more openly on their hypnotic experiences, and simulators generally indicated that they really could not remember, attributing their recall to viewing the tape. Simulators performed the same as initially amnesic subjects on the behavioral measures, showing the presence of demands for not recalling, but they did not stop the tape (recognition memory) as often as either the amnesics or the nonamnesics, suggesting that the real subjects were not responding to demands that called for not stopping the tape.

However, the differences between "simulators" and "reals" in their frequency of stopping the tape cannot be readily taken as indicating a special characteristic of hypnosis. The demands on simulators of being exposed if they are suspected as fakers are quite different from the demand on real subjects who are told to experience whatever happens. It is therefore not very surprising that simulators acted as they did when viewing the tape. They were cautious not to stop the tape too often, or to comment very freely when they did stop it. Real subjects had little reason not to show what they experienced.

In sum, the video-cued recall manipulation is a fairly strong one insofar as it breaches amnesia. The McConkey and Sheehan (1981) results showed little evidence that the majority of initially amnesic subjects *cannot* remember. In fact, if stopping the video replay is taken as a valid measure of recognition memory, it must be concluded that nearly all subjects fail to maintain posthypnotic amnesia under recognition testing.

Amnesia During Hypnosis. Three studies have investigated breaching amnesia during hypnosis: Spanos, Radtke, and Bertrand (1984); Silva and Kirsch (1987); and Radtke, Thompson, and Egger (1987).

Spanos and Radtke (1982) hypothesized that good subjects do not breach amnesia because it strengthens their self-presentation as someone who is unable to remember and, therefore, someone who is deeply hypnotized. Spanos, Radtke, and Bertrand (1984) tested the hypothesis on eight very susceptible subjects who had consistently described their responses to suggestions as involuntary, and who had repeatedly failed to breach amnesia despite exhortations to be honest. They were hypnotized and told during hypnosis that their minds possessed two "hidden parts" that could be contacted by a cue. One "part" remained aware of everything in their left hemisphere, while the other remained aware of everything in their right hemisphere. Half had been told before learning that their right hemisphere stored concrete words and their left hemisphere stored abstract words; the other half had been told the opposite. They were also told that their hidden parts would know these things even though they could not consciously remember them. Subjects then learned a list of abstract and concrete words and later demonstrated high levels of suggested amnesia for them. However, before cancelling amnesia, the experimenter contracted the subjects' hidden parts and tested recall. All subjects recalled all of their right hemisphere words but none of their left when the right hidden part was contacted, and vice versa. That is, all subjects breached amnesia completely in a context where breaching supported a self-presentation of being deeply hypnotized. Spanos (1986b) concluded that even subjects who are very highly hypnotizable and amnesic retain voluntary control over their behavior: "it is inaccurate to describe these subjects as unable to remember" (p. 452).

Silva and Kirsch (1987) took a somewhat different approach from Spanos et al. (1984), but for similar reasons. Like Spanos, Silva and Kirsch view good subjects as striving to present themselves as deeply hypnotized, and the researchers postulated that their subjects' expectations for reinforcement largely determine the way the subjects will respond. However, Silva and Kirsch criticized the Spanos et al. (1984) procedure of presenting the expectancy manipulation (hidden parts) during hypnosis. They argued that giving the instructions during hypnosis could lead to two alternative interpretations of the results. For one, it could be argued that the instructions temporarily created two dissociated cognitive subsystems, as Hilgard's neodissociation theory might claim (Hilgard, 1974, 1977a, 1977b). Two, and more parsimoniously, the instructions could be interpreted as hypnotic suggestions and responded to for the same reasons that subjects respond to other hypnotic suggestions.

Silva and Kirsch (1987) preselected subjects for high susceptibility and post-hypnotic amnesia. Before being individually hypnotized, all were told that while they were hypnotized, they would be given an amnesia suggestion for a list of words. The subjects would be tested for remembering the word list, then be put into a "very deep hypnotic state." Half were told that they would be able to remember even less in a deep state ("reduced"), and half were told that they would be able to remember even more in a deep state ("enhanced"). They learned a six-word list to two perfect recalls and then were hypnotized. Subjects were (1) tested for continued knowledge of the list, (2) given amnesia suggestion for the list, (3) tested for amnesia for the list, (4) given a procedure for deepening hypnosis, (5) again tested for memory of the list, (6) then had the amnesia suggestion cancelled, and (7) tested again for memory before they were brought out of hypnosis.

The results were almost 100 percent as predicted. Subjects in the two samples were equivalent when tested for learning, for amnesia, and after amnesia was removed. But, they were almost completely opposite when tested after deepening hypnosis. Eight of the ten "enhancement" subjects breached amnesia completely, recalling all six items, and eight of the ten "reduced" subjects remained completely amnesic.

Radtke, Thompson, and Egger (1987) used retrieval cues to breach amnesia during hypnosis. They employed a difficult learning task (forty-eight items: twelve categories, four items per category, one presentation) and forced recall (guessing) of all forty-eight items. All subjects were hypnotized, asked to learn the list, then tested on free recall, with instructions to draw a line under the last item they remembered, and then to fill in any of the remaining forty-eight spaces with guesses. One sample then received an amnesia suggestion while a comparison sample received only relaxation suggestions. A second forced, free recall trial was administered. Subjects were then given different answer sheets that contained the twelve category names with four lines below each, told to fill in all of the lines, and to place an "X" by any word that was a guess. A third recall was administered, after which the amnesia suggestion was removed from the amnesia sample (more relaxation for the comparison sample) and all were asked to recall again using the same procedure as the third recall.

Radtke et al. interpreted the results as showing complete breaching in amnesic subjects. Amnesics and nonamnesics, including controls, only differed on level of recall when amnesia was tested (recall 2). When force tested with retrieval cues, the amnesics increased their recall to the level of the nonamnesics and controls and did not gain more when tested after amnesia was lifted. The results were interpreted as support for a strategic enactment view of hypnotic amnesia. That is, subjects can avoid using retrieval cues in free recall by disattending to them, but when the cues are clearly present, as in recalls 3 and 4, it is difficult for subjects to use amnesia-producing cognitive strategies.

Taken together, the first two studies demonstrate the strong effects that instructions can have on breaching amnesia. All, or nearly all, high susceptible amnesic subjects breached under conditions meant to change their expectations about how deeply hypnotized subjects respond. The third study demonstrated the strong interfering effects that retrieval cues can have on maintaining hypnotic amnesia.

Spontaneous Recovery (Dissipation Hypothesis). Several studies have shown that some amnesic subjects who are not pressured to recall more, but are given two successive attempts to recall before amnesia is removed, recall more on the second trial (Ham, Radtke & Spanos, 1981; Kihlstrom, Easton & Shor, 1983; Kihlstrom et al., 1980; Sluis & Coe, 1987). Kihlstrom et al. (1980) hypothesized that amnesia tends to "wear away" naturally with time. Presumably, the postulated "amnesic barriers" wear down and the "dissociated" memories are allowed access to awareness.

Bertrand et al. (1983) and Spanos, Tkachyk, Bertrand, and Weekes (1984) tested the dissipation hypothesis. They gave amnesic and partially amnesic subjects a second recall after the challenge trial but varied the time interval between the initial recall and the second recall. In the Bertrand et al. (1983) study, the second recall was administered either 60 seconds or 120 seconds after the challenge (recall 1). In the Spanos et al. (1984) study, the second recall was administered immediately or 15 minutes after the first recall. In both studies, recall increased at the second recall, but the time between the two recalls made no difference. Thus, simply asking subjects to recall again is apparently the important variable in the dissipation of amnesia, not the passage of time.

Dubreuil et al. (1983) hypothesized that people expect to recall more on a second trial and that this expectation may be important with posthypnotic amnesia. Three samples were used to test the hypothesis. One was informed that people usually remember *more* on a second trial. A second sample was told that people usually recall *less* on a second trial, and the third sample was told nothing. The results supported their hypothesis. The samples recalled in descending order: "remember more" subjects, "no instruction" subjects, and "recall less" subjects.

Our series of studies on breaching (see above: Coe & Yashinski, 1985; Howard & Coe, 1980; Schuyler & Coe, 1984, 1987; Sluis & Coe, 1987) may shed some light on the issue of spontaneous recovery over time. In the first four studies, only one breaching recall was given after the challenge recall. Controls who were only asked to recall again (no breaching pressure) did not uniformly show increased recall at recall two. Generally, across the studies, subjects who had rated their first recall attempt as "mostly not in their control" (involuntaries) were not likely to recall more at the second recall. But, subjects who had rated their first recall as "mostly in their control" (voluntaries) were likely to recall more at recall two. In the Sluis and Coe (1987) study, control subjects were given three recalls after the challenge trial and before amnesia was removed. The voluntrary controls (no breaching pressures) recalled more items at each recall, and at a level equal to the voluntary or involuntary subjects in the breaching conditions. However, the involuntary controls did not increase their recall significantly until amnesia was lifted, even over about 45 mintues and three recall requests.

Thus, it may be accurate to say that without added pressures to breach, the amnesia of about half of the subjects who are initially amnesic dissipates over *recalls*. It remains to be tested, however, whether time alone is also an important factor. If time is important, then subjects given three post-challenge recalls over 45 minutes, would not show greater recall than subjects given only one post-challenge recall at the end of 45 minutes.

Taken together, our studies have suggested that, even with additional post-challenge recall requests, amnesia may be maintained for at least 45 minutes in subjects who view their amnesia as mostly out of their control. However, the fact that their involuntary counterparts who were under strong breaching pressures did not maintain amnesia qualifies the observation. They should not be viewed as having no control over remembering, because of inner cognitive workings like amnesic barriers or dissociated subsystems. When pressures to recall are added, they will be able to recall. Nevertheless, a subject's report of control-over-remembering may be an important variable to consider in future research on the spontaneous recovery of amnesia.

Enhancing Posthypnotic Amnesia

If hypnotic responding, and therefore posthypnotic amnesia, is primarily the result of a high dissociative capacity, as special process accounts predict, then highly responsive hypnotic subjects should be much more likely to experience posthypnotic amnesia than low responsive subjects (e.g., Hilgard, 1977a; Kihlstrom 1978, 1983). On the other hand, the response-strategy view predicts that the ambiguous and the conflicting demands in posthypnotic amnesia suggestions lead subjects to interpret and respond to them differentially. If so, Spanos (1986b) suggested that clarifying such demands "should substantially influence the amount of amnesia displayed by subjects" (p. 451).

Spanos and his colleagues conducted three experiments testing their hypothesis. Spanos, Stam, et al. (1980), using subjects unselected for susceptibility, explicitly instructed half of them to interpret the amnesia suggestion as a request to direct their attention away from the target items, even when challenged to recall. The other half were not told how to interpret the suggestion. Over 75 percent of the informed subjects, compared with 36 percent of the uninformed subjects, showed at least some amnesia.

Spanos, de Groh, and de Groot (1987) showed that low susceptibles who were trained on how to interpret the ambiguous aspects of test suggestions were significantly more amnesic than either lows or highs who were not trained. Also, trained subjects were as likely as untrained highs to describe their experience as involuntary.

Spanos and de Groh (1984) gave hypnotized high- and low-susceptible subjects two successive amnesia suggestions for a word list composed of three taxonomic categories, e.g., birds, flowers, etc. One suggestion said that they would be unable to attend to, or recall, any of the words. The other said that they would be unable to attend to, or recall, the words from one category, but that they would be able to recall the word from the other two categories. Thus, both inattention and automaticity of responding were suggested in both instructions. High-susceptibles showed more amnesia than lows on both suggestions. However, both highs and lows who were given explicit instructions without hypnosis on how to direct their attention away from target items in order to meet the demands for forgetting showed as much amnesia on both tasks as had the hypnotic highs, and more amnesia than the hypnotic lows. Clarifying the task as one that required a strategy, rather than a happening, created equal responsiveness for lows as for highs who were, or were not, hypnotized.

The above studies suggest that task ambiguity is an important factor in posthypnotic amnesia. Amnesia in low-susceptibles can be enhanced substantially when ambiguity is reduced, and the resulting experience is interpreted as involuntary. Spanos (1986b) views the findings as "consistent with the hypothesis that amnesia reflects response strategies" (p. 451).

Computer Analogies of Memory and
Posthypnotic Amnesia

Current theorizing in cognitive psychology has employed the computer analogy to study memory. Two areas of research have lapped over into the study of posthypnotic amnesia, information processing, and directed forgetting.

Information Processing. Heusmann, Gruder, and Dorst (1987) tested an information-processing model of posthypnotic amnesia. Because the amnesia suggestion occurs after learning and the cue releasing the amnesia almost entirely reverses it, posthypnotic amnesia cannot be the result of changes in encoding, organization, storage, a permanent structural change, or an ablation of the material. The to-be-forgotten (TBF) material is clearly available, though perhaps *not* accessible (Tulving & Pearlstone, 1966).

Heusmann et al. (1987) recognized the important finding that "the to-be-remembered items, which subjects report not being able to recall, still remain active in the cognitive system" (p. 36). As noted earlier, hypnosis investigators have called such findings the "paradox" of posthypnotic amnesia.

Huesmann et al. (1987) interpreted current theories of posthypnotic amnesia in terms of how closely they postulate the mechanism of amnesia to be from the point of final output. For instance, the postulated mechanism is farthest from output in Hilgard's *neodissociation theory* (Hilgard, 1976, 1977a). According to Hilgard (1977), various cognitive components become separated from one another such that they function with relative autonomy. That is, executive control of retrieval routines are turned over to the hypnotist. The TBF material is held in an area of storage that is unavailable to direct awareness. However, the material is still available to other memory functions, accounting for the paradoxical characteristics of posthypnotic amnesia.

Next farthest from output is Evan and Kihlstrom's theory of *disrupted search* in posthypnotic amnesia (Evans & Kihlstrom, 1973; Kihlstrom, 1977; Kihlstrom & Evans, 1976, 1979). They hypothesized that the search function is disrupted, or blocked, by the executive program when subjects try to recall the forbidden (TBF) material. The cue lifting amnesia frees the search function and the material is then recalled.

Huesmann et al. interpreted Spanos' early position as a *distracted attention* theory (Spanos, 1986b; Spanos-Radtke-Bodorik & Stam, 1980). Subjects' working memory and attention are directed away from the TBF material and directed instead toward material not associated with cues that might activate the TBF material. With the "lifting" cue, subjects direct their attention and working memory to the material.

Spanos, however, has more recently focused on his "strategic enactment" theory, which is an *output inhibition* position similar to other positions placing the "forgetting" mechanism closest to output (Coe, 1978, 1980; Sarbin & Coe, 1979, Spanos, 1986b). The TBF material is searched for and retrieved into working memory where it is processed as forbidden or not-forbidden. If labelled "forbidden" it is denied output and perhaps also access into awareness. The reversal cue then allows access and the material is recalled.

Huesmann et al. (1987) favored the output inhibition model because it avoided the knotty problem of explaining how forbidden material can be selectively denied retrieval. To decide not to process material, requires processing that material to some extent. The output inhibition model, on the other hand, allows the information to enter working memory where it is *then* denied output. Is the subject aware of such information? The evidence from postexperimental reports is that some subjects are aware but simply do not output it. Many others, however, appear not to be aware of having retrieved it. Furthermore, other subjects who are aware of the material report that, they could not say it no matter how hard they tried (Coe, 1978; Kihlstrom et al., 1980; Spanos, Radtke-Bodorik & Stam, 1980).

Huesmann et al. (1987) conducted two experiments to test more definitively the output inhibition theory of psthypnotic amnesia. They employed tasks that they believed would require the TBF material to enter working memory, but not necessarily awareness. The tasks were presented as examples of "active" processes. That is, the material is "used generatively," rather than passively as it is in retroactive and proactive interference.

Luchin's (1942) water jar problems were used in the first experiment. Two hypnotic groups and two unhypnotized control groups were examined. The hypnotic subjects were hypnotized then given "practice" problems where a problem-solving set was created. They were then given a posthypnotic amnesia suggestion for the problem solving. One group had the amnesia suggestion lifted (hypnotic-release group) before the "test" problems were administered; the other group was left amnesic. One control group was given the same problem-solving set without hypnosis. The other controls had no previous learning experience.

All groups were then given four test problems. The first two problems and the fourth problem could be solved by either the "set" solution or a shorter solution. The third problem could only be solved by the shorter (nonset) solution. The ways the groups solved the problems were then compared.

According to Huesmann et al., the results supported the output-inhibition theory. The "no set" controls used only the shorter nonset solution on all four problems. The "set" controls used the set solution completely on the first two problems, changed to the short solution on problem three, then almost half reverted back to the "set" solution for problem four. The amnesic subjects responded almost identically, indicating that they had actively retrieved the "set" solution. The amnesia-release subjects performed the same as the amnesic subjects, but they did not show amnesia for having learned the set solutions.

Huesmann et al. conducted a second study to test between two hypotheses about how TBF "tags" can be utilized at retrieval time. In one assumption individual items are tagged as forbidden in episodic memory. The tag would be detected during retrieval and the item would not be allowed access into working memory. The competing hypothesis was that large semantic structures are tagged and forbidden in episodic memory. Tags are not attached to items during search and they are therefore retrieved into working memory. Items are then tagged as forbidden, if appropriate, and output is suppressed.

Five groups of hypnotized subjects listened to one of three stories. Two of the stories used the same words but in different contexts, e.g., "bat" was introduced in one story about a visit to a baseball game, and in another story about the exploration of a cave; the word "diamond" was similarly treated. The third story contained no critical words.

Two groups heard the 'baseball' story and two groups heard the 'cave' story. Posthypnotic amnesia was suggested to all four groups, but it was lifted for one group of each story before a word associate task was administered. The fifth group heard a neutral story and remained amnesic for it during the critical task. The experimental task was to generate three close associates to ten critical homographs.

The results showed high levels of word associates in the expected direction for the baseball and cave stories while the associations of the neutral subjects were not biased. There were no differences between the still amnesic subjects and those whose amnesia had been lifted. That is, amnesia did not inhibit the output of forbidden items in another context (associations versus direct recall). Huesmann et al. (1987) concluded as follows:

> The subject attempts to associate "forbidden" tags with the material in memory. Such tags may be associated with individual items in episodic memory or with sets of items connected in lists or semantic structures. However, tagging will be imperfect both because of imperfect interpretation of the hypnotist's instructions and difficulties in interpreting the tags. When memory access is attempted during the posthypnotic period, activation of memory, search and retrieval into working memory proceeds unhampered. Therefore, the forbidden material may be employed actively by the information-processing system, may influence new learning, and may reveal itself indirectly through its effect on behavior. However, forbidden material cannot be explicitly reported, because it is tagged as forbidden and the output routines check for such tags. Unless the tag was not inserted or is not detected or obeyed at output time, the forbidden material will not be reported. (p. 54)

In sum, the Huesmann et al. (1987) results support an output inhibition accounting of posthypnotic amnesia.

Directed Forgetting (DF). In directed forgetting, subjects are told to learn one set of materials and led to believe they are not required to remember another set, even though they have learned it. For example, one list is learned, then subjects are told it was for practice and they can now forget it. Another list is learned and then subjects are asked to recall *both* lists. Cues can also be given for individual items, telling subjects to "forget" or "remember" after each item.

Because the "remember" (R) items were recalled at higher levels than the "forget" (F) items, the early work on DF focused on analyzing the role of diferential rehearsal (e.g., Bjork, 1972; Bjork & Geiselman, 1978). However, a shift of interest to disrupted retrieval occurred after Geiselman, Bjork, and Fishman (1983) evaluated the effects of DF instructions on words that subjects had no reason to rehearse.

Subjects were instructed to "judge" the pleasantness of some words and to "learn" others. Both types of words were presented before and after the "forget" instruction. They reasoned that the "judge" words would not be rehearsed, and therefore, any DF effects that could be attributed to differential rehearsal should be eliminated. The results showed that both "judge" and "learn" words were affected in the same way in regard to the forget cue. That is, words of either class that followed the forget instruction were recalled at a higher level than were words of that class that preceded the forget instruction.

The "learn" words were still recalled at a higher level than the "judge" words in either half of the list, indicating more rehearsal for the "learn" words, as assumed. However, because differential rehearsal presumably could not account for the recall pattern of "judge" words, disrupted retrieval processes were postulated. As was discussed earlier, disrupted retrieval mechanisms have also been postulated in accounting for posthypnotic amnesia (Kihlstrom & Evans, 1979; Coe, 1978). Geiselman and his colleagues therefore postulated that the process of retrieval inhibition might underlie both DF and posthypnotic amnesia, or PHA (Geiselman & Bagheir, 1985; Geiselman & Panting, 1985; Geiselman, Rabow, et al., 1985; Geiselman, Bjork & Fishman, 1983; Geiselman, MacKinnon, Fishman, Jaenicke, Larner, Schoenberg & Swartz, 1983).[7] Kihlstrom (1983), while tentatively agreeing, indicated that final acceptance of the similarities "awaits comparisons of the two types of instructed forgetting within a common experimental paradigm" (p. 73).

Posthypnotic amnesia and DF had not been examined in the same paradigm until a recent study by Coe, Basden, Basden, et al. (1988). However, Geiselman, MacKinnon, et al. (1983) came close. Subjects were hypnotized in a first session on the Harvard Group Scale of Hypnotic Susceptibility (HGS) (Shor & Orne, 1962), which included a posthypnotic amnesia suggestion. In a second session subjects were administered an item-by-item DF task, i.e., items were randomly assigned a "forget" or "remember" instruction and administered intermixed. Amnesia score and DF scores correlated significantly with F-item-recall level, but not R-item-recall. That is, the fewer amnesia items recalled before the releaser cue, the lower the level of F-item-recall, and, the greater the recall after the amnesia releaser cue, the greater the F-item-recall. The researchers concluded: "These findings indicate that the forgetting processes in both paradigms are related and the implication is that some of them are the same" (p. 633).

There appeared to be two problems with the study. First, since subjects were tested for hypnotic susceptibility before participating in a directed forgetting experiment, they might have attempted to respond as if amnesic in the DF condition. They may have interpreted the forget cue as an amnesia cue and inhibited their output, accounting for the positive correlation between amnesia score and F-item-recall. Second, it is difficult to equate the DF item-by-item cueing procedure with the posthypnotic amnesia procedure. The amnesia suggestion is given for the entire set of items, not individual items. It seems unlikely that the processes used to tag individual items as to-be-forgotten would be similar to those used for entire sets of items. Since the processing requirement of the tasks are dissimilar, similar responding could reflect a tendency to withhold responses on both tasks. If so, the common processes Geiselman, MacKinnon, et al. (1983) identified could have had more to do with demand effects than with memory processes.

Coe, Basden, Basden, et al. (1988) compared posthypnotic amnesia and DF in a midlist cueing task. That is, subjects were instructed to forget all of list one before learning list two. Hypnotic susceptibility was also manipulated in order to determine its effects, if any, on directed forgetting.

The DF procedure was as follows: Subjects were first given the task of learning a list of words, then told, "You can forget that list, it was only for practice." They then learned a different word list, after which they were asked to recall all of the words from *both* lists. Finally, to be consistent with the amnesia paradigm, the first recall was followed by the amnesia releaser cue ("You can remember the words from the first list") and a second recall trial.

Three studies were conducted, each included preselected highly susceptible hypnotic subjects who demonstrated posthypnotic amnesia and low susceptible hypnotic subjects who did not show amnesia. Two thirty-six-item word lists (six categories, six items per category), presented individually, at a rate of five seconds per word, were used as the learning material.

In the first study, high and low susceptibles were administered (1) DF instructions or (2) PHA instructions while hypnotized. After item ten of the SHSS:C, subjects—still hypnotized—were requested to learn a list of words (list 1). After its presentation they were given either the DF instruction ("Stop learning, the list is completed. Close your eyes again and relax. [Subject closes eyes.] This first list was just for practice. You can forget the words you have learned on that list.") or the amnesia instruction (Same as above until after the subject's eyes close, then, "You have learned the words on the first list, but you will not be able to remember any of those words until I tell you later that 'you can remember the words from the first list.' Even if I ask you to recall some of the words from the first list, the words will simply be gone from your memory. You will not be able to remember any of these words until I tell you later, 'you can remember the words from the first list.'").

For the remainder of the session, all subjects were treated the same. They were asked to learn another list with the same number of words but with different categories (list 2). After list 2 was presented, the awakening instructions for SHSS:C were administered and subjects were then asked to "recall all of the words that you have learned from both lists while you were hypnotized" (test 1). After completing recall 1, the posthypnotic cue for lifting amnesia was administered to *all subjects*. They were again asked to recall all the words that they could remember from both lists (test 2).

The results showed that low susceptible subjects responded as expected under posthypnotic amnesia, i.e., they were *not* amnesic. They recalled lists 1 and 2 equally well at test 1 and at test 2. They showed no significant increase across recalls (reversibility), and they recalled the TBF list (list 1) at test 1 at a marginally higher level than did the high-susceptible amnesics. The low-susceptible directed-forgetting subjects responded as expected. They recalled the TBR list (list 2) at a higher level than the TBF list (list 1) at test 1 and marginally higher at test 2. High-susceptible posthypnotic amnesia subjects recalled as expected, with marginally lower recall for list 1 than list 2 at test 1 (posthypnotic amnesia), and again in recall on list 1 after amnesia was lifted (reversibility). The high-susceptible DF subjects showed a pattern some place in between the results of the low-susceptible DF subjects and the high-susceptible PHA subjects. They responded similarly to both the low-susceptible DF subjects and the high-susceptible amnesic subjects in that at test 1 they recalled list 1 at a marginally lower level than list 2. At test 2 they also responded like both the low-susceptible DF subjects and the high-susceptible amnesic subjects, but for different reasons. Like the DF subjects, but unlike the amnesic subjects, they did *not* show a significant increase of the recall of list 1. Like the amnesic subjects, but unlike the DF subjects, they showed no significant difference at test 2 on the levels of recall for list 1 and list 2.[8]

Since susceptibility level interacted with type of instruction, the processes involved in directed forgetting did not appear to be the same as those involved in posthypnotic amnesia, at least not when the two were compared in the same paradigm. The results suggested that the effect of the PHA instruction was a temporary retrieval deficit, since list 1 was recalled at a higher level at recall 2 than at recall 1. On the other hand, when lows were given directed-forgetting instructions, the superiority of list 2 over list 1 recall was maintained on both trials. Further, the fact that list 1 recall was not lower in this condition than in the other two conditions suggests that the DF instruction altered (increased) storage of list 2 but had relatively little effect on the storage of list 1.

The highly susceptible subjects showed recall levels somewhere in between the usual posthypnotic-amnesia response and the usual DF response. This suggests that these subjects were unsure about whether or not to interpret the DF instructions as calling for posthypnotic amnesia, perhaps a compromise responding. Low susceptibles, on the other hand, had no investment in presenting themselves as hypnotized, and therefore responded to the DF instructions in the same way as they would have in a nonhypnotic context. Trying to understand the effects of context on high susceptibles in the DF paradigm led to our second study. We attempted to evaluate more closely the effects of expecting hypnosis on DF with high-susceptible subjects.

Being administered the DF task during hypnosis had an effect on high-susceptibles. The unhypnotized samples showed an enhanced recall effect for the TBR list while hypnotized subjects showed the same level of recall for both lists without the enhancement effect for the TBR list.

The question remained as to what accounted for differential responsiveness of subjects while hypnotized. Was it a characteristic of high-susceptibles (a trait), or was it the interaction of susceptibility level with the hypnotic context (relaxed, expectations, etc.)?

Our third study attempted to answer the foregoing question. We tested both high- and low-susceptibles on DF outside the context of hypnosis. If highs and lows differed, the trait hypothesis was supported. If they did not, the interaction hypothesis was supported.

We found that recall performance in the DF groups did not differ as a function of susceptibility level. Both the highs and lows demonstrated directed forgetting outside the hypnosis context. Since highs and lows did not respond differently to DF instruction outside the context of hypnosis, but did respond differently within the context, we concluded that high susceptibility alone did not produce the "confused" pattern of recall obtained in experiments 1 and 2.

Some of the highs and lows in this experiment were given neither amnesia nor DF instructions. The uninstructed highs did not differ significantly from uninstructed lows when tested during hypnosis. However, the uninstructed highs recalled list 2 better than list 1. Recall from the two lists was equal for the uninstructed lows, indicating that the difference in recall found for the highs was not a function of list order or other list characteristics. Higher recall of list 2 than of list 1 for uninstructed highs must have been a function of hypnotic context. Our hypothesis was that the high subjects were probably still engaged in fulfilling the demands of the hypnosis scale, relaxed, etc., and failed to store adequately the items from list 1.

The three experiments demonstrated that the mechanisms involved in posthypnotic amnesia and directed forgetting were not the same. The two types of instructions produced different patterns of recall for low-susceptible and high-susceptible subjects depending upon the context in which they were tested.

In conclusion, it does not appear that posthypnotic amnesia and DF can be accounted for in terms of the same memory processes. Nor does it appear that the effects of hypnosis on memory can be explained by information-processing models alone. The context of hypnosis interacts importantly with susceptibility and must be delineated before a viable accounting can be formulated.

Episodic/Semantic Dissociation Hypothesis

Special process theorists have long recognized that amnesic material is not functionally ablated from memory, as shown, for example, in studies of proactive and retroactive interference and other paradoxical findings (e.g., Coe, Basden, Basden & Graham, 1976; Dillon & Spanos, 1983; Huesmann et al., 1987). However, it was not until recently that a special process theorist attempted a theoretical accounting. Kihlstrom (1980) relied on Tulving's (1972) differentiation between the semantic and episodic components of memory. Episodic memories are associated with specific episodes of one's experience, e.g., a list you learned in an experiment, or the trip you took last summer. Semantic memories are free of context, facts one knows without recall of where or when they were learned, e.g., $4 \times 2 = 8$ or fish live in water.

According to Kihlstrom (1980), posthypnotic amnesia disrupts episodic but not semantic memory. For example, subjects learn two word lists while hypnotized and amnesia is suggested for one list. Subjects are subsequently unable to recall the specific list words, but their proactive or retroactive effects are still shown in the recall of the other list. Kihlstrom postulated that the forgotten list was stored in episodic memory. However, semantic memory still contains the associations of the words on both lists. Unlike episodic memory, semantic memory has not been dissociated by amnesia. Thus, interference effects occur because the semantic associates of the to-be-forgotten words were "primed" during learning, and there remains a "residual priming effect" that interferes with the recall of the nonamnesic words.

Kihlstrom (1980) tested his hypothesis by giving amnesic subjects both an episodic and a semantic memory task. Forgetting a previously learned word list was the episodic task. A word association test (WAT) was the semantic task; i.e., subjects were to free associate to words. The WAT words were chosen as common associates of the forgotten words, e.g., if "needle" was a forgotten word, "pin" was presented on the WAT. Subjects amnesic for the recall of the word list (episodic task) were not affected on the WAT (semantic task). They even responded with the "forgotten" words more often than controls who learned a different list, suggesting a "residual priming effect" for the forgotten list. After the WAT, another free recall showed that the subjects were still amnesic for the list. Thus, the amnesics' memory impairment appeared to be limited to episodic tasks.

Two studies have since raised doubts about Kihlstrom's hypothesis. Spanos, Radtke, and Dubreuil (1982) modified the amnesia instructions to imply subtly that subjects would not only fail to recall the words, but that the words would also not be shown on other tasks. These subjects were compared to subjects who received Kihlstrom's more explicit instructions that they would not be able to recall the words. Spanos et al. postulated that Kihlstrom's instructions had led his subjects not to construe the semantic task as relevant to their amnesic performance, and that the modified instruction would produce a different response strategy. The results confirmed the researchers hypothesis. High-susceptibles with the altered instructions showed impairment on both the recall test and on the WAT. The subjects who received Kihlstrom's more explicit instructions showed impairment on only the recall task.

DeGroh and Spanos (1986) took a somewhat different approach. According to Kihlstrom's priming hypothesis, subjects who are amnesic for episodic material should respond in the same way to a semantic task as subjects who are not amnesic for the same material. That is, even though they cannot remember the material, its residual priming effects will not affect a semantic task to which the material is associated.

Three subject samples learned the same three personality traits belonging to a hypothetical person. Two of the samples also learned that the person was "sociable." One of these samples was given the suggestion that its participants would be amnesic for the sociable trait. Before amnesia was removed, all subjects were requested to rate the person on twelve new traits, three of which had been associated with "sociable" in previous research. After amnesia was lifted for the one sample, all subjects again rated the traits.

The results did not confirm Kihlstrom's residual priming-effect hypothesis. On the first rating, the amnesia sample rated traits related to sociable as significantly *less* true of the person than did subjects who had not learned sociable at all (controls), and even further "less true" than subjects who had learned it but were not amnesic. At recall two, after amnesia was lifted, amnesic subjects changed their sociable trait ratings to a level equal to that of the nonamnesics, and significantly "more true" of the person than the controls.

Not only was a priming effect absent, but the amnesic subjects also went toward the opposite extreme (comparison with controls). De Groh and Spanos interpreted the amnesics' response as indicative of response strategies based on their interpretations of the setting. Because the episodic task (learn traits) and the semantic task (rate different but associated traits) were similar, subjects were likely to connect them. In turn, they employ a strategy that will present themselves as unable to remember.

In sum, the episodic/semantic dissociation hypothesis for posthypnotic amnesia does not appear to be passing the test of time. To explain the de Groh and Spanos findings in terms of dissociations and memory processes is most difficult. Instead of amnesia being associated with "residual priming" effects, to explain the performances of the de Groh and Spanos subjects amnesia would have to be associated with "pumping the well dry" effects. That is, amnesia makes the trait even less accessible than it normally would be without instruction.

CONCLUSION

I have gone to some lengths to argue the desirability of a contextual, interactionist view in understanding posthypnotic amnesia. This chapter began by delineating some objective, empirical referent as a criterion for credible posthypnotic amnesia. The answer led to subjects' phenomenal experiences of amnesia. Being unable to observe phenomenal experience, we must settle for an indirect measure, the subjects' verbal report. Because the validities of verbal reports are difficult to evaluate, the task becomes one of trying to understand them without simply accepting or rejecting them as valid reflections of inner experiences. A number of variables were postulated that may be useful in investigating what leads persons to say what they say about their experiences, what leads us to believe them, and what leads them to believe themselves.

The point was stressed that understanding the total context is important, and the context within which posthypnotic amnesia takes place is complex. It is the task of scientists to operationalize theoretical concepts, and many were provided, but it is also the scientists' task to adopt a productive frame of reference for guiding their observations. In my opinion, the frame of reference should be broad. I have tried to show how a contextual view provides one.

The major differences between social psychological (contextual) theories and special process theories were examined. The latter view posthypnotic amnesia as something that "happens" to subjects. Posthypnotically amnesic subjects are seen as having little or no control over remembering, as in other usual examples of forgetting. They are persons to whom something happens; dissociated cognitive subsystems are an example. On the other hand, social psychological proponents view subjects as actively involved in their role of good hypnotic subject. They are "doing" things that result in their behaviors and experiences.

The two views part ways in their emphasis on which variables are the most important ones to be studied. Special process views emphasize the subject's inner cognitive workings as sufficient to understand their behavior and reports. They also tend to view hypnosis as a special phenomenon that cannot be accounted for with the same concepts that are used to study behavior in other social situations.

Social psychological positions emphasize the interactions of the context with the subjects' characteristics. Understanding such interactions is believed to provide a more accurate accounting of hypnotic behavior. Hypnosis is viewed in the same way as other social situations. No special concepts are needed.

Research phenomena were evaluated next. Three had been reviewed in 1978: source amnesia, disrupted retrieval, and breaching. New studies in these areas were included in this chapter.

Source amnesia still does not appear to be a hypnosis-specific phenomenon. More recent studies indicate that it can best be understood as one of several possible strategies of dealing with an ambiguous test situation.

Disrupted retrieval findings still suffer from methodological weaknesses, the primary one being that really amnesic subjects cannot be included in the data. Studies claiming differences between partial amnesics and nonamnesics in seriation of recall have not always been replicated. New flaws in seriation studies were also pointed out. The most telling problem was that seriation differences have been related to hypnotizability rather than amnesia: More recent studies have shown that high-susceptibles show less seriation than low-susceptibles even when they *are not* amnesic. Other studies using simulators who showed "partial amnesia" suggested that low seriation may be the result of experimental demands rather than amnesia.

Studies that have examined disruptions in category clustering at recall have produced the most consistent results. However, the data here indicate rather clearly tht disorganized recall is not specific to hypnosis or to high susceptibility. They reflect instead that (1) subjects are not attending to the list words during recall, or (2) they are being compliant.

Information on *breaching* posthypnotic amnesia has been supplemented by a number of studies. Studies increasing the pressures on subjects to breach have produced near-100 percent breaching in initially amnesic subjects. Others have shown that recognition testing and instructional variations produce near 100 percent breaching in amnesics, both after and during hypnosis. There seems little doubt that most amnesic subjects will breach amnesia given the proper characteristics of the setting.

Four phenomena not reviewed earlier were also examined: spontaneous recovery, enhancing posthypnotic amnesia, computer analogies (information processing and directed forgetting), and episodic/semantic recall.

No firm conclusions have been found to demonstrate that posthypnotic amnesia is *spontaneously recovered* over time. It appears that about half of the subjects who show initial amnesia gradually regain the material with additional recall trials before the lifting cue. It remains to be shown that amnesia dissipates over time alone, i.e., without recall tests. The recall tests may be the important factor in so-called spontaneous recovery.

Several studies have demonstrated that posthypnotic amnesia can be *enhanced* in low-susceptible subjects. When the ambiguity of the posthypnotic task was reduced, low-susceptibles showed a considerable amount of amnesia and rated it as involuntary.

A study analyzing theories of posthypnotic amnesia in *information processing* terms showed that amnesia appears to occur at the point of output inhibition. The to-be-forgotten material is retrieved into working memory, but perhaps not awareness, where it is searched for tags. Output is then suppressed for material with forbidden recall tags, although the material is still available for generativity uses.

Information processing accounts of posthypnotic amnesia were also considered in comparing directed forgetting with posthypnotic amnesia. The two phenomena do not appear to be the result of similar processes. Directed forgetting seems primarily a problem related to poor storage while posthypnotic amnesia is not. Further, directed-forgetting instructions appear to interact with hypnotic susceptibility in the hypnotic setting. High-susceptibles are confused when administered directed-forgetting instructions during hypnosis and do not show the usual directed-forgetting response. Instead, they appear to be responding to the unclear demands of the hypnotic setting and trying to meet these demands as they are perceived.

The hypothesis that posthypnotic amnesia has differential effects on *episodic and semantic* memory seems inviable. Recent studies indicate that differences in recall of the two can be explained more parsimoniously as (1) a function of the degree of similarity between the two memory tasks and/or (2) the specificity of the posthypnotic-amnesia instructions.

All in all, as more research becomes available, posthypnotic amnesia appears to be most parsimoniously understood in the framework of role enactment. Responsive hypnotic subjects can be viewed as engaged in strategic enactment to fulfill the role of good hypnotic subject as they perceived it.

NOTES

1. Portions of this chapter were taken from Coe (1978).

2. We have pointed out elsewhere (Sarbin & Coe, 1972) that the same criterion, that is, the report of believed-in imaginings, is also taken to demonstrate the presence of an altered state of consciousness, or trance. Our analysis of a specific report ("I could not remember.") is therefore applicable to a more general understanding of hypnotic responsiveness.

3. The reader may confuse the following analysis with dissimulation and faking. This is not the intention. The interested reader will find a discussion of dissimulation in some detail elsewhere (Sarbin & Coe, 1972; Coe & Sarbin, 1977).

4. Parenthetically, it is rare for subjects to report with complete conviction that they could not remember anything, or that they did not in some way actively try to prevent themselves from remembering or from reporting.

5. The reader should be alerted at this point lest he or she begin to believe that contextualists view the inner workings of persons as unimportant. This is not at all the case. Peoples' phenomenal experiences, beliefs, expectations and so on may be of value in understanding their actions, but by themselves and out of contexts, they have little meaning in regard to understanding the complexity of human conduct. Elsewhere, we have delineated a number of concepts relating to cognitive processes besides role skills, e.g., role expectations, role location, and self (Sarbin and Coe, 1972; see also, Shor, Pistole, Easton & Kihlstrom, 1984, for some agreement from more cognitive oriented investigators).

6. To be sure, persons who favor hypnosis as special continue to refer to posthypnotic source amnesia as one of the special phenomena of hypnosis. Such claims are to be expected when there are important nonscientific reasons for hypnosis to be thought of as unusual and special. That empirical findings do not support the special relationship between source amnesia and hypnosis is simply ignored. See Coe (1983, 1987a, 1987b) for more detail on the effects of sociopolitical factors in hypnosis.

7. The Huesmann et al. (1987) study reported above, plus Spanos's (1986b) review and research, suggests that the disorganization in recall claimed by Kihlstrom and Evans (1979) should not be taken as a defining characteristic of posthypnotic retrieval. If so, a disrupted retrieval process is fortuitous.

8. Space does not permit a reporting of other results involving category recall and item-per-category recall. Suffice it to say that they were essentially the same as total list recalls.

6

Methodological and Theoretical Considerations in the Study of "Hypnotic" Effects in Perception

William J. Jones and Deborah M. Flynn

Research on the topic of hypnosis has traditionally assumed that the phenomena subsumed under hypnosis are outside of our ordinary range of experience, that the abilities demonstrated by subjects "under hypnosis" are out of the common run. Our aim here is to show that the modifications of perceptions that have frequently been shown to occur in experiments using hypnosis are better understood as examples of the normal ability of experimental subjects to vary their performance according to the context of the experiment. As we shall see, this is tantamount to the claim that we need not invoke any special "state of hypnosis" to explain enhanced or decreased perceptual abilities (cf. Erickson, Rossi & Rossi, 1976; Orne, 1959; Hilgard, 1975).

For some theorists perceptual distortions are a defining feature of hypnosis. At least one author, Naish (1983), has argued that individual differences in hypnotic susceptibility are explicable as variations in criterion placement (in the signal detection theory sense, e.g., Green & Swets, 1966), and authors of virtually all theoretical persuasions have studied perceptual distortions as a means of exemplifying their particular theoretical concerns. Consequently the methodology of these studies is of overriding concern in deciding between competing theories.

Moreover, the perceptual distortions that have been induced in hypnosis experiments are often thought to imply genuine practical advantages. Thus, Bowers (1976), in his popular book *Hypnosis for the Seriously Curious*, argues that the apparent finding by Graham and Leibowitz (1972) that hypnotic suggestions may enhance visual acuity in myopic persons is one of the more important manifestations of the applied value of hypnosis research. Similarly, it has been widely claimed that hypnotic techniques may be applied with success to the control of pain (see, e.g., Hilgard & Hilgard, 1975).

In addition to relatively narrow theoretical and practical concerns, we believe that the study of suggested perceptual changes may have wide implications beyond the apparently narrow focus of this chapter for the pursuit of psychology as a scientific enterprise. At the least, the field is, or should be, the junction point of sensory psychology and social psychology. Close study of the field may reveal broad implications for the conduct of psychophysical experiments and for the conduct of social psychology experiments.

Unavoidably, this chapter must concern itself with detailed methodological issues if only because the precise way in which a hypnosis experiment is carried out is crucial to an interpretation of its results in the light of conflicting theories. In our view, method and theory are inextricably intertwined. Methodological squabbles are ordinarily disguised theoretical debates. A methodological critique of an experiment does not, and cannot, proceed on some theoretically neutral ground. To take one relevant example, signal detection methods in psychophysics were not merely alternative procedures to the traditional methods of threshold estimation. The use of the new methods implied a radically different account of the nature of the threshold. Similarly, the psychophysical scaling procedures advocated by Norman Anderson and his colleagues (e.g., Anderson, 1974, 1975) are not simply improvements from a mathematical point of view on the influential procedures advocated by S. S. Stevens (e.g., 1971). Anderson's so-called "functional measurement" approach is based on a profoundly different view of the meaning of the context in psychophysical experimentation. (Perhaps not surprisingly, Anderson has also made important contributions to social psychology [e.g., 1982].)

THEORIES OF HYPNOSIS

We begin by sketching the broad theoretical ideas that are current in the field before we move to a discussion of experimental findings.

Theories in this area, with due account of differences of detail, may be conveniently classified as one of two types. A number of labels have been used for the two theories, for example, "credulous" and "skeptical" (Sutcliffe, 1962), as "special state" and "non-state" theories. We shall use the terms "state theory" and "social psychological theory" to distinguish the two camps (cf. Spanos, 1982, 1986a, 1986b). On one side there is a set of state theories associated with such writers as Erickson (e.g., 1964, 1967; Erickson, Rossi & Rossi, 1976), Orne (1959, 1971), Hilgard (1965, 1975), and Bowers (1976). More or less sharply contrasted with these views we have a set of social psychological theories associated in recent times with Barber (1969), Sarbin and Coe (1972), Spanos (1982, 1986a, 1986b), and Wagstaff (1981, 1986). As may already be evident to the reader, we place ourselves unequivocally in the social psychological camp. We shall be more concerned in this summary exposition to contrast the two classes of theory. We shall not try to highlight differences of detail between the two broad theories, nor shall we do much to point up the areas of overlap between the two.

State Theories of Hypnosis

The state theories are characterized by a reliance on the notion of a trance as an explanatory variable. They tend to insist that the effects obtained in hypnosis experiments are specific to this trance state. Thus, the state theorist is likely to find it useful to try to identify unique features of hypnotic responding, patterns of responding that do not hold in so-called "waking" consciousness (e.g., Orne's emphasis on what he calls "trance logic" as the distinguishing mark of hypnotic behavior, Orne, 1959). The overarching construal of the hypnotic subject on this view is as passive and involitional.

The Trance State. State theorists consistently attribute explanatory or descriptive power to the notion of trance or, as it is sometimes described, to an "altered state of consciousness," often said to be analogous to sleep. Subjects "fall into" or "slip into" a trance, some altered state of consciousness that is specific to hypnosis. Orne (1959) writes explicitly that the assumption of an altered state of consciousness is a necessary feature of any complete theory of hypnotic responding:

> The third aspect of hypnosis, the altered state of consciousness presents the greatest problem for investigation, yet it has been felt necessary to include the concept in all attempts to explain the phenomenon. The residual aspect which remains after increased motivation and role-playing are accounted for, may be regarded as the "essence" of hypnosis, with reference to which increased motivation and role-playing appear as artifacts (p. 227).

Entry into this altered state is at least part of the explanation for a subject's purportedly transcendent ability to modify his or her perceptions.

The Involuntary Nature of Hypnosis. Importantly, the subject's behavior in the trance is typically seen as involuntary or passive. Numerous examples may be found in the work of E. R. Hilgard, who argues that hypnosis involves processes of "dissociation" "that occur in response to simple suggestions, when the only modification of consciousness is in the automatization of a simple act that is otherwise performed voluntarily" (1982, p. 38).

The work of Hilgard and Hilgard (1975) on the hypnotic relief of pain is so shot through with a belief in the involuntariness of hypnotic responding that they present no explicit argument for this position. They note simply that difficulties may arise if we find a subject "who so much wants to be hypnotized that 'he helps out' by doing voluntarily what is supposed to occur involuntarily" (p. 9). Similarly, Erickson, Rossi, and Rossi (1976), while careful to argue against the popular media stereotype of the hypnotized subject as an automaton, note that "Trance is thus an *active process of unconscious learning* [italics theirs], somewhat akin to the process of latent learning or learning without awareness" (p. 298). Throughout their text these authors view "trance" and "hypnosis" (used more or less synonymously) in terms of what happens to a person rather than in terms of what a person does.

Status of Subjective Reports. Theorists of the state persuasion are more likely to accept that the subjects' verbal reports constitute an adequate criterion that subjects have entered a trance or have modified their perceptions.

> If an *S* responds and describes the experience of hypnosis, he must be considered as having been hypnotized regardless of the manner in which this experiment was brought about. If he fails to respond behaviorally and reports no alterations in his experience, he must be considered as having been awake regardless of the hypnotist's activities. (Orne, 1971, pp. 190–191)

If the subject reports that he or she cannot hear following a suggestion for deafness, this will be taken by the state theorist as sufficient to establish that subject was deaf. Hence Sutcliffe's characterization of such theorists as "credulous" in contrast to "skeptical" theorists who are less likely to take verbal reports at face value. In this reliance on the subject's testimony, the state theorist can be seen to follow a rarely questioned Cartesian tradition that each of us has privileged access to logically private mental events. From time to time some psychologists have questioned this attitude, arguing that the subject in a psychological experiment has no special knowledge that is not available to the experimenter (e.g., Nisbett & Wilson, 1977). The strongest attack on the theory of privileged access is, of course, Wittgenstein's *Philosophical Investigations* (1958).

Social Psychological Theories of Hypnosis

In contrast to state theories, the social psychological accounts view the hypnotic subject as responding to social cues to modify behavior in an active and often highly cognitive fashion. The tendency of social psychological accounts is to focus on the social and cognitive strategies that the subject may be said to enact in order to give particular perceptual reports. For example, Spanos, McNeill, Stam, and Gwynn (1984; see also Farthing, Venturino & Brown, 1984) have argued that distraction may be an effective strategy for reducing experienced pain in the laboratory. Theorists of this stripe are likely to pay close attention to the precise wording of suggestions, and to the interaction between suggestions and prior attitudes and beliefs. Possibly, the social theorist has more to say about the behavior of those who do *not* pass many of the suggestions on a test of susceptibility, as the state theorist is likely to view as interesting only the supposedly transcendent behavior of the hypnotized subject.

Status of Verbal Reports on the Social Psychological View. There is much less tendency among social psychological theorists to grant any special status to the subjects' avowals. A theorist like Wagstaff (1981, 1986) explicitly considers the behavior of hypnotic subjects in terms of compliance, which he takes to be exemplified in such situations as a subject feeling pain while reporting that no pain is experienced following a suggestion for analgesia. It follows, therefore, that the subjects' descriptions of their experiences cannot be accepted at face value. Spanos (1986b) writes:

> From a social-role standpoint one does not assume that subjects' reports are always honest or that they are dishonest . . . the problem is instead to determine the conditions under which it is theoretically useful to treat such reports as accurate reflections of experience and the conditions under which it is not useful to do so. As Wagstaff (1981) has emphasized, there are many social circumstances in which dishonest subjective reports are routinely expected and proffered. (p. 489)

In practice, as Spanos and his colleagues (Spanos, Bridgeman, Stam, Gwynn & Saad, 1982-83; Spanos and Radtke, 1981-82) have implied, much confusion in the area of suggested hallucinations may be generated by the experimenter taking literally the subjects' claims that they "saw" something (cf. Zamansky and Bartis, 1985).

In their study, Zamansky and Bartis (1985) gave highly susceptible subjects suggestions for anosmesia and for a negative visual hallucination. Five out of sixteen passed at least one of the suggestions, in the sense that they reported either that they could not smell ammonia and/or that they could not see a digit written on a card. When these subjects were given a variant of Hilgard's "hidden observer suggestion" (see Hilgard, 1977) that some hidden part of the mind knows what is going on, ten of the eleven subjects now correctly reported the stimuli. The authors conclude that prior to the hidden observer suggestion the subjects could not consciously perceive either the odor or the digit though "Clearly it is possible for some hypnotized individuals to monitor the state of events while experiencing a variety of perceptual distortions" (p. 246). We find this tortuous to say the least and particularly surprising in a study that was intended to take some of the wind out of the the skeptics' sails. There simply is no warrant in the experiment for the claim that the subjects experienced perceptual distortions of any kind other than the subjects' own avowals. Unfortunately, the veracity and the accuracy of such avowals are precisely what is at issue in experiments of this kind.

In this context we should also consider the controversy over whether or not the hypnotic subject's behavior should be construed as involuntary. In part, state theorists give as their warrant for the assumption of involuntariness statements by the subjects that this was how they experienced the events during the hypnotic session.

> For example, when an arm has been paralyzed as the result of suggestion, the subject perceives the arm in the same way as an arm paralyzed by stroke would be perceived. "When I try to bend it, I am unable to bend it, no matter how hard I try." The contracture was produced involuntarily, but the voluntary trying may be perfectly normal and genuine, often accompanied by surprise that the arm does not bend. (Hilgard, 1982, p. 34)

It is clear that the criterion for "genuine" here is an oral report, including expressions of surprise, accepted at face value.

At this point the social theorist will point out that hypnotic induction procedures frequently state explicitly and emphatically that events in the session are supposed to "just happen" to the person. Moreover, popular stereotypes of hypnosis, whether clinicians accept them or not, continue to be based on a belief in automatic behavior. Hence it is not difficult to see that the role of a "good" subject requires at least the report of involuntariness. Some social theorists argue that in fact the subject comes to construe his or her own actions as involuntary (e.g., Spanos, 1986a). Others such as Kirsch (1986) argue that the subject only reports involuntariness when in fact his or her behavior was experienced in this way. Neither position is altogether clear. How may we here distinguish compliance from a genuine belief (or experience) that one's own actions were involuntary? What would the structure of such a belief (or experience) be like? Much needs to be done at this point to convince the outright skeptic that the subjects who report involuntariness are not merely compliant. As Wittgenstein (1980) asks, "If someone were to tell us that with him eating was involuntary—what evidence would make one believe this?" (p. 137)

One possibility is that suggestions, and in particular hypnotic suggestions, have something like the same cultural properties as alcohol. The "hypnotized" person, like the drunk, is able to produce a socially acceptable account of what may normally be seen as socially inappropriate acts (Fellows, 1986). This account is reasonable up to a point. Our problem is that the behaviors said to be involuntary in a hypnosis experiment are such normally unexceptionable behaviors as lifting one's arm, and so on. We think the following possibility is worth consideration. Assuming that some of those subjects who describe their actions as involuntary are not merely complying with an implicit or explicit demand of the experimenter, we believe that it is plausible to characterize their statements as examples of philosophical confusion. The related concepts of voluntary and involuntary movement are by no means simple to sort out, and researchers themselves sometimes disagree on conceptual grounds. It is of interest that in criticizing what he takes to be Kirsch's (1986) account of involuntariness, Spanos (1986b) makes a conceptual point about the distinction between actions and happenings that is familiar in the philosophical literature. We invite the reader to consider this remarkable passage from Wittgenstein (1980):

> How could I prove to myself that I can move my arm voluntarily? Say by telling myself "Now I'm going to move it" and now it moves? Or shall I say "Simply by moving it"? But how do I know that I did it, and it didn't move just by accident? Do I in the end feel it after all? And what if my memory of earlier feelings deceived me, and these weren't at all the right feelings to decide the matter?! (And which are the right ones?) And then how does someone else know that whether *I* moved my arm voluntarily? Perhaps I'll tell him: "Tell me to make whatever movements you like, and I'll do it in order to convince you."—And what *do* you feel in your arm? "Well the usual feelings." There is nothing unusual about the feelings, the arm is not e.g., without feeling (as if it had "gone to sleep"). (p. 150)

We take Wittgenstein to be making his central point that the criteria for "voluntary" cannot be found in private sensations. However, we cannot pretend to find this passage easy to understand and that, in a way, is our point here. The distinction between voluntary and involuntary action involves a profound conceptual analysis that, perhaps not surprisingly, the typical subject in a hypnosis experiment may not be equipped to make. We do not presume to add to the philosophical debate on the nature of voluntary action literature. Our point is the social psychological one that if professors can disagree as to the nature of voluntary and involuntary, the student-subject is not likely to be in a better position to solve the philosophical problems.

The Meaning of the Social Context

It should be emphasized that no theorist doubts that subjects are responsive in some sense to the social context of the experiment. The state theorist tends to believe that it is possible with the appropriate methodology to distinguish "genuine" hypnotic responding from simple compliance or faking induced by the social context (see Sheehan & Perry, 1976). Orne's simulation design (e.g., Orne, 1971) has been particularly influential. In our view, the popularity of this design often reflects an implausibly simple view of the effects of social context.

As is well known, Orne, who certainly believes in the explanatory value of the trance concept, coined the expression "demand characteristics" to refer to the pervasive influence of implied social demands in *any* psychological experiment (see Orne, 1962). Yet how does the social context function for Orne or for Bowers (1966). The utility of the simulator design (Orne, 1971) for these writers is informative here. In this procedure, one group of subjects, drawn from those who have tested low in hypnotic susceptiblity, is instructed to try to deceive the experimenter into believing that they are genuinely hypnotized. Presumably this deception must be based on the way in which the simulator believes that a good hypnotic subject would respond. The simulators are then compared to subjects who "really experience" hypnosis. Notice that the logic here takes it for granted that some subjects, the highly susceptible, may enter a special state of hypnotic trance. Orne (1971) writes:

> When the deeply hypnotized *S* behaves differently [i.e., from the simulating subject], his actions are counterexceptional and can no longer simply be attributed to his effort to play the role of a hypnotized individual; his behavior must involve some other mechanism and reflect some of the processes which are the essence of the hypnotic phenomenon. (p. 207)

For Orne this "essence" is, as we have seen, an "altered state of consciousness." Sometimes the result of the simulation experiment is that the simulators "overplay the role" (see, e.g., Orne, 1979), though there are numerous experiments in which the behaviors of "real" hypnotic subjects and of simulators are indistinguishable (see, Sheehan and Perry, 1976, 199–205; see also, Miller & Leibowitz,

1976; Leibowitz, Lundy & Gruez, 1980, for examples of perception research in which simulators and hypnotized subjects showed the same patterns of responses to suggestions). When the two groups do differ, it is tempting for the state theorist to conclude that the behavior of the "reals" is influenced by variables other than faking, including the possibility that the behavior of the hypnotic subjects was determined by the hypnotic trance. Bowers (1966), for example, assumed that the simulator design allowed a direct contrast of two explanations of hypnotic responding, demand characteristics on the one hand, and trance state on the other.

One example must suffice. Harvey and Siprelle (1978) gave subjects suggestions for color blindness in one of two conditions. Either the suggestions were accompanied by a hypnotic induction procedure or the subjects were asked to "pretend" that they were hypnotized. On a Stroop test only the subjects instructed to pretend showed evidence of "color blindness." While this flatly contradicted the authors' view that hypnotic suggestions would induce color blindness, they were at least able to make the claim that "pretending" led to overplaying the role of a hypnotic subject. They argued that this result indicated that hypnotic responding must therefore be distinct from role playing or responding to experimental demand characteristics.

All of this is reasonable provided we assume that the only important implicit demand contained in the social context of the hypnosis experiment is to fake the presumed behavior of a "good" hypnotic subject. The effects of the social context may then in principle be distinguished from the effects of hypnosis in itself, hypnosis, as it were, independent of context. In our view, this is equivalent to holding that the social context is a "nuisance" or "background" variable that may be easy or difficult to "filter out" according to circumstance. This position is familiar in psychophysics in the work of Stevens (e.g., 1971), who attempted to demonstrate that a specific power-law relation would hold between stimulus energy and psychological judgments regardless of the context. Here, too, it has been cogently argued that this position seriously misconstrues reality. Most psychophysicists would now argue that context is an integral part of the process of psychophysical judgment (e.g., Anderson, 1974, 1975; Birnbaum, 1974, 1982; Helson, 1964; Mellers & Birnbaum, 1982; Parducci, 1974). It is no longer useful, if it ever was, to speak of the context of judgment as a "nuisance" (Stevens, 1971). Psychophysical theory must rest on a theory of the context, and the experimental approach in psychophysics must be to manipulate systematically the context of judgment (cf. Spanos, 1982, 1986a, 1986b).

A theorist who assumed hypnotic responding to be context specific would argue that both simulating and "genuine" responding are different kinds of socially influenced behavior. On this account, the effect of context is not inherently separable from the phenomena in themselves. It follows that no single experimental control can be of value in distinguishing hypnosis from other contexts. An appropriate experimental strategy must be to demonstrate the intimate connection between phenomena and contextual manipulations (see in particular the work of Spanos and his students reviewed in Spanos, 1982; and Spanos, 1986a,

1986b). It follows equally that no single experiment, or even group of experiments, is likely to persuade a follower of one of the two camps to change sides. Although some empirical claims may be contradicted by the data (for example, the claim that a ritual hypnotic induction will modify the effects of suggestions), the conflict between the two sides is deep-rooted conceptually as much as empirically. It concerns the very nature of contextual effects.

METHODOLOGICAL CONCERNS

Many of the methodological concerns that we shall now discuss are at least implied by our statement of our theoretical persuasion. Some of our concerns relate to the conduct of any perceptual experiment; some are more specific to the study of hypnosis.

For convenience, let us begin with an idealized schema of an experiment on the modification of perception through hypnosis. First, subjects are selected for hypnotic susceptibility on the basis of one of the available screening instruments. Frequently subjects at extremes of the range of responding on the pretest, i.e., subjects "high" and "low" in hypnotic susceptibility, will be compared in the experiment. Both theories predict differential effects of suggestions for "highs" and "lows." The preselected subjects may then be divided at random into "Hypnosis" and "No Hypnosis" groups. Both groups will receive suggestions of some kind for perceptual enhancement or degradation, the difference being that in the "Hypnosis" group these suggestions are preceded by an additional set of suggestions that define the situation as one of hypnosis. Typically, the subject is told that he or should relax, become sleepy, and enter hypnosis.

The effect of the suggestion for perceptual change is usually assessed by reference to a baseline "No Suggestion" condition. The hypnosis manipulation and the manipulation of suggestions may function as either within-subject or between-subject variables. For reasons that will become evident, we prefer to see both sets of variables manipulated between subjects, unless, of course, the specific purpose of the experiment is to examine "carry-over effects" (see, Poulton, 1973, 1975, 1982; Poulton and Freeman, 1966) between conditions (see especially, Stam & Spanos, 1980).

Relevant Control Groups

The Baseline Condition. As the purpose of the experiment in this area is to determine the effectiveness of suggestions in enhancing or degrading perception, it follows that a comparison will ordinarily be made with a baseline condition in which is measured the subject's performance uninfluenced by explicit suggestions from the experimenter. A hidden premise here is that the subject in the baseline condition is performing as efficiently as possible. This premise may ordinarily be false. Watson and Clopton (1969) have shown that unpracticed subjects in psychophysical experiments may only rarely perform asymptotically. Rather, they appear spontaneously "to keep something in reserve." The demonstration by Spanos, Hodgins, Stam, and Gwynn (1984) that baseline reports of the perceived painfulness of ice water or pressure may depend upon the subject's knowledge of the structure of the experiment is of particular relevance here. We need to be aware that the baseline performance of our subjects may be just as crucially dependent upon contextual effects as their performance in the suggestion conditions.

Hypnotic and Nonhypnotic Conditions. Why build into the experiment a comparison of hypnotic and nonhypnotic responding? (In practice this comparison is by no means ubiquitous.) The reason is that otherwise the effects of the general suggestion to treat the situation' as one of hypnosis are confounded with the specific suggestion for perceptual change. This was perhaps first made clear in the important work of Barber (1969), though there had been a number of earlier demonstrations that effects attributed to the uniqueness of the hypnotic trance could be more easily obtained by suggestion alone or by specific instructions (see, Sheehan & Perry, 1976). In fact, contrary to the assertion by Hilgard and Hilgard (1975) "that subjects are found to be more responsive after an [hypnotic] induction than if given suggestions without an induction," the evidence is overwhelming that the general hypnosis suggestion is neither necessary nor sufficient to enhance or degrade perception with respect to a "No Suggestion" condition. If suggestions modify perceptual reports, they do so whether or not the situation is defined in terms of hypnosis (see, e.g., Graham & Leibowitz, 1972; Jones & Spanos, 1982; Jones & Spanos, 1987; see also the review in Spanos, 1986b).

Carry-over Effects

A number of concerns are not peculiar to the conduct of hypnosis experiments, though they may emerge with a sharper focus in this context. A concern in any perceptual experiment is the issue of "carry-over" effects, or what Poulton and Freeman (1966) call "asymmetrical transfer effects."

The notion of carry-over effects refers to the possibly unwanted range effects that may occur from condition to condition in a within-subject experiment because the subject learns a strategy in one condition and then tries to apply it in another where it may be less appropriate. Underwood and Shaughnessy (1975) noted that asymmetrical transfer is likely to be a particular problem in experiments in which the researcher wishes to manipulate the effects of instructions. Obviously, hypnosis research constitutes a paradigm case of instructional manipulation and the between-subject design will, therefore, ordinarily be more appropriate. A useful cautionary tale is provided by Stam and Spanos (1980). They showed that the degree to which subjects report pain when given suggestions for analgesia may crucially depend on the order in which the subjects experience the different conditions of a within-subject design. For example, subjects high in susceptibility reported less pain in a suggestion-only condition when they knew that a hypnosis-plus-suggestion condition was to follow than did "highs" who had no expectation that hypnosis was to follow.

Pretesting for Hypnotic Susceptibility. Along similar lines, we have already noted that the typical hypnosis experiment includes a pretest of suggestibility, sometimes explicitly designated as a test of "hypnotic" susceptibility and sometimes not. This aspect of experimentation also raises serious methodological concerns. There are a number of well-standardized instruments available to the experimenter. These include the Barber Suggestibility Scale (Barber, 1969), the Harvard Group Scale of Hypnotic Susceptibility (Shor & Orne, 1962), the Stanford Hypnotic Susceptibility Scale (Weitzenhoffer & Hilgard, 1959), and the Carleton University Responsiveness to Suggestions Scale (Spanos, Radtke, Hodgins, Bertrand, Stam & Moretti, 1983). (The reader will notice that theoretical differences are exemplified in the titles of these instruments.) Pretesting is carried out to determine the subject's "level of suggestibility," or "level of susceptibility," usually indexed as the number of suggestions that the subject carries out during the session.

Pretesting is always a controversial procedure. Some authors believe that pretesting is always likely to lead to "sensitization" to the experimental task (e.g., Campbell & Stanley, 1963), while others have argued that sensitization is limited to specific experimental paradigms such as memory and learning experiments (e.g., Lana, 1969; see, however, Rosnow & Suls, 1970, and Rosenthal and Rosnow, 1975). However the more general problem of pretesting is resolved, it is reasonable to ask whether or not pretesting for hypnotic susceptibility has discernible experimental effects, as the pretests of hypnotic susceptibility often require activities that will be manipulated in the experiment.

Data here are scanty as few studies have assessed suggestibility after, rather than before, the experiment proper. It is noteworthy that Spanos, Hodgins, Stam, and Gwynn (1984) did not find a correlation between suggestibility and reported reduction in pain following a coping suggestion when the suggestibility measure was taken *after* the experiment, though such an effect has frequently been reported when suggestibility is tested *before* the experimental sessions (see, e.g., Evans & Paul, 1970; Spanos, Radtke-Bodorik, Ferguson & Jones, 1979).

These results suggest that the normal habit of pretesting for hypnotic susceptibility prior to an experiment should lead to some caution in the interpretation of results. The otherwise interesting findings by Wallace and his colleagues (Wallace, 1979; Priebe & Wallace, 1986; Wallace and Patterson, 1984; see also, Wallace, 1984) of perceptual differences between subjects who had pretested as high or low on the Harvard Group Scale may be more ambiguous than appears at first sight. Wallace (1979) found that "highs" reported more illusory direction changes and more persistent after-images than "lows" after both groups had viewed light flashes in the dark. Similar results were observed after subjects had viewed a black dot for two minutes. The effect of initial susceptibility disappeared in a third experiment in which "highs" and "lows" were told to focus their attention on the black dot. Wallace argues that highly susceptible individuals are better able to focus their attention selectively on the relevant features of a visual array. An alternative possibility is that pretesting for hypnotic susceptiblity leads to both "highs" and "lows" construing the situation as related to hypnosis. For "lows" this construal may be a strongly negative one (Jones

& Spanos, 1982, 1987; see also, Christensen, 1977; Weber & Cook, 1972) leading to less willingness to report after-images or illusory perceptions. Wallace himself suggests that "an after-image does not really endure longer for highs; they only report it as such" (p. 685). The Wallace theory that "highs" are better able to focus attention is also contradicted by findings that "highs" are sometimes less accurate than "lows" in discrimination experiments (Jones & Spanos, 1982, 1987). More efficiently focused attention should lead to the reverse finding that "highs" are ordinarily more sensitive than "lows."

Repeated Testing of the Same Subjects

Poulton (1982) has criticized the practice in some psychophysical laboratories of relying upon the same group of individuals to serve as subjects in experiment after experiment. This may be a particular problem in hypnosis experiments. Thus Blum throughout his work has candidly noted that subjects in his laboratory are highly trained in hypnosis—"hypnotically programmed" is how he puts it— and are used in numerous studies. The difficulty is to know just what the subjects have learned. In one case Blum (1975) claimed to have induced "tubular vision," sometimes known as "tunnel vision," in one subject in a way that was highly reminiscent of the hysterical clinical phenomenon and extremely difficult to break through; i.e., the experimenter could not demonstrate that the subject could see anything outside the narrowly focused "tube." This subject had served for three years as a subject in Blum's laboratory. He argued that the subject was unlikely to have faked tubular vision as, among other things, she had given evidence of veracity in earlier studies. This amounts to little more than an assertion by an experimenter that the subject responded honestly. We are reminded of Popper's story about Adler who easily explained, on the basis of his "thousand-fold experience" a case that seemed exactly counter to Adlerian theory. Popper rejoined that Adler's experience must now be "a thousand-and-one-fold" (Popper, 1963). Evidence of veracity in experiment after experiment may be no more than evidence that the subject has early learned that it is undesirable to appear anything other than honest. Whatever we think about this particular experiment, it must surely be concluded that the development of a "semi-professional" corps of subjects is unwise if only because theorists of a rival persuasion are then licensed to claim, and with some reason, that subjects in a particular laboratory learn to comply with the theoretical requirements of the experimenter. In general we believe that a situation in which the subject is relatively well informed and the experimenter rather naive is as likely a priori as the reverse situation of omniscient observer and naive subject.

In practice the very difficulty that Blum experienced in "breaking through the tube" may tell against his interpretation. Theodor and Mandelcorn (1975) using a two-alternative, forced-choice procedure have shown that it may not be difficult to demonstrate that the subject can see when she claimed to be blind. In fact it may be plausible to consider the "extreme" behavior of Blum's subject as an example of that "overacting" characteristic of the "pretending" subject.

Blum's subject showed, for example, a chance level of responding to events outside the tube, while the Theodor and Mandelcorn subject responded significantly below chance to events in the same area.

Issues of Measurement

The literature on hypnotic effects in perception, like the cognate clinical literature, is sometimes difficult to interpret because the psychophysical methods used by the experimenters are more controversial and less theoretically neutral than is sometimes immediately apparent. In particular, in studies of sensory scaling, often of painful events, in response to suggestions, it is troublesome that little attention is paid to the psychophysical properties of the derived scales. Similarly, the use of threshold estimation techniques to assess perceptual modifications induced by suggestions is especially disquieting.

The Scaling Problem. In many studies of the effects of suggested analgesia the researchers attempt to show how the subjects' number responses are functionally related to the intensity of the same noxious stimulus. One common technique, so-called cold pressor pain, involves the subject in immersing an arm in ice water. Most subjects report that the experience is increasingly painful over the first minute or so of immersion. The problem is how may we measure the effectiveness of suggestions in alleviating painfulness? This implies that we can measure painfulness in two conditions, in a baseline condition without direct influence of suggestion, and in an experimental condition in which analgesic suggestions of some kind are provided to the subject.

Probably the majority of studies rely on threshold measurement or on tolerance. The threshold measure is the point in time at which the subject reports that the situation is first experienced as painful. Tolerance is the length of time that the subject is willing to keep his or her arm in the ice water (e.g., Wolff, 1971). In some studies, the researcher obtains a single category rating of painfulness either at the time the subjects remove their arms from the water (Avia and Kanfer, 1980), or at some predetermined point, e.g., after sixty seconds' immersion. This technique has been extensively used by Spanos and his associates in their studies of the effects of contextual manipulations upon reported pain (see Spanos, 1986a).

Some of the problems with threshold measurement will be dealt with below. Suffice it to say that the measure gives us no information about pain growth in relation to time. One of the first studies to try to derive such information was carried out by Hilgard, Ruch, Lange, Lenox, Morgan, and Sachs (1974). These investigators asked the subjects to report the magnitude of experienced pain every five seconds by means of a category scale labeled from 1 to 10, the upper category meaning the subjects wished to remove their arm from the water. If subjects reached this point on the scale, they were exhorted to keep their arm in the water, endure the pain, and to count, in some manner, beyond ten as the pain continued to grow. Hilgard et al. refer to this procedure as "magnitude estimation," in the sense used by Stevens (e.g., 1975, 1977). In fact, the procedure combines category scaling at the lower end with a procedure that may or may not be magnitude estimation at the upper end of the time scale. This would depend upon what rule the subjects used to assign numbers after ten. Stam, Petrusic, and Spanos (1981) conclude, rather charitably, "that it is unclear whether meaningful magnitude scales can be obtained from these procedures" (p. 612)."

In a magnitude estimation experiment, the subject is given instructions to assign to some initial stimulus a number that represents the magnitude or intensity of the stimulus. Numbers are then to be assigned to further stimuli in proportion to the first. For example, the subject might be told that if a stimulus is judged to be "twice as intense" as the first, assign a number that is twice as great as the original response value. This procedure is clearly very different from that of Hilgard et al. (1974).

Stevens (e.g., 1975,1977) ordinarily assumed that the magnitude estimation procedure led to a validated ratio scale of sensation. He argued that "prothetic" or intensive sensory systems always be characterized by a power function in log-linear form,

$$\log R = \log b + a\log S,$$

where $\log R$ is the log of geometric mean magnitude estimates; $\log S$ is the log of the stimulus intensity; a, the exponent of the power rule, is a rate parameter; and b is a constant reflecting some arbitrary choice of a scale unit. For Stevens the value of a was crucial, as this parameter was thought to represent the specific rate of sensory transduction in a given channel. It should be said at once that many theorists do not share Stevens's assumptions either that the procedure results in a validated ratio scale (see, e.g., Anderson, 1975) or that a fixed constant independent of context may be obtained for each sensory system (see, e.g., Birnbaum, 1982). Nevertheless, it may be useful to examine the behavior of magnitude estimation parameters under certain contextual manipulations such as suggestions for analgesia (e.g., Spanos, Jones, Brown & Horner, 1982; Stam, Petrusic & Spanos, 1981; Stam & Spanos, 1980).

Several problems of interpretation were raised by Stam et al. (1981). They found that linear functions gave better fits to the data than power functions (see also, Spanos, Jones, Brown & Horner, 1983), which makes the assumption of a universal psychophysical power law difficult to justify. There was some tendency for subjects to choose lower magnitude estimates, reflected in lower values of b, in analgesia suggestion conditions. This can be interpreted conveniently in terms of a fairly simple compliance mechanism. However, rates of pain growth, if this is what is indexed by a, were comparable for suggestion and no-suggestion conditions. The authors note that individual differences in a, which were considerable, are almost impossible to interpret. At any rate the power-law exponent, a, cannot easily be interpreted as simple sensory transduction, though it may be of interest that once again hypnosis and simple suggestions have comparable effects on a psychophysical parameter.

The authors argued that *a* may vary so much between individuals because subjects confuse affective and sensory components of the experience when asked to judge the intensity of pain. We doubt that "confuse" is the right word here. What else are subjects to do? Most theorists take it for granted that pain judgments are complex and multidimensional (e.g., Gracely, 1980; Rollman, 1983). Consequently, a unidimensional procedure such as magnitude estimation may fail to capture important features of pain perception. An alternative procedure, Anderson's functional measurement (e.g., 1975), is founded on the assumption that judgments are complex, multidimensional, and contextually based. Moreover, this procedure offers the advantage that under certain conditions it is possible to derive validated equal-interval scales from subjective judgments.

Suppose subjects are required to judge the combined or the average painfulness of the intensities of two electric shocks presented in sequence. An algebraic model of the stimulus integration might be

$$R_{ij} = w_i s_i + w_j s_j + e, (w_i + w_j = 1)$$

where R_{ij} is the mean response on a rating scale to pairs of stimuli; s_i and s are subjective values associated with the first and second stimuli, respectively; w_i and w_j are similarly associated weights; and e is a random error term with zero expectation. Anderson calls this an example of a psychological rule that reflects both an integration process and a valuation process. He shows how the goodness-of-fit of this law may be tested and, assuming an adequate fit, how a psychophysical rule may be derived from the data (see also, Jones, 1980; Jones & Gwynn, 1982).

It is central to Anderson's position that a uniform psychophysical law is *not* assumed. Rather, the experimenter examines how variables combine in a given context to determine perceptual judgments. This approach has considerable advantages as a model of psychophysical judgment in a context of suggested perceptual distortions. The researcher has, in principle, a means of untangling subjective values associated with stimulus intensities from the weighting or evaluation of the stimuli.

To date there appears to be only one attempt to assess the effects of analgesic suggestions using functional measurement techniques. Jones, Spanos, and Anuza (1987) compared the effects of no suggestion, suggestion alone, and suggestion combined with a hypnotic induction on the integration of painful electric shocks. The same additive psychological rule held in all three conditions. The derived psychophysical functions showed that the rate of growth of painfulness as a function of stimulus intensity was virtually identical across conditions. Suggestions, at least in this case, were not effective in moderating painfulness.

Threshold Measurement and Signal Detection Theory. It is now widely believed that the sensory detection threshold confounds sensitivity to the stimulus with criterion placement, the subject's decisional rule with respect to the amount of evidence required to report the presence of the stimulus. In a threshold experiment every trial, except for a small number of "catch" trials, involves the presentation of some level of stimulus energy. In the method of limits, these levels are either systematically increased or decreased. The subject reports whether or not the stimulus has been detected. Customarily the threshold is stated as the energy level, measured in decibels, for example, at which the subject reports the presence of the stimulus with some probability, often 0.5. In one version of the signal detection experiment, on the other hand, the subject's task is to distinguish "noise" on which no stimulus or "signal" is presented from "signal plus noise" trials in which the event to be detected is embedded in the random noise. According to the theory, the subject must choose on each trial between two hypotheses: either the signal was presented or only the noise was presented. To make this choice the subject must apply a statistical decision rule that will depend upon the goal he or she wishes to achieve. Suppose the subject receives a relatively large monetary reward each time he or she makes a "hit," i.e., correctly reports that the signal was presented, and pays only a small forfeit for a "false alarm," or incorrectly reporting the presence of the signal. Here it is in the subject's best interest to be biased to report the presence of the signal even when the evidence favoring the hypothesis that the signal was present is relatively weak. If, on the other hand, the reward for a hit is small relative to the penalty for a false alarm, the subject is likely to develop a stringent criterion for the presence of the signal, indicated by a bias-to-respond "noise" in order to minimize the penalty associated with a false alarm. It is a priori plausible that the effects of suggestions, whether or not they are defined as hypnotic, may be to shift the typical subject's criterion in the direction of a bias-to-respond "signal" if the suggestion is for perceptual enhancement, or toward "noise" if the suggestion is for perceptual degradation. The criterion shift may occur in place of or in addition to a shift in perceptual sensitivity.

To point up the practical problems of interpretation of threshold changes, we take an example from an area in which similar problems arise without the problem being complicated by a host of other variables. In experiments on hearing in relation to age, we typically find that older subjects have higher loudness thresholds than younger subjects for the detection of pure tone (see, e.g., Potash & Jones, 1977). Is this because the older subject is less sensitive to the tone as a result of inevitable physiological deterioration in the auditory system? Or does the older subject set a more stringent, more conservative, criterion for the hypothesis that the signal is present? In practice, both effects may occur. The older subject may be both more conservative and less sensitive than the younger (Potash & Jones, 1977).

The parallel with hypnosis research is evident. If subjects have a higher threshold for the detection of a tone after a suggestion for hypnotic deafness, have the suggestions produced a change in sensitivity or have the subjects changed their criterion for detection? Or have both effects occurred? Clearly the threshold experiment is silent on this issue as the threshold confounds sensitivity and criterion placement.

It may be important here to enter a caveat about the value of signal detection procedures in hypnosis or social psychological research. The utility of these procedures in understanding perceptual distortions in hypnosis experiments is, in our view, derived from the general utility of these procedures in perception. We would make no stronger case. We do not subscribe, for example, to the tempting view that a change in response bias or criterion placement is a simple index of motivational and situational factors, while change in an index of perceptual sensitivity reflects systemic variables. To be sure, indices of criterion placement can be shown to be influenced by motivational factors (e.g., Glanater & Holman, 1967). This is not, however, to say that motivational factors never influence sensitivity. In practice, as we have argued following Watson and Clopton (1969), it is perfectly reasonable to believe that a well-motivated, better-focused observer will respond more accurately in the sense that he or she will make more correct responses and avoid making errors. In the end the responses made by individuals in a signal detection experiment are verbal reports subject to the same problems of interpretation (compliance, etc.) as any other verbal reports.

Nor do we believe that perceptual distortions in hypnosis experiments can be characterized entirely in terms of criterion shifts as Naish (1985, 1986) has argued. Naish characterizes the hypnotic session as "an exercise is misperceiving." We would have no difficulty with this were it not for the fact that Naish believes that misperceptions, including hallucinations, arise from criterion shifts. This part of the theory appears to be based on a rather eccentric interpretation of signal detection theory. As Gregg and Whiteley (1985) have commented, criterion placement reflects the subject's willingness to respond "signal" or "noise"; a shift in response bias is not treated in signal detection theory as a shift in what is experienced, in what is seen, heard, or felt. Naish makes two empirical points: that the more susceptible the subject is to hypnotic induction procedures, the more likely he or she is to experience wide shifts in criterion placement; and, that there is a reasonable correlation between hypnotic susceptibility and the choice of a decisional strategy in a signal detection experiment.

In the first case, while we would accept the premise of Naish's account that suggestions and instructions have effects on criterion placement, such effects do not seem limited only to highly susceptible subjects. Jones and Spanos (1982, 1987) have found differential effects of suggestions on criterion placement for both "highs" and "lows." Further, the confirming evidence adduced by Naish with respect to the second point has not always been replicated. Naish refers to the finding by Farthing, Brown, and Venturino (1982) that highly susceptible subjects made more false alarms or, to put it another way, adopted a more relaxed criterion in a detection experiment. However, Graham and Schwartz (1973) found no differences in baseline criterion placement for auditory signal detection between subjects who had scored high (10 or more) and subjects who had scored low (4 or less) on the Harvard Group Scale. Jones and Spanos (1982, 1987) also found that highly susceptible subjects were indistinguishable from those who were low in susceptibility for both an auditory detection experiment (1982) and a visual discrimination experiment (1987). Thus, there is reason to question Naish's view that highly susceptible subjects are spontaneously more likely than others to adopt a looser decisional criterion and hence, somehow, see or hear "things which aren't there."

Nonetheless, we would emphasize, as does Naish, that when we claim that the principle indication of a response to suggestion is to shift criterion, or change response bias, we are not implying that the effect of the suggestion was in some sense spurious or uninteresting. Rather we are claiming that the subjects were able to modify voluntarily their pattern of responding in a way that is reasonably well understood in order to achieve some goal such as maximizing pay-offs. Equally, we would not assume that a demonstration that suggestions serve to modify sensitivity is, in itself, evidence that the hypnotic subject has experienced some involuntary change of state. Modifications in sensitivity may be due to a number of voluntarily manipulable factors including focusing of attention, etc. As we have emphasized, the assumption that subjects perform at their normal asymptotic level in any experiment is difficult to sustain.

Some Illustrative Experiments

To illustrate our methodological and theoretical concerns to this point, it will be useful to treat a number of experiments in some detail. We shall concentrate on three studies to which we have already referred: Graham and Leibowitz (1972), and Jones and Spanos (1982, 1987).

Graham and Leibowitz, 1972. Bowers (1976) argues that "Graham and Leibowitz have demonstrated beyond any reasonable doubt that visual acuity can be improved through hypnotic suggestions" (p. 56). How reasonable is this conclusion? Graham and Leibowitz carried out three interrelated experiments. In the first, they selected nine subjects who had achieved the maximum score on the Barber Suggestibility Scale. Of this group three were highly myopic, three slightly myopic, and three showed no myopia. These subjects were compared to two control groups of $n = 5$ and $n = 4$, to determine in principle, respectively, the effects of memorization of the acuity chart and the effects of motivation on improvements in visual acuity. In the experimental sessions the subject without glasses was asked to read an acuity chart made up of nineteen rows of ten Landolt's "Cs" until he or she made fewer than 50 percent correct responses on a line of the chart. Essentially the task required the subject to detect a progressively smaller gap in the "C." Upon meeting the criterion of fewer than 50 percent correct responses, the subject was asked to replace his or her glasses, and a hypnotic induction procedure was administered that stressed relaxation of the muscles of the eye. The acuity-testing procedure was then repeated without glasses. Prior to "awakening from hypnosis," the subjects were given a "post-hypnotic" suggestion that they now knew how well they could see and that their ability depended upon relaxation of the eye muscles that they could practice in the week prior to the next session. In all, the experimental subjects were tested in three sessions over a period of three weeks. One control group was tested over a period of three days, with a relaxation session substituted for the hypnotic induction. This group was intended to control for any apparent tendency to show gains in visual acuity from memorizing the chart. The second control group was tested over the same three-day period but told only that subjects could improve their acuity with practice.

The results were that the two myopic experimental groups showed a lowering of threshold visual angle over sessions, with both groups showing the lower thresholds in the hypnosis condition. Both control groups showed similar small gains in acuity over the three days of the experiment, though improvement in the hypnosis groups was significantly greater. There was also an indication that two of the three highly myopic experimental subjects showed some transfer of the experience gained in the laboratory to testing in an optometrist's office.

The second experiment was similar to the first. Here two groups of myopic subjects, one high (*n* = 5) and one low (*n* = 4) in suggestibility, were compared. The subjects had not been tested in the first experiment. The most important change from the first was that here the subjects were not exposed to a hypnotic induction procedure after the pretest. Both groups were told that being hypnotized was not a prerequisite for gains in acuity, and memory cues were limited by only allowing the subjects to view the acuity chart with their glasses off. In short, this was a "suggestion only" experiment. Over the three-week period suggestible subjects showed a significant decline in threshold visual angle. This effect was not significant for the nonsuggestible subjects. The author asserted that they found no transfer to the optometrist's office in this experiment. Unfortunately, they provided no data on this point so that claim is impossible to assess.

The third experiment involved five highly suggestible myopic subjects who were tested in three sessions over a period of days. The results showed a strong positive rank-order correlation between the initial degree of myopia and the apparent improvement in visual acuity. Importantly, the authors also established using a laser scintillation technique that any improvements could not be associated with changes in the refractive power of the eye.

A number of comments on these results are in order. First, can the effective decline in threshold visual angle be attributed to hypnotic induction, as Bowers (1976) would appear to have claimed? The conclusion must be that relaxation by itself was about as effective in lowering thresholds as relaxation combined with hypnotic induction; we find suggestible myopic subjects showing comparable changes in threshold visual angle in both experiments 1 and 2. Second, it is difficult to tell what role memorizing the chart played in the results. The relevant control group showed a smaller decrease in threshold visual angle, but this group also had less opportunity to practice between sessions. Moreover, the two groups almost certainly differed in suggestibility (cf. Sheehan, Smith, and Forrest, 1982). Third, we find in both experiments 1 and 3, that threshold declines are more strongly associated with extreme myopia. This raises the possibility that the initial degree of myopia evidenced by the subjects may be to some extent motivational in nature. Finally, it is important to note that the threshold measure may confound visual acuity per se with the subjects' decisional criterion for the gap detection task (cf. Sheehan et al., 1982).

Sheehan et al. varied the procedure of Graham and Leibowitz by, among other features, the use of a signal detection method, a two-alternative forced-choice procedure, to measure acuity. On each trial the subject viewed two stimuli in sequence, one an unbroken horizontal line, and the other a horizontal line with a gap in it. The task was to report whether the line with the gap had been presented first or second. Subjects were matched for suggestibility and compared in two conditions, one in which the subjects listened to a fifteen-minute set of relaxation suggestions, and a second, control condition in which the subjects listened to a passage of music for the same length of time. The authors claim that the effect of suggestion was to improve acuity independent of response bias. Unfortunately, as Wagstaff (1983) has already pointed out, the difference between "before" and "after" sensitivity for the relaxation group was nonsignificant.

All in all, the case that hypnotic suggestions for relaxation or such suggestions by themselves lead to an improvement in visual acuity must be regarded as not proven. Of course, one might always argue that the fifteen-minute session used by Sheehan et al. was too brief, or one might point out that the mean suggestibility level attained by their subjects, at 3.9 out of 8, would not ordinarily be regarded as high. Rather than speculating further at this point, we turn to two experiments by Jones and Spanos (1982, 1987) in which some of the issues raised by Graham and Leibowitz are examined.

Jones and Spanos, 1982. These authors argued explicitly that the behavior of subjects in the psychophysical experiment is influenced by the role demands associated with particular self-presentations. Highly suggestible subjects invest strongly in the role of the "good" hypnotic subject following an induction procedure that defines the situation as one of hypnosis (cf. Coe and Sarbin, 1977; Dolby and Sheehan, 1977; Stam and Spanos, 1980). The role demands for enhanced sensory acuity are quite obvious; the subject should increase accuracy of responding. Less obviously, the subject may choose to interpret the suggestion as an implicit instruction to minimize "misses," failures to report the signal when it has been represented. In other words, the highly suggestible subject given a suggestion for enhanced ability to detect a signal may respond appropriately to the suggestion by exhibiting a bias to respond "signal" (cf. Naish, 1985, 1986). Analogous predictions may be easily derived with respect to suggestions for decreased sensitivity.

What of subjects who test low in suggestibility? A number of studies in the literature show that some subjects will respond counter to what they take to be the experimenter's wishes, particularly if they perceive themselves as being manipulated (e.g., Christensen, 1977; Weber & Cook, 1972). Subjects who are low in suggestibility may resent attempts to control their behavior in a hypnosis experiment, as this is, after all, a paradigm case of manipulation in the popular view. In fact, Spanos has found that subjects who are relatively unsuggestible are considerably more likely than "highs" to report they were deliberately uncooperative (Spanos, 1973; Spanos and Bodorik, 1977). There is even physiological data to confirm that "lows" sometimes respond counter to a suggestion. Galbraith,

Cooper, and London (1972) recorded visual and auditory evoked responses under conditions of selective attention—the subjects were instructed to count flashes or clicks in a train of stimuli. Subjects high in hypnotic susceptibility showed large evoked potentials in response to the stimuli to which they were instructed to attend. "Lows" showed the reverse pattern of responding: larger evoked potentials for the stimulus that they were instructed to ignore. In terms of response bias, these considerations suggested that subjects low in suggestibility may behave in a counterdemand fashion by setting a more stringent criterion for reporting a signal.

In experiment 1, Jones and Spanos randomly assigned ninety-six subjects, evenly divided into "highs" and "lows," to six cells of a 2 (Hypnosis vs. No Hypnosis) × 3 (Standard Instructions, Standard Instructions plus a Suggestion for Increased Sensitivity, Standard Instructions plus a Suggestion for Decreased Sensitivity), completely randomized design. Thus, the design allowed for comparisons of the effectiveness of hypnotic and nonhypnotic suggestions in differentially suggestible subjects. The subjects' task was to detect the presence of a 1200 Hz, 30db pure tone embedded in a 30-db white-noise burst under the various conditions. The subjects responded by categorizing each stimulus presentation in terms of a six-point rating scale. This procedure allows the derivation of a "receiver operating-characteristic curve" for the subject and, hence, of signal detection parameters of sensitivity and bias.

Contrary to some other studies (e.g., Graham and Schwarz, 1973; Wallace, 1979), "lows" were on average more sensitive than "highs" across conditions. For "highs" either suggestion was associated with increments in sensitivity and a decrease in individual differences between subjects. The more interesting findings were undoubtedly in terms of response bias. As predicted, "highs" showed an increased bias to respond "signal" when given a suggestion for enhanced acuity and a slight shift toward responding "noise" given a suggestion for decreased sensitivity. Low suggestibles exposed to a hypnotic induction, on the other hand, responded in a clear counterdemand fashion; they developed a strong bias to respond "noise." These findings for "lows" were confirmed in detail in a second experiment using a more difficult auditory discrimination.

Clearly, these results are counter to numerous reports that highly suggestible subjects will show at least partial deafness when given a suggestion for hearing loss (e.g., Black and Wigan, 1961; Crawford, Macdonald & Hilgard, 1979; Erickson, 1938a, 1938b; Korotkin, Pleshkova, and Suslova, 1969). The results are, however, consistent with the large body of data (Barber, 1969; Spanos, 1986a) showing that a hypnotic induction procedure is not a necessary condition for responsiveness to suggestions. The study also illustrates an advantage of the social psychological formulation in contrast to the state theory. It is possible, in at least some conditions, to develop predictions about the perceptual responsiveness of subjects who are low in suggestibility.

Jones and Spanos, 1987. This study followed the design of Jones and Spanos (1982). The subjects' task was to discriminate a masked visual signal (the upper-case letter N) from masked "noise" letters (upper-case M, W, or X) using the same signal detection rating-scale procedure. In this case, 144 subjects evenly divided between "highs" and "lows" were randomly assigned to the six cells of the design. The results were comparable to those of the earlier study. Once again, "lows" were more accurate than "highs." Sensitivity did not vary as a function of hypnosis or as a function of suggestions. However, both "highs" and "lows" showed variations in response bias in a manner predictable from the earlier study.

Taken together, these studies show the importance of appropriate experimental design in hypnosis research and the importance of appropriate measurement of the dependent variable "sensitivity." It may be that suggestions for perceptual change exert a powerful effect on the subjects' rational choice of decision rules in acuity experiments. The effect on acuity per se appears to be somewhat harder to demonstrate.

INDIRECT MEASURES OF SUGGESTED PERCEPTUAL EFFECTS

So far we have dealt with direct attempts to quantify sensory enhancement or degradation by determining such parameters as rate of growth of sensation, thresholds, signal detection estimates, and so on. A different approach to the problem of how suggestion affects perception also has a long history. This consists of examining some concomitant of a suggested response that is assumed to be outside of the subject's direct control or that, at least may reasonably be assumed to be outside of his or her experience. For example, some physiological correlates of a response, such as galvanic skin response or evoked potentials, are often assumed to be beyond the subject's control. Other phenomena may be the normal, involuntary concomitants of an activity or may involve some knowledge of perceptual processing that a subject is presumed to possess. The logic of these studies is based on a desire to obtain indications of perceptual processing distinct from the subject's verbal avowals and less liable to be thought of as consciously compliant responses. This logic is summarized carefully by MacCracken, Gogel, and Blum (1980). An observer's perceptions

> can be measured indirectly by having the observer respond to some dimension other than the one of interest in the experiment, with the relation between the response dimension and the dimension of interest in the experiment known to the experimenter but not obvious to the observer. . . . The method of indirect measurement avoids the influence of cognitive variables which may come into play in direct measurement. Since the observer is unaware of the relation between the perception required by the experimental task and the perception being indirectly measured, it is unlikely that the observer will be able to modify the response in an effort to meet the demands of the experiment. (p. 562)

Physiological Correlates of Hypnotic Perceptions. We shall deal only briefly with what is quite a large literature. On the face of things, it is tempting to believe that our problems would be solved were we to find some neural marker, some physiological measure or set of measures associated with hypnotic responding. After all, evoked potentials and other physiological responses are unlikely to be under the voluntary control of the subject. Were subjects to exhibit all of the usual behavioral signs of hypnotic deafness and at the same time all of the physiological signs of normal hearing, we might wish to conclude that their overt behavior reflected compliance. Unfortunately, things are not just that simple. In the first place, the literature on evoked potentials and hypnosis is extremely inconsistent—Weitzenhoffer (1982) commented regretfully that efforts to detect physiological counterparts of hypnosis had "failed miserably." Secondly, and perhaps more importantly, physiological responses are never self-explanatory. These data are as susceptible as any other to interpretation in the light of our competing theories.

If some studies find physiological differences between hypnotized and non-hypnotized subjects, others do not. If some studies find differences between "highs" and "lows," again others do not. Thus, Serafetinides (1968), for example, recorded EEG, EKG, GSR, and respiratory rates from a subject with "a proven capacity to develop a trance quickly" in a hypnosis session and in a nonhypnotic control condition. No differences were observed between the two conditions. Wilson (1968), on the other hand, claims that the photic arousal response in the EEG discriminates between subjects "under hypnosis" and the same subjects in the "waking" state.

The difficulty in establishing firm details here is not as serious in our view as the problem of interpretation. To illustrate the problem, we refer to two studies, one by Barbasz and Lonsdale (1983) and one by Spiegel, Cutcomb, Chen, and Pribram (1985). Barbasz and Lonsdale compared four high susceptibles with five subjects low in susceptibility who were asked to simulate hypnosis. The subjects were exposed to a standard induction procedure, following which suggestions for anosmia were administered. The test stimulus was a strong concentration of eugenol. In "waking" conditions highs and lows did not differ in terms of evoked potentials. However, after exposure to the hypnotic induction "highs" showed significantly higher late-component (P300) amplitudes in response to the odor than did the simulators. The authors take these findings to mean that hypnotized subjects are engaged in filtering out incoming signals "that are not to be admitted to full awareness." This is not implausible, though other explanations suggest themselves without difficulty. Perhaps the hypnotized subjects were in fact focusing attention on the odor and perceiving the stimulus in the normal way. This is consistent with the usual interpretation of late components of evoked potentials as correlated with shifts in attention. Simulators, on the other hand, would have no need to focus attention. Possibly, too, the late-component amplitude reflects a conflict on the part of the subject who detects the odor as usual but is required to play the role of the "good" hypnotic subject and pretend to anosmia. Again, no such conflict would be likely in the case of the simulators. Finally, we note that the experimental design confounds the effects of the hypnotic induction with the specific suggestions.

Similar remarks may be made about the Spiegel et al. study. Again the authors claim variations—this time suppression—in late-component evoked potentials in highly susceptible, hyponotized subjects. In this case the subjects were said to be experiencing visual hallucinations. The problem here is to know just what the subjects were experiencing. The verbal reports and behavioral indications of hallucinating are in no way confirmed by the physiological data. One might as well argue that the late-component suppression is the physiological manifestation of compliance. In practice, we would support the view that the subject who claims to be hallucinating is more likely to be engaged in imagining (cf. Spanos et al., 1982-83).

In short, physiological measures do not and cannot provide the kind of indirect measure that would help in the interpretation of perceptual distortions. In the end the physiological measures must always be correlated with behavior such as verbal reports. How this behavior is understood depends upon the observer's theoretical standpoint.

Indirect Measures Specific to the Perceptual Phenomenon

Hypnotic Deafness. A number of investigators have used delayed auditory feedback to assess deafness. This technique involves playing back the speaker's own voice with a brief lag. The effect is invariably to seriously disrupt speech in normal individuals. Consequently, if the "hypnotically deaf" individual suffers the normal disruptions of speech during conditions of delayed auditory feedback, the parsimonious conclusion is that the individual can hear normally. Other manifestations of deafness may then be attributed to compliance. In practice we find that, indeed, susceptible subjects who have been exposed to a suggestion for deafness show speech patterns that are disrupted by delayed auditory feedback (Barber and Calverley, 1964; Sutcliffe, 1961).

A rather difficult indirect test of hypnotic deafness was devised by Spanos, Jones, and Malfara (1982). In this study "highs" and "lows" listened to a dichotic tape that simultaneously represented word pairs, one member of the pair to each ear. The subjects were exposed to a hypnotic induction followed by two sets of suggestions in a randomized order. One set of suggestions was for deafness in one ear. The second set was to attend selectively to one ear. A forced-choice recognition paradigm was employed that required the subject to indicate by circling on a printed list the items that they could remember hearing following presentation of a word list. The lists included all of the items presented to the subject, i.e., the material from the "deaf" or the "non-attended" ear as well as the material that the suggestions allowed the subject to hear.

Two dependent measures were employed. Subjects were asked to rate on a ten-point scale the extent to which they had been deaf following the suggestion. The number of intrusions from the deaf and the nonattended ears was also counted. High susceptibles rated themselves as significantly more deaf than did low susceptibles. However, the two groups did not differ in terms of the number of intrusions. If anything, the hypnotically deaf subjects tended to hear slightly more from the "deaf" ear. The two sets of suggestions also produced comparable effects.

These results show that verbal reports of deafness match the explicit demands of the experiment that the hynotized subject experience deafness. An objective, albeit indirect, index of the adequacy of the subject's hearing following a deafness suggestion showed clearly that the apparently deaf subject picked up auditory information with the same efficiency as the low susceptible who was less likely to report that he or she experienced deafness. As in the Jones and Spanos (1982) study, we find no objective evidence that suggestions for deafness reduce auditory acuity.

The Perception of Egocentric Distance. An ingenious experiment by Mac-Cracken et al. (1980) used the fact that subjects will make a concomitant lateral motion of the head in association with the apparent movement of an object. Two highly susceptible observers served in the experiment. Although the details are complicated, the experiment is simple enough in concept. The subjects were given a suggestion that a stimulus light would posthypnotically appear "near," "middle," or "far." During testing with stimuli at distances of two, four, or six feet, it was clear that the posthypnotic suggestion influenced the verbal reports of the distance of the stimulus to a considerable extent. However, concomitant head movements, on which judgments about egocentric distance are based, were modified by the physical distance of the stimulus, but not by the posthypnotic suggestion. The conclusion must be that "the apparent distance of the point of light was immune to posthypnotic suggestion" (p. 567). Once again we observe a serious discrepancy between a verbal report and a behavior that is not under the subject's immediate control.

Color Vision and Suggested Colorblindness. Highly susceptible individuals given suggestions for colorblindness will frequently claim to be unable to discriminate hues, say, red from green (see, Barber, 1969). Yet, these individuals cannot in any ordinary sense be said to be colorblind. When exposed to the Isihara "malingering" card, they will not report that they can see the number in the array that can be seen by all genuinely red-green blind individuals (Harriman, 1942). The conclusion we draw is that verbal reports are easily adjusted to the demands of the experimenter. However, the subject cannot mimic the indirect defects that accompany colorblindness (see also, Cunningham and Blum, 1982, who rather oddly argue that subjects posthypnotically "experience colorblindness" even though their responses are readily distinguishable from those of congenitally colorblind individuals).

Hypnotic Suggestions Concerning the Ponzo Illusion. Miller, Hennessy, and Leibowitz (1973), using a simulator design, gave subjects suggestions to "ablate" the radiating lines of the Ponzo configuration. The authors again wished to find an objective measure of the effects of suggestion independent of verbal report. They argued that the use of a partially ablated illusory figure provided such a test as, unlike in the case of the typical suggested negative hallucination, the effects of the suggested ablation would be subtle and beyond the subjects' immediate awareness. The results were clear-cut. The suggestion had no effect whatsoever on the magnitude of the Ponzo illusion as measured by an objective technique.

CONCLUSIONS

We draw ambiguous conclusions from our review. There is no evidence of any perceptual distortion, whether enhancement or degradation, that may be attributable to some special state of hypnosis. When distortions are demonstrated in well-designed experiments, the hypnotic induction procedure is neither necessary nor sufficient to produce the effects. There is good evidence in this field as in others that subjects, particularly highly suggestible subjects, will strategically adjust their behavior to meet the demands of an experimenter for perceptual enhancement or degradation. We have discussed a number of well-known procedures that subjects may use to achieve their voluntary ends.

We realize that it is always possible to save any theory. One may always argue that each of the results obtained by the application of indirect methods of measurement is a special case. Perhaps the Ponzo illusion is simply resistant to suggestion, etc. The problems are not insurmountable for the state theorist. They are merely pointlessly onerous. In contrast, the ease with which the social psychological formulation can explain these findings is noteworthy. There is simply no need to resort to more or less poorly defined "altered states" to explain behavior. Nor do we need to face the task of specifying why behaviors that we ordinarily judge to be voluntary should be regarded as involuntary. Our ordinary knowledge of the social world is as sufficient as it is necessary to explain our behavior in hypnosis experiments.

7

Hypnosis and Time Perception

Richard St. Jean

Interest in hypnotic time perception dates back to the early mesmerists who frequently claimed that their subjects experienced an enhanced ability to estimate accurately the passage of time. Many of these early studies, often no more than anecdotal reports, were reviewed and criticized by Moll ([1890]1958). Moll's analysis led him to hypothesize that subjects' typically employed specific strategems, such as counting or attending to time markers, and that their vaunted ability was no greater in the hypnotic than the waking context. Bramwell (1903) reported a large number of experiments on time appreciation, initiated by Delbouef in 1886 and continued by Bramwell from 1889 to 1902. Most of these involved giving a responsive subject a posthypnotic suggestion to carry out a particular task after a specified interval of time. The errors in temporal accuracy, according to Bramwell's report, were exceedingly small, a fact that Bramwell attributed to the enhancing effect of hypnosis on the ability to appreciate the passage of time. Unfortunately, the studies of Delbouef and Bramwell lacked even the most minimal of controls. In none of the cases cited was the subject's timing ability measured under normal waking conditions.

Loomis (1951) reviewed a number of studies conducted between 1930 and 1950 in which observations were made under somewhat more controlled conditions. Stalnaker and Richardson (193), working in Hull's laboratory, tested the ability of nine subjects to judge numerous short intervals under counterbalanced waking and hypnotic conditions. No reliable differences were found. However, their subjects uniformly reported that they had done better in the hypnotic trials. Sterling and Miller (1940) confirmed both observations. Eyesenck (1941), however, reported data from two subjects indicating greater accuracy in the hypnotic than the waking trials. Loomis (1951) concluded his review quite cautiously, citing the need for additional controlled investigations.

Interest in the hypnotic investigation of time was renewed by the 1954 appearance of Cooper and Erickson's book, *Time-Distortion in Hypnosis.* Cooper and Erickson reported a series of studies in which highly responsive subjects were given hypnotic suggestions that they would experience alterations in their subjective experience of time. All of their subjects were given preliminary training, involving practice with starting and stopping signals, concentration on suggested imaginary activities, and the reporting of subjective durations. The experimenter made a point of informing the subjects that time distortion was occurring whenever the reported subjective duration departed from the actual elapsed time. As the training progressed, the actual allotted time for a particular task would gradually be decreased while the suggested personal duration remained constant. Only those subjects who reported successful training experiences were retained for the experimental series. In all of the experiments a hypnotic induction was followed by the assignment of a cognitive activity (for example, counting the flowers during an imaginary walk through the park), together with a suggested personal duration far in excess of the actual time alloted. Overall, subjects reported experiences that were more consistent with the suggested than the actual time. For example, one subject reported being able to design elaborate dress patterns during very brief test intervals. Another subject was apparently able to learn a list of paired-associate nonsense syllables in less time using hypnotic time distortion than was required during waking trials. Since waking comparisons were occasionally, although rarely, made and since experiential reports were given with great conviction, Cooper and Erickson (1954) concluded that their results were not due to deliberate falsification but instead reflected a genuine increase in the speed of thought resulting from hypnotic suggestion.

Despite the major inadequacies in their research designs and experimental procedures, Cooper and Erickson's speculations have proved irresistible to a new generation of researchers. In the succeeding thirty years, two rather distinct lines of inquiry have developed. In one, a variety of attempts have been made to document effects of suggested time distortion on measures of behavioral performance. In the other, the concern has been to compare estimates of subjective duration in hypnotic and waking contexts. The remainder of the chapter will review the research in these two areas.

SUGGESTED TIME DISTORTION

The majority of the studies investigating suggested time distortion have employed some measure of verbal learning as their major dependent variable. A few studies, in an attempt to assess subjective experience, have employed other measures not directly related to learning or performance.

Learning Measures

The first systematic attempt to determine whether time-distortion suggestions would influence performance was reported by Barber and Calverley (1964). They selected sixteen subjects who had achieved high scores on the Barber Suggestibility Scale (BSS, Barber, 1969) and compared their performance with two samples of subjects who had not been tested on the BSS. Following a hypnotic induction their high-suggestible subjects were given explicitly worded time-distortion instructions. They were repeatedly told "everything is slowing down, seconds are stretching out into hours" (p. 211). One of their control groups was given the same instructions without hypnosis, while the other control group received neither hypnosis nor time distortion. All subjects were presented with a list of twelve nonsense syllables and given a 5-minute study period followed by a two-minute test interval. The two time-distortion groups were informed that the study period would be experienced as 5 hours in length. Their results showed that the hypnotic time-distortion group actually learned fewer nonsense syllables than either of the nonhypnotic comparison groups. Nevertheless, in contrast to the no-distortion control, both time-distortion groups reported the study duration to be far longer than the allotted 5 minutes.

Two similar studies appeared shortly after the Barber and Calverley (1964) report. Casey's (1966) procedure was a close replica of Cooper and Erickson's (1954) in that his subjects were given extensive prior training in time distortion, some in a hypnotic context and others in a waking context. On both learning and experiential measures the hypnotic subjects were indistinguishable from the waking controls. Edmonston and Erbeck (1967) selected eight subjects who had scored above the mean on the BSS and assigned four to a hypnotic and four to a waking control treatment. The hypnotic, but not the control, subjects received individual training in time-distortion techniques. All subjects proceeded through a series of 15-second learning trials until a list of nonsense syllables had been learned to criterion. The hypnotic subjects were given prior instructions that each trial would be experienced as 3 minutes; the control subjects were given no special instructions. A comparison of the number of learning trials required found no reliable difference between hypnotic and control subjects.

Surprisingly, the results of these three studies did not lay the matter to rest. Krauss, Katzell, and Krauss (1974), in a complex design comprising eight independent groups of subjects, reported a dramatic learning enhancement in their hypnotic time-distortion subjects. All of their subjects were presented with a written list of sixty categorized nouns. Five groups were allotted 3 minutes of study time, and the other three groups were allotted 10 minutes.

The time-distortion manipulation consisted of the instruction that the internal time scale could be altered by suggestion and, further, that the subject would experience the study period as 10 minutes, regardless of what the actual duration might be. Subjects in the hypnotic time-distortion group recalled more words than any of the 3-minute comparison groups, including a waking-time distortion group, a placebo group, a hypnotic non-time-distortion group, and a no-instruction waking group. In addition, their level of recall was only slightly, but not significantly, less than that of three other comparison groups with an actual 10-minute study period. Krauss et al. (1974) noted that their results were discrepant from those of previous investigators and suggested that further research was warranted.

Johnson (1976) replicated a portion of the Krauss et al. (1974) design, but tested subjects in a large group setting rather than individually. Despite the use of identical time-distortion instructions as well as the same word list, a very different pattern of results emerged. Although not statistically reliable, subjects in the hypnotic time-distortion group recalled fewer words than did the two waking control groups. The level of recall obtained in the two 10-minute groups was substantially higher than that of any of the 3-minute groups, and also higher than that reported by Krauss et al. for their 10-minute groups.

Wagstaff and Ovenden (1970), again using the Krauss et al. word list and the same set of instructions, found that their hypnotic time-distortion group recalled significantly fewer words than both the 3-minute and the 10-minute waking control groups. Hypnotic depth estimates were also collected and found not to be related to level of recall.

In a review of the hypnotic time-distortion and learning literature, St. Jean (1980) noted that previous researchers had not adequately controlled for hypnotic responsiveness. In the studies by Krauss et al. (1974), Johnson (1976), and Wagstaff and Ovenden (1979), unselected subjects were employed, rendering it impossible to determine whether time-distortion instructions might be uniquely effective for highly responsive subjects. Treatment condition and hypnotic responsiveness were potentially confounded in Barber and Calverley's (1964) study. In addition, the form of the time-distortion instructions varied across studies. Barber and Calverley (1964) used explicitly worded suggestions that time was slowing done and stretching out. Krauss et al. (1974), as well as Johnson (1976) and Wagstaff and Ovenden (1979), used implicitly worded suggestions that a unit of time would be experienced as defined by the experimenter, regardless of its actual length.

To assess the effects of these variables, St. Jean (1980) compared the effectiveness of explicit, implicit, and no-time-distortion treatments for subjects selected for their high (8–12) or low (0–4) scores on the Harvard Group Scale of Hypnotic Susceptibility (HGSHS; Shor & Orne, 1962). All subjects were tested individually on a modified version of the Stanford Hypnotic Susceptibility Scale, Form C (SHSS:C; Weitzenhoffer & Hilgard, 1962). The experimental procedure was embedded between SHSS:C items. All subjects were given 3 minutes to study a list of forty common nouns. Those receiving the time-distortion suggestions were told that they would have an experienced time of 10 minutes. Subjects in the no-distortion control groups were accurately informed of the 3-minute limit. Overall, subjects recalled approximately eighteen words, and this level did not vary as a function of either instructional treatment or level of hypnotic responsiveness.

In a second study, St. Jean (1980) attempted to focus the time-distortion suggestion on a smaller unit of time. Words were projected on a viewing screen at a constant 2-second rate and, on various counterbalanced trials, subjects were given explicit or implicit suggestions that the word would appear for 6 seconds. Recall on the time-distortion trials did not exceed that for the no-distortion trials and was significantly less than that for the original waking trial. On a postexperimental questionnaire subjects high in hypnotic susceptibility indicated that they experienced a slowing of time during both time-distortion trials. However, these experiential reports failed to correlate with the performance data.

In summary, only one study, that of Krauss et al. (1974), has found an enhancement in learning associated with suggested time distortion, while seven others have failed to find such an effect. Wagstaff and Ovenden (1979) speculate that the apparent enhancement reported by Krauss et al. (1974) may be due to an exceptionally low level of performance in their control groups. None of their 3-minute control groups recalled more than 14.5 words, a level of performance that falls considerably below that reported by Johnson (1976), St. Jean (1980), and Wagstaff and Ovenden (1979) for any of their comparison groups. In fact, the mean recall score of 20.4 in the hypnotic time-distortion group of Krauss et al. (1974) is on a par with the level of recall reported for both the time-distortion and the control groups in the various replication studies. It appears now that the research in time distortion and learning can be added to the growing literature demonstrating that hypnotic suggestions do not, in general, enhance performance beyond maximal waking levels (e.g., Barber, Spanos & Chaves, 1974; Smith, 1983).

Time Distortion and Subjective Experience

Several of the studies reviewed in the previous section included measures designed to assess experiential effects. Following the suggestion that a 5-minute period would be experienced as 5 hours, Barber and Calverley (1964) asked their subjects to rate how quickly time had passed and to provide an estimate of how much time had actually passed. Time-distortion subjects reported that time passed much more slowly than usual. Those in the hypnotic group estimated 89.1 minutes and those in the waking time-distortion group 46.9 minutes (a nonsignificant difference). The estimate of 4.2 minutes in the no-treatment control group was reasonably accurate and reliably lower than both time-distortion groups. St. Jean (1980) also found ratings and estimates to be influenced by suggested time distortion, but only for hypnotically responsive subjects.

Weitzenhoffer (1964) attempted to provide evidence for subjective time distortion using a very different procedure. His subjects were asked to produce 10-second intervals, commencing with the experimenter's start command, while listening to a metronome. During hypnosis subjects were instructed that the metronome was set for 60 beats/minute. However, the actual setting was some multiple or fraction of this. On some occasions it was set at 30 beats and on others at 120 beats. If subjects use the metronome beat as a basis for their estimates, then a 30-beat rate, if experienced as a 60-beat rate, should result in estimates approximately twice as great as the actual duration. Weitzenhoffer (1964) reported that, after a series of trials, the results approached predicted levels, providing evidence for an underlying change in the rate of subjective time. Such a conclusion, however, is not permitted by the study's design. A total of only four subjects was used, and one did not give expected results. Of the remaining three, one had been instructed to simulate hypnosis, and his results were equally as good as those of the two remaining hypnotic subjects. The fact that estimates gradually approached the expected level of performance over a series of trials seems more consistent with an experimenter-shaping effect than with a fundamental alteration in time perspective.

Zimbardo and his colleagues have conducted two studies in an effort to provide objective indicators of subjective time experiences. In the first (Zimbardo, Marshall & Maslach, 1971), a high-susceptible hypnotic group and two other comparison groups were given the suggestion that the present was expanding, and that the past and future were receding. A fourth group was not given these suggestions. All subjects were high in hypnotic responsiveness as assessed by the Stanford Hypnotic Susceptibility Scale, Form A (SHSS:A; Weitzenhoffer & Hilgard, 1959). Dependent variable tasks included writing stories for two TAT (thematic apperception) pictures, listening to an old radio "bloopers" program, and building with clay. Various changes in the behavior of the hypnotic group, such as laughing out loud to the radio tape and not washing the clay from their hands, were interpreted as attesting to the subjective reality of an altered temporal perspective. Although changes also occurred in the behavior of simulating subjects, they were not as extensive as those in the hypnotic group. On this basis, the authors felt that an interpretation in terms of demand characteristics or role behavior could be eliminated. These conclusions, however, are not justified. Prior to the start of the experiment the hypnotic subjects, but not those in the various comparison groups, received 10 hours of hypnotic training, particularly concentrating on the ability to dissociate and to produce vivid images. Such training may well have biased subjects toward producing behavior that could be interpreted as dissociated or fantasy oriented. That is, the role behavior expected of these subjects, and especially their training in such roles, may have encouraged them to present themselves as living in an expanded present. Utilizing the cognitive skills that they learned during the training period may have enabled them to give a particularly convincing performance. This analysis does not rule out the possibility that participants may have indeed convinced themselves that they were experiencing an expanded present. Instead, the point is simply that the procedures of Zimbardo et al. (1971) do not give direct evidence of an alteration in temporal perspective.

In their second study (Zimbardo, Marshall, White & Maslach, 1973) a more quantitative index of hypnotic time distortion was sought. High-susceptible subjects were assigned to a hypnotic, a simulating, or a no-treatment control group. Subjects were taught to tap a telegraph key at different rates in order to illuminate various target lights. If the key were tapped at a rate faster or slower than the current target rate, other lights in the array were activated. On a particular trial, for example, a subject would learn to tap at the rate of 3 per second to keep a red light on. Following such a trial hypnotic and simulating subjects received suggestions that time was slowing down or, on counterbalanced trials, speeding up. Control subjects received no suggestions. Half of the subjects in each group continued to receive feedback from the light array, while the lights were extinguished for the other half. In the no-feedback condition both hypnotic and simulating subjects altered their tapping rate in accord with the direction, either faster or slower, of the time-distortion suggestions. However, in the continued-feedback condition only the hypnotic subjects altered their tapping rate. According to Zimbardo et al. (1973) the continued-feedback condition poses a difficult conflict for those who are motivated to change their behavior voluntarily. This conflict, between the demand to comply with the experimenter's suggestion and the demand to complete the task, should be resolved in the direction of the most salient reinforcer, feedback from the target. For hypnotic subjects, who presumably experience a genuine alteration in their time sense, there should be no conflict, but simply an inability to complete the task.

There are several problems with this analysis. First, hypnotic subjects changed their response rate to a greater degree in the no-feedback condition, indicating that perhaps there was some conflict in the feedback condition. Second, as in their previous study, the authors gave the hypnotic group extensive training in hypnotic responding. Such training involves practice in the enactment of counterfactual suggestions (e.g., "you are a young child" or "your body is floating away"). Successful enactment demands that the subject learn to attend away from, or ignore, current environmental input. Thus, the hypnotic subjects have been trained in skills that are relevant to the successful performance of the critical feedback trials, while the comparison groups have not. Again, this does not rule out the possibility that hypnotic subjects may have convinced themselves that they were experiencing an alteration in subjective time flow.

This section has reviewed a number of attempts to explore subjective concomitants of time-distortion suggestions. Due to procedural biases and other methodological limitations, none of these studies is able to present convincing evidence of changes in subjective time experiences. On the other hand, presently available data do not rule out such changes. A tentative interpretation of these data, based on Spanos's (1982) strategic enactment hypothesis, can be offered. Hypnotic subjects learn and, in the appropriate context, enact behaviors that present, the subjects themselves as experiencing a distorted time orientation. By successfully enacting such behaviors, and by focusing attention on thoughts incompatible with a normal time orientation, hypnotic subjects may indeed convince themselves that their normal experience of time has changed. Time estimates compatible with the time frame suggested by the experimenter are not, by this analysis, motivated by simple compliance, but instead reflect an honest assessment of the subject's experience.

INTERVAL ESTIMATION

Accuracy of Estimation

In the years since Loomis (1951) reviewed the research on the accuracy of hypnotic time perception, the data base has only marginally increased. Schubot (1964) compared hypnotic with waking time estimates, using the method of production, for both high- and low-susceptibility subjects. The experimenter instructed the subject to produce intervals of 8, 32, and 64 seconds. The subject's task was to indicate the onset and offset of each interval. Word association tasks were carried out during the intervals to prevent counting. High-susceptibles in the hypnotic condition produced relatively accurate estimates. All other groups significantly overestimated the intervals.

A similar, but methodologically weaker, study was reported by Tebecis and Provins (1974). A group of high-susceptible subjects was asked to produce an interval of 131 seconds on three different occasions, twice in the hypnotic context and once following waking imagination instructions. A comparison group consisting of subjects significantly lower in susceptibility produced the same interval on only one occasion, in a waking imagination context. No reliable differences in estimates between groups or conditions were found. All subjects tended to underproduce (i.e., overestimate) the interval, by about 40 percent.

Bowers and Quan (1978) compared time estimates of high-and low-susceptibility subjects made while listening to absorbing short stories. All estimates were made in a normal waking context. For one story subjects were asked to produce 2-minute intervals. For the other, subjects provided retrospective estimates of a series of 3-minute intervals. The production data revealed a slight tendency to overproduce (i.e., underestimate) by about 1.1 percent. The estimation tasks yielded estimates nearly identical to the actual 3-minute interval. Time estimates were related to neither hypnotic susceptibility nor ratings of listening involvement.

Given the paucity of research in this area, it is impossible to improve on Loomis's (1951) statement that no conclusion is warranted. Hypnosis may increase the accuracy of time perception, as Schubot (1964) claims, or it may not, as Tebecis and Provins (1974) claim. It is difficult, however, to conceive of any variables associated with either the hypnotic context or hypnotic responsiveness that would increase the accuracy of time estimation beyond normal, nonhypnotic levels.

Estimation of Hypnotic Intervals

A related question has focused not on the accuracy of time estimation, but instead on the subjective experience of time during periods of hypnotic involvement. The issue here is different because the concern is not with the operation of a temporal motive, as Doob (1971) has defined it, but rather with the subject's retrospective assessment of the passage of time.

Schwartz (1978) appears to be the first researcher to have asked his subjects to estimate the length of the hypnotic period retrospectively. High-susceptible hypnotic subjects were compared with unselected waking controls who responded to the SHSS:C items without a prior hypnotic induction. At the completion of the scale, but before the formal alerting procedure, subjects were asked to provide a verbal estimate of elapsed time. The responses of the hypnotic subjects were, on the whole, much more variable than those of the controls. In a follow-up study, Schwartz (1980) confirmed these findings and reported that whether the estimates were collected just prior to or just after the formal termination of hypnosis made little difference. Unfortunately, neither study reported the actual magnitude of the estimates. In the alter study, Schwartz (1980) reported that the general tendency was to underestimate the duration of the scale but did not report the extent of this tendency. Limitations in the design of both studies prevent us from determining whether time estimation varied with experimental condition or level of hypnotic responsiveness.

Bowers and Brenneman (1979) provided data that addressed both questions. They tested a large sample of subjects on the HGSHS and, immediately following the alerting instructions, asked them to estimate how much time in minutes had passed since the beginning of the induction. The data indicated an overwhelming tendency for subjects to underestimate, by about 40 percent, the actual time of 27 minutes. Contrary to expectation, no relationship was found between time estimation and the number of items passed on the HGSHS. Several weeks later, a subset of the original sample was asked to estimate an identical interval embedded in a lecture period. These waking estimates were substantially more accurate. However, since the hypnotic and waking contexts differed considerably in content, and since the treatments were not counterbalanced, a number of alternative interpretations are possible. For example, it is not unlikely that undergraduate subjects would find a group-hypnosis procedure more interesting and involving than the typical lecture period.

A replication study (Bowers, 1979) employing the individually administered SHSS:C confirmed the underestimation finding. In this study, degree of underestimation was found to be strongly related to susceptibility level; high-susceptibles underestimated to a greater degree than low-susceptibles. However, this relationship emerged only after a small group of overestimators had been removed from the data pool. Bowers's (1979) explanation is that hypnotic subjects, especially those who possess high ability, become imaginatively absorbed in the proceedings, and that such absorption leads to a perceived shortening of the duration.

An alternative explanation is based on Ornstein's (1969) theory of perceived time. According to this theory, the more events processed and stored during a given interval, the longer the temporal judgment of that interval will be. Ornstein (1969) hypothesized that the storage of an interval might be altered by a posthypnotic suggestion to forget the events of that interval. Thus, if a subject is amnesic for some or all of the events of a hypnotic session, that session may appear briefer in retrospect. In this view the relationship between susceptibility and time estimation that Bowers (1979) reported occurs because of the correlation between hypnotizability and response to the amnesia suggestion.

This amnesia hypothesis was rejected by Bowers (1979). He reported that when some of his subjects were asked to provide estimates before the amnesia suggestion was given, the correlation with susceptibility was unaltered. However, this conclusion does not necessarily follow. It seems possible that the high-hypnotizables in this group, although not receiving a formal amnesia suggestion, were functionally amnesic in the sense that they were attending to immediate experience when asked for time estimates and not focusing on, or attempting to recall, past events. In addition, a comparison of this group with a sample tested following the amnesia suggestion revealed an even greater degree of underestimation in the latter group.

St. Jean, MacLeod, Coe, and Howard (1982) tested the amnesia hypothesis in a straightforward manner. During an administration of the HGSHS their subjects were asked to provide two time estimates, one while the amnesia suggestion was in effect and a second following its removal. If underestimation is due to amnesia, then the second estimates should be considerably more accurate. In addition, subjects' response protocols were scored for degree of amnesia, using several different indexes, to determine whether amnesic recall was related to time estimation. As predicted by the amnesia hypothesis, second estimates were higher than initial estimates. However, correlations between amnesic responding and time estimates hovered around zero. It appeared that the increase in second estimates could reasonably be attributed to a repeated-testing artifact. Control subjects who made postamnesic estimates only showed approximately the same degree of underestimation as occurred on the first estimates of the amnesic sample. St. Jean et al. (1982) concluded that the underestimation effect could not reasonably be attributed to amnesia.

The absorption hypothesis proposed by Bowers (1979) was tested by St. Jean and MacLeod (1983). They attempted to manipulate absorption by having subjects listen to two taped story narrations selected to represent opposite extremes of interest and involvement. Sixty subjects, thirty high- and thirty low-susceptibles selected on the basis of their HGSHS scores, were asked to provide retrospective estimates of the tapes' durations in either a waking or a hypnotic context. Overall, time estimates were shorter for the involving than the non-involving tape, and high-susceptible subjects tended to give shorter estimates than their low-susceptible counterparts. However, the only substantial underestimation of the actual 8.5-minute duration occurred when the high-susceptible subjects listened to the involving tape in the hypnotic context. This pattern fits well with the notion that as the hypnotic subject becomes absorbed in the proceedings, little or not attention is paid to the passage of time and, in retrospect, time seems to have passed quickly. Nevertheless, St. Jean and MacLeod (1983) pointed out that their absorption manipulation may have produced a confounding with other variables. The stories employed in their study differed not only in involvingness, but also in theme complexity, and encodability. Since the low-involving tape contained a large number of unfamiliar terms and did not possess a recognizable plot, subjects may simply have paid little attention to it. Thus, it is possible that differences in attentional processing, rather than, or in combination with, absorptional differences, played a critical role.

In a conceptual replication, St. Jean and Robertson (1986) attempted a different manipulation of absorption, one designed to eliminate confounding with story style and content. All subjects listened to the high-involving story employed by St. Jean and MacLeod (1983). Half of the subjects were given preliminary instructions designed to facilitate an absorptive set, while the other half received instructions to listen in an attentional manner. The absorption subjects were simply told to relax and to listen to an interesting story. In the attention condition the experimenter explained that hypnosis is sometimes used to enhance memory, and that this ability was to be tested by determining how accurately subjects could recall the number of sentences and the occurrences of a particular name. A postexperimental questionnaire contained manipulation checks on the level of absorption and attention. The instructional manipulation failed to produce differences in reported absorption but, as indicated by the memory scores, did produce differences in level of attention. Subjects in the attention condition, but not those in the absorption condition, significantly underestimated the story's duration.

Although absorption was not manipulated, the absorption hypothesis was indirectly assessed through the pattern of correlations relating time estimates to hypnotic susceptibility and absorption ratings. None of these correlations was significantly different from zero. Brown (1984) has also reported a finding of no relationship between time estimation and absorption as measured by the Tellegen and Atkinson (1974) Absorption Scale.

An alternative means of manipulating absorption was reported by Mc-Cutcheon (1985). The general strategy was to have subjects listen to the concluding portion of a highly involving story. In the high-absorption condition subjects received a capsule introduction structured to maximize interest and involvement in the story's conclusion. An analysis of verbal and written ratings indicated that the manipulation successfully varied absorption. Time estimates, however, did not vary between conditions. Contrary to Bowers's (1979) findings, high-susceptible subjects gave higher estimates that low-susceptibles.

St. Jean and Robertson (1986) suggested that the underestimation effect is not due to absorption per se but instead is a by-product of the systematic attentional processing of meaningful material. This interpretation is buttressed by some of the recent experimental and theoretical work in the time-perception literature. Michon and Jackson (1984) have proposed, and presented evidence in support of, the notion that temporal information processing is deliberate, rather than automatic. If attention is viewed as a limited-capacity process (Kahneman, 1973), then tasks that draw on this capacity reduce processing resources that might otherwise be allocated to temporal information. Indeed, Curton and Lordahl (1974) found that time estimates were lower when subjects performed an attention-demanding task than when they were engaged in a task designed to focus attention on the passage of time. Further, Tsao, Wittlieb, Miller, and Wang (1983) showed that subjects underestimated the duration of a secondary event when they were attentively engaged in a demanding primary task.

In the St. Jean and Robertson (1986) study, the attention subjects were asked to estimate the duration of a secondary event, the entire story, while attentively engaged in the primary task of attempting to keep track of sentences and names. The cognitive demands of being fully engaged in this task reduced the subject's ability to process temporal cues in the story, thereby resulting in retrospective underestimates.

This hypothesis can also be applied to the St. Jean and MacLeod (1983) study. Their initial instructions differed in a potentially critical manner from those employed in St. Jean and Robertson's (1986) absorption condition. Subjects were told that after listening to the tape, they would be answering questions about it. The effect may have been to elicit an attentional set, inducing subjects to keep track of names and events, rather than an absorptive set as initially intended. The boring tape, which subjects overestimated, contained many difficult names and no recognizable plot, thereby rendering it difficult to process in any systematic manner.

Several recent investigations (Karlin, 1979: Wallace & Patterson, 1984) have suggested that hypnosis may lead to an increase in active, attentional processing. In his strategic-enactment theorizing, Spanos (1982) has emphasized attention deployment as a major cognitive strategy that subjects employ to produce hypnotic phenomena. If, as seems increasingly likely, hypnosis involves active attentional processing of environmental information, then it seems reasonable to propose that the cognitive demands imposed by hypnotic tasks mediate the underestimation effect. By this interpretation, then, the underestimation effect is not causally related to the hypnotic context but instead occurs because the tasks presented as part of the hypnotic session tend to fully engage attentional processing. Indeed, Fraisse (1984), in concluding his recent review of time perception, has proposed that whenever an interval is filled by a demanding and/or interesting task, that interval will be relatively underestimated. Hypnosis would seem to be such an interval.

8

Trance Logic, Duality, and Hidden Observer Responding

Hans P. de Groot and Maxwell I. Gwynn

Since the eighteenth century, the topic of hypnosis has been associated with the idea that hypnotic induction rituals produce an altered state of consciousness that is reflected in the behavior of the hypnotized subject. Orne (e.g., 1959) is an influential contemporary spokesman for this perspective, and over the last twenty-five years, has devoted much of his research toward isolating an "essential" aspect of hypnosis that cannot be accounted for in terms of subjects' preconceptions or the demands of the experiment. One early result of this research program was the trance logic hypothesis. According to the trance logic hypothesis (Orne, 1959), hypnotized subjects show a marked tolerance for situations that they would experience as disturbingly incongruous in normal "waking" life. For Orne, this uncritical acceptance of the logically incongruous suggests a basic discontinuity between hypnotic and nonhypnotic behaviors.

Orne (1959) originally derived support for the trance logic hypothesis using an experimental design known as the real/simulating technique. In this design, subjects previously determined to be either high or low in hypnotic susceptibility are compared on their responses to suggestions. Low-susceptible subjects, prior to meeting the main experimenter, are instructed by an assistant not to become hypnotized during the session, but instead to try to fool the experimenter by "acting as if [they] were entering a trance" (Orne, 1959, p. 287) or "to simulate being a very good hypnotic subject" (Orne, 1979, p. 533). In other words, these lows (or "simulators") are asked to fake deep hypnosis. They are further instructed to use anything they know about hypnosis and any information they can glean from the situation to present themselves convincingly as deeply hypnotized. High-susceptible subjects (or "reals") are given no such instructions prior to the hypnotic session.

In Orne's (1959) original experiment with this design, subjects sat facing the principal experimenter and his assistant. During the sessions, subjects were asked to close their eyes and receive an hypnotic induction. As the hypnotist administered a suggestion to visually hallucinate the assistant sitting opposite them, the assistant rose and quietly moved behind the subjects. Orne reported that when the subjects were asked to open their eyes and to interact with their visualization, some of the reals but none of the fakers spontaneously indicated that they could see both the image of the assistant and the chair through his image at the same time. This pattern of reporting was labeled the transparent hallucination response. When the hypnotist pointed to the actual assistant standing behind the subjects, almost all of the reals did a "double-take" and indicated that they were perceiving both the actual and the hallucinated assistant at the same time. When subjects were queried about their experience, they tended to give "bland" responses by ascribing the dual presence of the assistant to such factors as mirrors or a trick. In contrast, only two of thirty simulators indicated seeing two assistants. The majority of these subjects either failed to identify the assistant or reported that their hallucination had disappeared. Reports of seeing both the actual and the hallucinated co-experimenter simultaneously were labeled by Orne (1959) as the double hallucination response.

Orne (1959) concluded that the transparent and double hallucination responses indexed a cognitive process that was the "essence" of hypnosis. Specifically, he argued that these responses violated the everyday logical principles that solid objects are opaque and that objects can only occupy a single location at any one time. Consequently, these responses reflected the operation of a type of logic unique to hypnosis. He defined this unusual type of logic, or "trance" logic, as

> the ability of the [highly susceptible hypnotic] subject to mix freely his perceptions derived from reality with those that stem from his imagination and are perceived as hallucinations. These perceptions are fused in a manner which ignores everyday logic. . . . The absence of expression of a need for logical consistency seems, at this point, to be one of the major characteristics of hypnosis. (Orne, 1959, pp. 295–96).

Over the last twenty-five years, the trance logic hypothesis has been subjected to steady criticism. Part of this criticism stems from failures to replicate Orne's (1959) original findings, and part from questions concerning the underlying assumptions of the real/simulator design. Orne's (1959) formulation was based on two underlying assumptions: first, that hypnotic responding was composed of both an artifactual component involving experimental demands, and an "essential" component involving the effects of the "hypnotic state" per se; second, that exposing reals and simulators to the same hypnotic testing situation caused them to be exposed to the same demands, and thereby to be equated on the artificial component. Given exposure to the same demands, behavioral differences between these treatments could be attributed to the one variable that purportedly distinguished them: the presence of a "hypnotic state" in the reals and its absence in the simulators. However, several studies have suggested that instructions to simulate hypnosis may contain demands that are different from those to which reals are exposed. These studies question not only Orne's (1959) interpretation of real/simulator differences, but also his underlying concept of hypnosis as involving an underlying or "essential" trance component.

In this paper, we present a critical review of the trance logic literature. This review will involve a consideration of the issues raised above. More importantly, however, we will attempt to develop an alternative interpretation of trance logic responding. According to this alternative, cognitive-social psychological account (Spanos, 1982, 1986b), reliable real/simulator differences reflect the divergent demands to which these two groups of subjects are exposed. In particular, we shall develop the argument that simulating instructions "set" subjects to enact ideal or complete responses to even the most difficult hypnotic suggestions.

Replication Failures

Since the publication of Orne's (1959) report, at least nine studies (Blum & Graef, 1971; Johnson, Maher & Barber, 1972; McDonald & Smith, 1975; Obstoj & Sheehan, 1977; Peters, 1973; Sheehan, Obstoj & McConkey, 1976; Spanos, de Groot & Gwynn, 1987; Spanos, de Groot, Tiller, Weekes & Bertrand, 1985; Stanley, Lynn & Nash, 1986) have failed to replicate his original finding of a higher frequency of double hallucination responding among reals than simulators. Nevertheless, Kihlstrom (1985) and Orne and Hammer (1974) suggested that these replication failures are not inconsistent with the trance logic hypothesis. Orne and Hammer (1974) argued that previous investigators had failed to obtain significant real/simulator differences on the double hallucination response because they had unwittingly cued simulators to give this response. To test this hypothesis, Sheehan et al. (1976) exposed reals and simulators to two levels of cuing for the double hallucination response. Hallucinating subjects in the high-cue condition were asked to look at the location of the actual stimulus object and describe what they saw; those in the low-cue condition were simply asked to look around the room and describe anything they saw. Interestingly, although high-cue subjects gave the double hallucination response more frequently than low-cue subjects, no differences emerged between reals and simulators on this measure. Thus, even under the supposedly optimum (low-cue) testing conditions specified by Orne and Hammer (1974), the double hallucination response failed to discriminate between reals and simulators.

More recently, Kihlstrom (1985) argued that although the double hallucination results fail to attain conventional levels of statistical significance, studies have typically revealed a trend toward real/simulator differences on this index. However, even a cursory examination of the available findings fails to support this contention. To the contrary, not one of these studies reported probabilities even approaching conventional levels of statistical significance (all ps — .10), regardless of the explicitness of cuing for this response (Sheehan et al., 1976).

In contrast to these recurrent failures to replicate Orne's double hallucination results, studies (Johnson et al., 1972; McDonald & Smith, 1975; Peters, 1973;

Sheehan et al., 1976; Spanos, de Groot, et al., 1985; Spanos, de Groot, et al., 1987; Stanley et al., 1986) have consistently reported that reals were significantly more likely than simulators to give the transparent hallucination response. Moreover, the transparent hallucination response has been elicited over a variety of stimulus objects, e.g., styrofoam cups, elaborate vases, stuffed toys, as well as actual persons. The only apparent inconsistency in these findings concerns discrepancies across studies in the rates of transparency reporting by reals and simulators. Although the cause of these discrepancies has not been investigated systematically, these differences may reflect variations in the criteria used to assess transparency, as well as variations in the extent to which this response was cued by investigators (cf. Orne, Dinges & Orne, 1986; Peters, 1973; Sheehan et al., 1976; Spanos, de Groot et al., 1985).

Orne (1959) originally implied that spontaneous (i.e., uncued) transparency reports were absolutely diagnostic of real hypnosis. In line with this report, several studies (McDonald & Smith, 1975; Peters, 1973; Sheehan et al., 1976; Stanley et al., 1986) have found that spontaneous transparency reports emerge only among hypnotic subjects. However, spontaneous transparency reports are quite rare even among reals. No more than 40 percent of these subjects proffered this response in any of these studies, and in two studies none of the reals or simulators exhibited spontaneous transparency. On the other hand, studies in which subjects were explicitly asked if their hallucinated images were transparent found that the majority of reals as well as some simulators proffered this response (Johnson et al., 1972; Spanos, de Groot, et al., 1985; Spanos, de Groot, et al., 1987; Stanley et al., 1986). Orne et al. (1986) have criticized the latter studies for not providing optimum assessments of the transparency response. According to them, the emergence of this response among simulators reflects demands produced by explicitly asking subjects about transparency.

However, cuing for transparency can have two possible effects. Although cuing may lead to compliance, it may also lead subjects to report accurately about some aspect of their experience that was not salient to them and therefore not reported spontaneously. Several considerations indicate that cuing tends to have the latter effect. Thus, two studies (Johnson et al., 1972; Spanos, de Groot, et al., 1985) relied exclusively on cued reports to discriminate between subjects, because this response failed to emerge spontaneously even among hypnotics. The difference between these studies and those that obtained spontaneous reports appears to lie primarily in the extent of the interview procedure and on the emphasis placed on querying subjects about the phenomenological properties of their image. Specifically, studies that failed to obtain spontaneous reports of transparency typically provided minimum questioning about phenomenological experience by restricting their queries to only one or two questions. These questions simply asked subjects to describe the appearance and actions of their hallucination. For instance, Johnson et al. (1972) simply asked subjects to describe their hallucination (of the co-experimenter, Joe) as follows: "Describe Joe. What is he doing?" In contrast, studies that obtained spontaneous transparency reports appear to have engaged in a more extensive questioning of subjects and/or asked subjects to compare and discriminate between their actual and suggested images. Stanley et al. (1986) asked subjects, "How does the cup on the right look to you? How does the cup on the left look to you? Compare the two cups for me. Do they look alike, or can you tell them apart? [If they can tell them apart, ask how]" (pp. 449–50). Taken together, these considerations suggest that extensive or perhaps even leading questions about the phenomenological properties of the hallucinatory experience may be necessary if the dimension of transparency is to become salient enough for subjects to mention "spontaneously."

Interestingly enough, although cuing appears to enhance the transparency reporting of hypnotic subjects, most simulators respond as if they were perceiving a solid object even under conditions of high cuing. Spanos (1986b) has interpreted these data as indicating that querying subjects about transparency may actually expose simulators to demands for reporting opaque rather than transparent hallucinations. According to this idea, simulators tend to interpret an affirmative response to a question like "Can you see the background through the object?" as an admission of imperfect hypnotic ability. Therefore, to avoid detection by the hypnotist, these subjects tend to report a solid rather than a transparent hallucination. Recently, Stanley et al. (1986) obtained findings consistent with this interpretation. They attempted to elicit reports of transparency among reals and simulators by asking subjects about an unusual quality of their image ("shininess") before assessing them for (cued) transparency. Although significant proportions of both reals and simulators reported shiny images, only one of fifteen fakers subsequently reported transparency. These data suggest that even when subjects are set to report unusual aspects of their hallucinations, queries for transparency actually expose simulators to demands for reporting solid rather than transparent images.

The notion that reals and simulators are affected differentially by queries about transparency is consistent with a large body of literature (Spanos, 1986a) that indicates the existence of reliable treatment effects associated with simulating instructions. The presence of such effects suggests caution before interpreting reliable real/simulator differences as due to factors unique to hypnosis. These effects also suggest the advisability of including nonsimulating (real) subjects in any real/simulator design.

Simulation Treatment Effects

Orne (e.g., 1959; 1962) originally argued that real/simulator differences reflected the effects of hypnosis per se in high-susceptible subjects. However, more recently, Orne (1979) has recognized that real/simulator differences may reflect treatment effects associated with simulation instructions and should, therefore, be interpreted with caution. Several studies support this argument. These studies (e.g., Lynn, Nash, Rhue, Frauman & Sweeney, 1984; Sheehan, 1970, 1971; Spanos, de Groot, et al., 1985; Spanos, et al., 1987; Williamsen, Johnson & Ericksen, 1965) suggest two reliable patterns of responding by simulators. Importantly, these two patterns appear to vary as a function of the degree of explicitness of the experimental demands.

Several studies (e.g., Lynn et al., 1984; Sheehan, 1970; Sheehan, Grigg & McCann, 1984) have reported a tendency by simulators to show relatively moderate levels of responding when contextual demands do not provide clear information concerning what is expected from an excellent, deeply hypnotized person. Thus, relative to reals, simulators (*a*) showed changes on some sentence completion tasks before being hypnotized (Sheehan, 1970); (*b*) were more likely to follow the hypnotist's instructions when previously instructed to resist suggestions (Lynn et al., 1984); and (*c*) were found to incorporate less misleading information into memory during a test of eyewitness recall (Sheehan et al., 1984). These data indicate that when confronted by a situation in which they cannot determine how a good hypnotic subject would respond, simulators tend to adopt a conservative strategy of only responding to a moderate degree. Such a strategy involves avoiding extreme responses and might be perceived by these subjects as minimizing the probability of their being detected as fakers by the hypnotist (Sheehan, 1971).

A second characteristic pattern of simulator behavior emerges when the demands of the experiment are more explicit. Under these conditions simulators appear to interpret their instructions to fake deeply hypnotized behavior as a mandate to give ideal or complete responses to suggestions. Thus, simulators have been found to outperform reals by showing higher levels of suggested amnesia (Spanos, de Groot, et al., 1985; Williamsen et al., 1965), by "passing" more initial hypnotic suggestions (Spanos, de Groot, et al., 1985; Spanos, de Groot, et al., 1987), and by reporting higher levels of experiencing suggested effects (Spanos, de Groot, et al., 1985; Spanos, de Groot, et al., 1987). These findings are consistent with the notion that when suggested demands are explicit, simulators interpret their instructions as indicating that faking the behavior of a very good hypnotic subject entails giving "ideal" responses, i.e., behaving as if they fully experienced suggested effects.

Advisability of Testing Nonhypnotic Reals

Several investigators (e.g., Barber et al., 1974; Johnson et al., 1972; Spanos, 1986a) have questioned the use of simulators as the sole control group in hypnosis experiments. These investigators have advocated the use of nonhypnotic subjects (imagination controls) matched for susceptibility to hypnotic subjects. Although imagination controls are equivalent to hypnotic subjects in pretested susceptibility, they do not receive an hypnotic induction. Instead, they are simply instructed to think with and imagine the suggestions to the best of their ability. Thus, unlike simulators who simply fake hypnosis or reals who receive an hypnotic induction, imagination controls represented a nonhypnotic, nonsimulating group of subjects. A number of studies (e.g., McPeake & Spanos, 1975; Spanos, Bridgeman, Stam, Gwynn & Saad, 1983; Spanos, Mullens & Rivers, 1979; for a review and discussion of these findings see Spanos & Radtke, 1981–82) compared the responses of hypnotic and imagination control subjects to suggestions for visual hallucinations. These studies consistently failed to find any differences in performance between these two groups of subjects. Thus, in terms of overt criteria, both imagination controls and hypnotics are equally likely to "pass" these difficult suggestions. More importantly, reals and imagination controls report similar types of subjective experiences to visual hallucination suggestions: the two groups are equally likely to describe their visualizations as vague, fuzzy, varying in intensity, and non-lifelike. Significantly, when reals and imagination controls are given the opportunity to rate their experience on the dimensions of "seeing" versus "imagining," subjects in both of these groups typically indicate that they had imagined rather than seen the suggested object. These findings suggest that hypnotic subjects who report "seeing" an object are actually using perceptual language metaphorically to describe their imaginings. Presumably, such a metaphorical use of the perceptual idiom reflects the operation of an implicit and contextually supported analogy between actual and suggested experience.

These findings suggest the following interpretation of real/simulator differences on the transparent hallucination response: Reals who are administered a suggestion for visual hallucination typically respond by generating and attending to an image of the suggested object. However, because imagining with open eyes is a relatively difficult task for most individuals, these subjects tend to experience hallucinations that lack vividness and stability (Rhue & Lynn, 1987). When these subjects are subsequently queried about their visualization, they tend to report honestly on their failure to fully align their subjective experience with the implicit demand of the suggestion to generate a lifelike (i.e., opaque) visualization. In this respect, querying subjects about transparency can be viewed as providing reals with the opportunity to acknowledge their inability to enact a complete response to the visual hallucination suggestion. Simulators, on the other hand, are set by their instructions to give ideal rather than honest reports. To give an ideal report implies reporting phenomenological characteristics that would be present if the subject were actually seeing the suggested object, i.e., stability, vividness, and opaqueness.

Several studies (Johnson et al., 1972; Spanos, Bridgeman, et al., 1983; Spanos, de Groot, et al., 1985; Spanos, de Groot, et al., 1987) have reported findings that are consistent with this differential demands interpretation of real/simulator differences on the transparent hallucination response. These studies tested imagination control subjects along with hypnotic reals and simulators. No differences in transparent hallucination responding were found between reals and imagination controls. However, subjects in these two groups reported transparent hallucination significantly more frequently than simulators. These findings are consistent with the notion that, in order to escape detection by the experimenter, simulators simply follow suggested demands and report "hallucinations" with all the phenomenological attributes of the actual stimulus object.

The finding that transparency responding is not hypnosis specific is clearly inconsistent with the trance logic hypothesis as originally formulated. However, Orne et al. (1986) have attempted to explain this apparent anomaly by arguing that the imagination controls in these experiments were actually hypnotized. According to this "inadvertent hypnosis" argument, defining a situation as being hypnosis is not essential for eliciting hypnotic experience and behavior. Rather, such aspects of the situation as the imaginal and suggestive nature of test items may interact with subjects' suggestibility to produce the hypnotic "state" in the absence of a formal hypnotic induction procedure. In effect, imagination controls report transparent hallucinations because they "slip" into hypnosis.

The inadvertent hypnosis argument involves serious difficulties. To begin with, the notion that persons who respond like hypnotics are necessarily hypnotized provides no means for distinguishing hypnosis from other alterations in experience that may produce similar behaviors. More importantly, the inadvertent hypnosis argument implies that any type of activity involving either imaginal and/or persuasive factors will lead to persons quietly slipping into hypnosis. As Spanos (1986b) has indicated, this implication suggests that in daily life, persons are often unwittingly hypnotizing or being hypnotized by others. In effect, such mundane activities as conversing with others, watching television, or undergoing psychotherapy would lead to people quietly "slipping" into hypnosis.

The inadvertent hypnosis argument also contradicts the available experimental evidence. For instance, Spanos, Bridgeman, et al. (1983) asked their real, imagination control, and simulating subjects to rate how deeply hypnotized they were during a visual hallucination suggestion. In contrast to the predictions of the inadvertent hypnosis hypothesis, they found that imagination controls gave significantly lower depth ratings than either hypnotic or simulating subjects. Similarly, Obstoj and Sheehan (1977) asked groups of hypnotic and imagination control subjects if they had experienced any effects of hypnosis during trance logic testing. They reported that only one of thirty-six imagination controls indicated experiencing any effects of hypnosis. Nevertheless, the hypnotic and imagination control subjects showed similar rates of trance logic responding. These findings are inconsistent with the notion that imagination controls inadvertently "slip" into hypnosis. They are, however, consistent with a large body of data (cf. Barber et al., 1974) that indicates that the definition of the situation as involving hypnosis is a potent factor in shaping subjects' attributions about their experience and behavior.

Additional Trance Logic Tests

Since Orne's (1959) original report, a number of additional indicators of trance logic have appeared in the literature (cf. Hilgard, 1965; Peters, 1973; Obstoj & Sheehan, 1977). The two most frequently used of these more recent indicators are the negative hallucination and incongruous writing tests. A test of the negative hallucination response usually involves suggesting to subjects that an object (e.g., a wastebasket) placed directly in front of them has disappeared. Subjects are then instructed to walk across the room to some point behind the wastebasket. Subjects who pass this suggestion and subsequently walk around (rather than bump into) the "missing" object are considered to show trance logic. Similarly, subjects who accept a suggestion for age regression and subsequently write correctly a complex sentence that would be impossible for a child to write (e.g., "I am participating in a psychological experiment") are scored as showing the incongruous writing response to trance logic.

Several studies (e.g., Obstoj & Sheehan, 1977; Peters, 1973; Spanos, de Groot, et al., 1985; Spanos, de Groot, et al., 1987) have tested subjects on a number of trance logic tests. Interestingly, besides the transparent hallucination index, only the incongruous writing test has shown any success at differentiating reals from simulators. However, even this item failed to discriminate between real and simulating subjects in all of the studies in which it was used. Thus, although Nogrady et al. (1983), Obstoj and Sheehan (1977), Spanos, de Groot, et al. (1985), and Spanos et al. (1987) reported significantly higher frequencies of incongruous writing by reals than simulators. Lynn et al. (1985) and Peters (1973) reported no significant difference between their subjects on this index. Although the reason for these inconsistencies remains to be addressed, the lack of replicable findings for this criterion calls into question its utility as an indicator of supposed real/simulator differences.

Kihlstrom (1985) suggested that although individual trance logic tests often fail to differentiate between reals and simulators, significant gains in discriminative power can, nonetheless, be achieved by summing subjects' responses to a number of trance logic indicators. Kihlstrom (1985) based this contention on earlier findings reported by Peters (1973). Peters (1973) tested real and simulating subjects on a variety of purported trance logic measures. Although, when taken individually, a significant real/simulator difference only emerged on the transparency index, Peters (1973) reported significantly higher scoring by reals than simulators on a sum of their individual trance logic responses. Importantly, however, Peters (1973) did not assess the ability of his trance logic aggregate to discriminate reals from simulators once the critical transparency item had been removed from the index. Because the transparency test differentiated reals from simulators when taken individually, Kihlstrom's (1985) claim for the greater discriminative power of trance logic batteries can only be evaluated by removing this test from these aggregates. Recently, Stanley et al. (1986) performed just such a test. Using a battery of trance logic tests, they reported that removing the transparency item from their computation of an overall trance logic score resulted in a failure to find a significant real/simulator difference.

Another problem associated with summing across trance logic indicators is that these indicators typically fail to intercorrelate. For instance, Spanos, de Groot, et al. (1985) performed an analysis of Peters's (1973) data and failed to obtain any significant associations among items. Similarly, Obstoj and Sheehan (1977) reported only a "sporadic" pattern of association among the various tests in their trance logic battery. Importantly, Spanos, de Groot, et al. (1985) and Spanos, de Groot, et al. (1987) reported that even trance logic tests that discriminated between reals and simulators failed to intercorrelate significantly. These findings call into question the procedure of summing across purported trance logic indicators. They are also inconsistent with the idea of trance logic as a cognitive dimension underlying trance logic test performance.

In his original report, Orne (1959) indicated that trance logic responding was positively related to hypnotic susceptibility. Obstoj and Sheehan (1977) tested this hypothesis by administering several trance logic tests to subjects who had previously undergone hypnotic susceptibility testing. In line with Orne's (1959) prediction, Obstoj and Sheehan (1977) reported a significant positive correlation between subjects' susceptibility scores and a sum of their responses to the trance logic tests. Although this finding indicates support for the trance logic hypothesis, the procedure used by Obstoj and Sheehan (1977) most likely confounded trance logic responding with susceptibility. Typically, trance logic testing involves a two-stage procedure: Subjects must first pass a suggestion before they can be tested for a trance logic response. However, because most trance logic tests involve difficult suggestions, it is unlikely that low- or medium-susceptible subjects will pass these initial suggestions, let alone show trance logic. Nonetheless, in calculating the aggregate trance logic scores for their subjects, Obstoj and Sheehan (1977) simply summed the number of trance logic responses without taking into account the number of suggestions subjects passed. One probable consequence of this procedure may have been that only high susceptibles showed trance logic, because only these subjects passed a sufficient number of the initial suggestions.

In fact, it would be difficult to test for a relationship between susceptibility and trance logic. The difficulty of most trance logic suggestions implies that only a truncated range of susceptibility scores would be available for testing this relationship. The only practical alternative involves assessing subjects on dimensions that are related to susceptibility but usually yield a wider range of scores. According to the trance logic hypothesis, trance logic should be associated with a high degree of hypnotic responsiveness. Therefore, trance logic responding should be positively associated with measures of the extent to which subjects report experiencing suggested effects. In contrast to this prediction, but consistent with the differential demands hypothesis, Spanos, de Groot, et al. (1987) found that measures of the intensity with which subjects experienced suggestions were inversely related to measures of incongruous writing and transparency reporting.

Taken together, these findings pose serious problems for the trance logic hypothesis. This hypothesis simply cannot provide an explanation for the superior discriminative power of the incongruous writing and transparency tests over other purported measures of trance logic. The validity of the trance logic construct is also jeopardized by findings that trance logic items fail to intercorrelate in any meaningful fashion across studies. Finally, the trance logic hypothesis is contradicted by findings that the performance of hypnotic subjects on trance logic items that discriminate reals from simulators is negatively rather than positively related to the intensity of subjects' experience of these suggestions.

Although these findings are inconsistent with the trance logic hypothesis, they can be parsimoniously explained in terms of the differential demands hypothesis. According to this hypothesis, real/simulator differences emerge on the transparency and incongruous writing tests because these items actually measure incomplete responding to difficult suggestions. Unlike most purported trance logic measures, the criterion for scoring these responses involves a failure to fulfill suggested demands completely. For instance, under conditions of low demands for correct spelling, a hypnotically age-regressed subject's response of writing like a child but spelling like an adult would reflect his/her inability to fully retain the perspective of being a child for the entire duration of the age-regression suggestion. The notion that transparency reporting and incongruous writing actually tap incomplete responding is consistent with findings that these tests are inversely related to the intensity of subjects' experience of these suggestions. The incomplete responding account is also supported by reports that imagination controls also show incongruous writing (e.g., Spanos et al., 1985; Spanos et al., 1987).

Although responses to other trance logic measures might conceivably involve an element of incomplete responding also, the differential demands hypothesis suggests that their failure to discriminate between real and simulating subjects reflects their contamination by such potentially extraneous factors as situational demands and/or interference from intervening tasks. For instance, during a test of the negative hallucination response, subjects who passed the suggestion are typically asked to look around the room and describe everything they see. Subjects are then given a suggestion that an object beyond the negatively hallucinated stimulus (e.g., a wastebasket) is becoming too heavy for them to lift. Finally, after this series of intervening tasks subjects are assessed for the negative hallucination response when they go to pick up the "heavy" object. At this point, their response of walking around the wastebasket (the trance logic response) might reflect an incomplete response, simple forgetting, or an attempt to avoid the noise and embarrassment of kicking the basket over.

The differential demands hypothesis also suggests a possible explanation for the failure of the incongruous writing and transparent hallucination indexes to intercorrelate. Specifically, the failure of these tests to intercorrelate may reflect the moderating effects of the difficulty of these two suggestions. Thus, subjects who respond incompletely to the easier suggestion would also be likely to respond similarly to the more difficult item. However, those who enacted a complete response to the easier suggestion might respond completely or incompletely to the more difficult one depending on their ability to generate the requisite subjective experiences.

Duality in Age Regression

In an early paper, Orne (1951) reported that during suggested age regression to early childhood, some subjects exhibited noticeable shifts in perspective between the experience of feeling like a child and adult experiences. Orne labeled this pattern of responding "dualism." According to Orne, dualism is related to trance logic, because these phenomena both reflect a suspension of everyday logical functioning in hypnotized subjects.

Orne (1951) did not investigate dualism in any systematic fashion. However, this pattern of responding has recently received much attention from Perry and his co-workers (Laurence & Perry, 1981; Nogrady et al., 1983; Perry & Walsh,

1978). In their studies, dualism (relabeled "duality") in age regression was defined as an alternating or simultaneous experience of being both a child and an adult during a suggestion for age regression to childhood. Perry and Walsh (1978) compared the performance of reals and simulators on a variety of purported tests of contralogical responding during age regression. They reported that only the duality index was diagnostic of high susceptibles: Whereas five of nine reals reported duality, not one simulator gave such a response. This finding was subsequently replicated by Laurence and Perry (1981) and Nogrady et al. (1983). These three studies consistently found that about half of reals, but none of the simulators, reported shifts in experience during age regression to childhood.

Two recent studies performed in our laboratory (Spanos, de Groot, et al., 1985; Spanos, de Groot, et al., 1987) augmented a conventional real/simulator experimental design with a group of high-susceptible imagination control subjects. Consistent with the earlier reports by Perry and his associates, we found that reals were more likely than simulators to report duality. However, we also found that imagination controls proffered duality reports as frequently as hypnotics, and more frequently than simulators. Thus, like transparency responding and incongruous writing, real/simulator differences in duality reporting may also reflect the unusual demands associated with the simulation instructions. Moreover, these findings also suggest that, like transparency reports, reports by reals that they felt both like a child and an adult during age regression may be honest admissions by subjects that they failed to completely fulfill the demands of this suggestion. The fact that simulators do not report duality is consistent with their tendency to give complete responses to even difficult suggestions. In this instance, attempts to simulate a complete response to the age-regression suggestion would involve reports by simulators that they felt like a child for the full duration of the suggestion.

Taken together, the results obtained in studies that assessed trance logic and duality responding fail to support the idea that hypnotic responding is associated with unique, hypnosis-specific or "essence like" alterations in cognitive functioning. However, these findings can be parsimoniously explained in terms of the differential demands to which real and simulating subjects in these studies were exposed. Specifically, these findings are consistent with the idea that real/simulator differences in measures of duality and trance logic reflect a failure by reals to fulfill suggested demands completely.

A recent study (Spanos, de Groot, et al., 1987) explicitly tested the hypothesis that real/simulator differences in duality, incongruous writing, and transparency reporting are attributable to incomplete responding by reals. The study involved two independent experiments. In the first experiment, reals and simulators were administered suggestions to regress to age five and to experience positive hallucination of a stuffed toy. Subjects were tested for duality, incongruous writing, and transparency. According to the differential demands hypothesis, these tests discriminate between real and simulating subjects because they measure incomplete responding to suggestions. Following each of the suggestions, subjects rated the extent to which they experienced suggested effects and the extent to which they had been absorbed in suggestion-related imaginings. Finally, subjects were interviewed and their testimony rated for the extent to which they indicated belief in the reality of each suggested effect.

As in previous trance logic studies (e.g., Spanos, de Groot, et al., 1985) reals were more likely than simulators to exhibit duality, incongruous writing, and transparency. However, in contrast to the trance logic hypothesis, but consistent with the differential demands hypothesis, trance logic responding among hypnotic subjects was inversely related to intensity of suggested experience. Thus, reals who indicated belief in the suggested effects were *less* likely than nonbelievers to show duality, incongruous writing, and transparency. This relationship was also reflected in the absorption and subjective experience ratings of reals. For reals, ratings of subjectively experiencing suggested effects and of being absorbed in the suggestions covaried *negatively* with trance logic responding.

In experiment two, we supplemented the real/simulating design with both a high-susceptible imagination control group and a high-susceptible simulating condition. Subjects were tested for both trance logic and incomplete responding. These tests were grouped into three different categories: tests that assessed trance logic exclusively (double and negative hallucination indices); tests that are considered to assess trance logic but that were hypothesized to be measures of incomplete responding (incongruous writing and transparency); and, finally, tests that are not measures of trance logic but that directly assess incomplete responding during age regression, negative hallucination, positive hallucination, and recall amnesia suggestions. The criterion for incomplete responding to these suggestions involved a failure to fulfill suggested demands completely. For instance, subjects were scored as showing incomplete responding during age regression if they indicated at any point during the suggestion that they had failed to maintain the suggested perspective of being five years old. Similarly, reports by subjects that the wastebasket did not vanish completely, vanished intermittently, and the like were scored as incomplete responding to the negative hallucination suggestion. Subjects in this experiment also rated the extent to which they had experienced suggested effects following each suggestion.

Once again, results supported the differential demands hypothesis. To begin with, no differences in performance were found between hypnotic and imagination control subjects (collectively called nonsimulators). Further, no differences were found between low- and high-susceptible simulators. Importantly, no differences emerged between nonsimulators and simulators on measures that assessed trance logic but not incomplete responding (i.e., double hallucination and avoiding the "missing" object). However, nonsimulators were more likely than simulators to respond positively to items that confounded trance logic with incomplete responding (i.e., incongruous writing and transparency). Moreover, nonsimulators exhibited higher levels of incomplete responding to each of the four suggestions (scored independently of trance logic) than simulators. An aggregate incomplete response measure was also devised and intercorrelated with each of the trance logic tests. The overall measure involved scoring subjects' responses to suggestions using a trichotomous rating scale that ranged from no response (subject failed the suggestion), to incomplete responding, to a complete response (subject fulfilled suggested demands completely). As predicted, aggregate incomplete responding was associated with trance logic responding to those trance logic tests that were hypothesized to assess incompleteness (incongruous responding, transparency) but was not associated with responding to tests that assess trance logic but not incompleteness (double and negative hallucination tests).

Taken together, these findings support the idea that reliable real/simulator differences in trance logic actually reflect a failure on the part of nonsimulating "reals" to fulfill suggested demands completely. Thus, only trance logic items that were hypothesized to assess incomplete responding by reals, but none of the remaining trance logic items, discriminated between reals and simulators. In addition, the trance logic items that assessed incomplete responding, but none of the remaining trance logic items, correlated with aggregate measures of incomplete responding to suggestions. The trance logic hypothesis predicts that duality, incongruous writing, and transparency responses reflect high levels of responsiveness to hypnotic suggestions. Instead, our findings indicated that these responses reflected a failure on the part of subjects to remain absorbed in and to completely experience the suggestions.

DUALITY, TRANCE LOGIC, AND HIDDEN OBSERVER RESPONDING

Recall that several studies (e.g., Nogrady et al., 1984; Perry & Walsh, 1978; Spanos et al., 1987) found real/simulator differences in duality reporting. Laurence and Perry (1981) and Nogrady et al. (1984) also reported an association among high hypnotics between duality reports, trance logic responding, and so-called hidden observer responding. Specifically, they reported that subjects who exhibited a hidden observer response during suggested analgesia almost invariably proffered duality reports. During age regression, these subjects also showed incongruous writing of a complex sentence significantly more frequently than did highs who failed to show a hidden observer. Importantly, this pattern of responding only emerged for highs: Nogrady et al. (1983) reported that no simulators showed duality or hidden observer responding. Based on their findings, Laurence and Perry (1981) suggested the existence of "different methods of cognitive processing and different analgesia mechanisms [among high-susceptible hypnotic subjects]" (p. 342).

The "Hidden Observer" in Hypnosis

The "hidden observer" is a metaphor employed by Hilgard (e.g., 1974, 1979) in the context of his neo-dissociation theory of hypnosis. According to Hilgard, consciousness is composed of a number of (usually) interacting cognitive subsystems. During hypnosis, these subsystems may become dissociated to the extent that subjects' awareness of the actual situation may become virtually inaccessible to their hypnotic awareness. Hilgard used the term "hidden observer" to denote that "part" of subjects' awareness that becomes dissociated from immediate consciousness during hypnosis. In particular, this metaphor has often been used in the context of hypnotic analgesia studies to denote an unconscious "part" of subjects that continues to experience high levels of pain during suggested analgesia (see chap. 9, Spanos).

Typically, subjects being tested for hidden observer responding are tested on baseline, analgesia, and hidden observer trials that involve exposure to a noxious stimulus of gradually increasing intensity (e.g., immersion of a hand in ice water or finger pressure over several seconds). During analgesia testing these highly susceptible subjects usually report substantial decrements in reported pain. Following analgesia testing, subjects are informed that they possess a hidden "part" that can experience high levels of pain during analgesia and that can be contacted by the hypnotist with a prearranged cue (e.g., placing his/her hand on subject's shoulder). Results (e.g., Knox, Morgan & Hilgard, 1974; Spanos & Hewitt, 1980) have consistently indicated that a significant proportion of susceptible hypnotically analgesic subjects report near-baseline levels of pain following the administration of hidden observer instructions. In other words, the analgesic "part" of these subjects reports relatively low levels of pain while the purported hidden "part" reports high levels of pain.

The hidden observer procedure employed by Laurence and Perry (1981) and Nogrady et al. (1983) marks a distinct departure from conventional assessments of this phenomenon. Thus, unlike conventional hidden observer instructions that clearly explicate to subjects the pattern of responding that is expected, the item used by these investigators is vague and ambiguously worded. This item does not inform subjects that they have a hidden "part," but, instead, it simply implies that they may have a hidden "part." In addition, unlike conventional tests of the hidden observer that employ a stimulus that produces a gradual buildup of painful sensations, the Laurence and Perry procedure utilizes a punctate electric shock of unspecified intensity. Nonetheless, despite these procedural differences, these investigators as well as Hilgard (1983) argue that this unconventional item taps the same underlying dissociative process as that tapped by the more conventional assessment procedure.

Failures to Replicate

Spanos, de Groot, et al. (1985) and Gwynn, de Groot, and Spanos (1988) administered items assessing duality, incongruous writing, and hidden observer responding to real and simulating subjects, but we failed to replicate Laurence and Perry (1981) and Nogrady et al.'s (1983) hidden observer findings in two important respects. First, we tested subjects for their responses to both an explicit and a more ambiguously worded hidden observer suggestion but failed to obtain a significant real/simulator difference in the frequency of hidden observer responding with either suggestion. In addition, we failed to detect any associations between explicit or ambiguous hidden observer responding and either duality or incongruous writing during age regression. The reasons for our failure to replicate the results of Perry and his co-workers even when using an ambiguous hidden observer item remain unclear, but may be related to the fact that our studies employed long-acting pain stimuli whereas their studies always involved punctated stimuli. When simulators are confronted with an ambiguous or confusing situation and have little time to rehearse or determine what manner of response is called for in such a position, they may do their best not to appear foolish or give themselves away as a faker by adopting a conservative response. The finding that real/simulator differences, and associations between hidden observer responding and measures of trance logic, appear to represent contextually bound phenomena calls into question the validity of the hidden observer as an indicator of a dissociated cognitive subsystem during hypnosis.

TRANCE LOGIC IN COURT

The use of trance logic measures has not been confined exclusively to laboratory settings. In at least one documented case (cf. Orne, Dinges & Orne, 1984), trance logic indicators were used in a forensic context to evaluate the credibility of a defendant. The case of the so-called Hillside Strangler (Watkins, 1984) serves to illustrate the difficulties associated with the assessment and interpretation of trance logic in a practical context. It also serves to point out some basic ambiguities in Orne's (1959) original formulation.

In 1979, K. Bianchi was arrested for his suspected involvement in the murder of several women in the Los Angeles area. Prior to his trial, Bianchi was remanded for a psychiatric evaluation, and during a hypnotic interview, the clinician elicited evidence that he considered to be consistent with a diagnosis of multiple personality. However, given the weight of evidence against Bianchi, and the possible advantages that might accrue by his faking a multiple personality, the prosecution expressed doubt at this diagnosis (cf. Orne et al., 1984). In order to discredit Bianchi's self-presentation as a multiple, the prosecution appealed to Orne as an expert witness.

Orne (Orne et al., 1984) reasoned as follows: If it could be demonstrated that Bianchi was faking hypnosis, then the credibility of his self-presentation as a multiple would also be seriously undermined. Furthermore, if it could be shown that Bianchi faked hypnosis, then testimony given by him during the hypnotic session that implicated his cousin as an accomplice in the murders could be admitted as evidence in his cousin's trial. To determine if Bianchi was in fact faking hypnosis, Orne (Orne et al., 1984) conducted several trance logic tests to discriminate between actual and simulated hypnotic conduct. Included in this battery were the double and transparent hallucination indicators originally used by Orne to infer trance logic. During hypnotic testing, Orne suggested to Bianchi that the latter's attorney was sitting in front of him. He then pointed out the actual attorney in the room and noted Bianchi's response. According to Orne et al. (1984), Bianchi looked back and forth between the actual and hallucinated images and appeared to acknowledge the simultaneous presence of both. In other words, Bianchi clearly exhibited the double hallucination response that according to Orne (1959) serves as an indicator of hypnosis. Despite this response, Orne et al. (1984) argued that Bianchi was faking. As evidence of faking Orne et al. (1984) pointed out that Bianchi did not show "blandness" of response but instead became excited during the hallucination suggestion. They also indicated that Bianchi reported that his hallucination vanished after he had identified the actual attorney.

Watkins (1984) criticized the conclusions reached by Orne et al. (1984). He argued that Bianchi's failure to show "blandness" or "undue concern" is not inconsistent with his having been really hypnotized. Watkins (correctly) noted that there exist no experimental data to verify the notion that "undue concern" over apparent incongruities is related to trance logic responding, or that it differentiates between reals and simulators. Orne has never specified criteria for assessing "bland" responding. Indeed, apart from the enumeration of a few anecdotal examples in his original report (Orne, 1959), his only description of "blandness" is that it resembles "la belle indifference" shown by hysterical patients (Orne et al., 1984).

As indicated above, simulators typically report that their hallucinations appear clear and lifelike. Contrary to this response, Bianchi reported that his image had been "unclear" and "like looking at a strobe light" (Orne et al., 1984; Watkins, 1984). Nonetheless, Orne et al. (1984) discounted this response as evidence of hypnosis because it did not emerge spontaneously during the suggestion. However, as was also indicated above, the fact that Bianchi failed to spontaneously report unlifelike imagery is not inconsistent with the spontaneous responses of highly susceptible "real" hypnotic subjects.

The controversy regarding the reality of Bianchi's hypnotic enactment illustrates the problematic nature of the trance logic construct. Although Orne and Watkins both agree on the existence of trance logic, and the possibility of measuring it with the double and transparent hallucination tests, they apparently cannot agree on exact criteria for scoring these responses. One solution to this dilemma assumes that because Orne originated the trance logic hypothesis, his criteria should be used to assess trance logic responding. Unfortunately, several of the criteria used by Orne et al. (1984) simply do not square with either common practice or with Orne's own past practice. For instance, despite the importance attributed by Orne et al. (1984) to the purported failure of Bianchi to respond blandly, studies that tested the trance logic hypothesis experimentally never used blandness of response as a criterion. With respect to blandness, it is instructive to note that Peters (1973) did not assess his subjects for "undue concern" when testing the trance logic hypothesis. Peters (1973) himself acknowledges that Orne advised him on the selection and construction of his trance logic battery.

Assuming that these issues could be resolved, the fact remains that a sizable proportion of real subjects fail to show trance logic on any particular test or on any combination of such tests. For instance, transparency responding differentiates reals from simulators more consistently than any other trance logic test. However, even with this relatively reliable criterion, a failure to cue subjects for this response can result in the complete absence of transparency reports among reals (cf. Johnson, de Groot, et al., 1972; Spanos, de Groot, et al., 1985; Spanos et al., 1987). Furthermore, even those studies that obtained some level of uncued transparency reports from reals always reported that *most* reals failed to exhibit this response. Even when reals are explicitly asked about transparency, up to 30 percent of them report solid rather than transparent images. More importantly, even when cuing for tranparency is extremely low, simulators occasionally proffer such reports (cf. Spanos, de Groot, et al., 1987). The finding that even the most reliable trance logic test fails to provide unambiguous diagnoses of subjects in carefully controlled experimental contexts argues against its application in a more practical context, such as the identification of a potentially malingering criminal. Indeed, in any given individual case, the diagnostic value of this test or any other trance logic test appears to be virtually nil.

A further problem in all of this concerns the validity of the "hypnosis" construct itself. The notion of hypnosis as an entity, state, or process is, of course, not a denotable "thing," but instead a hypothetical construct of dubious scientific utility. In other words, terms like "hypnotic state," "trance," "hypnosis per se," and so on refer to a scientific fiction that according to some (e.g., Orne, 1959) has heuristic value and according to others (e.g., Barber, 1969; Spanos, 1986b) is both unnecessary and misleading. However, California law reified the fiction of hypnosis-as-entity by ruling that testimony from hypnotized witnesses was inadmissible in court. Purportedly, hypnosis (tacitly viewed as a denotable state or condition into which the person is placed) could cause the memories of witnesses to become unreliable (Udolf, 1983). Since Bianchi had implicated his cousin during testimony given in a hypnotic session, that testimony would become inadmissible as evidence against the cousin unless it was demonstrated that Bianchi had not "really" become hypnotized when he testified. Thus, in order to circumvent a legal ruling that itself was based on the fiction of hypnosis-as-entity, the prosecution chose to treat the fiction as real and then constructed a rather elaborate scenario that would legitimize placing Bianchi's hypnotic testimony outside the bounds covered by the legal ruling that concerned the fiction. To do this the prosecution employed the trappings of scientific objectivity (e.g., expert testimony concerning the performance of the defendant on "scientific trance logic tests" that can "diagnose" the presence or absence of "hypnosis-as-entity").

To examine Bianchi's behavior in terms of whether or not he was really "hypnotized" is to treat the hypothetical construct "hypnosis" as though it were a denotable entity. Beginning with Sarbin (e.g., 1950) over a quarter-century of research has demonstrated not only the circularity involved in the application of constructs such as "hypnosis," or "trance," but also how unnecessary and misleading these constructs can be in attempting to explain suggested behavior. Instead, as Barber (e.g., 1979; Barber et al., 1974) has so cogently argued and demonstrated, suggested responding can be parsimoniously explained as involving situationally specific and attributions and behaviors made by subjects who are both willing and able to assume the identity of an hypnotic subject. From this perspective, it makes little sense to ask whether or not Bianchi was "really hypnotized," because the construct "hypnosis" has little utility as a scientific account of hypnotic responding.

CONCLUSION

Historically, investigators have tended to account for the apparently extraordinary conduct of hypnotized persons in terms of equally extraordinary explanatory constructs. Thus, the claim has been made that hypnosis reflects an altered state of consciousness, or that susceptible hypnotic subjects are qualitatively different from less susceptible individuals. To support their claim, investigators have traditionally appealed to reports of such unusual cognitive phenomena as posthypnotic amnesia, clairvoyance, or, more recently, trance logic, duality, and hidden observer responding. Although often separated in time, these phenomena are related by the underlying notion that there exists a fundamental discontinuity between hypnotic responding and more everyday social conduct.

In time, however, many of these unusual concomitants of hypnotic responding have either disappeared from the repertoire of hypnotic subjects or have been parsimoniously explained using constructs drawn from cognitive and social psychology. Similarly, there is increasing evidence that such phenomena as trance logic and hidden observer responding can be accounted for in terms of contextually generated meanings and interpretations that shape subjects' responses to the hypnotic test situation. In contrast, ideas such as an altered state of consciousness, "trance," or dissociation, besides producing conceptual confusion, appear peculiarly inept at explaining the many subtle variations in subjects' responding as a function of changes in the experimental context. Thus, like other controversies in hypnotic research before it (cf. Ellenberger, 1970), empirical work aimed at resolving the trance logic controversy has served to reinforce the notion that hypnotic behavior is essentially social psychological in nature.

9

Experimental Research on Hypnotic Analgesia

Nicholas P. Spanos

Much contemporary research in hypnosis is organized around two major theoretical paradigms. The older of these paradigms has traditionally been associated with the ideas that hypnotic responding differs in fundamental ways from nonhypnotic (i.e., waking) behavior, that it results from an altered or "trance state" of consciousness, involves the operation of unusual or special psychological processes, and/or requires abilities or capacities that are restricted to only a relatively few individuals (Barber, 1969, 1979).

Elsewhere this traditional paradigm has been labeled as the special process view of hypnotic responding (Spanos, 1986b). At the core of special process formulations is a view (often tacit rather than explicit) of hypnotic subjects as passive in relation to the genesis of their own behavior, and a view of hypnotic responding as a set of behavioral happenings or events that are no longer under the subject's personal control (Coe & Sarbin, 1977; Spanos, 1986c). For example, hypnotic subjects given suggestions for limb rigidity and amnesia are typically described as being *unable* to bend their arms and *unable* to recall target information (Hilgard, 1977; Kihlstrom, Evans, Orne & Orne, 1980). From this perspective hypnotic responses are not the achievements of sentient agents. They are, instead, events brought about by psychological processes over which people retain little control.

The alternative cognitive-behavioral or socio-cognitive paradigm conceptualizes hypnotic responding as continuous with other types of complex social action. From this perspective social behavior in general, and hypnotic behavior in particular, is seen as meaningful goal-directed action that is tied to subjects' understandings of the context they are tested in. Hypnotic subjects are seen as actively engaged in interpreting the communications they receive and in presenting themselves in a manner that is congruent with their interpretations and with the social impression they wish to convey (Spanos, 1986c; Wagstaff, 1981, 1986).

In order to avoid misunderstanding, it is worth noting that the emphasis placed by socio-cognitive theorists on notions like role enactment and self-presentation does not imply that public enactments are always viewed as being at variance with private experience (Coe & Sarbin, 1977; Sarbin & Coe, 1979; Spanos, 1986b; Wagstaff, 1986). For instance, to describe a man as enacting the role of "concerned husband" does not imply that the man's displays the concern are necessarily feigned. By the same token, the socio-cognitive view does *not* hold that hypnotic subjects who report lessened pain following an analgesia suggestion must be experiencing higher levels of pain than they report, or that those who fail to report target items covered by an amnesia suggestion must be privately rehearsing the very items they fail to divulge. On the contrary, the socio-cognitive perspective attempts to account for how, and under what circumstances, hypnotic subjects come to convince themselves as well as others that they are unable to remember, unable to bend their arms, and the like (Coe & Sarbin, 1977).

The remainder of this chapter will address the topic of hypnotic analgesia. The bulk of the chapter will contrast Hilgard's (1973, 1977a, 1977b, 1979) dissociation theory of hypnotic analgesia with a socio-cognitive account of the same phenomenon. Hilgard's account has been singled out because it is the most influential special process account currently available and has been articulated in more detail than other special process accounts. Furthermore, the ideas that form the basis of Hilgard's account of analgesia have been employed by him (Hilgard, 1977a) and by others (e.g., Erdelyi, 1985) to account for hypnotic phenomena in general as well as for a wide range of cognitive phenomena (e.g., psychogenic amnesia) in nonhypnotic settings.

For better or for worse, contemporary theories of hypnotic analgesia have been formulated and tested almost exclusively on healthy subjects who were administered relatively transient noxious stimulation under laboratory conditions. Consequently, our literature review will be largely restricted to experimental studies. For the most part special process and socio-cognitive theorists have employed similiar pain testing and assessment procedures. Typically, subjects in these experiments are exposed over several trials to some harmless but painful source of noxious stimulation. The most commonly employed stimuli include limb immersion in circulating ice water or heavy pressure from a tapered wedge lowered onto a finger (e.g., Brown, Fader & Barber, 1970). Ischemia (suppression of blood flow) induced by limb occlusion and punctated electric shock have also been employed from time to time (e.g., McGlashin, Evans & Orne, 1969; Laurence & Perry, 1981). The first stimulation trial is usually employed to obtain pretreatment (baseline) estimates of painfulness. A variety of procedures for measuring pain are available (see Jones & Flynn, this volume), but the most commonly employed in this area are pain tolerance (usually measured as the length of time the subject is willing to undergo the stimulation) and category ratings of pain intensity. Following the baseline trial subjects are usually exposed to one of several treatment conditions (e.g., hypnotic induction plus analgesia suggestion; analgesia suggestion without induction) or to a no-treatment control condition, and are then reexposed to the noxious stimulation.

TWO THEORETICAL APPROACHES TOWARD HYPNOTIC ANALGESIA

The Dissocation Account of Hypnotic Analgesia

Hilgard's (1973, 1977a, 1977b, 1979, 1987) formulation of hypnotic analgesia is based on the notion that people vary widely in their capacity for experiencing dissociations between cognitive subsystems. Purportedly, hypnotic responding occurs when the "part" of the person that responds to suggestions is partially split off or dissociated from the "part" associated with normal consciousness. This splitting of cognitive subsystems implies that incoming perceptual information is processed in parallel by the two subsystems. Moreover, an amnesic barrier constructed between the subsystems prevents the "conscious part" of the person from gaining access to the information in the dissociated subsystem.

For reasons that Hilgard never specifies, many subjects are thought to experience dissociation to only a slight degree if at all, and such people remain unresponsive to hypnotic procedures and to suggestions that call for reality distortion (e.g., suggestions for amnesia, hallucination, analgesia). On the other hand, in subjects who have the capacity, dissociation is supposedly facilitated by the administration of hypnotic induction procedures. Highly hypnotizable subjects are capable of profound dissociation and, for this reason, respond easily to a wide range of suggestions, including suggestions for pain reduction. On the other hand, low hypnotizables have little capacity for dissociation and, consequently, should be unable to respond effectively to suggestions that purportedly require this capacity.

A Two-component Theory. According to Hilgard (1977a, 1979), hypnotic analgesia involves two psychological components. The first component is available to all subjects regardless of their level of hypnotizability and includes such conscious strategies for pain reduction as self-distraction and relaxation. Also included in this first component is any pain reduction produced by placebos (Hilgard & Hilgard, 1983). Importantly, this first component is thought to be relatively ineffective and, at best, to lead to only small reductions in the magnitude of felt pain.

The second component of hypnotic analgesia purportedly involves the dissociation of pain from conscious awareness. According to this idea, a dissociated "part" of the subject continues to experience high levels of pain. However, this dissociated pain is, for the most part, separated from the conscious part of the subject by an amnesic barrier. Consequently, the conscious part of the subject feels and reports little pain.

The Hidden Observer in Hypnotic Analgesia. It is assumed by Hilgard (1977a, 1979) that hypnotically analgesic subjects continue to feel high levels of pain at an unconscious level, but no longer have access to this dissociated pain. One of the most controversial aspects of Hilgard's formulation holds that, in at least some highly hypnotizable subjects, the experimenter can, literally, talk with the dissociated part of the subject and obtain numerical estimates of pain intensity from that part. Along these lines Hilgard and his associates (Hilgard, Hilgard, Macdonald, Morgan & Johnson, 1978; Hilgard, Morgan & Macdonald, 1975; Knox, Morgan & Hilgard, 1974) conducted a series of experiments in which hypnotically analgesic subjects were taught to give two types of pain ratings. Supposedly, overt ratings reflected the amount of pain consciously experienced by the "hypnotized part" of the person (i.e., the part that responded to the analgesia suggestion), while hidden (sometimes called covert) ratings reflected the amount of pain felt by the hidden or dissociated part. Many of the highly hypnotizable subjects in these studies reported higher hidden than overt pain during hypnotic analgesia trials. Hilgard (1979) interpreted these findings as providing support for his contention that hypnotically analgesic subjects experience reductions in consciously felt pain while simultaneously experiencing high levels of dissociated pain.

The Socio-Cognitive Paradigm

From the socio-cognitive perspective the subject is viewed as an active agent who can engage in cognitive activities of various kinds in order to ameliorate the effects of noxious stimulation. A good deal of work carried out within this framework indicates that treatment procedures designed to encourage the use of such coping strategies as self-distraction, positive imagery, cognitive reinterpretation or transformation of noxious input, and positive self-statements (e.g., "this isn't so bad") produce significant decrements in reported pain and/or significant enhancements in pain threshold and pain tolerance (Barber & Cooper, 1972; Beers & Karoly, 1979; Chaves & Barber, 1974; Chaves & Doney, 1976; Dubreuil, Endler & Spanos, 1987; Grimm & Kanfer, 1976; Friedman, Thompson & Rosen, 1985; Horan, Hackett, Buchanan, Stone & Demchik-Stone, 1980; Jaremko, 1978; Johnson, 1974; Klepac, Hauge, Dowling & McDonald, 1981; Scott & Barber, 1977; Scott & Leonard, 1978; Spanos, Brown, Jones & Horner, 1981; Thelen & Fry, 1981; Turk, 1977; Worthington, 1978). Although these studies often differed from one another in terms of the specific strategies or combination of strategies assessed, their underlying rationale was based on the assumption that subjects can gain at least partial control over their level of discomfort by controlling and directing their cognitive activity.

Direct support for this assumption has been found in studies that assessed relationships between indexes of ongoing cognitive activity and pain ratings. For instance, a number of studies (Genest, 1978; Genest, Meichenbaum & Turk, 1977; Spanos, Brown, et al., 1981) found that even before exposure to treatment, subjects who coped with noxious stimulation by "spontaneously" using such strategies as self-distraction and the generation of pleasant imagery (i.e., copers) reported lower levels of pain and exhibited higher pain tolerance than subjects who focused on and exaggerated the noxious aspects of the stimulation (i.e., catastrophizers). Subjects continued to exhibit wide variability in cognitive activity even after they had been explicitly instructed to use particular strategies. Importantly, however, decrements in pain were correlated with increments in strategy use (Spanos, Brown, et al., 1981; Spanos, Ollerhead & Gwynn, 1986).

Expectations and Reductions in Reported Pain. The socio-cognitive perspective places emphasis on the fact that experimental pain testing occurs in a social situation, and that subjects' responses in that situation are influenced by their understandings of the situation and its requirements, and by their expectations concerning their abilities to cope effectively in that situation (Spanos, 1986b). For instance, Neufeld and Thomas (1977) manipulated subjects' expectations about their ability to cope with noxious stimulation. Subjects were first informed that relaxation enhanced pain tolerance. Those in one group were then provided with false feedback that indicated that they were relaxing during noxious stimulation, while those in another were given feedback indicating that they were not relaxing. Controls did not receive feedback. On a later test trial those who received the positive feedback exhibited significantly higher pain tolerance than either the controls or those given negative feedback. Importantly, none of the groups differed significantly on either physiological or verbal report indexes of relaxation. Thus, changes in pain tolerance resulted from subjects' appraisals of their coping abilities rather than from actual changes in relaxation.

In a related study Marino, Gwynn & Spanos (1988) instructed subjects to use a distraction strategy on one trial and an imagery strategy on another. Subjects in one group were given bogus feedback from personality questionnaires informing them that they had the ability to use distraction effectively but not imagery, while those in a second group received the opposite information about their abilities. A third (neutral) group was instructed to use each strategy on separate trials without any information concerning efficacy. Distraction and imagery were equally effective in reducing reported pain for subjects in the neutral group. In the other conditions distraction was either less effective or more effective than imagery depending upon the expectancy information imparted to subjects. Moreover, in all conditions, subjects' stated expectations closely matched their pain ratings. Those who believed that distraction would produce little benefit reported little pain reduction when using this strategy, those who believed distraction would be effective reported large pain decrements, and so on. Interestingly, the provision of positive expectancy information for a strategy did not produce any greater decrements in reported pain than the same strategy under the neutral condition. On the other hand, negative expectancy information markedly lowered the degree of rated pain reduction relative to the reductions obtained for the same strategies in the neutral conditions. In short, negative expectations concerning the ability to use specific strategies interfered selectively with the use of those strategies and with the extent of reported pain reduction.

Although the findings of Neufeld and Thompson (1977) and Marino et al. (1988) underscore the importance of expectations on psychologically induced pain reduction, they do not imply that expectation is the only important variable in this regard. For example, two studies (Reese, 1983; Spanos, Perlini & Robertson, 1988) found that both placebos and cognitive strategies were effective in enhancing expectations for pain reduction in experimental subjects. In both studies, however, the placebos failed to produce significant decrements in rated pain that matched the significant increments in expectation. On the other hand, cognitive strategy treatments that were effective in enhancing expectations always produced corresponding decrements in reported pain. In a related study, Devine and Spanos (1988) found that four cognitive strategy conditions and a nonstrategy expectancy-enhancing procedure were all equally effective at enhancing subjects' expectations of pain reduction. Nevertheless, significant decrements in rated pain were found for the strategy conditions but not for the expectancy-without-strategy condition.

Taken together, these findings suggest that cognitive activities that lead subjects to reinterpret and/or attend away from noxious aspects of stimulation produce decrements in the felt magnitude of experimentally induced pain. Subjects who hold strong negative expectations about their ability to use strategies for pain control are relatively unlikely to make sustained use of those strategies even when the strategies are available. Instead, these subjects tend to focus on and sometimes to even exaggerate the noxious aspects of the stimulation. Consequently, they report little pain reduction.

Subjects who develop positive expectations about reducing their pain may or may not exhibit such reduction depending upon how their expectations affect the manner in which they deal with the noxious stimulation. For example, experimental subjects whose expectations have been raised by administration of a placebo are likely to believe that pain reduction will occur automatically. Consequently, these subjects are likely to focus on (rather than away from) the noxious stimulation while waiting for the pain reduction to "just happen." Because of this attentional focus these subjects are likely to continue experiencing high levels of pain despite heightened preexposure expectations for pain reduction. On the other hand, people who develop positive expectations about their ability to use cognitive strategies are relatively likely to make consistent use of those strategies and thereby to experience some reduction in felt pain (Bandura, 1977).

Subjects' expectations and their understandings concerning what is required from them are sometimes influenced by relatively subtle aspects of the test situation. For instance, the extent to which subjects implement coping strategies for pain control can be greatly influenced by the tacit assumptions they make concerning what constitutes appropriate responding in the test situation. Along these lines Spanos, Hodgins, Stam, and Gwynn (1984) found that subjects who had not been given by the experimenter explicit permission to cope with the pain to which they were exposed often refrained from doing so. These subjects later demonstrated the ability to generate and use cognitive strategies for effective pain control. However, in the absence of explicit permission to cope, they deemed the use of such strategies as inappropriate. For some subjects permission to cope was given along with instructions to use specific imaginal strategies. Other subjects were encouraged to cope but were given no information concerning the use of cognitive strategies (i.e., do whatever you can to reduce the pain). Subjects in these two groups exhibited equivalent reductions in reported pain. These findings suggest that coping instructions produce much of their effectiveness *not* by providing subjects with new strategies, but instead, by inducing them to employ strategies already in their repertoires.

Implications for Hypnotic Analgesia. The implications of the work outlined in this section for a socio-cognitive account of hypnotic analgesia are relatively straightforward. From this perspective hypnotic procedures do not possess intrinsic properties that lead to a "splitting of consciousness," "heightened suggestibility," or the like. Instead these procedures constitute meaningful cultural rituals that define the situation as hypnosis by unfolding in a manner consistent with subjects' conceptions of what constitutes hypnosis. Attitudes and preconceptions concerning hypnosis vary widely (Spanos, Brett, Menary & Cross, 1987). Consequently, defining a situation as hypnosis may enhance motivation and self-efficacy in subjects who are favorably disposed to hypnosis, while decreasing cooperativeness and feelings of efficacy in those who are negatively disposed (Hendler & Redd, 1986; Jones & Spanos, 1982). Analgesia produced by hypnotic suggestions and analgesia produced by nonhypnotic suggestions are basically similar. In neither case does pain reduction occur automatically through the unconscious construction of "amnesic barriers," and in both cases, felt pain is reduced when motivated subjects engage in goal-directed cognitive activity that functions to reinterpret or deflect attention away from noxious aspects of the stimulation. Consequently, the socio-cognitive perspective, unlike the dissociation perspective, suggests that hypnotic analgesia is intrinsically no more effective than nonhypnotic procedures that enhance subjects' motivations and expectations for active cognitive coping.

From the socio-cognitive perspective hypnotizability does not reflect a "stable dissociative capacity." Instead, individual differences in responsiveness to test suggestions are conceptualized in terms of differences in subjects' attitudes and expectations concerning hypnosis and hypnotic responding, differences in the tacit interpretations that subjects apply to the demands of test suggestions, and differences in the ability and willingness of subjects to become absorbed in generating and implementing imaginal or other strategies that are congruent with the aims of test suggestions (Spanos, 1986a). By changing the attitudes, expectations, and interpretations of low hypnotizables, it should be possible to substantially enhance their responsiveness to suggestions—including suggestions for analgesia. This hypothesis is, of course, at variance with the contention of dissociation theory that low hypnotizables lack the capacity to exhibit high levels of suggested analgesia.

DISSOCIATION VERSUS SOCIO-COGNITIVE APPROACHES:
THE EMPIRICAL EVIDENCE

In a number of important respects Hilgard's dissociation theory and the socio-cognitive formulation make different empirical predictions. In this section the available evidence concerning these divergent predictions will be reviewed.

Hypnotic and Nonhypnotic Analgesia

According to Hilgard (1977a, 1977b, 1979), hypnotic analgesia is more effective than nonhypnotic (suggestion alone) analgesia. Two types of studies have addressed these issues. In the first type (between-subjects studies) subjects were assigned at random to either a hypnotic suggestion treatment or a nonhypnotic suggestion treatment. In the second type (within-subject studies) the same subjects received both treatments: a nonhypnotic suggestion on one trial and a hypnotic suggestion on a different trial. These two types of studies have typically yielded different findings and, therefore, they will be described separately.

Between-Subjects Studies. Eleven experiments have compared the degree of analgesia attained by subjects who were randomly assigned to either hypnotic suggestion or nonhypnotic suggestion treatments. Four of these studies (Evans & Paul, 1970; Girodo & Wood, 1979; Sapanos, Barber & Lang, 1974; Spanos, Ollerhead & Gwynn, 1986) tested subjects who were unselected for hypnotizability, while the remainder used only highly hypnotizable subjects, or subjects who had been stratified in terms of hypnotizability (Barber & Hahn, 1962; Jones, Spanos & Anuza, 1987; Spanos, de Groot, Tiller, Weekes & Bertrand, 1985; Spanos & Katsanis, 1988; Spanos, Kennedy & Gwynn, 1984; Spanos, Radtke-Bodorik, Ferguson & Jones, 1979; Van Gorp, Meyer & Dunbar, 1985). Only one of these studies (Van Gorp et al., 1985) found that hypnotic analgesia was associated with larger reductions in reported pain than nonhypnotic analgesia, and interpretation of these findings is problematic because hypnotic and nonhypnotic subjects were administered different analgesia suggestions. In all of the remaining studies hypnotic and nonhypnotic analgesia produced equivalent reductions in reported pain. Four of these studies provided postexperimental interview or rating scale data about the cognitive strategies used by hypnotic and nonhypnotic subjects (Spanos, Kennedy et al., 1984; Spanos & Katsanis, 1988; Spanos, Ollerhead, et al., 1986; Spanos, Radtke-Bodorik, et al., 1979). None of these studies found differences between the hypnotic and nonhypnotic subjects in the length of time spent using coping strategies, degree of absorption in those strategies, or in the number of such strategies used. In short, the evidence from between-subjects studies consistently failed to support the hypothesis that hypnotic analgesia is more effective than nonhypnotic analgesia.

Within-subjects studies. A number of experiments have compared hypnotic and nonhypnotic analgesia when both of these treatments were administered to the same highly hypnotizable subjects (Hilgard, Macdonald, Morgan & Johnson, 1978; Spanos, Voorneveld & Gwynn, 1987; Stacher, Schuster, Bauer, Lahoda & Schulze, 1975). In each of these studies reductions in reported pain or increases in pain tolerance were greater in hypnotic than in nonhypnotic subjects.

Hilgard (1977a, 1977b) has interpreted the results of within-subjects studies as indicating that hypnotic analgesia is intrinsically more effective than nonhypnotic analgesia. He has suggested two reasons for why differences in hypnotic and nonhypnotic analgesia have not been found in between-subjects experiments. The first reason is based on the hypothesis that hypnotic procedures facilitate dissociation (and thereby high levels of analgesia) only in high-hypnotizable subjects. Several between-subject studies used subjects who were unselected for hypnotizability. There are relatively few high hypnotizables in samples of unselected subjects. Therefore, the facilitative effects of hypnotic procedures on the few high hypnotizables may be averaged out because between-subjects statistical analyses are insensitive to treatment effects when there is wide variability within the treatments.

Hilgard's (1977a, 1977b) reasoning implies that the superiority of hypnotic to nonhypnotic analgesia will become evident even in between-subjects experiments if variability in pain reduction scores is lessened by comparing only the highly hypnotizable subjects in the two treatments. Contrary to this hypothesis, the between-subject studies that compared only high hypnotizables consistently reported equivalent decrements in rated pain for hypnotic and nonhypnotic analgesia treatments (Barber & Hahn, 1962; Spanos & Katsanis, 1988; Spanos, de Groot, et al., 1985). These consistent findings make it highly unlikely that some small but real pain decrement due to hypnotic induction is being masked by statistical insensitivity.

Hilgard's second hypothesis for why high-hypnotizable hypnotic and nonhypnotic subjects display equivalent levels of analgesia holds that the nonhypnotic subjects may have inadvertently slipped into hypnosis. According to this hypothesis high hypnotizables tend to "drift into hypnosis" even in the absence of formal hypnotic induction procedures. Hence, the pain reductions exhibited by these nominally nonhypnotic subjects actually result from inadvertent hypnotic analgesia. This hypothesis is unable to account for both the equivalence of hypnotic and nonhypnotic analgesia in between-subjects experiments and the superiority of hypnotic analgesia in within-subjects experiments. If high hypnotizable nonhypnotic subjects drift into hypnosis in between-subjects experiments they should presumably drift into it as well in within-subjects experiments. Two recent experiments (Spanos, MacDonald & Gwynn, 1988; Spanos & Katsanis, 1988) also provide strong evidence against the "drift into hypnosis" hypothesis. However, we will delay examination of these studies until we look in more detail at the issue of carry-over effects in hypnotic analgesia studies.

Carry-over Effects and Hypnotic Analgesia. From the socio-cognitive perspective the superiority of hypnotic to nonhypnotic analgesia found in within-subject experiments resulted from a carry-over of expectations produced by testing the same subjects with and without a hypnotic induction procedure. This account is based on the idea that high-hypnotizables are invested in presenting themselves to the experimenter in a favorable light, and in hypnosis experiments this usually means presenting themselves as good *hypnotic* subjects. One implication of this self-presentation is that they should be more responsive when "hypnotized" than when awake. Consequently, testing high-hypnotizables under both a nonhypnotic and a hypnotic analgesia treatment is likely to produce the expectation that they should feel less pain during hypnotic than nonhypnotic analgesia.

To test these ideas, Stam and Spanos (1980) varied whether or not high-hypnotizables who received nonhypnotic analgesia were first informed that they would later receive a hypnotic analgesia trial. Hypnotic analgesia turned out to be as effective, less effective, or more effective than nonhypnotic analgesia depending upon the expectations conveyed to subjects by the order of treatment administration. For instance, subjects who received nonhypnotic analgesia while knowing that hypnotic analgesia was to follow seemed to perform less than optimally during nonhypnotic analgesia, so as to leave room for improvement when later tested with hypnotic analgesia. These subjects reported smaller pain reductions during nonhypnotic analgesia than did corresponding subjects who received nonhypnotic analgesia with no anticipation of a later hypnosis trial. Moreover, subjects who received nonhypnotic analgesia with no expectation of later hypnosis reported as much pain reduction as subjects who received hypnotic analgesia.

Subjects in the Stam and Spanos (1980) study seemed to meet implicit expectations for different amounts of pain reductions by selectively using coping strategies that led to the desired results. When treatment demands called for high levels of pain reduction, subjects spent much time engaged in coping imagery and reported low levels of pain. When implicit demands called for only small pain reductions (despite the explicit requests of the analgesia suggestion), subjects engaged in little coping imagery and reported high levels of pain.

The findings of the Stam and Spanos (1980) study are similar to the findings of those nonhypnotic studies (Marino et al., 1988; Spanos, Hodgins et al., 1984) that indicated that subjects were highly sensitive to and often moderated their pain reports and strategy usage in terms of the demands conveyed by relatively subtle aspects of the test situation. Taken together, the findings of the Stam and Spanos (1980) study and the nonhypnotic pain studies (Marino et al., 1988; Spanos, Hodgins, et al., 1984) underscore the important role of contextual factors in guiding subjects interpretations of the test situation, as well as the role of motivational factors in leading subjects to perform in terms of those expectations.

Carry-over Effects and "Drifting into Hypnosis." Hilgard, it will be recalled, explained the equivalent pain reductions found in hypnotic and nonhypnotic treatments by suggesting that highly hypnotizable nonhypnotic subjects inadvertently "drift into hypnosis" when given analgesia suggestions. Hilgard and

Tart (1966) further suggested that subjects can tell when they have "drifted in." Consequently, high-hypnotizables should be explicitly admonished *not* to slip into hypnosis during analgesia testing. Furthermore, as a check on whether or not they "slipped in," subjects can be instructed to rate the level to which they became hypnotized (i.e., hypnotic depth ratings) during analgesia testing. Hilgard (1977b) has outlined these ideas as follows:

> Highly hypnotizable persons readily drift into hypnosis when given any kind of suggestions, so that a comparison of waking and hypnotic condition is inappropriate if the comparison is made of waking and hypnotic suggestion without correcting for drifting into hypnosis in the so-called waking condition . . . . [Highly hypnotizable subjects] if not advised against it will use their hypnotic abilities when given suggestions in the waking state, especially if confronted with something unplesant such as a pain.

In short, Hilgard's (1977b) recommended procedure for analgesia testing involves informing high-hypnotizables that they will be tested under both non-hypnotic and hypnotic conditions and then admonishing them to not "slip into hypnosis" during the nonhypnotic treatment. Embedded in all of this is the assumption that degree of analgesia and degree ("depth") of hypnosis are inextricably intertwined. Because high hypnotic depth (i.e., dissociation) is seen as a requirement for high levels of analgesia, subjects should be *unable* to experience high degrees of analgesia unless they attain high hypnotic depth (i.e., unless they dissociate).

From a socio-cognitive perspective, Hilgard's (1977b) testing procedures are tantamount to informing high-hypnotizables that they should refrain from exhibiting high levels of analgesia on the nonhypnosis trial so that they can perform maximally and thereby "shine" on the hypnosis trial. However, the socio-cognitive perspective also suggests that the relationship between hypnotic depth ratings and degree of analgesia is context dependent and related to subjects' expectations. For this reason it should be possible to create situations in which high hypnotizables respond counter to Hilgard's (1977b) hypothesis, situations in which these subjects report high levels of analgesia while, at the same time, rating themselves as not hypnotized.

Two recent experiments addressed this issue. Spanos, MacDonald, et al. (1988) first tested highly hypnotizable subjects for hypnotic analgesia and then tested these same subjects on a nonhypnotic analgesia trial. Information given to subjects in one treatment admonished them against drifting into hypnosis and implied that they would experience little analgesia on the nonhypnotic trial. Subjects in a second treatment were also admonished against slipping into hypnosis on the nonhypnotic trial. However, these subjects were explicitly informed that they were likely to reduce pain at least as much if not more on the nonhypnotic trial and were provided with a legitimating rationale for why such an effect was likely.

Subjects who were informed that hypnosis was the more effective treatment exhibited larger increments of pain tolerance and higher ratings of hypnotic depth on the hypnotic than on the nonhypnotic trial. Subjects informed that nonhypnotic analgesia was at least as effective as hypnotic analgesia also reported much higher hypnotic depth on the hypnotic than on the nonhypnotic trial. Despite this, however, these subjects exhibited equivalent increments of pain tolerance on the two trials. In a related study, Spanos and Katsanis (1988) also provided high-hypnotizable nonhypnotic subjects with a rationale that justified their experiencing high levels of suggested analgesia while remaining unhypnotized. These nonhypnotic subjects exhibited as much analgesia as corresponding hypnotic subjects. Despite these equivalent levels of analgesia, the nonhypnotic subjects reported much lower levels of hypnotic depth than the hypnotic subjects.

Taken together the findings of Spanos, MacDonald, et al. (1988) and Spanos and Katsanis (1988) support the contention that hypnotic analgesia is no more effective than nonhypnotic analgesia and underscore the importance of contextual factors and expectations in determining when hypnotic and nonhypnotic treatments will yield equivalent levels of analgesia and when they will yield different levels. Contrary to Hilgard (1977b), these studies also indicate that there is no intrinsic relationship between "hypnotic depth" and degree of suggested pain reduction. High-hypnotizables need not be seen as "slipping into hypnosis" when exhibiting large pain reductions in nonhypnotic settings. On the contrary, when given an appropriate legitimating context, high hypnotizables in nonhypnotic conditions report high levels of analgesia even when they have been explicitly admonished against slipping into hypnosis, and when they rate themselves as unhypnotized.

Interpretational Sets and Cognitive Strategies. In a recent study, Miller and Bowers (1986) acknowledged that nonhypnotic instructions were as effective as hypnotic suggestions at producing analgesia. They argued, however, that the psychological mechanisms underlying pain reduction differed in the two cases. From their perspective nonhypnotic analgesia results from subjects' use of cognitive strategies, while hypnotic analgesia results from the operation of an unconscious dissociative mechanism.

Miller and Bowers (1986) compared subjects who were administered stress inoculation procedures with those administered hypnotic analgesia. Unfortunately, the study contained a number of methodological and statistical inadequacies that make many of its findings unclear and difficult to interpret (cf. Nolan & Spanos, 1987, for a critique of that study). Nevertheless the findings relevant to our present purposes were relatively clear-cut. Miller and Bowers (1986) claimed that subjects who reported reduced pain following stress inoculation usually reported that they used cognitive coping strategies during the analgesia test trial. For instance, these subjects stated that they attempted to ameliorate their pain by distracting themselves, imagining events inconsistent with pain, and so on. Supposedly, however, subjects who reduced pain with hypnotic analgesia did not report the use of cognitive coping strategies. Miller and Bowers (1986) took the absence of reported strategies by the hypnotic subjects as evidence that pain reduction during hypnosis occurred automatically and unconsciously and, therefore, did not require the use of coping strategies.

Miller and Bowers's (1986) contention that hypnotic subjects failed to use coping strategies was particularly surprising because a very similar study (Spanos, Ollerhead, et al., 1986) found that subjects treated with hypnotic analgesia and those given stress inoculation rated themselves as using equivalent levels of cognitive coping and also as reported equivalent levels of reported pain. Nolan and Spanos (1987) suggested that Miller and Bowers (1986) employed an inappropriate definition of cognitive strategies that led them to selectively underestimate the strategy use in their hypnotic subjects.

In the Miller and Bowers (1986) study, subjects were counted as using a cognitive strategy only if they explicitly indicated that they *deliberately* carried out cognitive activity to reduce their pain. Subjects who reported the use of coping imagery, but did not describe their imagery as deliberate were counted as *not* using a strategy. For instance, the hypnotic analgesia suggestion used by Miller and Bowers (1986) instructed subjects to imagine that their arms felt as if they had turned into blocks of wood or stone. However, statements from subjects like "My arm felt like it turned into a piece of wood" were *not* classified as instances of strategy use because such statements do not explicitly indicate deliberateness on the subject's part.

The importance of Miller and Bowers's (1986) restrictive definition of strategy use becomes apparent when it is kept in mind that their study compared hypnotic analgesia against a nonhypnotic *stress inoculation* treatment. Stress inoculation refers to a set of procedures that explicitly and repeatedly emphasize to subjects that they can reduce pain and distress by deliberately carrying out imaginal and other cognitive strategies. Furthermore, subjects are usually given repeated practice at carrying out their preferred strategy, and repeated encouragement for defining themselves as purposive agents who can control pain and distress through their own cognitive efforts (Turk, Meichenbaum & Genest, 1987).

Unlike stress inoculation procedures, hypnotic analgesia instructions implicitly define pain reduction as an event that happens to subjects automatically. Even suggestions to cope are typically phrased in a passive voice that implies that cognitive and perceptual alterations are occurrences that happen automatically rather than achievements that are actively self-produced (e.g., your arm is growing numb and insensitive, like a piece of wood).

From a socio-cognitive perspective, subjects in both hypnotic and stress inoculation treatments reduce distress through their use of cognitive coping strategies. However, the instructions and procedures associated with these two treatments set subjects to interpret and describe their experiences in very different ways. The emphasis on active doing that pervades stress inoculation procedures leads subjects to develop a schema for interpreting their coping cognitions and pain reduction as self-generated and deliberate activities. Alternatively, the emphasis on passivity and automaticity that typically runs through hypnotic procedures leads subjects to interpret their coping cognitions and pain reductions as events that occur automatically and without their active efforts.

On the basis of these ideas, Spanos and Katsanis (1988) hypothesized that both hypnotic and nonhypnotic subjects could be led to interpret their suggestion-induced coping imagery and their pain reductions as *either* deliberate and self-generated *or* as automatic and effortless, depending upon the instructional sets administered to them. To test these ideas, highly hypnotizable subjects were administered either a hypnotic or a nonhypnotic analgesia treatment. The analgesia suggestion given to all subjects asked them to imagine a heavy glove that protected their hand from the painful stimulation. For half of the hypnotic subjects and also for half of the nonhypnotic subjects, all instructions were worded in the passive voice and implied that their imagery and pain reductions would occur automatically and without their active participation. The remaining hypnotic and nonhypnotic subjects were administered instructions that implied that coping imagery and pain reduction required their active, self-generated efforts.

The findings of the Spanos and Katsanis (1988) study were inconsistent with the variants of dissociation theory proffered both by Hilgard (1977a, 1977b) and by Miller and Bowers (1986). Contrary to Hilgard (1977b), hypnotic and non-hypnotic high-hypnotizables reported equivalent pain reductions, even though the hypnotic subjects rated themselves as much more deeply hypnotized than did the nonhypnotic subjects. Contrary to Miller and Bowers's (1986) ideas, hypnotic and nonhypnotic subjects were equally likely to report the use of coping imagery and equally likely to rate their pain reductions as effortless. In fact, whether subjects described their pain reductions as effortless or as effortful was unrelated to whether they received a hypnotic treatment, unrelated to their ratings of hypnotic depth, and unrelated to their use of coping imagery. As predicted by the socio-cognitive hypothesis, however, ratings of effortless pain reduction were very strongly related to whether subjects received passively worded or actively worded treatment instructions. Hypnotic and nonhypnotic subjects who received passive instructions were much more likely than those who received active instructions to rate their pain reductions as occurring automatically and without active effort. In short, the available data fail to support the hypothesis that suggested analgesia in hypnotic and nonhypnotic subjects results from different psychological mechanisms. On the other hand, these findings suggest that contextual variables play a very potent role in effecting the attributions of causality that both hypnotic and nonhypnotic subjects apply to their suggestion-induced pain reductions.

Hypnotizability and Suggested Analgesia

Recall that in Hilgard's (1977a, 1979) formulation hypnotizability, to a large degree, reflects dissociative capacity, and low-hypnotizables are conceptualized as lacking the capacity to dissociate. From this perspective, low-hypnotizables should be unable to experience high levels of suggested analgesia in either hypnotic or nonhypnotic contexts. A number of studies have reported significant correlations between pretested hypnotizability and degree of suggested analgesia both in hypnotic subjects (Hilgard & Hilgard, 1983; Price & Barber, 1987; Spanos, Ollerhead, et al., 1986) and in nonhypnotic subjects (Farthing, Venturino & Brown, 1984; Spanos, McNeil, Gwynn & Stam, 1984; Spanos, Stam & Brazil, 1981).

Moreover, several studies found that the strength of the relationship between hypnotizability and degree of suggested analgesia was of approximately the same magnitude in hypnotic and nonhypnotic subjects (Evans & Paul, 1970; Spanos, Radtke-Bodorik, Ferguson & Jones, 1979). These correlational findings are, of course, consistent with Hilgard's (1977a, 1979) dissociation hypothesis. However, they are equally consistent with a socio-cognitive perspective.

Our socio-cognitive formulation suggests that both high- and low-hypnotizables may possess cognitive abilities that are helpful in ameliorating pain and distress. However, low hypnotizables may come to view themselves as unwilling or unable to respond maximally to the kinds of suggestions associated with hypnosis (Spanos, 1986a). As we saw in the previous section, suggestions for analgesia are often phrased in the passive voice to imply that pain reductions will occur automatically, and furthermore, they often ask subjects to experience specific patterns of imaginings. In both of these respects analgesia suggestions closely resemble the suggestions employed on the standardized scales commonly used to assess hypnotizability (Spanos, 1986a). Subjects who obtain low scores on these scales often hold relatively negative attitudes toward hypnosis and relatively low expectations concerning their own hypnotic responding, even before they undergo hypnotizability testing (Barber, 1969; Spanos, Brett, Menary & Cross, 1987; Katsanis, Barnard & Spanos, 1988). Poor performance during hypnotizability testing is likely to strengthen the view these subjects already have of themselves as unwilling or unable to respond to hypnotic procedures. Low-hypnotizables who notice the similarities between analgesia suggestions and the suggestions used to test hypnotizability are likely to transfer their negative attitudes and expectations concerning hypnosis to the analgesia test situation. Consequently, they are likely to define themselves as unwilling or unable to respond effectively to suggestions for analgesia. These considerations suggest that the commonly obtained correlation between pretested levels of hypnotizability and degree of suggested analgesia may be context dependent and likely to break down unless the two testing situations are implicitly or explicitly defined as related to each other. Relatedly, these ideas also imply that it should be possible to create situations in which low-hypnotizable subjects exhibit as much suggested analgesia as high-hypnotizable hypnotic and nonhypnotic subjects.

Analgesia in Low-Hypnotizables. Support for the above ideas has been obtained in a number of recent studies. For instance, Spanos, Hodgins, et al. (1984) found a significant correlation between hypnotizability and suggested analgesia in nonhypnotic subjects when hypnotizability testing preceded the analgesia-testing session. However, when analgesia testing preceded hypnotizability testing the correlation between these variables dropped to nonsignificance. Somewhat relatedly, Spanos, Ollerhead, et al. (1986) compared reductions in reported pain in subjects who received hypnotic analgesia, or brief nonhypnotic instructions to "do whatever you can" to reduce the pain, or nonhypnotic stress inoculation. The three procedures were equally effective in reducing reported pain. Nevertheless, pretested hypnotizability correlated significantly with degree of analgesia *only* in the hypnotic treatment. In the "do whatever" and stress inoculation treatments high- and low-hypnotizables reported pain reductions of equivalent magnitudes.

Two experiments compared the degree of pain reduction reported by high- and low-hypnotizables assigned to external distraction (shadowing words) or suggested analgesia conditions (Farthing et al., 1984; Spanos, McNeil, et al., 1984). Both studies found that highs reported less pain than lows with suggested analgesia. With distraction, however, both highs and lows reported as much pain reduction as the highs given suggested analgesia, and more pain reduction than the lows given suggested analgesia. These findings are inconsistent with Hilgard's (1977b) hypothesis that conscious distraction is a less effective pain reducer than dissociation (supposedly induced by suggestion in highs), and with his hypothesis that low-hypnotizables are unable to match the pain reductions obtained with suggestion in high-hypnotizables who have not been instructed against drifting into hypnosis.

In two other studies (D'Eon & Perry, 1983; Spanos & O'Hara, 1988) subjects were allowed to choose between a distraction (shadowing letters) or an imagery strategy, and then to employ the strategy of their choice in an attempt to reduce pain. In both studies, hypnotizability failed to predict which strategy subjects chose. More important, hypnotizability also failed to predict degree of reported pain reduction either in subjects who chose imagery or in those who chose distraction.

Spanos, Lush, and Gwynn (1988) exposed low-hypnotizables to a one-session training program designed to enhance hypnotizability by teaching subjects appropriate attitudes, imagery strategies, and interpretations of suggested demands. Training or practice in suggested analgesia was *not* part of the training program. As in other studies that have employed this training package (e.g., Gorassini & Spanos, 1986; Spanos, Robertson, Menary & Brett, 1986), about half of Spanos, Lush, et al.'s (1988) low-hypnotizables scored in the high-hypnotizability range following training. These "created highs" were then compared on a test of suggested analgesia to subjects who attained high scores without training (i.e., natural highs), as well as to low-hypnotizables who did not undergo training. The created highs and the natural highs reported equivalent reductions in pain, and more pain reduction than the low-hypnotizable controls. Both the finding that low hypnotizables exhibited large gains on hypnotizability scales and the finding that these subjects then exhibited as much suggested analgesia as high-hypnotizables contradict Hilgard's (1977a) dissociation formulation.

The findings of Spanos, Lush, et al. (1988) should not be interpreted to mean that training for the enhancement of hypnotizability is required ·before low-hypnotizables can match the suggested analgesia of high-hypnotizable hypnotic subjects. On the contrary, two studies (Spanos, Kennedy & Gwynn, 1984; Spanos, Voorneveld & Gwynn, 1987) have now demonstrated that low-hypnotizables given no training and no externally administered distraction can reduce reported pain to the same degree as hypnotic high hypnotizables. Spanos, Kennedy, et al. (1984) gave hypnotic and nonhypnotic subjects brief, actively worded instructions to try their best to reduce pain. The usual significant correlation between hypnotizability and reported pain reduction was found in the hypnotic group. In this group, hypnotizability also correlated significantly with increments in the use of cognitive coping strategies. In the nonhypnotic instruction group, however, hypnotizability failed to corrrelate significantly either with reported pain reduction or coping increments. Importantly, the low-hypnotizables given the nonhypnotic instruction reported (*a*) significantly larger pain reductions than the low-hypnotizables given the hypnotic instruction, and (*b*) pain reductions as large as those shown by the high-hypnotizable hypnotic subjects.

In a related study, Spanos, Voorneveld, et al. (1987) first tested high- and low-hypnotizables with a hypnotic analgesia suggestion. As expected, the highs under these circumstances reported larger pain decrements and higher ratings of hypnotic depth than the lows. Subjects were then tested in a final pain trial. One group of highs and lows was readministered the hypnotic analgesia suggestion and, once again, the highs reported greater pain reduction and higher hypnotic depth than the lows. However, for a different group of lows the hypnotic procedures were terminated. These subjects were then informed that low-hypnotizables like themselves are often put off by hypnosis because they are independent-minded and resent being treated as gullible and easily led. These subjects were further informed that they possessed the natural ability to control their own minds and, now that they no longer had hypnosis to worry about, they could use their natural abilities to the fullest in order to reduce pain on their upcoming trial. The lows who received these instructions reported substantially more pain reduction than they had reported only moments before under hypnotic analgesia. Moreover, the reported pain reductions following these "natural ability" instructions were as large as those reported by the highly hypnotizable hypnotic subjects. Despite their large reductions in reported pain, lows given the "natural ability" instructions continued to rate themselves as unhypnotized. In short, nonhypnotic low-hypnotizables reported as much pain reduction as high-hypnotizable hypnotic subjects, and the large pain reductions of the lows cannot be explained in terms of these subjects "slipping into hypnosis."

Hypnosis, Placebos and Hypnotizability. Recall that Hilgard and Hilgard (1983) conceptualized placebos as effecting the first component in their two-component model of hypnotic analgesia. To support their contention Hilgard and Hilgard (1983) cited a well-known study by McGlashin, Evans, and Orne (1969) that compared hypnotic and placebo analgesia in high- and low-hypnotizables exposed to ischemic pain. All subjects received both a hypnotic analgesia trial and a placebo trial, and the placebo trial was always administered last. McGlashin et al. (1969) claimed to find the following: (*a*) Placebo analgesia produced a small increment in pain tolerance that was of equal magnitude for high- and low-hypnotizables. (*b*) Hypnotic and placebo analgesia produced equivalent increments in pain tolerance for low-hypnotizables, but hypnotic analgesia produced larger tolerance increments than placebo analgesia in high-hypnotizables. (*c*) Hypnotic analgesia produced a larger increase in pain tolerance for high than for low-hypnotizables.

Placebo administration is, of course, a form of influence communication aimed at altering subjects' expectations. Consequently, McGlashin et al. (1969) interpreted the superiority of hypnotic to placebo analgesia in their high-hypnotizables to mean that hypnotic analgesia cannot be accounted for in terms of subjects' expectations and motivations or, by implication, in terms of other social-psychological variables. The account offered by Hilgard and Hilgard (1983) is similar; the small placebo effect purportedly reflects the first component of pain reduction, and the larger-than-placebo tolerance increments of the high-hypnotizables reflects dissociation.

Unfortunately, the results of the McGlashin et al. (1969) experiment are less clear-cut than secondary accounts sometimes suggest. For instance, Wagstaff (1981, 1987) offered numerous trenchant criticisms of McGlashin et al.'s (1969) methodology, pain assessment procedures, and statistical analyses. To cite but one example, Wagstaff (1981, 1987) pointed out that when conventional criteria of statistical significance are applied to the treatment means reported by McGlashin et al. (1969), then high- and low-hypnotizables did *not* exhibit significant differences in tolerance increments during hypnotic analgesia. Relatedly, Stam and Spanos (1987) pointed to serious artifacts in McGlashin et al.'s (1969) procedures for assessing pain tolerance. When Stam and Spanos (1987) used a more appropriate procedure for assessing tolerance to ischemic pain, they found that the effects of hypnotizability on placebo and hypnotic analgesia were complex and moderated by order effects. High-hypnotizables administered the placebo trial before the hypnotic analgesia trial exhibited a significant increase in tolerance from placebo to hypnotic analgesia. Low-hypnotizables showed no change in tolerance from placebo to hypnotic analgesia. Under the reverse order (hypnosis first-placebo second) neither highs nor lows showed significant tolerance changes from hypnosis to placebo.[1]

The reasons for the complex order effects obtained by Stam and Spanos (1987) remain unclear but were perhaps related to the fact that ischemic pain grows much more slowly and is less predictable than pain induced by more commonly employed laboratory stimuli such as ice water and finger pressure.

In order to eliminate some of the difficulties found in earlier studies that compared hypnotic and placebo analgesia, Spanos, Perlini, and Robertson (1988) used finger pressure as the pain stimulus and assessed category ratings of pain magnitude rather than pain tolerance. However, the main purpose of the Spanos, Perlini, and Robertson (1988) study was to examine the implicit assumption of Hilgard and Hilgard (1983) and McGlashin et al. (1969) that placebo administration constitutes an adequate means of controlling for the effects of social psychological variables in experiments of hypnotic and suggested analgesia.

Following a baseline pain-stimulation trial Spanos, Perlini, and Robertson (1988) administered a placebo (described as a topical anesthetic that would numb the finger) and a second pain trial to high- and low-hypnotizables. Before a final pain trial one group of highs and lows was administered a hypnotic analgesia suggestion. However, a second group of highs and lows was administered an actively worded instruction asking them to cognitively cope with the pain.

As in the McGlashin et al. (1969) study, both highs and lows exhibited only very small and equivalent reductions in reported pain following the placebo. Moreover, highs reported much larger pain reductions following hypnotic than placebo analgesia, whereas lows did not. These findings are consistent with those reported by McGlashin et al. (1969) and consistent with the speculations of Hilgard and Hilgard (1983).

On the other hand, the results obtained with the active, nonhypnotic suggestion ran counter to the theorizing of Hilgard and Hilgard (1983) and McGlashin et al. (1969). Both high- and low-hypnotizables reported larger pain decrements with the nonhypnotic suggestion than with the placebo. Moreover, lows who were given the nonhypnotic suggestion reported as much pain reduction as highs given either hypnotic or nonhypnotic suggestion, and significantly more pain reduction than lows given the hypnotic suggestion. Spanos, Perlini, and Robertson (1988) also found that subjects' levels of cognitive coping corresponded to their pain ratings. Both highs and lows reported little cognitive coping on their placebo trial, highs but not lows reported high levels of coping during hypnotic analgesia, and both highs and lows reported high levels of coping during nonhypnotic suggested analgesia.

The findings of Spanos, Perlini, and Robertson (1988) indicate very clearly that higher-than-placebo levels of analgesia shown by high-hypnotizables do *not* mean that hypnotic analgesia requires the positing of special psychological processes unique to high-hypnotizables or that social psychological accounts of hypnotic analgesia are incomplete or inadequate. On the contrary, the finding that both highs and lows showed higher levels of analgesia with the nonhypnotic suggestion than with the placebo, and the finding that lows showed as much suggested analgesia as highs in one context and less suggested analgesia than highs in another, underscore the inadequacies of dissociation accounts of hypnotic responding.

In summary, a significant relationship between pretested levels of hypnotizability and degree of hypnotic analgesia has been replicated in several independent laboratories. This relationship, however, is much more context dependent than dissociation theory allows. The relationship tends to break down when subjects are tested for suggested analgesia in contexts that are unrelated to hypnosis. Low-hypnotizables tested in such contexts reported as much pain reduction as high-hypnotizables given either hypnotic or nonhypnotic analgesia suggestions. Furthermore, the use of distraction strategies by low-hypnotizables was as effective as either suggestion or distraction given to high-hypnotizables. Suggestions for analgesia and placebo treatments do not necessarily produce similar results in low-hypnotizables. On the contrary, when given actively worded suggestions in a nonhypnotic context, low-hypnotizables show as much greater-than-placebo analgesia as highly-hypnotizable hypnotic subjects. Moreover, the analgesia effects reported by both the high-and low-hypnotizables appear to be mediated by cognitive coping. These findings very clearly contradict the notion that high levels of suggested analgesia require dissociative capacities that are available only to high-hypnotizables. On the other hand, these findings highlight the social psychological nature of the analgesia test situation, and the importance of subjects' attitudes, expectations, and interpretations in determining the degree of cognitive coping and pain reduction that occurs in that situation.

The Hidden Observer Phenomenon

The findings most frequently cited in support of dissociation theory come from a series of "hidden observer" experiments begun in Hilgard's laboratory (Crawford, MacDonald & Hilgard, 1979; Hilgard, Hilgard, et al., 1978; Hilgard et al., 1975; Knox et al., 1974), and more recently continued in the laboratories of several other investigators (Laurence & Perry, 1981; Nogrady, McConkey, Laurence & Perry, 1983; Zamansky & Bartis, 1985). Although most of these studies dealt with hypnotic analgesia, the hidden observer phenomenon has also been examined in the context of hypnotic deafness and hypnotic suggestions for negative visual hallucinations. All of these studies are premised on the contention that a dissociated part of hypnotic subjects can, in some literal sense, be contacted and communicated with by the experimenter. Regardless of the dependent variable under investigation, the basic design in all of these experiments is similar. In order to understand the criticisms leveled against Hilgard's (1979) interpretation of these experiments, we will examine the design of those that dealt with hypnotic analgesia in some detail.

Hilgard's Hidden Observer Studies. The three experiments from Hilgard's laboratory that examined hidden observer responding during hypnotic analgesia employed highly hypnotizable subjects (Hilgard, Hilgard, et al., 1978; Hilgard et al., 1975; Knox et al., 1974). Typically, these subjects received a baseline pain stimulation trial during which they verbally reported the intensity of their pain at repeated intervals. Afterwards, subjects were administered a hypnotic induction procedure and explicitly told that a hidden part of them remained aware of experiences of which their "hypnotized part" was unaware. For instance, "When I place my hand on your shoulder, I shall be able to talk to a hidden part of you that knows things that are going on in your body, things that are unknown to the part of you to which I am now talking. The part of you to which I am now talking will not know what you are telling me" (Knox et al., 1974, p. 824).

In some of these studies subjects also practiced performing two tasks simultaneously, one in and one supposedly out of awareness. On one task, for example, subjects verbally named colors while "unconsciously" tapping out a pattern on a key-tapping device. Later, during hypnotic analgesia, these subjects were instructed to give verbal (i.e., overt) reports indicating the degree of pain felt by the conscious part of them (i.e., the hypnotized part), and hidden reports (numbers tapped out in a key-pressing code) that supposedly indexed the degree of pain felt by their "hidden part." Both an overt and a hidden report were requested by the experimenter at repeated intervals. Many of the high-hypnotizables exposed to this testing sequence reported relatively low levels of overt pain (i.e., they showed hypnotic analgesia), but relatively high levels of hidden pain. Typically, the open-ended posttest testimony of these subjects corresponded to their pattern of pain reporting. They described having a hidden part that remained aware of high levels of pain (Hilgard et al., 1975; Knox et al., 1974).

Part of the controversy surrounding these findings stems from Hilgard's (1977a, 1979) repeated assertion that hidden pain reports do *not* result from suggestion or from other demands in his experimental procedures. In fact, it is assumed that hypnotically analgesic subjects experience high levels of pain regardless of whether the experimenter gives them instructions for accessing a hidden part. In the absence of such instructions the hidden pain is separated by an amnesic barrier, and both the subject and the experimenter remain unaware that a hidden part of the subject is experiencing high levels of pain. According to Hilgard (1979), explicit hidden observer instructions like those cited above do *not* provide subjects with the idea that they possess a hidden part or with the idea that hidden reports and overt reports should be different. Instead, these instructions are viewed as simply creating a channel that allows the preexisting hidden pain to come to light. For instance, Knox et al. (1974, p. 841) stated that the instruction to elicit hidden reports "permits access to a cognitive system of which the hypnotically anesthetic subject is not normally aware . . . felt pain is reported by the (hidden) system when the apparently more open conscious system is reporting no pain."

On the face of it, the idea that a substantial number of highly hypnotizable hypnotic subjects would *not* pick up and respond in terms of the rather transparent demands contained in the kinds of explicit hidden observer instructions cited above seems difficult to believe. These subjects are, after all, invested in presenting themselves as "deeply hypnotized" and are attuned to cues in the test situation that enable them to self-present as such. The fact that Hilgard (1977a, 1977b, 1979, 1987) has so consistently failed to examine or even consider the obvious social demands inherent in his hidden observer testing procedures underscores the extent to which his formulation views hypnotic subjects as passive responders who no longer regulate their own behavior, and who exhibit little understanding of what is occurring to them.

Varying the Direction of Hidden Reports. The socio-cognitive alternative to dissociation theory views highly hypnotizable hypnotic subjects as cognizing agents who are actively involved in using contextual information as it unfolds in the ongoing experimental test situation to continuously shape and reshape a self-presentation that is congruent with their understandings of the role they have tacitly agreed to enact. This perspective suggests that ratings of hidden pain and reports of experiencing a "hidden self" reflect the interpretations that subjects place on the instructions used in hidden observer experiments (Coe & Sarbin, 1977; Spanos, 1983, 1986; Wagstaff, 1981). Two experiments on hypnotic analgesia obtained support for the socio-cognitive view by demonstrating that the direction of hidden reports varied with the expectations conveyed by hidden observer instructions (Spanos & Hewitt, 1980; Spanos, Gwynn & Stam, 1983).

Spanos and Hewitt (1980) exposed eight highly hypnotizable subjects in one treatment condition to the procedures used by Hilgard et al. (1975) to elicit hidden reports. These instructions were similar to those cited above. They implied to subjects that a hidden part of them continued to feel high levels of pain while their hypnotized part responded to the analgesia suggestion by experiencing reduced pain. High-hypnotizables in a second treatment condition were exposed to similar procedures with one important difference. These subjects were informed that their hidden part was so deeply hidden that it would be even less aware of what was being experienced by their body than their hypnotized part. Subjects in the two treatments exhibited "hidden observers" with opposite characteristics. Subjects given Hilgard's "more aware" hidden observer instructions reported higher levels of hidden than overt pain (the same results obtained in the Hilgard experiments). Importantly, however, subjects given the "less aware" instructions reported lower levels of hidden than overt pain.

Spanos and Hewitt's (1980) findings clearly indicate that hidden observer responding is strongly influenced by the demands conveyed in hidden observer instructions. These findings do *not* demonstrate that hidden observer responding is necessarily faked (i.e., that subjects' private beliefs about what they experienced are necessarily different from their public avowals). For instance, subjects may have met demands to report both relatively high and relatively low levels of pain by sequentially shifting attention away from and back to the noxious stimulation. Oscillations in pain experience produced by such contextually cued attentional shifts might then have been interpreted as emanating from different "parts" or "levels" of consciousness. Interpretations of this kind are common in our culture. For example, people often express ambivalence metaphorically with statements like "I was of two minds about the issue" and "One part of me wanted to do it, but another part held me back." Given instructions that encouraged and legitimated such linguistic usage, and given a strong investment in appearing hypnotically responsive, many of the subjects who participated in hidden observer experiments may well have come to define themselves as possessing mental parts that experience events differently (Spanos, 1986b).

Spanos, Gwynn, et al. (1983) also informed hypnotically analgesic subjects that they possessed a hidden part that could report pain intensity. Initially, however, these subjects were given no information concerning the relative magnitudes of overt and hidden pain (i.e., low-cue condition). If the only function of hidden observer instructions is to access an already-existing cognitive subsystem that "holds" high levels of pain behind an amnesic barrier, then specific information about the relative magnitudes of overt and hidden pain should be unnecessary. When accessed, the "hidden part" should simply report the higher-than-overt level of pain that "it" experiences. Contrary to the dissociation hypothesis, subjects reported no differences in the levels of overt and hidden pain. Later in the test session these same subjects were given "more aware" hidden observer instructions on one pain trial and "less aware" instructions on another. As predicted by the socio-cognitive formulation, these subjects reported higher hidden than overt pain on the "more aware" trial and lower hidden than overt pain on the "less aware" trial.

Simultaneous or Sequential Reporting? According to Hilgard (1979), the conscious and dissociated "parts" of hypnotically analgesic subjects operate in parallel and, therefore, experience their respective pain intensities simultaneously. In support of this contention, Hilgard and Hilgard (1975) stated that hypnotically analgesic subjects give their overt and hidden reports simultaneously. Relatedly, Knox et al. (1974) stated that overt reports and hidden reports occurred "simultaneously or almost simultaneously" (p. 842). Unfortunately, these contentions were not supported with quantitative data. On the other hand, both Spanos and Hewitt (1980) and Spanos, Gwynn, et al. (1983) did provide such data. Both studies found that overt and hidden reports almost never occurred simultaneously. In almost every case, the two types of report followed one another in succession and were separated by an interval of at least .5 seconds. These findings suggest that overt and hidden reports reflect the operation of sequential rather than simultaneous information processing activity. For instance, sequential changes in the degree of felt pain might have been achieved by subjects rapidly shifting attention to and away from the painful stimulation whenever they were instructed to give such reports.

The Hidden Observer in Nonhypnotic Subjects. According to Hilgard (1977b), the hidden observer phenomenon does not occur unless subjects are first "hypnotized." Reports of higher hidden than overt pain were not obtained from high-hypnotizable nonhypnotic subjects. However, these same subjects reported higher hidden than overt pain during hypnotic analgesia (Hilgard, 1977b). Given the carry-over of expectations that we already documented as regular occurrences in within-subjects hypnosis experiments, Hilgard's (1977b) findings are easily explicable from a socio-cognitive perspective. After all, if experimental demands lead high hypnotizables to believe that higher hidden than overt pain is a hypnosis-specific phenomenon, it is not surprising that they respond so as to confirm that expectation. Spanos, de Groot, Tiller, Weekes, and Bertrand (1985) examined these issues by testing highly hypnotizable hypnotic and nonhypnotic subjects for hidden observer responding in a between-subjects suggested-analgesia experiment. Contrary to Hilgard's (1977b) hypothesis the hypnotic and nonhypnotic subjects were equally likely to report higher hidden than overt pain. Moreover, the two groups reported equivalent levels of overt pain and also equivalent levels of hidden pain.

Differing Rates of Hidden Observer Responding. The proportion of subjects reporting higher hidden than overt pain when given conventional "more aware" instructions has varied from study to study (Spanos, 1983). Different experiments have used different instructions and procedures for eliciting hidden reports, as well as different hypnotizability criteria for selecting subjects. Both of these variables have probably influenced the between-study variability in hidden observer reporting. For instance, the clarity and explicitness of the instructions used to elicit hidden reports appear to be particularly important variables in this regard

(Spanos, 1986a). The instructions used by Knox et al. (1974) and by Spanos and Hewitt (1980) were fairly explicit and, in both studies, subjects were also given practice at performing several "hidden tasks" before analgesia testing. Eighty-seven percent of the subjects in each of these studies exhibited a hidden observer effect. On the other hand, Laurence and Perry (1981) used ambiguous instructions that did not clearly specify that higher hidden than overt reports were called for. Only 39 percent of Laurence and Perry's (1981) subjects showed the hidden observer effect. In the low-cue condition, Spanos, Gwynn, et al.'s (1983) subjects were given no information concerning expected levels of hidden and overt pain. Only 14 percent of the analgesic subjects (two people) in that condition reported higher hidden than overt pain, and an equal proportion reported lower hidden than overt pain. The percentage of Spanos, Gwynn, et al.'s (1983) subjects who reported higher hidden than overt pain jumped to 58 percent when high-cue instructions implied that such a pattern of responding was called for. As indicated in earlier sections, several studies (e.g., Gorassini & Spanos, 1986) demonstrated that responsiveness to suggestions can be substantially enhanced by clarifying ambiguous aspects of the test situation and providing practice and affirmative feedback for correct responding. The Spanos, Gwynn, et al. (1983) findings indicate that similar procedures will also enhance hidden observer responding.

Although most hidden observer studies have preselected subjects for high hypnotizability, they employed criteria for high hypnotizability that differed in stringency. Although it is not unreasonable to suppose that subjects will respond to demands for hidden observer responding as a function of their hypnotizability, only one study directly assessed this hypothesis. Not surprisingly, Crawford et al. (1979) found that hidden observer responding was positively correlated with hypnotizability when all subjects received explicit hidden observer instructions.

Studies critical of the Socio-Cognitive View. In numerous publications, Hilgard has indicated that he is aware of the criticisms leveled against his ideas (Atkinson, Atkinson & Hilgard, 1987; Hilgard, 1987; Hilgard & Hilgard, 1983). Nevertheless, in none of these publications has he directly addressed or attempted to counter any of these criticisms. His only response has been to cite two experiments (Nogrady et al., 1983; Zamansky & Bartis, 1985) that he contends have effectively answered the criticisms leveled against his interpretation of hidden observer studies. Therefore, we will examine each of these studies.

In different ways, Nogrady et al. (1983) and Zamansky and Bartis (1985) address issues raised by the socio-cognitive perspective by attempting to reduce the influence of situational demands on hidden observer responding. Nogrady et al. (1983) compared highly hypnotizable hypnotic subjects with low-hypnotiz-ables who had been explicitly instructed to fake behaving like excellent hypnotic subjects. Both groups were administered ambiguous hidden observer instructions that hinted, but did not explicitly indicate, that higher hidden than overt reports were called for. A minority of the hypnotic subjects but none of the simulators given these ambiguous instructions reported higher hidden than overt pain. Nogrady et al. (1983) made the assumption that their hypnotic subjects and simulators were exposed to the same situational demand characteristics. Consequently, they concluded that the higher rate of hidden observer responding in hypnotic subjects than in simulators could not be explained in terms of situational demands.

Contrary to the assumption made by Nogrady et al. (1983), the available evidence now indicates rather clearly that hypnotic subjects and simulators are *not* exposed to the same situational demands. Instead, the explicit instructions to fake hypnosis given to simulators leads these subjects to interpret later test demands in a very different light from that of hypnotic subjects who have not been instructed to simulate (Spanos, 1986b). Furthermore, the differences that are sometimes found in the performance of hypnotic and simulating subjects can usually be accounted for in terms of the different demands to which these groups are exposed (see chapter 8 for a review of simulation studies). For instance, when exposed to ambiguous test situations, simulators often respond more conservatively than hypnotic subjects in order to avoid being "found out" by the experimenter (Sheehan, 1970). Nogrady et al.'s (1983) hypnotic/simulator differences may simply indicate that simulators responded to the ambiguous hidden observer instructions used in that study somewhat more conservatively than the hypnotic subjects. Because those ambiguous instructions did not make clear whether higher hidden than overt pain was the "correct" response, simulators may have been less likely than hypnotic subjects to experiment with a response option that could risk their being exposed as fakers.

The most interesting finding in the Nogrady et al. (1983) study was not the uninterpretable hypnotic/simulator difference, but the fact that more than half of the hypnotic subjects given only a subtle hint for hidden observer responding failed to show a hidden observer effect. When Spanos, Gwynn, et al. (1983) went further and removed even the subtle hint for higher hidden than overt pain, the hidden observer effect was practically eliminated. Taken together, the findings of the Nogrady et al. (1983) and Spanos, Gwynn, et al. (1983) studies are inconsistent with Hilgard's (1979) hypothesis that a nonsuggested subsystem that "holds" high levels of pain invariably accompanies hypnotic analgesia. On the other hand, the findings of these studies are consistent with the notion that the rate of hidden observer responding is influenced by the degree of ambiguity in hidden observer instructions.

Zamansky and Bartis (1985) acknowledged that hidden observer responding in the Hilgard studies was influenced by situational demands. However, they also conducted an experiment of their own that purportedly reduced the impact of situational demands on hidden observer responding. Because hidden observer responding continued to occur in their ostensibly low-demand experimental situation, they concluded that their findings helped "to place the notion of the hidden observer on a substantially more secure footing" (p. 246).

Zamansky and Bartis (1985) used negative hallucination rather than analgesia suggestions. For instance, on one task it was suggested to subjects that when they opened their eyes they would see only a blank page. However, the page shown to subjects had printed on it a highly visible number (e.g., the figure

8). Hypnotic subjects "passed" this suggestion if they reported seeing nothing on the page. The page was then withdrawn and these subjects were given explicit hidden observer instructions informing them that their "hidden part" remained aware of all they had experienced during the suggestion period. When their "hidden part" was instructed to respond, all of these subjects correctly reported the number that had been on the page. Zamansky and Bartis (1985) contended that these subjects had not consciously seen the number on the page, but that their hidden part had unconsciously seen and stored this information. Supposedly, this hidden part was not influenced by situational demands. Instead, "it" simply reported what "it" had seen when instructed to do so.

On the basis of their findings, Zamansky and Bartis (1985) concluded that "the interpretation that the hidden observer report is simply a creation of experimental demands becomes much less tenable" (p. 244). How Zamansky and Bartis (1985) justified this conclusion on the basis of their experimental findings is difficult to fathom. They provided no evidence whatsoever to support the contention that their experimental procedures minimized or controlled for the impact of contextual demands on hidden observer reports. On the contrary, their use of very explicit hidden observer instructions seemed guaranteed to make contextual demands crystal clear.

In order to examine the role of situation demands in the Zamansky/Bartis paradigm, Spanos, Flynn, and Gwynn (1988) gave highly hypnotizable hypnotic subjects a negative hallucination suggestion and then showed them a page with the number 18 printed on it. Half of those who reported that the page was blank were given standard hidden observer instructions implying that their hidden part knew the number that had been on the page. The remaining half of these subjects were informed that their hidden part reversed everything that it saw. Because the page with the number had been removed before administration of hidden observer instructions, subjects in the reversal condition could give the correct response only by knowing that the page contained an 18, knowing that the reverse of 18 is 81, and responding to demands for the reversed number. All of the subjects in the standard and reversal conditions responded in terms of their respective situational demands. Those in the standard condition all reported having seen an 18 while all in the reversal condition reported having seen an 81.

Many of Spanos, Flynn, et al.'s (1988) subjects failed the initial negative hallucination suggestion (they reported seeing the 18 on the page). These subjects were informed that they possessed a part so deeply hidden that "it" would be unable to see what their "hypnotized part" had seen. Despite initially failing the suggestion, 46 percent of these subjects gave hidden reports indicating that the page had been blank.

In summary, subjects exposed to Zamansky and Bartis's (1985) supposedly low-demand experimental paradigm exhibited not one but three patterns of hidden observer responding. Depending on the demands under which they were tested, these subjects gave hidden reports indicating that they saw what was there, saw the reverse of what was there, or did not see what was there. Obviously, the Zamansky/Bartis paradigm does nothing to reduce the impact of situational demands on hidden observer responding. On the contrary, Spanos, Flynn, et al.'s (1988) findings using this paradigm are consistent with all of the other literature that underscores the critical role of contextual cuing in hidden observer responding.

More broadly, the experimental work on the hidden observer phenomenon clearly highlights the limitations of dissociation theory. A formulation that views subjects as passively acted upon by nonsuggested, unconscious cognitive events outside their sphere of control is simply unable to account for the range, flexibility, and context specificity of hidden observer responding. The available data make it obvious that such responding is shaped by the social demands that constitute the hidden observer test situation. The manner in which the high-hypnotizables in these studies continually modified their responding in conformance with unfolding test demands underscores the importance of viewing hypnotic subjects as agents involved in creating hypnotic behavior rather than as passive responders who somehow "relinquish control" and suffer the experiences imposed upon them by suggestions.

OTHER ISSUES

Without doubt, the dissociation/socio-cognitive controversies have served as the major pivot around which hypnotic analgesia research has been organized for over a decade. Nevertheless, a number of issues that are unrelated or only tangentially related to these controversies have also been addressed. These will be reviewed briefly in the remainder of the chapter.

Hypnotic and Acupuncture Analgesia

A number of studies have explored relationships between hypnotic analgesia and acupuncture-induced analgesia. Two issues have been addressed: the comparative effectiveness of the two treatments, and a possible correlation between hypnotizability and degree of acupuncture analgesia. When compared in experimental settings, hypnotic analgesia has consistently produced larger reductions in reported pain and larger pain tolerance increments than acupuncture analgesia (Knox & Shum, 1977; Knox, Shum & McLaughlin, 1978; Knox, Gekoski, Shum & McLaughlin, 1981; Li, Ahlberg, Lansdell, Gravitz, Chen, Ting, Bak & Blessing, 1975; Stern, Brown, Ulett & Sletten, 1977). Findings concerning a possible relationship between hypnotizability and acupuncture analgesia have been mixed. Some studies found that high-hypnotizables reported greater acupuncture analgesia than low-hypnotizables (Katz, Kao, Spiegel & Katz, 1974; Kapes, Chen & Schapira, 1976; Knox & Schum, 1977; Knox et al., 1978; Moore & Berk, 1976). Even in these studies, however, the high/low hypnotizability differences in acupuncture analgesia did not always reach statistical significance, were invariably quite small by absolute standards, and sometimes occurred for only some noxious stimuli and not others (e.g., cold pressor versus ischemic pain; Stern et al., 1977). Several other studies reported no differences between high- and low-hypnotizables on acupuncture analgesia (Berk, Moore & Resnick, 1977; Clark & Yang, 1976; Knox et al., 1981).

Physiological Concomitants of Hypnotic Analgesia

Since the 1930s, an extensive series of studies has assessed relationships between hypnotic analgesia and a large number of physiological variables (see reviews by Barber, 1959, 1970; Hilgard & Hilgard, 1983; Shor, 1967). In most of these studies the primary concern was to legitimize hypnotic analgesia by providing physiological evidence of pain reduction that was more "objective" than subjects' verbal reports. Since the mid-1970s, however, the focus in some of this work has shifted toward attempting to identify neuro-chemical mediators of hypnotic analgesia.

Autonomic Correlates of Hypnotic Analgesia. The issue underlying much of the early work in this area can be phrased as follows: If hypnotic analgesia really reduces pain, and is more than just a verbal sham, it should also produce reductions on autonomic indicators of pain that are not under subjects' voluntary control. The autonomic indexes of pain most commonly employed have been galvanic skin response (GSR), heart rate, and blood pressure. Although all of these indexes correlate significantly with intensity of noxious stimulation, these correlations are rarely more than moderate in magnitude and are consistently lower than the correlations between stimulus intensity and verbal report indicators of pain magnitude (Hilgard, 1969). Early studies in this area contained extensive methodological shortcomings that preclude the drawing of reliable conclusions (see Shor, 1967 for a critical review). Although more recent studies are not all without methodological problems, most have consistently pointed to the conclusions that (*a*) neither hypnotic nor nonhypnotic suggestions for analgesia produce reductions on autonomic measures, and (*b*) the degree of suggested analgesia in hypnotic and nonhypnotic subjects (as indexed by verbal report) is unrelated to changes on autonomic measures (Barber & Hahn, 1962; Evans & Paul, 1970; Hilgard, MacDonald, Marshall & Morgan, 1974; Hilgard & Morgan, 1975; Shor, 1962; Sutcliffe, 1961).

Hilgard (1979; Hilgard & Hilgard, 1983) has interpreted the discrepancy between autonomic and verbal report indicators of pain during hypnotic analgesia as support for his dissociation hypothesis. Purportedly, autonomic indexes remain uneffected by hypnotic analgesia suggestions because they reflect subjects' high levels of "hidden pain." This hypothesis has difficulty with the fact that autonomic/verbal report discrepancies occur to the same extent in nonhypnotic-suggested analgesia (which supposedly does not involve dissociation) as in hypnotic analgesia (Barber & Hahn, 1962; Evans & Paul, 1970). Moreover, given the serious theoretical inadequacies of the dissociation hypothesis documented throughout this chapter, there seems little point in using it to account for autonomic/verbal report discrepancies.

At least two other hypotheses have been advanced to account for autonomic/verbal discrepancies. One of these suggests that hypnotic analgesia reflects compliance. This account holds that hypnotic analgesia suggestions do not reduce pain, they simply pressure subjects into reporting such reductions. Since subjects are unable to voluntarily influence autonomic indexes, these indexes continue to register the high levels of pain that are actually experienced (Wagstaff, 1981). As a partial account of hypnotic analgesia this hypothesis is not without merit and deserves more serious consideration than it is typically afforded. We will return to it later.

A final hypothesis suggests that autonomic indexes like GSR, heart rate, and blood pressure are not valid indexes of felt pain. For instance, subjects sometimes exhibit equivalent autonomic changes to painful stimuli and to intense but nonpainful stimuli. As well, subjects simply asked to imagine pain and also subjects anticipating forthcoming pain often show autonomic changes that are similar to those that accompany actual noxious stimulation (Barber & Hahn, 1964; Hilgard et al., 1974; Hilgard & Morgan, 1975; Levine, 1930; Shor, 1967). The generally low correlations between autonomic indexes and the intensity of noxious stimulation mentioned earlier, along with generally low correlations between the various autonomic variables themselves (e.g., Pennebaker, 1982) call into question the validity of these measures as indexes of felt painfulness. In short, changes on autonomic variables like blood pressure and heart rate are a complex function of a great many factors other than felt pain. Consequently, there is nothing incongruous about the possibility that felt pain might be reduced without corresponding reductions on autonomic measures.

Endogenous Opiates and Hypnotic Analgesia. In the last decade, the discovery of endogenous opiates (i.e., endorphins) and receptor sites in the brain for those opiates (Goldstein, 1976) stimulated the speculation that hypnotic analgesia might be mediated through the release of these opiates. This hypothesis gained credence when still-controversial studies implicated endogenous opiates in both placebo and acupuncture analgesia (Gracely, Dunbar, Wolskee & Deeter, 1983; Grevert, Albert & Goldstein, 1983; Levine & Gordon, 1984; Levine, Gordon & Fields, 1978; Mayer, Price & Rafii, 1977; Sjolund & Eriksson, 1976). Direct measurement of endorphin levels is both difficult and expensive and, therefore, the usual procedure in this area is to determine whether administration of the opiate antagonist naloxone eliminates the pain-reducing effects of the analgesic under consideration. For example, suppose that in a double-blind experiment subjects administered naloxone and subjects administered a placebo were given an analgesia suggestion and then assessed for pain reduction. Evidence that sugggested analgesia was opiate mediated would be obtained if the placebo plus suggestion group exhibited a larger analgesia effect than the naloxone plus suggestion group (Grevert & Goldstein, 1985).

Frid and Singer (1979) reported that naloxone partially reversed hypnotic analgesia when subjects were exposed to high stress plus painful stimulation, but had no effect on hypnotic analgesia for subjects in a low stress plus pain stimulation condition. Frid and Singer (1979) did not test nonhypnotic subjects given analgesia suggestions. Recently, however, Bandura, O'Leary, Taylor, Gauthier, and Gossard (1987) reported that, under at least some circumstances, naloxone partially reversed suggested analgesia in nonhypnotic subjects. In contrast to Frid and Singer (1979) and Bandura et al. (1987), a large number of studies indicate that naloxone administration had no effect on hypnotic analgesia (Barber & Mayer, 1977; de Beer, Fourie & Nichaus, 1986; Domanque, Margolis, Lieberman & Kaji, 1985; Goldstein & Hilgard, 1975; Spiegel & Albert, 1983).

It is important to understand that the reversal of hypnotic or suggested analgesia by naxloxone does not necessarily mean that the analgesia effect was opiate mediated. Naloxone can influence the perception of pain independently of its effects òn the opiate system (Grevert & Goldstein, 1985). Consequently, the few positive findings in this area should be viewed with caution. Moreover, the endogenous release of opiates produces systemic effects. However, suggested analgesia can be limited to any body part specified in the suggestion (e.g., the ring finger of the right hand) and can be reversed and reinstated easily and repeatedly with verbal cues (Spanos, Hodgins, et al., 1984). Effects of this kind are inexplicable in terms of endorphin mediation but are easily understandable in terms of cue-produced attentional shifts. In short, the role of endogenous opiates in hypnotic and nonhypnotic suggested analgesia requires further study. Nevertheless, the available data indicate that opiate mediation is unlikely to account for the analgesia effects obtained in typical laboratory experiments that employ intense but relatively transient stimuli under conditions of relatively low anxiety.

What Is Reduced in Suggested Analgesia

Experiments on suggested/hypnotic analgesia have usually used unidimensional category rating scales to assess pain magnitude. For instance, during arm immersion in ice water subjects might be asked to periodically report their level of pain on an 11-point scale, where 0 indicates "no pain" and 10 indicates "excruciating pain" (e.g., Spanos et al., 1979). Frequently, such ratings are made both before and after administration of treatment instructions designed to reduce pain. In addition to or instead of category ratings, it is also common to assess baseline-to-posttest changes in pain tolerance. Despite widespread use, substantial controversy exists concerning the inferences that can legitimately be drawn about subjects' experiences when suggestions produce decrements in pain ratings or enhancements in pain tolerance. At least three hypotheses can be advanced with respect to these issues.

Decreased Perceptual Sensitivity. Perhaps the attentional/cognitive activities induced by suggestions temporarily reduce the ability of subjects to perceptually discriminate levels of noxious stimulation. According to this hypothesis, category ratings of pain intensity and indexes of pain tolerance accurately mirror reduced perceptual sensitivity produced by suggestions. There is, in fact, little evidence to support this hypothesis. Both category-rating procedures (e.g., Poulton, 1979) and pain tolerance indicators (e.g., Mikael, Vendeursen & von Baeyer, 1986; Scott, 1980) are subject to a number of systematic biases that preclude their use as accurate indexes of pain sensitivity (see also chapter 6). Relatedly, the use of alternative scaling procedures, some of which were specifically designed to separate perceptual sensitivity from decisional biases, provide little support for the reduced sensitivity hypothesis. For instance, neither hypnotic nor non-hypnotic suggested analgesia appears to be consistently related to reductions in pain sensitivity when sensitivity is measured with signal detection procedures (Clark, 1974; Clark & Goodman, 1974), functional measurement procedures (Jones, Spanos & Anuza, 1986), or magnitude estimation/magnitude production procedures (Clum, Luscomb & Scott, 1982; Spanos, Jones, Brown & Horner, 1983; Stam, Petrusic & Spanos, 1981). In short, the hypothesis that suggestion-induced increments in tolerance or decrements in category ratings reflects reductions in perceptual sensitivity to noxious stimulation has as yet received little support.

Pain Reduction as Reinterpretation. A second hypothesis holds that cognitive variables influence the manner in which subjects interpret and report their sensory experiences but leaves their ability to discriminate intensities of sensory stimulation unchanged. This hypothesis does not imply that subjects are lying when they rate their pain as reduced following suggestion. Instead, it indicates that the intensity of sensory events may remain unchanged, but the manner in which those events are defined to the self (e.g., the pain level assigned to them) has changed. For example, sensory events previously labeled "painful" may now be categorized in some other way, e.g., "intense but not painful," "numb," "very cold," "prickly" (Rollman, 1977; Spanos, Brown, et al., 1981; Spanos, 1982). This hypothesis holds that subjects who report pain reductions reevaluate their experiences and in this sense feel less pain. However, this hypothesis does not imply that these subjects are less able to discriminate between different intensities of noxious stimulation, i.e., they are not necessarily less sensitive to pain.

With respect to the typical ice-water experiments used to assess hypnotic analgesia, the reinterpretation hypothesis suggests that the sensory experiences of subjects during immersion are ambiguous as well as intense. Such experiences involve a complex of diverse and changing sensations (e.g., cold, ache, throbbing, prickliness) that subjects are forced to categorize periodically along a painfulness dimension with a restricted range of numbers. Suggestion-induced changes in rated painfulness may, in part, reflect attentional shifts to different facets of the sensory complex. These ratings involve the integration of diverse and changing sensory events and the expression of the integration as a single number (or successive set of numbers). This integration may involve weighing various facets of the sensory complex differently under suggestion and no-suggestion conditions. For example, changes in the relative weight given to "cold" and "ache" sensations before and after an analgesia suggestion may be one factor leading a subject to conclude that the water is cold, "but not as painful as before."

In a tolerance experiment such a conclusion might well enhance a subject's willingness to increase the duration of the immersion.

Category ratings of pain are likely to be influenced by nonsensory (as well as sensory) information. In hypnotic analgesia experiments two of the most salient pieces of nonsensory information are expectations of pain reduction created by the suggestion and self-observations of reacting to the noxious stimulation either by coping or by catastrophizing. These ideas suggest that category ratings of pain intensity may involve an attribution process. Because their sensory experiences are ambiguous and not easily classifiable in terms of the available category-scale units, subjects' pain ratings may be influenced by their observations of their own responses to the noxious situation. For instance, those who observe themselves behaving in a manner inconsistent with feeling high levels of pain (e.g., remaining clam, engaging in coping cognitions) are likely to infer (and rate themselves as feeling) relatively little pain. Alternatively, those who observe themselves catastrophizing are likely to infer relatively high levels of pain, and those who observed themselves catastrophize on the baseline test but cope after the suggestion are likely to conclude that the suggestion (or hypnosis) reduced their posttest pain (Spanos, 1982).

A number of studies that employed category-rating procedures during noxious stimulation are consistent with the reinterpretation hypothesis (Bandler, Madaras & Bem, 1968; Kopel & Askowitz, 1974; Lanzetta, Cartwright-Smith & Kleck, 1976; Nisbett & Schachter, 1966). For instance, it is well known that the intensity of noxious stimulation is reflected in subjects' facial expressions (e.g., Prkachin & Craig, 1985). This suggests that during noxious stimulation, feedback from the facial musculature that reflects expression may serve as a source of information for inferring level of painfulness. Along these lines, Lanzetta et al. (1976) induced subjects to display behavioral expressions of either suffering (e.g., wincing) or calmness during the administration of electric shocks. Despite being exposed to identical shock levels, those who displayed suffering rated themselves as feeling higher levels of pain than those who displayed calmness.

As indicated earlier, levels of autonomic arousal (e.g., heart rate) are moderately correlated with the intensity of noxious stimulation (Hilgard, 1969). Interestingly, Nisbett and Schachter (1966) found that subjects' judgments concerning pain intensity were influenced by the attributions they made about the sources of their own autonomic arousal. Subjects were first administered a placebo and then a series of mild electric shocks. Those who were led by experimental instructions to attribute signs of autonomic arousal (e.g., flushing) to the placebo rated the shock as less painful and exhibited higher tolerance for the shock than those who were led to attribute their arousal to the effects of the shock. In short, category ratings of painfulness may be determined at least in part by attributions based on subjects' self-observations of their own behavior, as well as by the magnitude and complexity of the sensory effects produced by the noxious stimulation.

Hypnotic/Suggested Analgesia as Compliance. Hypnotic and nonhypnotic suggestions for analgesia contain very clear demands for reductions in reported pain and/or increased tolerance of the noxious stimulation. Moreover, it is clear from casual observation in everyday life, as well as from the findings of numerous psychological experiments (e.g., Asch, 1958; Crutchfield, 1955; Milgram, 1975; Miller, 1986), that people frequently respond to social pressure by doing and saying the things that authority figures demand of them. Considerations of this kind have been raised for well over a century in support of the hypothesis that hypnotic analgesia may be explicable in terms of compliance (Wagstaff, 1981). In its strongest form this hypothesis holds that hypnotic suggestions do not in any sense reduce the experience of pain or induce subjects to reinterpret or relabel noxious stimulation. Instead, suggestions simply pressure subjects into falsely reporting lower levels of pain than they actually feel and/or pressure them into enduring more pain than they endured on the baseline trial.

Several studies (Gelfand, 1964; Sternback & Tursky, 1965; Wolff & Horland, 1967) do, in fact, indicate that simple requests or mild coaxing without any strategy provision can enhance pain tolerance. As mentioned in an earlier section, the compliance hypothesis can easily account for the verbal/autonomic discrepancies typically found during hypnotic analgesia. Moreover, Wagstaff (1981) described in some detail how this hypothesis can also account for the equivalence of hypnotic and nonhypnotic analgesia in between-subjects experiments, the typical superiority of hypnotic to nonhypnotic analgesia in within-subjects experiments, and the discrepancies between overt and hidden pain reporting in hidden observer studies. By making the reasonable assumption that, in any standard context, there are likely to be individual differences in the extent of complying, then a compliance hypothesis could easily be generated to account for the typical correlation between hypnotizability and hypnotic analgesia.

Despite all of this, a number of considerations suggest limits to the compliance hypothesis. It is important to emphasize that suggestions always call for changes in experience as well as changes in overt behavior. By implication, behavioral change in the absence of corresponding experiential change is defined as cheating. Furthermore, psychological experiments are typically defined as serious scientific enterprises that place a premium on accuracy and honesty. Thus, while experiments may sometimes contain pressures toward compliance, it is important to keep in mind that they also contain pressures against engaging in compliance. These ideas suggest that subjects will often attempt to generate the experiences that legitimize their making the requisite overt responses. After all, the combination of subjective experience plus overt response fully meets suggested demands and avoids any guilt that might be associated with violating implicit norms for honest and accurate reporting (Spanos, 1986a; Wagstaff, 1981, 1983).

Compliance is likely to become a regnant consideration for subjects who are invested in meeting role demands, but are unable to generate the requisite subjective experiences (Spanos, 1986a; Wagstaff, 1983, 1986). Moreover, there is little doubt that compliance sometimes occurs under these circumstances. For instance, subjects who exhibit high levels of hypnotic amnesia sometimes confess to compliance during postexperimental interviews (Spanos & Bodorik, 1977), and many subjects admit to making the overt responses called for on hypnotizability tests when their corresponding subjective experiences were weak or nonexistent (Spanos, Radtke, Hodgins, Stam & Bertrand, 1983).

On the other hand, there are also data to indicate that many subjects respond overtly to test demands only when they first generate the requisite subjective experiences. For instance, recall that Reese (1983) created demands for pain reduction in both a placebo and a coping suggestion treatment. Moreover, both treatments produced equivalently high expectations for pain reduction. Nevertheless, placebo administration was associated with much less analgesia responding than the suggestion treatment. Given the equivalent levels of expectation produced by the two treatments, it is difficult to see how the resultant differences in analgesia responding can be accounted for parsimoniously in terms of compliance.

Perhaps the most unfortunate aspect of the topic compliance is that it has received very little systematic experimental attention in the hypnosis literature. With the notable exception of Wagstaff (1981, 1986), most investigators have either ignored the topic or attempted to treat compliance as an artifact rather than as a potentially important component in hypnotic responding (e.g., Orne, 1959). As a result, the role of compliance in hypnotic analgesia, and in hypnotic responding more generally, remains poorly understood.

Finally, it is important to note that the three hypotheses discussed above are not mutually exclusive. To differing degrees, in different subjects, and as a function of different stimulus conditions, decreased sensitivity, reinterpretation, and compliance might all occur during hypnotic analgesia. Determining which processes occur (and do not occur) under which circumstances requires much future research.

OVERVIEW

Hypnotic procedures have been employed since the nineteenth century to reduce pain. Until the seminal work of Sarbin (1950) and Barber (1969), however, hypnotic phenomena in general and hypnotic analgesia in particular were almost always conceptualized either as out-of-the-ordinary events produced in passive subjects by the induction of an unusual state of consciousness (special process views), or as deliberate faking. Of course, special process formulations did not remain static. Over time they changed by adopting the theoretical language that reflected the dominant scientific paradigms of the day. Mesmer, for example, adopted the language of fluids and forces common to eighteenth-century physics and biology, mid-twentieth-century theories of hypnosis were often framed in psychoanalytic jargon (e.g., regression in the service of the ego), and Hilgard's language is frequently drawn from contemporary information-processing models of cognition (e.g., cognitive subsystems, executive control systems, parallel processing). Despite such changes in terminology, however, the basic assumptions that hypnotic subjects are passive, that they "relinquish control" over psychological processes, and that hypnotic analgesia is something that happens to them rather than something that they do have all remained and are clearly reflected in theoretical notions like "amnesic barrier," "dissociated subsystem," and "hidden observer."

By and large, the socio-cognitive view of hypnosis grew out of symbolic interactionist and dramaturgical traditions in social psychology (Berger & Luckman, 1966; Goffman, 1959). These traditions provided the theoretical scaffolding used by Sarbin (1950; Sarbin & Coe, 1972) and Barber (1969) to challenge the fundamental assumptions of special process theories and to promulgate the alternative view of hypnotic responding as context-embedded goal-directed action.

This chapter has reviewed the manner in which these alternative perspectives conceptualize the phenomenon of hypnotic analgesia. In so doing, it has laid bare the serious limitations inherent in viewing human subjects as passive responders, and in deemphasizing the importance of contextual factors in guiding subjects' understandings, the impressions they seek to convey, and the identities they attempt to validate through reciprocal interaction with the hypnotist/experimenter. By viewing subjects as agents who develop plans, remain sensitive to implicit social norms, interpret and impose meanings both on their surroundings and on their own actions, the socio-cognitive formulation can account for (a) the equivalence of hypnotic and nonhypnotic analgesia in between-subjects experiments, (b) the carry-over of expectations that effects the levels of analgesia obtained in within-subjects experiments, (c) low-hypnotizables who exhibit as much analgesia as high-hypnotizable hypnotic subjects in some settings, but less analgesia than high-hypnotizables in other settings, (d) low-hypnotizables who show much higher levels of suggested analgesia than placebo analgesia, (e) context-dependent relationships between degree of suggested analgesia and reports of hypnotic depth, (f) hypnotic analgesia defined either as passively produced or as actively achieved, depending upon social context, and (g) "hidden observers" who report more overt than covert pain, less overt than covert pain, and no difference in overt and covert pain.

In contrast to socio-cognitive formulations, Hilgard's (1977a, 1979) dissociation theory assumes that hypnotic analgesia results from certain psychological changes that occur automatically and outside subjects' sphere of control. Moreover, the capacity to undergo these changes is purportedly restricted to only a relatively few people (high-hypnotizables). As a result of these restrictive and unnecessary assumptions, Hilgard's dissociation theory is simply unable to account parsimoniously for the flexibility that people demonstrate in response to changing social contexts.

Part Three

Hypnotic Procedures
in Applied Settings

10

Hypnotic Control of Clinical Pain

John F. Chaves

One of the benefits to emerge from the theoretical conflict between the special process view of hypnotic phenomena and the socio-cognitive perspective over the last several decades has been the evolution of a clearer understanding of the psychological aspects of pain perception and pain management. Not only have we enhanced our understanding of hypnotic pain reduction, but we have gained a much better understanding of the possible mechanisms underlying some related unorthodox pain reduction procedures as well. The present chapter provides a reexamination of the phenomenon of hypnotic control of clinical pain from the socio-cognitive perspective. Consideration is also given to related methods for pain reduction in which suggestion appears to play a significant role.

HYPNOTIC REDUCTION OF PAIN: A HISTORICAL PERSPECTIVE

Healing rituals that in one way or another resemble the hypnotic induction procedures employed by nineteenth- and twentieth-century investigators can be traced back as far as the ancient Hindus, Chinese, and Egyptians (Bernheim, 1891; Edmonston, 1986; Kroger, 1957; 1977). For instance, early rituals and mantras of the various Hindu Vedas contain elements that resemble contemporary hypnotic induction procedures. Some of these early rituals and incantations appeared to involve combinations of eye fixation and the laying on of hands that became essential elements in eighteenth- and nineteenth-century mesmerism and hypnotism. Early historical documents such as the Papyrus Ebers, which dates to 1550 B.C., provide detailed instruction for the laying on of hands for the control of pain. Similar practices were also conducted in the sleep temples of Egypt, Greece, and Rome after the fifth century B.C. (Edmonston, 1986).

Throughout the intervening centuries, a wide variety of related techniques for alleviating pain have been proposed, all of which can be traced to these historical antecedents. In the late eighteenth and early nineteenth century, interest became focused on mesmerism when it was observed that some patients appear to show a diminished response to surgical pain subsequent to a hypnotic (or mesmeric) induction procedure. Although hypnosis and mesmerism are frequently taken to be synonymous (e.g., Gravitz, 1988; Hilgard & Hilgard, 1983), early mesmerism differed from later hypnotic procedures in several important respects. Mesmerism typically involved making rhythmic passes over the patient's body and, at times, breathing over the patient's face and top of the head. This resembles the traditional practice of *Jar Phoonk,* which literally means stroking and blowing. This practice was well known in India and makes it likely that patients exposed to these procedures may have had specific expectations regarding the probable outcome of this treatment, although early workers, such as Esdaile, contended that they did not (Gibson, 1982). Sometimes, adjunctive devices such as wands, Mesmer's well-known baquet, and background music were employed to facilitate the process. It was not uncommon for mesmerists to conduct their procedures without explaining to the patient what was to be done, although it seems improbable that many did not come to know what to expect (Edmonston, 1986; Gibson, 1982; Wagstaff, 1981).

Hypnosis, on the other hand, became a primarily verbal procedure in which suggestions were administered to a subject who ordinarily was informed about what was being done. While mesmeric procedures could, at times, take hours or days (Chaves & Barber, 1976; Esdaile, 1950; Gibson, 1982), most hypnotic procedures, on the other hand, take only a matter of minutes. Another important distinction is that mesmeric procedures appeared to lead automatically to a state of analgesia, while hypnotic procedures did not ordinarily produce analgesia unless it was specifically suggested. Although these differences are in many ways very important, mesmerism clearly was the immediate precursor of the procedures we now label hypnotic (Gravitz & Gerton, 1984; Hilgard & Hilgard, 1983).

During the preanesthetic era, roughly prior to the 1840s, it was certainly understandable that any intervention that held out the slightest hope of diminishing surgical pain would stimulate interest. As Fülöp-Miller (1938) has noted, accounts of the barber surgeons of the Middle Ages and the records of modern hospitals prior to the middle of the nineteenth century conjure up images of horror:

> The patient, yelling with fear, was dragged to the operating table, was firmly held by as many as half a dozen stalwarts, feet and hands were tied. Then the surgeon could begin his cruel task, burning with a red-hot iron or cutting into the quivering flesh. The fully conscious patient watched the instruments in the hands of the tormentor, heard the instructions which the surgeon gave to the assistants, each order meaning fresh and yet more intolerable suffering. If the poor wretch could no longer endure this martyrdom, and tried to break away, the assistants would look to the security of the bonds and would hold him down yet more firmly with their restraining hands.

Even now, in the twentieth century, unorthodox procedures for pain control such as acupuncture analgesia and audioanalgesia have continued to attract a great deal of attention. The interest stimulated by these techniques reveals a fundamental truth: our triumph over both chronic and acute pain as well as our understanding of these phenomena is less than complete (Fülöp-Miller, 1938; Degenaar, 1979). Unorthodox procedures have generated interest not only because they hold out promise of clinical utility, but because it has been believed that the clinical success of these procedures might provide fresh insights and lead to a deeper understanding of the mechanisms underlying pain perception itself (Chaves & Barber, 1976).

The earliest claims for the hypnotic control of surgical pain appeared so dramatic that it is not surprising that it became virtually axiomatic that hypnosis itself must be a powerful and mysterious phenomenon to be capable of producing such a result. This assumption appears to have provided the initial foundation for traditional hypnotic state theory and it today remains a driving force behind "special-process" interpretations of hypnotic analgesia (Barber, Spanos & Chaves, 1974; Dingwall, 1967; Spanos, 1986b).

Although treatment of painful diseases occurred very early in the history of mesmerism, it is unclear who first tried somnambulism to render surgical operations painless. Early undocumented reports seem to indicate that M. Dubois performed a mastectomy in 1797. His example was followed in France by Recamier, an authority on cancer, and by Jules Cloquet, a professor of surgery who, in 1829, performed what appears to be the first documented surgical procedure with mesmerism. The operation was a mastectomy on a sixty-four-year-old woman suffering from cancer of the right breast (Chaves & Barber, 1976; Gravitz, 1988). During surgery, the patient's respiration and pulse were stable and there were no noticeable changes in her facial expression. When Cloquet reported his case to the French Academy of Medicine, Lisfranc, an eminent surgeon of that day, declared that Cloquet was either an impostor or a dupe, and Larrey, the former surgeon-in-chief of the Grande Armee claimed that Cloquet had been taken in by trickery. Additional reports appeared from time to time, documenting such procedures as tooth extractions, extirpation of tumors, and amputations performed with the assistance of mesmerism (Chaves & Barber, 1976; Gravitz, 1988).

Two of the most famous physicians to employ mesmerism for surgical pain were trained in Edinburgh, John Elliotson and James Esdaile. Elliotson was the first professor of medicine at the University of London. His technique involved the use of an elaborate and lengthy ritual (Fülöp-Miller, 1938). After first allowing his patients to rest for a while with eyes closed in a darkened room, Elliotson then made passes over the body, without actually making contact, and breathed onto the vertex. After about an hour, patients appeared to be sufficiently unresponsive so that surgery could begin. Elliotson was so convinced that this procedure would provide an effective means of producing painless surgery that he resigned his position rather than give up the practice in response to violent opposition from the Royal Medical and Chirurgical Society (Ellenberger, 1970).

Esdaile pursued his work in India, far from the din of skeptical colleagues. He reported thousands of minor surgical procedures as well as several hundred major surgical procedures, including the removal of very large scrotal tumors that were common among the natives. The favorable reports that emerged from Esdaile's hospital prompted workers in other countries to try to replicate his findings (Esdaile, 1950). Failures were reported by Strohmeyer in Vienna, by Nelation in France, and at the Massachusetts General Hospital by John Collins Warren, who later became the first physician to employ ether anesthesia in a public surgery. (Fülöp-Miller, 1938).

Esdaile's achievements were investigated locally by a commission of the Bengal government. Esdaile selected ten patients to be observed by the commission. He later excluded three of the ten patients because they appeared to be unresponsive to his technique. In the remaining seven cases, surgery was carried out while the patient was in a "mesmeric trance." In one case, involving the tapping of one side of a double hydrocele, the results were regarded as inconclusive. Although the patient tolerated the procedure without apparent pain, the other side of the hydrocele was tapped while the patient was completely awake and he still reported no pain. Moreover, the commission noted that numerous patients had tolerated this procedure while awake without apparent pain (Chaves & Barber, 1976)

The six remaining cases all involved more extensive surgery, including amputations and the removal of scrotal tumors. In each case, the patients testified that they had not felt pain during surgery. However, three of the six patients seemed to be in pain; the commission's report stated that they showed "convulsive movements of the upper limbs, writhing of the body, distortion of the features, giving the face a hideous expression of suppressed agony: the respiration became heaving, with deep sighs. There were, in short, all the signs of intense pain which a dumb person undergoing an operation might be expected to exhibit, except resistance to the operator." The remaining three patients did not show overt signs of pain, although two of the three showed erratic pulse rates during surgery. In short, although Esdaile's procedures may have been effective in diminishing anxiety and fear, the commission's report indicated that Esdaile's surgery was probably not as uniformly painless as has sometimes been supposed (Chaves & Barber, 1976).

With the discovery of the anesthetic properties of chloroform, ether, and nitrous oxide during the 1840s, there was a rapid decline in interest in mesmerism, although its staunchest advocates remained loyal, noting with satisfaction that not a single operative death could be attributed to mesmerism.

About fifty years later, there was a revival of interest in hypnosis, as it was called by this time. Bramwell (1903) reported that he could "sometimes induce anesthesia by suggestion, and from time to time occasionally perform surgical operations during hypnosis." However, all of the cases reported by Bramwell involved either dental extractions or other minor surgical procedures.

Moll (1889) took a more critical look at the use of hypnotic procedures in surgery, arguing that "a complete anesthesia is extremely rare in hypnosis, although authors, copying from one another assert that it is common." Moll also provided some examples, for instance: "I once hypnotized a patient in order to open a boil painlessly. I did not succeed in inducing analgesia, but the patient was almost unable to move so that I could perform the little operation without difficulty."

Throughout its early history, organized medicine expressed strenuous opposition to the use of hypnotic procedures for the relief of pain (Gravitz, 1988). For instance, the *Lancet,* one of the most influential medical weeklies in the world at this time, declared mesmerism to be preposterous and demanded that all of those who advocated its use be expelled from the profession as quacks and swindlers (Fülöp-Miller, 1938). Nevertheless, its use persisted and from time to time reports have continued to appear in the medical literature involving the use of hypnotic procedures in surgery (e.g., Butler, 1954; Finer & Nylan, 1961; Gheorghiu & Orleanu, 1982; Kroger & DeLee, 1957; Mason, 1955; Marmer, 1957; 1959; Rausch, 1980; Sampimon & Woodruff, 1946; Scott, 1975; Tinterow, 1960; Weyandt, 1976). Although these clinical reports have often been interpreted as supporting the use of hypnotic analgesia, detailed analysis typically reveals that these reported successes were not as uniformly pain-free as has sometimes been supposed (Barber, 1963; Chaves & Barber, 1976). Moreover, when reported pain has been less than might otherwise have been expected, it has not been clear that the hypnotic procedure itself was instrumental in attenuating pain.

Complicating the evaluation of hypnotic procedures for the reduction of pain were the underlying assumptions that were made about pain itself. The dominant conceptualization of pain for the past few hundred years can be summarized briefly: The experience of pain is precipitated by nociceptive stimuli impinging on pain receptors that, in turn, activate well-defined neural pathways that terminate in circumscribed pain centers in the brain (Mersky, 1980). The perception of pain is seen as the outcome of a linear transduction system that provides no obvious mechanisms for the attenuation of pain by psychological means (Melzack & Wall, 1965). While this traditional conceptualization of pain did not permit psychological factors to play a role in the perception of pain, a number of unorthodox procedures for treating pain in addition to hypnosis have been introduced over the last two hundred years. The success of these procedures seemed to be mediated, in large part, by psychological factors. In fact, hypnosis has sometimes been cited as an explanation for the success of these procedures. Let us look at a few examples.

RELATED UNORTHODOX PAIN-CONTROL METHODS

Perkins's Tractor

The device known as Perkins's tractors (Dingwall, 1967; Edmonston, 1986), was developed around 1800. The tractors consisted of two pieces of different kinds of metal, about three inches long, that were to be repeatedly drawn lightly over a painful or diseased area. Perkins was an American physician who annually presented to the public a collection of new cases and a list of eminent individuals who testified to their cures. Experiments with lower animals were cited to document that the tractors were more active with horses than cows and also established the immunity of sheep to the tractors, hypothesized to be due to the grease on their skin.

In 1801, Dr. J. Haygarth established the role of imagination and suggestion in understanding Perkins's reports. Haygarth experimented with imitation metallic tractors and found that these produced precisely the same results as those achieved with authentic metallic tractors. Haygarth stressed that imagination was a very potent factor in treating pain and disease (Dingwall, 1967).

The Blue Ray

About a century after Perkins was promoting his metallic tractors, an entirely new pain-control procedure, known as the "Blue Ray," was promoted by Camille Redard, a Swiss physician who practiced dentistry (Chaves & Rosenstiel, 1975). Redard was a prominent clinician who had established his reputation as a researcher with his studies of the analgesic properties of ethyl chloride and cocaine (Faulioner & Keys, 1965). In 1881, Redard was appointed Professor and Director of the Academy of Dentistry in Geneva.

The procedure advocated by Redard was simple: his patients were requested to look steadily at a blue incandescent lamp and were informed that if they did so, they would feel no pain during the subsequent dental procedure. It was thought important that patients keep their eyes wide open and persistently fixed on the lamp, which had to be equipped with a nickel-plated metal reflector. The distance between the lamp and the patients' eyes was between ten and fifteen centimeters. The whole apparatus, including the patient's head, was covered with a blue satinette cloth to exclude daylight. After two or three minutes of exposure to the blue light, analgesia was thought to be complete. When employing the blue ray for dental extractions, Redard reported a success rate of approximately 75 percent, although the criteria for success were never clearly spelled out. When failures did occur, they were taken as evidence that the patients failed to keep their eyes open, had high levels of preoperative nervousness, or were the types of persons who complained even when they felt nothing. Redard appeared to view his instructions to patients as merely a way of insuring that they would keep their eyes open. The dominant conceptualization of pain at the time probably precluded Redard's entertaining the notion that the expectations engendered by the instructions might play a role in reducing pain.

The analgesia resulting from the application of the blue ray was of brief duration, usually lasting from fifteen to thirty seconds. This was sufficient for a rapid extraction perhaps, but not much else. After Redard's initial report, confirmation of his findings began to appear in both the European and American literature (Anonymous, 1905; Hillard, 1905). Redard's followers rarely reported the same degree of success he appeared to enjoy; nevertheless, success rates of 50 percent were not unusual. Although some critics suggested that his results with the blue ray were due to hypnosis, Redard cited his failure to achieve similar success with lights of different hues as evidence that hypnosis was not an adequate explanation (Hodson, 1907; Turner, 1906). Redard and his contemporaries also appeared to assume that the percentage of patients who responded to the blue ray was much too high to be explained by hypnosis. Their analysis was probably based on the incorrect assumption that only a very small percentage of the population would respond to hypnotic suggestion (Barber, 1969; Barber, Spanos & Chaves, 1974).

As might be expected, Redard had a physiological explanation for the success of the blue ray. He postulated that the blue ray activated higher nerve centers through stimulation of the visual system, leading to analgesia. An alternative theory, suggested by Hillard, one of Redard's contemporaries, was that the analgesic effect was due to the patient rebreathing "vitiated air" (Hillard, 1905). Along with these theoretical debates, clinical reports continued to appear for about five years, although by 1910, interest in the blue ray had virtually disappeared (Raiche, 1908; Kuhnmeunch, 1908). Over the years, clinicians had become less and less enthusiastic about the procedure (Buckley, 1911). Among the factors contributing to this diminution of enthusiasm were (1) a lower success rate than originally reported by Redard, (2) a relatively long period of induction, (3) a very brief analgesic effect, and, finally, (4) growing realization that suggestion and expectation played an important role in producing the analgesia.

Before leaving the blue ray and Perkins's tractors, it is worth emphasizing several important themes that emerge from a review of these phenomena. First, both phenomena involve apparent attenuation of pain under conditions in which psychological factors were strongly implicated. Secondly, efforts were made to characterize and understand these phenomena as neurophysiological rather than psychological. Finally, when it became necessary to acknowledge the important role played by psychological factors in mediating these phenomena, they were abandoned as clinical techniques. It appears that the *Zeitgeist* simply did not permit the acceptance of psychological factors in pain perception and pain management. Perhaps for similar reasons, pain reduction with hypnosis was seen as involving a unique state of consciousness, radically different from the normal waking state. In any case, these same themes were seen again fifty years after the blue ray fell into disuse. This time, it was sound that was thought to suppress pain.

AUDIOANALGESIA

The phenomenon was audioanalgesia, first reported in 1959 by a dentist and an engineer (Gardner & Licklider, 1959; Licklider, 1961) to be effective in suppressing pain associated with a variety of dental procedures. The initial reports regarding this phenomenon were quite striking. A majority of dental patients were able to undergo normally painful procedures without difficulty and without chemical analgesics when exposed to intense auditory stimulation. Only about 10 percent of patients derived no benefit from audioanalgesia, and the vast majority reported no pain associated with their dental procedures. The discovery of audioangesia quickly led to the manufacture of a number of impressive-looking devices that were capable of presenting to patients either noises of varying intensity and bandwidth or music. The assumption seemed to be that the acoustic parameters were critical to the success of the procedure. The machines sold under various trade names, and with the fierce competition that developed, components of increasingly high quality were used and the prices of the equipment rose accordingly (Melzack, 1973c). Simultaneously, intensive research was conducted to determine the acoustic parameters of stimuli that were maximally effective in reducing pain. Elaborate neurophysiological models were constructed to explain the unexpected suppression of pain by sound (Licklider, 1961; Melzack, 1973c).

However, audioanalgesia did not always occur when expected. Laboratory studies in which audioanalgesia was used to reduce experimentally produced pain failed to demonstrate any effect on pain threshold (Carlin, Ward, Gershon & Ingraham, 1962). In 1963, Melzack and his associates demonstrated that audioanalgesia was effective in attenuating pains that had a gradual onset, but not those with an abrupt onset. It soon became apparent that the amount of pain tolerated by subjects was often determined by their expectation of future pain, rather than their currently experienced levels of pain. In a careful study, Melzack, Weiss, and Sprague (1963) found that intense auditory stimulation reduced pain only when it was accompanied by the strong suggestion that it should abolish pain. Suggestions alone and auditory stimulation alone appeared to be ineffective in reducing pain in this study, although other evidence indicates that suggestion and distraction may exert independent effects in reducing pain (Chaves & Barber, 1974a; Chaves & Duney, 1976; McCaul & Malott, 1984).

ACUPUNCTURE ANALGESIA

Acupuncture analgesia is probably the most recent unorthodox procedure for reducing pain in which psychological factors appear to be strongly implicated. The similarities between acupuncture analgesia for surgery and hypnotic analgesia for surgery seemed so striking that T. X. Barber and I (Chaves & Barber, 1973; 1974b) proposed a six-factor theory of acupuncture analgesia, incorporating many of the same factors that contribute to the apparent success of hypnoanesthesia for surgery. Although our theory was proposed in the early 1970s, subsequent data and clinical experience continue to support its basic tenets (Clark & Yang, 1974; Chapman, Beneditti, Colpitts & Gerlach, 1983; Galeano, Leung, Robitaille & Roy-Chabot, 1979; Lynn & Perl, 1977; Sweet, 1981). Although the theory is presented in detail elsewhere (Chaves & Barber, 1974b), a brief summary will be presented here because of its relevance to the understanding of the apparent success in using hypnotic analgesia for surgery.

The use of acupuncture as a surgical analgesic in China was first reported in 1959 (Hendin, 1972), although it has been used in other medical applications for thousands of years (Mann, 1972). Western attention became focused on surgical applications of acupuncture when James Reston, a *New York Times* reporter accompanying President Nixon on his visit to China, was treated for postoperative pain with acupuncture. Initial reports appeared to suggest that the Chinese routinely employed acupuncture as the analgesic of choice for major surgery, and that this procedure was routinely successful in making possible painless surgery without pharmacological agents of any sort while patients remained conscious throughout the procedure. Acupuncture analgesia captured the imagination of Western scientists and clinicians because its apparent success seemed to be completely inconsistent with existing theories of pain and contemporary strategies for its control in Western cultures.

Our six-factor theory (Chaves & Barber, 1973; 1974b; Chaves, 1975) attempted to show how the phenomenon of acupuncture analgesia could be understood in terms of principles that were already well known, although frequently over looked, by Western medicine. Let us review each of these factors in turn.

1. Patient Selection. Although early accounts seemed to imply that acupuncture was widely used in China, it soon became clear that it was used very selectively on a small minority of patients who had been carefully screened for their belief in the efficacy of the procedure, and their possession of an ideological zeal for Mao's thought-reform program (Diamond, 1971; Kroger, 1972; Sweet, 1981). The Chinese themselves collected data showing that acupuncture analgesia usually failed when these patient selection criteria were ignored (Chaves & Barber, 1973, 1974b; Knox, Shumy & McLaughlin, 1977). Surgical criteria were also employed in selecting patients for acupuncture analgesia. In general, acupuncture was avoided when high levels of muscular relaxation were required, or when surgery was done on an emergency basis. Even with careful patient selection, acupuncture analgesia could fail (Diamond, 1971). Moreover, the Chinese tend to use liberal criteria for judging the success of acupuncture in producing surgical analgesia. The mere tolerance of the procedure is generally taken as evidence of success. As He (1987) has noted, "Acupuncture cannot be expected to produce total abolition of pain perception and the best it can do is to lessen the sharpness of pain allowing certain operations." Patient comfort is not a requirement for judging the procedure to be successful (Chaves & Barber, 1974b). In a similar vein, hypnotic analgesia is sometimes said to be successful when it promotes patients' acceptance of their condition but does not lead to analgesia (Olness, 1981).

2. Adjunctive Chemical Analgesics and Sedation. Early accounts of acupuncture analgesia seemed to imply that it was normally the only analgesic needed to control surgical pain in China. A careful review of individual cases revealed, on the contrary, that in the vast majority of cases, chemical anesthetics, analgesics, and sedation were employed together with acupuncture to control pain (Chaves & Barber, 1973; 1974b; Sweet, 1981). It was not uncommon for surgical acupuncture patients to receive 50-60 mg. of meperidine hydrochloride (Demerol) through an intravenous drip, or 10 mg. of morphine injected subcutaneously. Some patients had local anesthetic infiltrated into the area of the incision, while others received sedative doses of barbiturates (Brown, 1972; Capperauld, 1972).

Since normal practice in China involves the simultaneous use of narcotic analgesics, sedatives, and local anesthetics together with acupuncture (Chaves & Barber, 1973; 1974b; Sweet, 1981), it is difficult to determine how much, if any, contribution to surgical pain relief is made by the acupuncture itself.

Similarly, the vast majority of surgical procedures accomplished with hypno-anesthesia are accompanied by adjunctive chemical analgesics, anesthetics, and sedation (Chaves & Barber, 1976). This confounding makes it difficult to evaluate the separate effects of the hypnotic procedure in these cases.

3. Pain of Surgical Procedures. Laymen frequently assume that surgical pain is proportional to tissue damage. However, surgeons are aware that the various tissues and organs of the body are not equally sensitive to the various forms of insult they are subjected to during surgical procedures. Thus, for example, while the skin is generally extremely sensitive to incisional pain, many other tissues and organs can be incised painlessly without benefit of acupuncture. For instance, hollow viscera, such as stomach and intestines as well as brain tissue, can be incised painlessly in waking surgical patients (Lennander, 1901, 1902, 1904, 1906a, 1906b). On the other hand, the internal viscera are extremely sensitive to distention and traction. Thus, some of the dramatic performances that have come to be associated with acupuncture analgesia are a good deal less impressive than they initially appear, particularly when the use of adjunctive local anesthetics and sedation are taken into account. This factor is also pertinent to the assessment of hypnotic analgesia for surgery.

4. Preoperative Preparation. Patients selected for acupuncture analgesia are routinely admitted to the hospital a few days prior to surgery. During this time they are provided with an elaborate preparatory procedure that includes discussions with other patients who have undergone similar procedures, dress rehearsals of the operative procedures, and other experiences designed to minimize the patient's anxiety and engender positive attitudes and expectancies regarding the forthcoming procedure (Tkash, 1972). The value of even brief preoperative visits for surgical patients was clearly established in this country in the 1960s by Egbert and his associates (Egbert, Battit, Turndorf & Beecher, 1963; Egbert, Battit, Welch & Bartlett, 1964). Patients who visited not only were calmer prior to surgery but also required less medication for postoperative pain and even left the hospital sooner than nonvisitor controls. Clinical studies of hypnotic analgesia also frequently incorporate specific and elaborate preoperative preparation protocols (e.g., Hilgard & LaBaron, 1984).

5. Suggestion. The period of preoperative preparation and the surgical procedure itself provide an opportunity for the effective use of suggestion for acupuncture patients. Acupuncturists make extensive use of suggestion (Rhee, 1972). Of course, acupuncture patients are selected, in part, because of their positive attitudes and expectancies regarding acupuncture analgesia. These attitudes and expectancies are further strengthened during the procedure itself. As we shall see, suggestions of analgesia, administered independently of any hypnotic procedures or acupuncture, can significantly reduce pain.

6. Distraction. When acupuncture is used to control surgical pain, the needles are not simply inserted, but they are also stimulated either thermally, electrically, or manually. As a consequence of this stimulation, the acupuncture needles themselves produce painful sensations and serve as a counter irritant that we know can effectively reduce pain (Chen, 1972; Man & Chen, 1972). As James Reston (1972) noted, the needles "sent ripples of pain racing through my limbs and, at least, had the effect of diverting my attention from the distress in my stomach." Acupuncture patients are further distracted by breathing exercises (Warren, 1972). Evidence reviewed elsewhere indicates that distraction can exert a powerful effect in reducing pain (Levine, Gormley, & Fields, 1976; Lewit, 1979; McCaul & Malott, 1984).

Acupuncture analgesia continues to stimulate interest and debate regarding its mechanisms and clinical efficacy (J. Barber, & Mayer, 1977; Goldberger & Tursky, 1976; Melzack, 1973a, 1973b; Price, Rafii, Watkins & Buckingham, 1984; Richardson & Vincent, 1986; Vincent & Richardson, 1986). Taken together, however, the success of these diverse unorthodox procedures for pain control makes clear the enormous contribution of psychological factors to the perception and management of pain (Melzack & Chapman, 1973; Weisenberg, 1977). Studies that view psychological factors as artifactual or incidental to the effects of other variables are unlikely to help in identifying precisely which psychological variables are important, or in showing how these variables can be optimally combined into effective treatment packages. The variables that appear to play an important role in pain reduction during these unorthodox procedures also play an important role in hypnotic reduction of clinical pain. Let us turn now to contemporary reports on the use of hypnosis for the control of clinical pain.

CONTEMPORARY PAIN CONTROL WITH HYPNOTIC SUGGESTION

Throughout the early twentieth century, a number of clinical reports have appeared that involved the use of hypnosis for the control of acute and chronic pain (Barber, 1959). Many of the reports are anecdotal. Some, for example, report the use of hypnosis as the sole anesthetic for surgical procedures conducted under conditions of war, when chemical anesthetics were unavailable (e.g., Sampimon & Woodruff, 1946). Other reports involve special circumstances in which the patient was at high risk because of allergies or because of dire medical condition (Crasilneck, McCrainie & Jenkins, 1956). Rarely has hypnosis been used as the sole anesthetic for operative procedures (Chaves & Barber 1976). Almost always, as is the case with acupuncture, it has been accompanied by the use of adjunctive chemical anesthetics, sedation, or the use of local anesthetics to control incisional pain (Chaves & Barber, 1976).

Occasionally, very dramatic observations are reported. Sometimes these take the form of films and videotapes, such as those of Ralph August performing a caesarean section, or Kay Thompson's films of a rhinoplasty and dermabrasion with hypnoanesthesia. At other times, personal accounts of health-care personnel undergoing surgery with self-hypnosis have appeared (e.g., Gruen, 1972; Rausch, 1980; Reis, 1966). These observations are difficult to interpret because of the unique motivation of the individuals providing these accounts, wide variation in patients' ability to tolerate pain, and the complexity of the circumstances under which these surgeries have been performed. Perhaps the most notable systematic observations in recent years are those provided in J. Barber's dissertation (J. Barber, 1976), which appears to support the complete substitution of hypnosis for chemical analgesics for dental procedures. However, there are serious problems with the design of this research, and other investigators have been unable to replicate the finding (e.g., Gillett & Coe, 1984). Thus, while the introduction of chemical analgesics did not quite make hypnosis obsolete for that purpose (Ellenberger, 1970), it did relegate hypnosis to a distinctly minor role as the sole anesthetic for surgery. On the other hand, anecdotal evidence did appear to support the adjunctive use of hypnotic suggestion to facilitate preparation for surgery, as an adjunct for chemical analgesics and anesthetics, and in the management of post surgical pain (Hilgard & Hilgard, 1983). Moreover, increasing attention has begun to be focused on its application in chronic pain management (J. Barber & Adrian, 1982; Turk, Meichenbaum & Genest, 1983; Wain, 1986).

The nature of clinical research and the difficulties in controlling potentially relevant variables make it essential to approach the phenomenon of hypnotic reduction of clinical pain with some appreciation for what is known about this phenomenon from studies of the hypnotic reduction of experimental pain. Accordingly, let us now turn to review briefly some of the principle conclusions that have emerged from studies of the control of experimental pain by hypnotic suggestion.

Control of Experimental Pain by Hypnotic Suggestion

Traditional interpretations of hypnotic analgesia have viewed the hypnotic induction procedure and the hypothesized hypnotic state to which it is said to lead as essential features of hypnotic analgesia (Hilgard, 1975, 1977, 1986; Hilgard & Hilgard, 1983). Certainly, the vast majority of clinical accounts of hypnotic analgesia take this assumption as a point of departure. The hypnotic subject is seen as passive, with the analgesic phenomenon, in a sense, inflicted upon them. Within recent years, the traditional interpretation has been elaborated considerably, and attention has been focused on the cognitive mechanisms, such as dissociation, thought to underlie hypnotic analgesia (Hilgard, 1977, 1986). Research conducted within the socio-cognitive perspective, however, has established a body of data inconsistent with that view. As a consequence, a new view of hypnotic analgesia has emerged (Spanos, 1986b; Spanos, Gwynn & Stam, 1983).

Beginning in the early 1960s, T. X. Barber initiated a series of important studies that had as their purpose the identification and isolation of those variables within the hypnotic situation that were instrumental in producing the effects that had been attributed to the hypnotic state. Barber recognized the complexity of the hypnotic situation and the importance of identifying within the hypnotic intervention those factors that were instrumental in achieving such phenomena as hypnotic analgesia. Subsequent studies by Barber and his associates (e.g., Barber & Cooper, 1972; Barber & Hahn, 1962; Chaves & Barber, 1974a; Spanos, Barber & Lang, 1974; Spanos, Horton & Chaves, 1975), as well as studies conducted in other laboratories (e.g., Beers & Karoly, 1979; Wolf & Horland, 1967; Worthington, 1978), make possible a number of important generalizations regarding the reduction of experimental pain by hypnotic suggestion. While it is widely acknowledged that clinical and experimental pain differ in important ways (Beecher, 1946, 1959), the generalizations that have emerged from laboratory studies of experimental pain have relevance for understanding possible mechanisms underlying the reduction for many of these conclusions and more complete documentary support are provided elsewhere in this volume (see Spanos's chapter).

1. Suggestions for the attenuation of pain, whether preceded by a hypnotic induction procedure or not, are equally effective in reducing pain magnitude, decreasing pain threshold, and increasing pain tolerance (e.g., Barber & Cooper, 1972; Chaves & Barber 1974a; Chaves & Doney, 1976; Worthington, 1978).

2. Suggestions designed to encourage the use of such cognitive coping strategies as imagining pleasant events, self-distraction, transformation of the noxious stimulus, and positive self-statements produce significant reductions in reported pain or corresponding increases in pain thresholds and pain tolerance (e.g., Chaves & Barber, 1974a; Chaves & Scott, 1979; Spanos, Horton & Chaves, 1975; Spanos, Stam & Brazil, 1981).

3. Some subjects will utilize spontaneous coping strategies to deal with pain even if not explicitly asked to do so (e.g., Chaves & Barber, 1974a; Brown & Chaves, 1978, 1987; Spanos, Brown, Jones & Horner, 1981).

4. The ability to cope with noxious stimulation is influenced by subjects' expectations regarding the situation and belief in their ability to cope with it (e.g., Marino, Gwynn & Spanos, 1988; Neufeld & Thomas, 1977; Spanos, 1986b).

5. Under a wide variety of experimental conditions, low-hypnotizable subjects are able to diminish their experience of pain to the same degree as highly hypnotizable subjects (Spanos, Radke-Bodorik, Ferguson & Jones, 1979; Spanos, Hodgins, Stam & Gwynn, 1984; Spanos, Kennedy & Gwynn, 1984; Spanos, Ollerhead & Gwynn, 1986; Spanos, Voorneveld, & Gwynn, 1987).

6. The frequently replicated finding of a positive correlation between pretest levels of hypnotic susceptibility and hypnotic analgesia is highly context dependent and tends to break down when hypnotizability is assessed independently of the analgesia test (see Spanos's chapter).

The picture of hypnotic analgesia that emerges from these and related findings (Spanos, 1986b, 1983) places the phenomenon of hypnotic analgesia within the socio-cognitive perspective. This view emphasizes the role of the hypnotic subject as an active agent who responds to a variety of situational and contextual cues by engaging in a complex array of cognitive activities designed to attenuate pain. As we shall see, contemporary accounts of clinical applications of hypnotic analgesia, while less well controlled than those reviewed by Spanos, create a similar picture.

HYPNOTIC REDUCTION OF CLINICAL PAIN:
CONTEMPORARY ACCOUNTS

Within recent years, assessment of hypnotizability has become an integral part of the intake protocol for many chronic pain patients (Malyon, Harris, Griffin & Pinsky, 1978; Wain, 1980). Moreover, hypnotic procedure are frequently, employed in inpatient and outpatient pain-management programs (Fordyce, 1973). Recently, Brown & Fromm (1986) have presented a multimodal treatment protocol for the use of hypnosis in the treatment of several types of chronic pain. The use of hypnosis as but one component in a multimodal treatment program for chronic pain is particularly appropriate. It has become clear in recent years that chronic pain problems are exceedingly difficult to treat and that comprehensive, multidisciplinary treatment programs are more likely to be successful than highly focused, unimodal approaches (Margolis, Zimny, Miller & Taylor, 1984; Turk, Meichenbaum & Genest, 1983).

When hypnotic procedures are utilized in chronic pain management programs, which of these many variables associated with the procedure are instrumental in reducing reported pain and reducing other pain behaviors? This question, of course, is simply a variant of the same question raised by Barber (1969) regarding the reduction of experimental pain by suggestion. Let us consider some of the important variables in turn.

1. Definition of the Situation as Involving Hypnosis. The experimental literature indicates that simply defining the situation as hypnosis enhances suggestibility (Barber, 1969). However, it is equally clear that the administration of suggestions of analgesia reduces reported pain even in the absence of a hypnotic induction procedure (Spanos, 1986).

2. Assessment of Hypnotic Susceptibility. Many clinicians advocate an initial experience with some simple hypnotic suggestions to enhance expectations of success in treatment (Brown & Fromm, 1986; Frankel, 1976; Chaves, 1985a, 1985b), The risk of formal assessment of hypnotizability is that failed items may diminish the patient's expectation of clinical success. Reported correlations between hypnotizability and clinical outcomes may reflect the operation of this process (see Spanos's discussion in chapter 9).

3. Assessment of Pain Phenomenology. Patients' pain descriptions frequently provide a rich resource for later development of therapeutic suggestion. These descriptions frequently reveal an array of metaphors already understood and utilized by the patient. These might include mechanical metaphors ("my head feels like its in a vice," "it feels as if someone were squeezing my tongue with a needle-nose pliers,"); thermal ("it feels as though my leg is burning, on fire"), or electrical. At other times pains may be described as having synesthetic attributes that cross sensory modalities, such as a pain that evokes a color, e.g., hot red, icy blue, etc. Responses to the Melzack-McGill Pain questionnaire, which helps elicit a semantic map of the pain, frequently help to generate these descriptions.

4. Assessment of Spontaneous Coping Strategies. Just as patients bring their own phenomenology of pain experience to the clinical setting, they also may bring an array of spontaneous coping strategies or expectations about which coping strategies might be effective for them (Chaves & Brown, 1978, 1987). One patient, a twenty-five-year-old female, presented with pain associated with rheumatoid arthritis that had persisted for several years. Open-ended inquiry about her coping strategies revealed that the time that was most challenging to her was the morning. She found it extremely difficult each morning to go through the battle off combating her own urge to avoid confronting her pain and stiffness. To make the situation more manageable for herself, she decided to externalize the process by inventing an antagonist, appropriately enough called "Arthur." The patient found it much easier to fight "Arthur," than to fight herself. Finding it hard to improve on that strategy, we evolved some strategies that made "Arthur" a genuinely despicable character to help the patient mobilize her resources to fight her enemy.

Another patient, a sixty-five-year-old female presented with pain associated with widespread metastases from breast cancer. She was seeking hypnosis in order to have an "out of body experience." Although she had never had such an experience, she had read about them and was convinced that if she could have such an experience she could gain some control over her pain. Although pain was her chief presenting complaint, it became clear that she was having other difficulties as well. Her appetite was poor as a consequence of chemotherapy. She readily acknowledged being depressed, being less active than she would like to have been, and feeling that she was not doing her share of work at home. Success in working with these other symptoms, as well as her belief in the potential efficacy of out-of-body experiences, provided a useful approach in working with this patient that quickly led to symptomatic improvement.

It is typical for chronic pain patients seeking hypnosis to present with a variety of complaints in addition to their pain. Frequently, these subsidiary problems provide a useful focus for early clinical attention because they are usually more easily managed initially than the pain problem, and patients gain confidence in their ability to use these techniques effectively (Chaves, 1985a, 1985b).

One of the problems with using success with chronic pain management to evaluate clinical interventions like hypnotic suggestion is that we often have no independent way of assessing how much pain the patient is experiencing. Moreover, the etiology of the pain is often unclear. Let us now turn to the use of hypnotic suggestion in the management of pain associated with a variety of medical and dental procedures, where we often have a clearer appreciation for the etiology of the pain.

HYPNOTIC MANAGEMENT OF SURGICAL AND POSTSURGICAL PAIN

After the discovery of chemical anesthetics, interest in the use of hypnosis as the sole anesthetic for surgical procedures greatly diminished. Although isolated reports appeared, many of these observations were made under extraordinary conditions such as wartime (e.g., Sampimon & Woodruff, 1946; Cooper & Powles, 1945), and there was little sustained interest in the phenomenon.

However, beginning in the 1950s, a renaissance of interest in hypnoanesthesia developed (Chaves & Barber, 1976; Crasilneck & Hall, 1975), and a number of anecdotal reports involving surgical applications of hypnoanesthesia began to appear in the literature (e.g., Anderson, 1957; Bernstein, 1963, 1965; Bonilla, Quigley & Bowers, 1961; Bowers, 1966; Clawson & Swade, 1975; Doberneck, 1950; Finer, 1966; Goldie, 1956; Hoffmann, 1959; Jones, 1962; Kelsey & Barron, 1958; Kroger & DeLee, 1957; Lozanov, 1967; Marmer, 1956; 1957; Mason, 1955; Morse, 1975; Mum, 1966, Papermaster, Doberneck & Bonello, 1960; Raginsky, 1951; Schwarcz, 1965; Scott, 1975; Steinberg & Pennell, 1965; Stone, 1977; Taugher, 1958; Todorovic, 1959, Van Dyke, 1965; Werbel, 1965, 1967; Winkelstein & Levinson, 1959). The range of surgical procedures was quite broad and varied, from minor surgeries involving simple biopsy or incision and drainage, to major procedures including abdominal exploration, caesarian sections, phneumonectomies, skin grafting, thyroidectomies, hysterectomies, prostatectomies, hemorrhoidectomies, and mammoplasties. To these we must add the few first-person accounts that have been provided by individuals who have reported utilizing self-hypnotic procedures in conjunction with their surgeries (Gruen, 1972; Rausch, 1980; Reis, 1966).

Taken together, these accounts indicate that the use of hypnotic suggestion was accompanied by relative calmness during surgical procedures, with accompanying reductions in anxiety (Chaves & Barber, 1976). In most instances, analgesics and sedatives were employed together with the use of hypnotic suggestion, although in a small number of cases, hypnotic suggestion served as the sole anesthetic. In some of these cases, pain was experienced by the patient, although in other instances, patients appeared to experience little pain. Unfortunately, these are all case reports, which severely limits the conclusions that are possible.

An additional complication is that clinicians using hypnotic suggestion in medical settings frequently do not employ a formal hypnotic induction procedure (Chaves, 1986; Fredericks, 1980). This has been a general problem in evaluating the use of hypnosis in the control of clinical pain. As Wadden and Anderton (1982) have noted, "Frequently, investigators fail to describe therapeutic techniques in sufficient detail to differentiate a hypnotic treatment from a cognitive-behavioral intervention, except in name alone." Moreover, they go on to note that, "At present it is unclear from both a theoretical and practical standpoint what criteria are used to identify a treatment as uniquely hypnotic" (p. 215). It is clear that suggestions of anesthesia alone, without a formal hypnotic induction procedure, were sufficient for one surgeon to perform a herniorrhaphy with little pain (Lazanov, 1967). Earlier, Sampimon and Woodruff (1946) had noted that "the mere suggestion of anesthesia" was sufficient to perform minor surgery on soldiers in a prisoner-of-war hospital during World War II. Even earlier, Tuckey (1889) had noted the effectiveness of suggestion, without a formal induction procedure, in reducing surgical pain. The case involved a young female who was to undergo surgical removal of two sebaceous tumors. To the surprise of onlookers, the patient appeared to become unconscious when an empty ether bottle and mask were applied to familiarize her with the procedure. "After a few inspirations she cried, 'Oh, I feel it; I am going off,' and a moment after, her eyes turned up, and she became unconscious." Since the ether had not arrived and the patient appeared to be insensitive to pain, the surgeon proceeded and "the operation was successfully and painlessly completed" (Tuckey, 1889, pp. 725-26).

Although there is considerable disagreement to this day regarding the proportion of patients for whom hypnosis could serve as the sole anesthetic in major surgical procedures, there seems to be widespread agreement that this is not a primary clinical application of hypnosis (Crasilneck & Hall, 1975; Udolf, 1987). Udolf (1987) contends that complete substitution of hypnosis for chemical analgesics is possible 25 percent of the time with minor surgical procedures and 10 to 15 percent in more major surgical procedures. He argues that only time and skill in using hypnosis are limiting factors and lists a number of clinical indications for its use. These include: (1) when chemical agents might be dangerous such as when the patient is allergic to anesthetics or the patient is severely medically compromised; (2) during neurosurgical procedures when it might be advantageous not to use agents that would alter the EEG; (3) when chemical agents are not available, as in certain emergency situations; (4) when prolonged anesthesia is required; (5) when it is important to minimize postoperative complications of anesthetic agents, such as nausea and vomiting; (6) whenever it is desirable for the patient to be fully conscious to cooperate with the surgeon. Some additional advantages have been claimed by Fredericks (1980). These include diminished surgical bleeding, enhanced wound healing, and the lack of suppression of normal reflexes.

The success figures cited by Udolf (1987) do not appear to be derived from from any series of well-controlled studies and seem, without empirical justification, to be more optimistic than previous estimates by Kroger (1957, 1977); Lederman, Fordyce, and Stacey (1958); Marmer (1959); and Wallace and Coppolino (1960). Marmer (1959) argued for a 10 percent success rate in use of hypnosis as the sole anesthetic, while Wallace and Coppolino (1960) concluded that there was no body of evidence to support the oft-quoted 10 percent figure and decided that the correct figure must be much less than that.

Certainly many clinicians have concluded that complete substitution of hypnoanesthesia for chemical analgesia is rarely effective. Werbel (1967) noted that hypnosis waš ineffective for abdominal surgery. Yankovski and Bricklin (1967) reported an "at the time uncontrollable reaction that took place on an operating table while the patient's abdomen was open." Bernstein (1963) noted that hypnosis did not always produce anesthesia but did increase pain tolerance. Steffanoff (1961) stated that "Hypnosis was never intended to replace chemical anesthesia." Crasilneck and Hall (1975) appear to support this conclusion in noting that the use of hypnosis as the sole anesthetic is "seldom indicated." Moreover, a recent review of significant developments in medical hypnosis over the past twenty-five years fails to cite a single report of hypnoanalgesia, although its adjunctive role in surgery is acknowledged (Frankel, 1987).

While the complete substitution of hypnosis for chemical analgesics and anesthetics does not enjoy much support in the literature, the adjunctive use of hypnotic suggestion does appear to offer more consistent benefits to surgical patients (Kolouch, 1962, 1964, 1968). Kolouch (1968) reviewed the convalescence of 254 surgical patients who had been administered hypnotic suggestions to instill confidence and the expectation of easy recovery. While the results were encouraging, three factors appeared to diminish the contribution of hypnotic suggestions: (1) increasing difficulty and complexity of the surgery, (2) "personality defects" in the patient, and (3) postoperative surgical complications. Field (1974) was able to demonstrate differences between hypnotic and control patients in postoperative course, although depth of hypnosis did correlate positively with less anxiety on the day of surgery and increased speed of recovery.

Hypnotic suggestion has also been used with reported success to deal with surgically related symptoms other than pain. For example, there have been a number of anecdotal reports of the use of hypnotic suggestion to control operative and postoperative bleeding (Benson, 1971; Clawson & Swade, 1975; Crasilneck & Fogelman, 1957; Dubin & Shapiro, 1974; Erickson, Hershman & Sector, 1961; Stolzenberg, 1953). In one controlled pilot study, Chaves, Whilden, and Roller (1979) measured surgical and postsurgical blood loss in eight patients who were undergoing bilateral third-molar extractions. One extraction was done subsequent to the administration of a hypnotic procedure with a variety of suggestions designed to reduce bleeding; the other extraction was done on a different occasion without any special procedure. Preoperative hemoglobin values compared to the hemoglobin values of the fluids aspirated during and after surgery provided a stable estimate of the volume of blood lost. The reduction in bleeding with the use of hypnotic suggestion was more than 65 percent which was statistically as well as clinically significant even with the small number of patients in this study. The design of the study did not permit the assessment of the relative contributions of the hypnotic procedure and the suggestions for blood loss to the measured decrease in blood loss. Additional research will be necessary to clarify this matter and to evaluate alternative mechanisms, such as vasoconstriction or changes in blood chemistry that might be responsible for this effect.

Other benefits that have been associated with the use of hypnotic suggestion in surgery include enhanced preparation for surgery (Surman, Hackett, Silverberg & Behrendt, 1974), improved tolerance for prolonged positioning in a body cast (Wollman. 1964), and control of the postgastrectomy dumping syndrome (Leonard, Papermaster & Wangenstein, 1957). These and other benefits beyond those directly related to pain management have been reviewed by others (Crasilneck & Hall, 1975; Ewin, 1984; Udolf, 1987). While there seems to be a general acknowledgment that many of the benefits attributed to hypnosis can be achieved without it, there remains a widespread assumption, unsupported by controlled studies, that adding a hypnotic procedure enhances the clinical efficacy of the use of suggestion.

HYPNOTIC TREATMENT OF PAIN ASSOCIATED WITH DENTISTRY

The acute pain associated with a wide variety of dental interventions has also been managed with the use of hypnotic suggestion. The primitive conditions that prevailed during World War II often necessitated dental extractions being accomplished without benefit of chemical anesthetic (Moss, 1963). Under these conditions, hypnotic suggestion was sometimes employed to reduce pain. At times dramatic results were reported, mostly anecdotally (Hilgard & Hilgard, 1983). As is true of other forms of surgery, complete substitution of hypnotic suggestion for chemical analgesia is rare in dentistry. Hypnotic suggestion is more commonly employed to deal with incomplete pharmacological control of pain and other clinical problems including dental anxiety, gagging, bleeding, control of excessive salivation and tolerance for dental prostheses (Dublin, 1976; Finkelstein, 1984; Kleinhaus, Eli & Rubenstein, 1985; Stolzenberg & Kroger, 1961). Nevertheless, reports of its continued use in pain control still appear. These include endodontic treatment of vital teeth (Morse & Wickle, 1979), placement of a dental implant (Gheorghia & Orleanu, 1982), gingivectomies (Daniels, 1976b), and restorative dental procedures (Weyant, 1976). There have also been a few controlled studies of the use of hypnotic suggestion to control clinical pain in the dental setting within recent years. Let us examine these in some detail.

Gottfredson (1973) found that 9 of 12 highly hypnotizable patients were able to have routine dental working completed without chemical analgesia, while only 5 of 13 less susceptible patients were able to do so. This represents an overall success rate of 56 percent, with 75 percent success for the highly susceptible and 38.5 percent for the low-susceptible group. Moreover, Gottfredson found a significant negative correlation (r = 0.39) between pain ratings made during the dental procedures and hypnotizability, indicating that more susceptible patients reported less pain. J. Barber (1977), in a widely cited report based on his unpublished doctoral dissertation (J. Barber, 1976), claimed that ninety-nine out of one hundred patients who were unselected with respect to hypnotizability could undergo routine dental work without chemical analgesics (99 percent success). Barber attributed his extraordinary success to the use of a specialized hypnotic induction procedure, which he labelled Rapid Induction Analgesia (RIA). This procedure in its original form takes more than twenty minutes to administer and is characterized by the use of indirect suggestions (J. Barber, 1977; Gillett & Coe, 1984).

Gillett and Coe (1984), in a well-controlled study, attempted to replicate and extend Barber's findings. They studied sixty patients who were undergoing dental procedure that would have routinely called for the use of local anesthetic. Hypnotizability was assessed for all patients using the Harvard Group Scale (half assessed before dental treatment, the other half after). Patients were exposed to either a recorded version of Barber's RIA (1977), or to a shortened version (ten minutes in duration) that eliminated duplications. The primary dependent variable was whether or not the patient requested chemical analgesia. In addition patients completed several rating scales to assess their comfort during the procedure. The overall success rate was 51.7 percent roughly comparable to that found by Gottfredson (1973). There was no difference in the efficacy of the original and the abbreviated version of the RIA. Success, whether defined in terms of completion of the dental procedure without chemical analgesia, or in terms of rated discomfort, was independent of susceptibility level. When the dental procedures themselves were dichotomized into high- and low-discomfort levels according to dentist ratings, a somewhat different picture emerged. While the overall success rate was 51.7 percent, the success rate for high-discomfort procedures (e.g., extractions, root canal-vital tissue, pulp capping) was only 33 percent, while for low-discomfort procedures (e.g., crown buildup with post, filling, cementation of crown), it was 79 percent.

Although the Gillett and Coe (1984) study is not an exact replication of the Barber (1977) study, it does cast serious doubt on J. Barber's conclusions and emphasizes the need for careful scrutiny of exaggerated claims of clinical efficacy for hypnotic procedures in controlling acute dental pain. As Gillett and Coe (1984) point out, it may well be that simple reassurance may have been as effective as J. Barber's procedure in assisting dental patients to tolerate procedure involving only minimal discomfort. Some support for this conclusion was provided in a recent study that showed that the level of relaxation achieved with a hypnotic induction procedure prior to dental treatment was comparable to that achieved by contemplating an aquarium, when it was suggested that both procedures would lead to relaxation (Katcher, Segal & Beck, 1984).

The results of the Gillett and Coe (1984) study are also pertinent to Barber's (1977) conclusions regarding the special benefits of indirect hypnotic suggestions.

The superiority of indirect hypnotic suggestions over their direct counterparts has been asserted from time to time in the experimental and clinical literature (e.g., Alman & Carney, 1980; Barber, 1977; Frichton & Roth, 1985; Stone & Lundy, 1985). Moreover, indirect suggestions have come to be viewed as a hallmark of Ericksonian Hypnosis, although as Hammond (1984) has noted, the Ericksonian promoters err in claiming that Erickson relied primarily on the use of metaphor and indirect suggestion. Several studies have failed to establish the greater efficacy of indirect over direct suggestions (Lynn, Neufeld & Matyi, 1987; Mathews, Bennett, Bear & Gallagher, 1985; Stone & Lundy, 1985). Price and J. Barber (1987) have recently provided some data indicating that the conditions under which indirect suggestions are more effective than direct suggestions may be more restrictive than had previously been thought. Moreover, efforts have failed to extend J. Barber's (1977) extraordinary claims regarding the efficacy of RIA with the acute pain associated with dental procedures (Gillett & Coe, 1984) and podiatric surgery (Crowley, 1980) as well as with chronic pain (Snow, 1979). Indeed, there is evidence that RIA may be less effective than traditional hypnotic procedures for reducing experimentally produced pain (Van Gorp, Meyer & Dunbar, 1985).

In evaluating the role of hypnotic suggestion in diminishing anxiety and pain within the dental setting, it is important to acknowledge the role played by spontaneous, self-administered suggestions by patients who have not been exposed to a hypnotic induction procedure. Chaves and Brown (1978, 1987) studied the spontaneous coping strategies employed by dental patients who were undergoing a mandibular block injection prior to a restorative dental procedure on a simple dental extraction. Forty-four percent of the dental patients studied engaged in spontaneous coping strategies, including attention diversion and coping self-statements. One patient described his utilization of a distraction strategy as follows: "Just like placid thoughts, pictures, and stuff. You just tend to let your mind . . . wander. Just think of different things, like I look around and observe things in the room and let them bring my attention to them rather than what is going on in my mouth."

Another patient appeared to use a dissociation strategy: "Well, I just tried basically in a philosophical way not to identify with the body. You know it is just like a vehicle which is needing some repair and they are doing that mechanical repair and sort of not identifying with the body in that way."

Another patient seemed to benefit from adaptive self-talk: "I just try and prepare myself. You know it is going to hurt so I tell myself: 'Just be ready for it—think about something else.' And I tense up more or less when he puts it in and then I just relax, and that's about it."

The cognitive activity of our coping patients contrasted markedly from another group of patients we labeled "catastrophizers." Catastrophizing took several forms including negative self-statements, catastrophizing thoughts, and catastrophizing images. The nature of catastrophizing and its potential to amplify the fearful and worrisome aspects of the dental treatments can be seen clearly in the following: "How I hated it. I hate having an injection. I think 'Oh no, here we go again.' I hate it with a passion. Just to see that great big needle coming down at you, the next thing you know you start going bananas. It's so bad."

Consider the following patient, who actually seems to be trying to mentally negate the effects of the local anesthetic: "You wonder what it feels like actually if you didn't have any Novocain or any shots or anything like that. What would it feel like? You wonder if its going to hurt a lot after the injection is in . . . . You're concerned all right. Wondering if something is going to go wrong, if your teeth are going to be OK."

Or consider the plight of the following patient and her dentist: "Oh this is terrible because I'd like to kill him. I don't like him and I told him before, 'I didn't like dentists because most of the time I feel they don't care about me.' And I'm just a blah, and they can do anything they want. And I want them to say, 'Oh, I known this is going to hurt, but I have to do it.' But I just feel like any minute I'm going to receive a terrific, horrible pain."

Catastrophizing ideation was identified in 38 percent of these dental patients, while an additional 19 percent denied any cognitive activity during the procedure. Patients who employed spontaneous coping strategies rated their dental procedures as less stressful than those who catastrophized. Interestingly, however, patients who denied any mental activity during the procedure found the procedures no more stressful then the copers. This finding indicates that additional research is needed to investigate the ways in which catastrophizing may amplify anxiety and pain in clinical and nonclinical settings. This finding also points to the potential clinical value of any type of clinical intervention, hypnotic or not, that can disrupt catastrophizing.

HYPNOTIC MANAGEMENT OF ACUTE MEDICAL PAIN

Hypnotic suggestion has been employed with reported success in managing a wide variety of acute iatrogenic pain problems, some associated with medical treatments such as the reduction of dislocations (Kubiak, 1983); exacerbations of chronic pain problems (Van Nuys; 1977); improved tolerance of intravenous lines, tubes, and catheters (Udolf, 1987); electrocauterization (Golan, 1975); and, tolerance for bone marrow aspiration and lumbar puncture (Hilgard & LaBaron, 1984). Hypnotic suggestion has also been employed to assist in the management of acute clinical pain syndromes, particularly pain associated with burns (e.g., Crasilneck et al., 1955; Ewin, 1983, 1985; Hartley, 1968; Finer & Nylen, 1961). Let us examine each of these kinds of problems in turn.

Hypnotic Control of Iatrogenic Pain

It is not uncommon for medical procedures to involve varying amounts of discomfort that may be difficult for some patients to tolerate. This is particularly true when the procedure must be repeated frequently, as is the case with dressing changes and debridement for burn patients or bone marrow aspirations for patients under treatment for certain types of cancers. Although many anecdotal examples of the use of hypnotic suggestion to control these types of pain are available (e.g., Crasilneck. McCraine & Jenkins, 1956; Dehenterova, 1967; Ewin, 1986; LaBaw, 1973; Shafer, 1975), these reports are frequently sketchy and often do not provide reliable outcome measures (Nugent, 1985). Fortunately, more systematic controlled studies are beginning to appear that make it possible to begin to quantify the effects of the interventions attempted and make some inferences regarding which variables associated with the interventions are effective in producing clinical benefits.

Schafer (1975), for example, found that fourteen of twenty patients in a burn unit appeared to be able to benefit by the use of hypnotic suggestion. Pain ratings were made, although it is not clear how these were done. In addition, hypnotizability was assessed using the Orne and O'Connell Scale (Orne & O'Connell, 1967). Although the data were not analyzed in a quantitative fashion, there appeared to be a relationship between hypnotizability and response to suggestions for anesthesia and analgesia.

Wakman and Kaplan (1978) studied forty-two patients with burns covering up to 60 percent of the body. In all cases, patients were provided with emotional support and ad lib access to analgesic medications (such as injectable morphine or equipotent doses of other analgesics) up to a limit of 100 mg of morphine, or its equivalent per twenty-four hours. Half of the patients were also provided with a hypnotic treatment that included several different types of induction techniques as well as suggestions for improved comfort. Analysis focused on the amount of medication used by the hypnosis and control patients. Regardless of burn magnitude, less medication was requested by hypnosis than control patients. Moreover, younger patients (7-18 years of age) showed greater reductions in their analgesic use under the hypnosis condition than older patients, a finding consistent with the greater suggestibility of individuals in this age range (Barber, 1969; Gardner & Olness, 1981).

Zeltzer and LaBaron (1982) compared hypnotic suggestion to a control condition for patients undergoing bone marrow aspiration, lumbar puncture, or both procedures. Patients in the control condition were provided with supportive counseling, deep-breathing techniques, distraction, and encouragement to use self-control procedures. However, the use of imagery and fantasy was avoided with these patients. Hypnotic patients were provided with the same sorts of supports augmented by suggestions of pleasant, interesting images. Both groups of patients showed reductions in pain, but greater reductions were reported for the hypnosis group than the control condition. One design problem that limits the conclusions that are possible from this study and many other studies is the confounding of a hypnotic procedure with specific types of suggestions or cognitive strategies for pain management.

Kellerman, Zelter, Ellenberger, and Dash (1983) employed hypnotic suggestion to attenuate the pain of three procedures; bone marrow aspiration, lumbar puncture, and intramuscular injections. Hypnotic procedures appeared equally effective with these three different procedures.

In a preliminary investigation, Hilgard and LaBaron (1984) studied 24 children, aged 4 to 19 years, who were referred because of anxiety and pain related to bone marrow aspiration (16); placement of intravenous needles and dressing changes (5), pain secondary to ulceration (2), and pressure from tumor (1). Although the results were reported to be encouraging, the patient population proved too heterogeneous to make valid inferences regarding the role of hypnosis. Accordingly, a larger-scale study was initiated that focused on the bone marrow aspiration procedure and identified a group of 63 patients who were initially observed under baseline conditions to establish the level of discomfort experienced during normal treatment protocols. Pain ratings were obtained using projective or scale techniques as appropriate to each patient's age. Subsequently, invitations were issued for these children to participate in an investigation of the use of hypnosis to reduce pain associated with bone marrow aspiration. Twenty-four of the 63 patients accepted the invitiation. As might be expected, patients with higher pain ratings were more likely to accept the invitation to participate. One of the purposes of this study was to investigate the relationship between hypnotic responsiveness and suggested hypnotic pain reduction. Accordingly, all patient's were administered age-appropriate versions of the Stanford Hypnotic Clinical Scale (Morgan & Hilgard, 1979a; 1979b).

Among the most interesting observations made during the baseline period was that the 18 patients with the lowest pain levels all reported utilizing spontaneous coping strategies to deal with pain. The types of strategies employed were both cognitive (e.g., watching fantasized TV programs, imagining favorite food, and praying) and noncognitive (clenching or squeezing hands, distractive screaming—to distract from pain rather than because of pain—and conversation). Whether or not a hypnotic procedure has been employed, Hilgard and LaBaron conceptualize these strategies as "hypnotic" to the extent that they are characterized as involving "imaginative orientation" (p. 111). They also offer the interesting speculation that nonhypnotic strategies are not as profound, are fatiguing, and less successful in managing long-term pain, but no evidence is offered on these points. Adult medical and dental patients are also known to utilize spontaneous cognitive strategies to attenuate the pain and stress of clinical procedures (Chaves & Brown, 1978; 1987; Copp, 1974) without the necessity for preceding hypnotic procedures or suggestions to engage in specific coping procedures.

The 24 patients who agreed to participate in the Hilgard and LaBaron study underwent a dress rehearsal of the bone marrow procedure using hypnosis, followed by the actual procedure. Pain reports and pain behaviors were diminished under the hypnotic treatment as compared to the baseline. Moreover, when dichotomized according to hypnotizability, highly hypnotizable patients showed greater reductions in pain than those rated less hypnotizable. Anxiety was also reduced, but as Hilgard and LaBaron caution, these ratings are not independent. Five of the 24 patients whose hypnotizability scores were low failed to reduce pain during the initial session, as well as in a follow-up session conducted generally six weeks later. Of the remaining 19 patients, 10 reduced their reported pain by 3 or more points during the initial session, while 14 showed as large a decrement in pain during the follow-up session.

Although Hilgard and LaBaron attribute the diminished pain they observed to hypnosis, their study does not demonstrate that unequivocally. Their intervention was actually rather complex, including as it did the explicit efforts of clinicians who were concerned for their patients' well-being, dress rehearsals of the medical procedure, and instructions in the use of cognitive strategies for pain control, all together with a hypnotic induction procedure. While the total treatment package appeared to be effective in improving tolerance for the procedure and reducing discomfort, it is by no means clear that the hypnotic intervention itself was necessary, sufficient, or helpful in achieving that outcome.

HYPNOSIS IN CHRONIC PAIN MANAGEMENT

Although most of the early observations of hypnotic pain control were made under conditions of acute pain, within recent years there has been a growing interest in the potential application of hypnotic suggestion to the management of chronic pain syndromes (Barber, 1959; 1982). The ubiquity of chronic pain and the inadequacy of current treatment techniques contribute to the need to identify potentially helpful approaches to this problem (Kotarba, 1983; Turk, Meichenbaum & Genest, 1983). Moreover, many of the cognitive and biofeedback techniques currently employed in chronic pain management incorporate components that resemble those that have historically been associated with hypnotic pain management, although they are typically interpreted and described within other theoretical perspectives (McCaul & Marlott, 1984; Wadden & Anderton, 1982).

Beyond the benefits of hypnotic analgesia for control of pain, there are other potential benefits for the typical chronic pain patient, including the decreased reliance on medication and the development of a greater sense of self-efficacy (Bandura, 1977; Bandura, O'Leary, Taylor, Gauthier & Gossard, 1987).

Unfortunately, the evaluation of hypnotic treatment for chronic pain is no easier than its evaluation for acute pain. Well-controlled studies are lacking. Clinical reports often provide only the most general notion about the nature of the intervention and its impact (Nugent, 1985). Furthermore, many of the clinical studies are conducted by workers who are already convinced of the efficacy of the procedure. Accordingly, what details are provided relate to stylistic aspects of the hypnotic intervention, while the contribution of other potentially important variables, such as establishment of rapport and assessment of preexisting mechanisms for coping with pain, are not reported. This bleak picture is further confounded with a frequent failure to provide follow-up. With these severe limitations in mind, let us turn to examine some of the ways that hypnotic suggestion has been used in chronic pain management.

The range of chronic pain problems to which hypnotic suggestion has been applied is virtually as broad as the range of chronic pain itself. It includes phantom limb pain (Cedercreutz & Uusitalo, 1967; Siegel, 1979; Chaves, 1985a); systemic lupus erythematosus (Smith & Balaban, 1983); chronic low back pain (J. Barber,

1982; Crasilneck, 1979); headache (Andreychuck & Skriver, 1975; Carasso, Kleinhauz, Peded & Yehuda, 1985; Cedercreutz, 1978; Cedercreutz, Lahteenmaki & Tulikoura, 1976; Drummond, 1981; Harding, 1961; Healy & Dowd, 1986; Horan, 1953; Levendula, 1962; Stambaugh & House, 1977), causalgia (Finer & Graf, 1968), cancer pain (Butler, 1954; Cangello, 1961, 1962), postherpetic neuralgia (J. Barber, 1982), rheumatoid arthritis (Elton, Stanley & Burrows, 1983); reflex sympathetic dystrophy (Lewenstein, 1981); Reynaud's syndrome (Braun; 1979; Jacobson, Hackett, Surman & Silverberg, 1973). It is relatively rare that hypnotic suggestion is the sole treatment applied in any of these conditions. Rather, it is usually one component within a diverse, and usually multidisciplinary, effort to manage pain associated with the underlying medical condition (Melzack & Perry, 1975).

It also appears that hypnotic interventions are attempted rather infrequently for at least some of these syndromes. For example, Sherman and his colleagues (Sherman, Gall & Gormaly, 1979; Sherman, Sherman & Gall, 1980; Sherman, Sherman & Parker, 1984) found that although phantom limb pain was a much more prevalent and persistent pain problem than has generally been acknowledged, less than one percent of those phantom limb patients who sought treatment were provided with treatments that were explicitly labeled hypnotic. This seems particularly surprising in view of the fact that traditional medical/surgical interventions for phantom limb pain are largely ineffective, while clinically successful interventions continue to be reported in the hypnosis literature (Cedercreutz, 1978; Chaves, 1985a; Melzack, 1974).

A number of controlled and uncontrolled clinical studies document the use of hypnotic suggestion in the treatment of migraine headache (Anderson, Basker & Dalton, 1975; Andreychuck & Skriver, 1975; Daniels, 1976a; Friedman & Taub, 1982; 1984; 1985) as well as tension headache (Schlutter, Golden & Blume, 1980; Spinhoven, Van Dyck, Zitman & Linssen. 1985). Hypnotic intervention for migraine headache typically includes suggestions designed to achieve peripheral vasodilation and resulting warming of the extremities. However, peripheral temperature is often not measured, and when it is, often reveals an inconsistent relationship to clinical outcome (Friedman & Taub. 1982, 1984). Moreover, these suggestions are often accompanied by suggestions for muscular relaxation, time distortion, enhanced capacity to deal with stress, symptom displacement, and "ego-strengthening" suggestions. Suggestions designed to impact the vascular system appear to play less of a role in interventions aimed at reducing tension headaches (Spinhoven, 1988). Regardless of etiology, posthypnotic suggestions of decreased vulnerability to headaches and decreased severity are often administered together with learning self-hypnotic procedures (Brown & Fromm, 1987).

Suggestions for handwarming or for shrinking of cerebral blood vessels are thought to produce their effects by stabilizing the vasomotor response pattern rather than by altering regional blood flow (Brown & Fromm, 1987). However, some authors have suggested that the patient's perception of control or self-efficacy is the most critical aspect of all cognitive approaches to headache management(Grzesiak, 1977; Tan, 1982; Turk, Meichenbaum & Genest, 1983).

In any case, the clinical results achieved with hypnotic suggestion appear to be equivalent to those reported with such alternative interventions as biofeedback, relaxation therapies, and cognitive/behavioral approaches (Spinhoven, 1988).

The relationship between hypnotizability and clinical outcome for chronic pain has been a matter of some debate (e.g., J. Barber, 1980; Brown & Fromm, 1987; Spinhoven, 1988; Udolf, 1987). Although most clinicians seem to support the notion that there is at least a weak relationship between hypnotizability and clinical outcome, there also seems to be some agreement that a sizabile majority of pain patients can benefit from the use of hypnotic suggestions. Even those clinical studies that appear to document a relationship between clinical outcome and hypnotizability reveal significant clinical benefits, such as reduced reliance on medication, accruing to the less responsive patients (e.g., Cangello, 1961). Evidence indicating that the relationship between hypnotizability and response to suggestion may be highly context dependent raises considerable doubt about the significance of clinical observations that do not as easily permit effective control of context effects (Spanos, 1986b, 1988).

It has been proposed (Udolf, 1987) that hypnotic suggestion is most effective when an organic basis for the pain problem has been established. Presumably, this is at least in part due to the less conflicted motivational picture presented by those patients with a clear diagnosis. However, there are other differences between those patients who have and those who do not have clear diagnoses for their pain problems.

Brown, Chaves, and Leonoff (1981) investigated the pain-related cognitions of two groups of chronic pain patients. One group consisted of 49 patients who had been accepted for treatment at an outpatient multidisciplinary pain-treatment clinic. These patients typically presented with pain of at least several months duration, which had been unresponsive to management by a single clinical specialty. Treatment available at the clinic was multidisciplinary and included medication, biofeedback, physiotherapy, hypnotherapy, and psychotherapy.

The second group consisted of 25 patients who had been diagnosed as having rheumatoid or osteoarthritis and were being followed by a local rheumatologist on a bimonthly basis. Treatment for this group was primarily pharmacological. The proportion of patients who displayed spontaneous coping strategies was similar in these two groups of patients. Moreover, the proportion of copers catastrophizers was about equal in the arthritis group. However, in the pain clinic group, the ratio of catastrophizers to copers was almost two-and-a-half to one. Demographic and psychological variables, including trait anxiety, hypnotizability, and responses to the Melzack-McGill Pain Questionnaire, did not differentiate these two groups of patients, although they did differentiate the copers from the catastrophizers. Interestingly, 69 percent of the catastrophizers, but only 21 percent of the copers, were prescribed antidepressants, anxiolytic agents, or analgesics with anxiolytic components, suggesting that coping and catastrophizing may affect physician prescribing behavior. We speculated that, in the absence of other differences between these two groups of patients, a one potentially critical difference is that while the arthritis patients carry a clear diagnosis, the patients seen at the pain clinic typically did not. If catastrophizing amplifies pain, and analgesia suggestions diminish pain, in part, by inhibiting catastrophizing, greater reductions in pain might be expected in those cases where pain etiology is unclear and the base level of catastrophizing is higher. This hypothesis needs further testing.

Cognitive Strategies for Acute and Chronic Pain Management

Research pertaining to the suggested control of pain has pointed to the critical role of cognitive activity that accompanies painful stimulation. In naturalistic settings, some individuals engage in spontaneous coping strategies designed to minimize their pain and stress (e.g., Brown & Nicassio, 1987; Copp, 1974; Chaves & Brown, 1978; 1987; Hilgard & LaBaron, 1984). On the other hand, others engage in a pattern of thinking and imagining that we have labeled catastrophizing in which pain and the accompanying fears are amplified (Brown, Chaves & Leonoff, 1981; Chaves & Brown, 1978; 1987). Sometimes, catastrophizing provides a way of venting anger at health-care providers, such as the following words of a pain patient, "I think of the job I lost—I'll never be able to get it back . . . I picture myself with pain . . . I use to have thoughts about hanging myself. I think about killing the doctor who operated on me." Another wrote, "at night when the pain is too great to sleep, I would like to take a hammer and hit the doctor who ridiculed me when I complained of the pain . . . I would like to twist his neck and back as grotesquely as mine was in the accident and then offer him a faith-healer, as he did me."

Catastrophizing takes many forms, including pair-related imagery and self-talk. Similarly, coping strategies take many different forms, some cognitive and others noncognitive. Furthermore, cognitive strategies themselves may involve a variety of specific approaches to dealing with pain. Taking advantage of recent findings regarding the importance of suggested strategies for pain reduction, current texts (e.g., Brown & Fromm, 1987; Golden, Dowd & Friedberg, 1987; Udolf, 1987) have begun to advocate the use of suggestions designed to catalyze pain-coping strategies and antagonize catastrophizing. Some examples are as follows:

1. Direct suggestions for attenuation of pain.

2. Relaxation suggestions, often accompanied by deflection of attention to breathing.

3. Transformation of pain sensation, e.g., by reducing its size, by moving it to another part of the body where it is more benign, or by altering its quality.

4. Suggesting sensations incompatible with pain, e.g., numbness, insensitivity.

5. Performing a cognitive analysis of the pain sensation, resolving it into such components as pressure, heat, coldness, etc.

6. Dissociation, for example, thinking of one's body as a machine needing repair, or mentally amputating a painful body part.

7. Simple distraction: facilitating absorption in a pattern of thought that leaves less attention available to concentrate on the pain.

8. Time distortion: Altering the perception of time when pain is being experienced, e.g., suggesting that time pass with the speed of light.

9. Age-regression/progression suggestions: Suggestions to become reabsorbed in thoughts, ideas, and feelings that were enjoyable prior to the onset of pain or will be enjoyable in the future.

10. Transformation of the painful stimulus into a benign one.

11. Modification of catastrophizing ideation experienced by the patient.

The examples listed are a limited subset of the kinds of suggestions that can be employed either within a hypnotic context or outside of it. Obviously, many questions remain regarding the kinds of strategies that are optimally effective, as well as the conditions under which they are effective. Some generalizations are beginning to be possible. For example, some have suggested that distraction strategies are more effective at low-pain levels, while reinterpretation strategies many be more effective at higher pain intensities (McCaul & Malott, 1984). However, recent evidence fails to support this view and indicates that distraction strategies may be more effective than reinterpretation strategies under high levels of experimental pain (Dubreuil, Endler & Spanos, 1987).

Hilgard (1977, 1979, 1986) has proffered a two-component theory of hypnotic analgesia that asserts that some of these pain-reduction strategies, i.e., relaxation and distraction, are available to all subjects regardless of hypnotizability, while more profound levels of pain reduction require the use of different strategies, such as dissociation, that are only thought to be available to highly hypnotizable subjects. However, this conclusion has been criticized by Spanos (1986b, chap. 9 of this volume), on the basis of a large number of studies that demonstrate the equivalent efficacy of distraction strategies when compared with more traditional hypnotic strategies.

Much work remains to be done to establish optimal clinical protocols for the use of these strategies. Studies are beginning to look at the latent, structure of pain-coping strategies in order to examine important differences between strategy types. Wack and Turk (1984), for example, studied the way 32 college students grouped a list of 30 coping strategies that had been randomly selected from a larger pool of strategies employed by college students who had been experimentally exposed to either cold pressor pain or pain associated with muscle ischemia. Cluster analysis revealed eight strategy clusters: (a) behavioral activity, (b) pleasant imaginings, (c) rhythmic cognitive activity, (d) external focus of attention, (e) breathing activity, (f) pain acknowledging, (g) dramatized coping, and (*h*)neutral imaginings. The eight clusters were embedded *i* dimensional scale. The three dimensions were characterized as follows:

Dimension I—Sensation Acknowledging—Strategies that acknowledge pain and seek to transform it, as contrasted with those that deny or dissociate the pain.

Dimension II—Coping Relevance—Strategies on this dimension were differentiated according to the apparent relevance of the strategy to pain management (e.g., doing breathing exercises was seen as obviously relevant, focusing on an irrelevant visual display was assumed to be irrelevant).

Dimension III—Cognitive/Behavioral—Strategies on this dimension differed in the degree to which they were characterized as either cognitive (e.g., imagining being on a beach) versus behavioral (e.g., engaging in some motoric response).

The validity of this three-dimensional model was confirmed in a second experiment (Wack & Turk, 1984) using an additional 16 coping strategies selected from the pool of 250 strategies employed in the first experiment. Taken together the results of these studies suggest that the broad spectrum of possible coping strategies used with experimental pain can be described and differentiated within a three-dimensional space. Of course, the relevance of this model to the study of suggested analgesia with clinical populations still needs to be established. Nevertheless, this methodology may offer a powerful analytic tool for enhancing our understanding of how people cope with pain and suggest clinical approaches that can help optimize this capacity.

OVERVIEW

It seems clear that human beings have a greater capacity to control their response to pain than has generally been acknowledged. When circumstances have permitted investigators to observe this capacity in either the clinical or laboratory setting, researchers have tended to explain the observation away, by incorrectly attributing it to the influence of a special external agent, as was the case with Perkins's tractors, mesmerism, the blue ray, audioanalgesia, and acupuncture. In the case of hypnosis, some have sought to explain the phenomenon in terms of a "special process" within the patient. In either case, the result has been a failure to do justice to the complexity of the phenomenon, a failure to acknowledge the contribution of contextual factors, and a failure to recognize the active role played by patients and subjects in responding to and generating cognitive strategies for pain control.

With respect to clinical pain, it seems rather clear that many patients have benefited by the kinds of interventions that are subsumed under the rubric of hypnotic analgesia, although extreme, and insupportable, claims have been made from time to time. What is a good deal less clear is the role of the hypnotic "special process" in achieving these benefits. Additional research is needed to separate the effects of the hypnotic procedures themselves from suggestions designed to initiate and maintain cognitive coping activity, and from contextual effects that complicate the clinical situation. In addition, much more information is needed about the complex interplay between spontaneous and suggested strategies for pain control before these procedures can be used with optimum effectiveness in clinical settings.

11

Hypnosis in the Control of Labor Pain

Joyce L. D'Eon

The reduction of pain during childbirth has been sought for centuries. Yet, despite developments in modern medications to alleviate pain during labor and delivery, birth is still rated as extremely painful (Melzack, 1984; Melzack, Taenzer, Feldman & Kinch, 1981). Medication either can be ineffective in relieving the pain of childbirth or, when it is effective, the woman may have already experienced a great deal of pain. In addition, there is concern that even the most accepted medications can slow the progress of labor or make it difficult for the parturient to participate fully in the birth process, either of which can result in further obstetrical intervention or complications. While opinions remain divided, the effects of these medications and interventions on the health and well-being of both the fetus and the parturient have been increasingly addressed (Avard & Nimrod, 1985; Macfarlane, 1977; Moire, 1977; Pore & Foster, 1985; Pritchard & MacDonald, 1980). This concern has prompted health practitioners and concerned lay people to refocus their attention on various psychological methods as an aid in childbirth (Parfitt, 1980).

Hypnotic procedures appear to be among the earliest formally applied psychological techniques used to control childbirth pain. However, these procedures have received scant research attention compared to contemporary methods of prepared childbirth. In spite of this, hypnotic procedures are often applauded as a useful approach for a large percentage of parturients (e.g., Hilgard & Hilgard, 1975). The term "prepared childbirth" will be used in this chapter to refer to both Read's natural childbirth method as well as psychoprophylaxis, or the Lamaze method, given that these methods are not operationally distinguishable (Beck, Geden & Broulder, 1979).

This chapter will examine why hypnotic procedures are not as ubiquitous as prepared childbirth techniques. In addition, hypnotic procedures will be evaluated in their own right and in relation to other techniques as methods of pain control during childbirth. In order to provide a background for this discussion, the first part of this chapter will briefly describe the physiological process of childbirth and discuss the evaluation of labor pain and variables related to the experience of pain during childbirth. The next part of the chapter will examine and evaluate the literature on the efficacy of chemical anesthesia, prepared childbirth techniques and hypnotic procedures in affecting pain during labor and delivery. The last section of the chapter will critically compare hypnotic procedures with conventional methods of prepared childbirth, in the control of pain during labor.

THE PHYSIOLOGY OF CHILDBIRTH

It is as yet unclear what factors initiate labor. A current theory suggests that labor is initiated by the formation of prostaglandins in the amniotic fluid and uterine decidua vera (Pritchard & MacDonald, 1980). Labor is divided into three distinct stages. The first, and longest, stage involves the effacement and dilation of the cervix. In order to allow the head (or other presenting part) of the fetus to descend into the vagina, the cervix must dilate to approximately 10 cm in diameter. The process of dilation is estimated to vary from 8 to 13 hours for a primigravida and 5 to 7 hours for a multigravida but is highly variable (Pritchard & MacDonald, 1980). Labor begins when the uterine muscles involuntarily contract in a manner designed to dilate the cervix. Variations in estimates of labor length occur, in part, because operational definitions of when labor begins differ (Davenport-Slack, 1975; Davenport-Slack & Boyland, 1974). At the end of the first stage of labor, contractions may last up to 90 seconds and have an interim period of less than 60 seconds (Pritchard & MacDonald, 1980).

The second stage of labor begins when the cervix is completely dilated, and the contractions, combined with the physical pushing of the parturient, force the fetus into and down the vagina. This stage of labor can last from 50 minutes in a primigravida, to 20 minutes in a multigravida but, as with the first stage, is highly variable (Pritchard & MacDonald, 1980). This stage ends with the delivery of the infant. The expulsion of the infant may result in a tearing of the perineum and/or vagina, or the attendant may perform an incision (episiotomy), all of which require stitching after delivery. While the stretching of the perineum is often rated as quite painful, the episiotomy itself may not be painful, even when the incision is made without a local anesthetic. The pressure and extension of the perineum caused by the descent of the head of the fetus can make this area insensitive to pain (August, 1961; Parfitt, 1980). The third and final stage of labor involves the separation and usually painless expulsion of the placenta from the uterus.

ASSESSMENT OF LABOR PAIN

Pain, in general, tends to be a fairly complex experience and labor pain is no exception (e.g., Barber, 1959; Melzack & Wall, 1983). The causes of pain during labor are not definitely known, however, it has been hypothesized that the pain is due to one or more of the following: hypoxia of the contracted myometrium, compression of nerves in the cervix and lower uterus, and stretching of the cervix and overlying peritoneum (Pritchard & MacDonald, 1980).

Attempting to measure pain objectively has proven to be quite complex and difficult (Melzack, 1983). This is a particularly important issue in the present context because psychological variables are often implicated, explicitly or implicitly, as contributing heavily to the pain experienced by women in labor, often over and above physiological variables (e.g., Chertok, 1969; Kroger, 1977; Lamaze, 1958; Read, 1933). The number of studies attempting to evaluate labor pain systematically pales by comparison to the vast amount of energy, effort, and literature devoted to the examination of the psychological correlates of labor pain and methods of alleviating it (e.g., Beck, Siegel, Davidson, Kormeier, Breitenstein & Hall, 1980; Read, 1933; Lamaze, (1958).

The manner in which pain is assessed is an important consideration in evaluating studies of labor pain. In the experimental pain literature, the term "pain threshold" is used to indicate the point at which sensation is labeled as painful. The term "pain tolerance" is used to define the point at which the individual can no longer tolerate the pain. However, women in labor typically label contractions as painful as soon as they begin, and they become more painful as labor progresses. In labor, tolerance is often defined as the point at which a woman receives medication. However, as will be pointed out, a number of variables affect the administration of analgesic medication aside from the wishes of the parturient.

The time at which labor pain is measured is an important consideration when drawing conclusions from studies examining this type of pain. One study found that women who had been interviewed three weeks postpartum gave similar pain ratings two years after the birth (Bennett, 1985). However, a recent study demonstrated that there are discrepancies between the amount of pain reported during labor and the amount of pain and discomfort reported two days postpartum. Overall, subjects tended to deflate the intensity of both pain and discomfort, but more so the pain (Norvell, Gaston-Johansson & Frid, 1987). It is interesting that these two studies, which attempted to clarify the effect of retrospective ratings on reports of labor pain differed at the time at which these reports were assessed. While many researchers have relied on retrospective reports of pain during labor in their investigations, the validity of such reports warrants further study.

Early attempts to evaluate childbirth pain employed cross-modality matching procedures, in order to avoid relying on subjective pain reports. Unfortunately, these procedures suffered from ceiling effects in that the intensity of labor pain exceeded the upper limit of the measures used. In one study, thermal radiation was applied to the skin of women in labor and they were asked to compare the pain intensity of the contractions with that of the heat. As labor progressed, the intensity of the labor pain increased to the point that many women incurred second-degree blisters from the application of the heat. In addition, results indicated that parturients exhibited little variability in pain thresholds and that "no deviations were observed indicating a "high" or "low" pain threshold, contrary to often expressed opinions in this regard" (Javert & Hardy, 1951, p. 194).

In another attempt to measure the intensity of childbirth pain, women were requested to squeeze a gauge according to the degree of pain they experienced during contractions (Macfarlane, 1977). However, the assessment remained incomplete because women squeezed the pressure gauge as hard as they possibly could long before they reached the end of the first stage of labor.

Melzack, Taenzer, Felman, and Kinch (1981) assessed the intensity of childbirth pain in 141 women using the McGill Pain Questionnaire between contractions. This standardized self-report measure assesses pain intensity as well as the evaluative, affective, and sensory components of pain. One advantage of this instrument is that it incorporates a multidimensional conceptualization of pain and can be used to compare various pain types. Results indicated that labor pain was rated as one of the most intense pains assessed by the McGill Pain Questionnaire and as more intense than cancer and low back pain. This study also found that approximately 9 percent of the primigravidae and 24 percent of the multigravidae reported low levels of pain. A recent study administering the same questionnaire following delivery, reported similar results (Reading & Cox, 1985).

It is interesting that, while the women often rated their pain as a 4 or a 5 on the 5-point intensity scale, some women would not use the accompanying adjective that went with the rating (such as "horrible" or "excruciating") to describe their pain (Melzack et al., 1981). This reluctance was attributed to the degree to which the women felt the experience was positive, in spite of the pain. Thus, while a term such as "horrible" may have encompassed the sensation of the pain, for some women it did not encompass the experience. As noted, one study found that women reported their pain experience as less painful two days postpartum than they had during labor (Norvell et al., 1987). These investigators suggested that women may not want to admit that their labor was extremely painful within the context that birth is viewed as a positive experience and such reports would have negative social connotations (Norvell et al., 1987). Additional support for this contention comes from a study that compared investigators' observations of events during childbirth to the parturients' recollections. The women tended to forget or minimize negative aspects of their experiences (Standley & Nicholson, 1980).

Using visual analogue scales, Price, Harkins and Baker (1987) examined the intensity of pain senations (sensory component) and the degree of unpleasantness (affective component) reported by cancer and chronic pain patients, as well as patients exposed to experimental pain and women in labor. Women evaluated their pain during early and active labor, transition, and pushing. The cancer and chronic pain patients gave higher unpleasantness than sensory pain ratings, while labor patients and patients exposed to experimental pain gave lower unpleasantness ratings than sensory ones. The authors noted that these differences were consistent with the hypothesis that the unpleasantness dimension of pain is augmented by perceived degree of threat to health. The sensory component of the pain during the transition and pushing phases of labor were rated similarly and as significantly more painful than the early and active phases of labor. However, the unpleasantness dimension decreased significantly from the transition to the pushing phase. In addition, this investigation found that women who focused on the birth of the child, as opposed to their pain, reported lower unpleasantness ratings although their sensory ratings were not significantly different.

A number of studies have examined the relationship between observers' ratings of a woman's pain during labor and her own evaluation. This use of behavioral assessment stems, in part, from an attempt to assess pain objectively, as well as more recent emphasis on chronic pain as behavior that can be learned, measured, reinforced, and altered by general learning principles (e.g., Fordyce, 1983). However, this approach appears to be no more accurate than subjective pain reports and, in fact, appears consistently to underestimate intense levels of labor pain. In addition, this method cannot examine the various experiential dimensions of pain that are assessed with other measures, such as the McGill Pain Questionnaire, which have demonstrated that labor pain, like other painful experiences, is a multidimensional phenomenon.

A number of studies comparing self-report ratings with behavioral indices of labor pain found the self-report ratings to be more sensitive. Winsberg and Greenlick (1975) reported that women in labor uniformly judged their pain as more severe than did staff observers. In addition, ratings of patient cooperation were not highly correlated with the parturient's report of labor pain (r = .26). Cogan (1975) reported that Lamaze instructors, husbands and doctors consistently rated the woman's pain as lower during active labor and transition and higher during the delivery than did the women themselves. Nettelbladt, Fagerstrom and Uddenberg (1976) found that 56 percent of women in their sample who reported intolerable pain were not rated by their midwives as having severely painful deliveries. Bonnell and Boureau (1985) examined a behavioral index of labor pain in relation to women's subjective pain ratings. Initially, behavioral scores correlated highly with self-reported pain intensity. However, self-reported pain intensity values increased more steeply than behavioral ones as labor progressed. Consequently, correlations between self and observer ratings of pain were higher at the beginning (r = .68) than at the end of labor (r = .27). The authors noted that agitated behavior (a criterion for the most intense behavioral rating) was not demonstrated at the time when subjective pain intensity was rated at its highest. On the basis of these findings, a "self-control" index, defined as the difference between behavioral and self-ratings, was examined in relation to psychological preparation. This index was found to correlate with psychological preparation in the latter phases of labor. While psychological preparation did not affect women's evaluation of pain, it was related to the behavior they exhibited.

This latter study supports the findings of Price, Harkins and Baker (1987) and Cogan (1975) that the delivery is reported by women as not being as distressing as active labor and transition, even though it is as painful, or more painful, than earlier stages. These studies consistently indicate that observers' evaluations of a woman's pain are not always congruent with that of the individual experiencing the pain. However, there is a degree of consistency among women in the relative degree of pain intensity and distress ascribed to the various stages of labor.

It is interesting to compare these behavioral observations of women in labor with data from animal studies. While it is often assumed that lower animals have relatively painless deliveries, the results of a recent evaluation of 88 cases of captive and wild nonhuman primates from 29 species indicated that mild or severe discomfort (defined as straining, grimacing, writhing, doubling up, etc.) was found in 78 percent of the cases (Lefebvre & Carli, 1985). Moderate levels of vocalization, such as grunts and moans, were reported most frequently. The absence of vocalization was found more frequently than loud vocalizations. Given that behavioral indices of pain tend to underestimate the intensity of labor pain in women, it could be hypothesized that such observations would also underestimate the pain intensity in these animals given the importance of concealment for protection against predation. The authors concluded that in nonhuman primates, parturition is characterized by; a significant degree of pain and discomfort, while vocal responses tend to be subdued (Lefebvre & Carli, 1985). While it has been noted that the structure of the pelvis of the human female is such that birth is likely to be more complex than that of other animals (Melzack, 1984), pain also appears to characterize labor and delivery among nonhuman primates.

CORRELATES OF LABOR PAIN

Pregnancy and birth occur in a context that will be influenced by varying mixtures of socio-cultural, psychological, endocrinological, structural, and metabolic factors and changes. Physiological and structural differences among women and their fetuses contribute heavily to the variability on the intensity and duration of labor, as well as the extent to which obstetrical intervention is required (e.g., Istvan, 1986, Pritchard & MacDonald, 1980).

Physiological measures have demonstrated that, in most women, the perception of labor pain depends on the intensity and pattern of uterine contractions, rather than on their duration. Pressure tracing of the uterus during contractions has been related to subjective reports of pain, and parturients are able to identify the point at which contractions peak (Greenhill & Friedman, 1974). The presence of a contraction can be assessed objectively and correlated with subjective reports. In an attempt to evaluate the correlation between variations in uterine contractions and subjective estimates of pain, Carli, Grossi, Roma, and Battagliarin (1986) examined intensity, duration, and pattern of contractions with topographic tracings. These investigators assessed the second phase of the first stage of labor in 15 primiparous women. The women also made subjective evaluation of their pain on visual analogue scales. The pain associated with contractions fluctuated both within the same woman and between women, and reported pain was significantly correlated with the characteristics of the uterine contractions. This study also indicated that it was the intensity of the uterine pressure, as opposed to the duration of the contraction, which resulted in greater perceived pain. This may explain why, contrary to popular opinion, length of labor is not strongly correlated with reports of labor pain (Norr, Block, Charles, Meyering & Meyers, 1977; Reading & Cox, 1977).

Some consistent findings have been reported relating certain maternal background variables to reports of pain during labor. These studies used verbal reports as their principal measure of pain. First, labor was usually longer and more painful than second labor (Davenport-Slack & Boylan, 1974; Melzack et al., 1981). Reported menstrual difficulties and degree of labor pain were positively related and it has been proposed that this relationship is mediated by an excessive production of prostaglandins (Melzack, 1984; Melzack, et al., 1981). Perhaps, for similar reasons, length of labor has been found to correlate with painful or unpleasant first menstrual experience (Davenport-Slack & Boylan, 1974). However, the relationship between menstrual symptoms and pain has not always been supported (Norr et al., 1977). While a number of studies indicate a negative relationship between socioeconomic status and childbirth pain, the meaning of this relationship is not clear. Some studies have found a relationship between socioeconomic status and patient manageability rather than with actual pain reports (Beck et al., 1980). Age has also been found to correlate negatively with pain ratings (Davenport-Slack & Boylan, 1974; Melzack et al., 1981; Winsburg & Greenlick, 1975). It is difficult to draw conclusions from these relationships because age, parity, and socioeconomic status are also correlated, and the latter is related to attendance at prepared childbirth classes, and social support during pregnancy and childbirth (Melzack, 1984; Norr et al., 1977).

A number of reports implicate psychosocial factors such as anxiety and life changes in the etiology of pregnancy, delivery, and/or postpartum complications (e.g., Beck et al., 1980; Reading & Cox, 1985; Smilkstein, Helsper-Lucas, Ashworth, Montano & Pagel, 1984). Istvan (1987) critically examined and reviewed the research relating the roles of stress and anxiety in birth outcomes. Obstetric difficulty was operationally defined in a variety of ways in the studies examined. Typically, length of labor and various delivery complications were measured. Despite the prevailing belief that emotional factors contribute to obstetric outcome, Istvan (1987) found only weak evidence for effects of maternal stressors or anxiety on either obstetric outcome or neonatal status. Given the physical and psychosocial complexity of labor and the degree of variability in labor length noted, Istvan (1987) stressed that psychosocial factors have to be disentangled from obstetric risk factors before any definitive statements can be made about the independent contribution of these factors. In addition, it was reported that pregnant women tend to have mean anxiety levels that are comparable to, or lower than, the norms for their age group and they also report among the lowest mean number of annual stressful life events as compared to other sociodemographic groups. The author noted that the restricted range of psychosocial predictors chosen may have accounted for their weak results.

In summary, the available data indicate that extremely variable, but typically intense, pain tends to be characteristic of normal labor and delivery, while from 9 to 24 percent of women experience low levels of pain. Aside from supposition, there is no objective evidence that women vary greatly in their threshold for labor pain, although the difficulty in evaluating "threshold" and "tolerance" in this context is recognized. Certain maternal characteristics such as previous menstrual difficulties, gravida, and the parameters of the labor are associated with the amount of pain reported. The manner in which pain is assessed is an important consideration in evaluating studies of labor pain, and retrospective reports may be less valid than reports taken during labor. Cross-modality matching procedures have tended to suffer from ceiling effects. Behavioral assessments correlate significantly with self-report scores during the initial labor but, during the latter phases, self-report ratings exceed behavioral ones, indicating that parturients feel more pain than is rated by observers. These results indicate that self-report may be a more sensitive index of pain than behavioral ratings as labor progresses; in that verbal reports are more strongly correlated with the pattern and intensity of the stimulus. In addition, while the sensory component of labor pain is noted as being quite intense, women tend to refrain from labeling the experience as horrible or excruciating, and tend to forget or minimize negative aspects of their experiences. The intensity of pain during labor and the discomfort reported are somewhat independent, with women reporting the pain during the pushing phase of delivery as less unpleasant than transition even though its sensory intensity is equivalent. This latter finding points to the importance of evaluating the multidimensional aspects of pain and that the most sensitive pain measure in this context appears to be one that assesses both sensory and affective components of pain. The overall picture of women in labor is one of individuals experiencing intense pain; who tend to minimize the negative affect associated with this pain; and whose behavior, in the final stages, underrepresents the pain experienced.

THE SEARCH FOR PAINLESS CHILDBIRTH

Chemical Anesthesia/Analgesia

Illustrations of pain during childbirth have been recorded throughout history. In Western cultures, this pain was attributed to the curse of Eve (Beck & Hall, 1978). This belief was so prevalent in the Christian world that any attempts to relieve childbirth pain were considered sacrilegious. For instance, a Scottish midwife was burned to death in 1591 for attempting to relieve a laboring woman's pain with opium (Parfitt, 1980). It took another two-and-a-half centuries before any real dent was made in this religious doctrine. In 1853, Queen Victoria used chloroform for the delivery of her eighth child. While this caused a furor in the Christian world for the next hundred years, it started the era of medicated childbirth (Beck & Hall, 1978).

    In 1914, "twilight sleep" (the combination of scopolamine with other medications, usually morphine) was introduced to America, and childbirth was thought to have become both painless and unremembered (Kohl, 1962). Scopolamine is no longer recommended for childbirth pain because, while it works well as an amnesic agent, it has no analgesic properties and is potentially dangerous to fetal respiration (Kohl, 1962; Pritchard & MacDonald, 1980). Today, local anesthesia and analgesia have replaced general anesthesia for vaginal delivery, and there is a trend for caesarean sections to be medicated in this manner as well (Moir, 1977; Pritchard & MacDonald, 1980). The frequency of medicated births varies among hospitals, regions, and countries and ranges from 8 percent to 80 percent in Canada and the United States (Baruffi, Dellinger, Strobino, Rudolph, Timmons & Ross, 1984; Melzack, 1981).

In spite of the development and widespread use of medications in childbirth during the last seventy years, there have always been obstetricians and health professionals (as well as nonprofessionals) who have been concerned with the effects of these medications on the health of the parturient and fetus. While local medications are potentially less harmful than general anesthetics, each has its own particular problems and contraindications (Kohl, 1962; Kolata, 1979; Moir, 1977; Pritchard & MacDonald, 1980). In addition, even the most effective pain-relief procedures and agents, such as epidurals, are only partly effective in relieving pain in 5 percent of cases, and ineffective in 10 percent to 33 percent of cases (Avard & Nimrod, 1985; Melzack, Kinch, Dobkin, Lebrun & Taenzer, 1984; Melzack et al., 1981; Moir, 1977).

The focus of the controversy over the use of medication in labor has tended to be on the effectiveness and the medical risks associated with these medications. The responses of parturients to these interventions have rarely been examined. When evaluated, it has been reported that women find the numbness associated with the epidurals disturbing and that they sometimes feel divorced from the experience of giving birth (Oakley, 1983). One study found that participation in delivery was important for a positive birthing experience (Norr et al., 1977). These investigators also found that labor pain and enjoyment in childbirth emerged as two distinct, though related, dimensions of the birth experience. Such findings suggest that the assessment of women's satisfaction with their childbirth experience is as important as the assessment of the efficacy of medical interventions (Melzack, 1984; Oakley, 1983; Richards, 1982). While it is clear that women do not desire pain in labor, some researchers have found that it is important for many women to maintain a sense of mastery or control during labor and delivery, and that these factors are related to enjoyment in the birth, independent of the pain experienced (Norr et al., 1977; Oakley, 1983; Richards, 1982).

The totally effective, risk-free analgesic has yet to be developed, and despite the prevalence of medication in labor, prepared childbirth methods continue to be popular. In the United States, more than 70 percent of hospitals surveyed reported that 50 percent of the women who delivered at their institutions had received Lamaze preparation (Wideman & Singer, 1983). Women are continuing to educate themselves about childbirth, and continue to seek safe aids in dealing with the experience of labor and delivery.

Prepared Childbirth Techniques

Hypnotic procedures were used to control pain during childbirth long before any of the prepared childbirth techniques were developed (Kroger, 1977). While the "hypnosuggestive" method was popular in Russia in the 1930s, this method was altered slightly and relabeled "psychoprophylaxis" by Velvosky (see reviews by Beck, Geden & Brouder, 1979; Beck & Hall, 1978). It is this method that Lamaze studied. The numerous similarities between hypnotic techniques and the other methods of prepared childbirth (Beck et al., 1979; Davenport-Slack, 1975; Kroger, 1953; Mandy, Mandy, Farkas, & Scher, 1952) resulted in both Read (1933) and Lamaze (1958) having to deny that their methods were "hypnotic." Since the components of these methods are similar to components of hypnotic techniques, the development of these methods, their rationale, and their efficacy will be presented.

In 1933, Grantly Dick Read published a book that contained a new theory about pain in childbirth. Until then, there had been little controversy over whether or not the process of childbirth was or, in fact, should be painful. Instead, debate centered more on the manner in which the pain should be relieved. Apparently, from the report of one woman who had a painless labor, Read developed his thesis that childbirth was not inherently painful. Read proposed that cultural misconceptions, fears, and biases were passed along the generations to parturient women and resulted in resistance to the naturally painless process of childbirth. This resistance created the pain during labor and it was hypothesized that if this resistance was eliminated (through education regarding the nature of childbirth, muscle relaxation exercises, and breathing techniques), then the process itself would no longer be painful.

Read supported his argument with evidence drawn from two main sources. First, anthropological reports at that time indicated that women in "primitive" cultures did not appear distressed during childbirth. From this observation, and the assumption that the expression of pain reflected the intensity of pain, it was inferred that these women did not experience pain. As noted earlier, using pain behavior as the sole index of pain is problematic not only because pain expression is moderated by many social and cultural variables unrelated to the experience of pain (Craig, 1980; Javert & Hardy, 1951; Mandy et al., 1952; Winsberg & Greenlick, 1975), but also because behavior becomes subdued during intense levels of labor pain (Bonnell & Bourreau, 1985). While there is no valid evidence to indicate that any civilization (ancient, primitive, or contemporary) or any ethnic or racial group has painless childbirth (Freedman, 1963; Freedman & Ferguson, 1950; Macfarlane, 1977; Pesce, 1987; Wolff & Langley, 1968), early reports were often cited as support for Read's thesis.

Second, since labor is a "natural" physiological process, it was suggested that childbirth should not be painful. It was assumed that pain was a response to tissue damage and since most labors and deliveries involve little or no tissue damage, it was thought that it should not be painful. This proposition was a reflection of the theories of pain at that time, and it now is understood that tissue damage is neither a necessary nor a sufficient condition for pain perception (Barber, 1959; Beecher, 1946; Melzack, 1983).

Twenty-five years after Read, Lamaze wrote a book on the Soviet technique of psychoprophylaxis (the English translation being published in 1958) and this form of prepared childbirth was popularized. The rationale proffered for the pain during childbirth, according to this method, was somewhat more complicated than Read's. Cortical excitatory processes and imbalances were posited as explanations for childbirth pain that was caused by the parturient's negative emotions. Through a series of techniques such as education, breathing exercises, stroking and pressing of specific "pain points," plus timing contractions, it was suggested that childbirth would be painless (Beck et al., 1979).

Both Read and Lamaze insisted that childbirth was not inherently painful, and neither author attributed the alleged success of their methods to the introduction or manipulation of psychological factors related to pain perception. Success was attributed to the elimination of specific psychic stimuli that, in turn, reduced the physiological cause and sensation of pain during childbirth. Stating that these techniques resulted in physiological changes that reduced pain in childbirth was accepted as legitimate more readily than attributing the success to psychological changes. Nevertheless, stating that childbirth is not "naturally" painful and that the "unnatural pain" can be eliminated by a number of techniques is fundamentally different from saying that the process is "naturally" painful but pain can be alleviated by these same techniques. For example, while it is commonly accepted that fear and anxiety can increase pain, as Read suggested, the available data fail to support the proposition that the elimination of fear and anxiety will eliminate pain (Melzack, 1983; Weisenberg, 1977).

Prepared childbirth techniques implicitly put the onus for the pain experienced during childbirth on the woman herself. Thus, her experience of pain would sometimes be met either with denial by medical staff, or by a punitive attitude that it was "her own fault" (Lennane & Lennane, 1973). At times, women who received prepared childbirth instruction but then experienced pain during labor reported feeling frustrated or "weak" because they required medication in spite of the time they (and perhaps their coaches) devoted to the training (Hilgard & Hilgard, 1975; Kohl, 1962; Lennane & Lennane, 1973; Melzack et al., 1981; Moir, 1977). In fact, there is evidence to indicate that realistic expectations regarding the painfulness of various procedures (including the pain in childbirth) will lead to better coping behavior and less pain than unrealistic expectations (Astbury, 1980; also see review by Weisenberg, 1977).

Today, most proponents of Lamaze claim that the preparation is effective in alleviating pain, not in abolishing it, and the use of drugs is not discouraged. While this viewpoint is likely a more accurate reflection of what occurs, it is based on the assumption that "normal" labor, even among prepared women, is often painful, and this is not the position originally argued by Lamaze. It continues to be argued that Lamaze training makes childbirth a more controllable and positive experience (Wideman & Singer, 1984).

The benefits claimed for prepared childbirth techniques have ranged from better fetal adjustment in the nursery, to less pain (or no pain) during childbirth, to fewer caesarean sections (Beck & Hall, 1978) to the prevention of decreases in marital satisfaction after birth (Markham & Kadushin, 1986). Both an older review (Mandy et al., 1952) and a more recent review (Beck & Hall, 1978) provide scathing critiques of the rationales behind prepared childbirth training, and the literature supporting its apparent success. Beck & Hall (1978, p. 377) state that "it is important to note the absence of a single adequately controlled study." One of the major problems with the area of research has been subject selection, with patients using prepared childbirth techniques tending to differ from those who do not on a number of variables, such as socioeconomic status and age (Beck & Hall, 1978; Leonard, 1973; Melzack, 1984). As discussed, these variables are independently related to more positive attitudes, increased support, and reductions in pain during labor. A discussion of other methodological problems will be presented later in this chapter.

It is difficult to make conclusive statements regarding the efficacy of these techniques on childbirth pain because of a number of moderating and confounding variables (Beck & Hall, 1978) and because of conflicting results. Some studies that compared the effect of prepared childbirth training versus no training on reported pain during labor found small but significant effects (Beck et al., 1980; Charles, Norr, Block, Meyering & Meyers, 1978; Melzack et al., 1981). In these studies, women who had received prepared childbirth training reported less pain. All of the studies used verbal reports, however, and only the study by Melzack and his colleagues (1981) assessed pain during labor. In contrast, other studies that also used verbal reports, failed to find this relationship (Davenport-Slack & Boylan, 1974; Doering, Entwisle & Quinlan, 1980; Reading & Cox, 1985). In these studies, pain was assessed after, not during labor, and all of the parturients in the study by Davenport-Slack and Boylan (1974) received medication, with 40 percent of the sample receiving general anesthesia. In spite of the small or nonsignificant effects of prepared childbirth techniques on reported pain, most investigators noted other benefits of preparation, such as increased sense of control, husband and parturient participation, and so on.

Neither chemical anesthetics, analgesics, nor prepared childbirth techniques have been found to be completely adequate in controlling the pain of childbirth for most women. There are a number of conceptual difficulties with the rationale underlying prepared childbirth techniques. Unrealistic or overzealous claims regarding the efficacy of prepared childbirth methods in controlling pain have resulted in disappointing experiences for some women and initial claims have now been modified. Research assessing the efficacy of these techniques on the subjective experience of pain have been inconsistent; when demonstrated, such effects have been small or nonsignificant. In addition, conclusions have been difficult because of subject selection factors.

HYPNOSIS IN THE CONTROL OF LABOR PAIN

The use of hypnotic procedures for pain control has tended to wax and wane along with the general acceptance and use of hypnosis by the medical profession. In 1958 the American Medical Association recognized hypnosis as a treatment in medicine and dentistry (Plunkett, 1958). Hypnotic procedures have been used to treat a variety of gynecological and obstetrical disorders (for example, Fuchs, Paldi, Abamovici & Peretz, 1980; Hartmann & Rawlins, 1960; Leckie, 1964, 1965). However, these procedures have most commonly been used to make the process of childbirth more comfortable for parturients. While the numerous single-case studies in the literature are suggestive (for example, Crasilneck & Hall, 1973; Crasilneck, McCranie & Jenkins, 1956; Coulton, 1966; Samuelly, 1972; Weishaar, 1986), they lack the appropriate controls to be conclusive. Studies that report on multiple cases, some of which examined comparable cases from hospital records, will be presented and evaluated in the following section. Studies that employed more adequate comparison groups will then be discussed.

Multiple-Case Studies

Abramson and Heron (1950) gave 100 parturients an average of four sessions of hypnotic training and compared their responses to 88 patient records pulled randomly from the hospital files. Hypnotic subjects exhibited significantly shorter first stage labor and were administered less medication than the comparison group patients. While reduced discomfort was also reported in the hypnosis group, it does not appear that pain was directly measured and it is unclear as to how this was determined for the comparison group.

Michael (1952) reported on 30 parturients who received hypnotic training. The women were administered a hypnotic treatment alone on two occasions and then in groups of six for up to 11 sessions. "Depth of trance" was assessed on a 5-point scale; however, these data were not reported. A comparison group was drawn from women of similar parity who were admitted to the same hospital immediately after the women receiving hypnotic training. Length of second stage labor of the primigravidae who received hypnosis training was reported to be significantly less than that of the comparison subjects. It was reported that 73 percent of the parturients had painless labors. However, pain does not appear to have been directly assessed, but rather inferred by the amount of medication administered. The issue of pain was not addressed for the comparison subjects.

Kline and Guze (1955) investigated the effects of self-hypnosis on 30 selected parturients and reported that 17 of these women did not receive any medication throughout labor and delivery, while another 12 were rated by their obstetricians as using the same or smaller doses of medication than would normally have been expected. Callan (1961) reported a decrease in the medication requirements and the total amount of time in labor for 79 parturients delivered with hypnosis during 1959 as compared to 86 parturients who had delivered during 1956. Gross and Posner (1963) compared 200 parturients who had received group training with hypnosis to 200 cases (collected two years previously) who had not, and found a reduction in the amount of pain medication administered and a shortened first stage of labor for the hypnosis group compared to the nonhypnosis group. Schibly and Aanonsen (1966) reported success with 78 of 93 unwed mothers who had been trained in self-hypnosis. Although the criteria for success were not clearly specified, it appears that they were based on a decrease in the amount of nursing care demanded and on the impression that the parturients delivered without as much medication as would have been expected without hypnosis.

One particular survey deserves special mention, not only because of the number of cases involved, but also because of the great deal of detail provided with these cases. August (1961) presented data on 1,000 parturients, 85 percent of whom went through delivery with hypnoanesthesia. Although no fewer operative interventions and no shorter labors were reported for these 850 parturients, a marked decrease in medication was noted, compared to the 150 parturients who did not have hypnoanesthesia. In all cases, August was the obstetrician, the anesthesiologist, and the hypnotist. Almost half of the parturients who received hypnosis received no chemical analgesia or anesthesia, while all of the 150 parturients for whom hypnoanesthesia had not been attempted received anesthetics. In addition, more than half of the parturients receiving hypnoanesthesia had not been previously prepared by August for the delivery. That is, 463 (or 57 percent) of the parturients received hypnosis and hypnoanesthesia for the first time when they were in the hospital for the delivery.

None of the studies cited assessed the parturients' susceptibility to hypnosis with standardized scales. While a few of the studies note responsive individuals, susceptibility appears to have been determined post hoc, on the basis of the parturient's ability to tolerate obstetrical intervention, to go without pain medication (August, 1961; Schibly & Aanonsen, 1966) or by some unspecified criteria (Callan, 1961; Michael, 1952). The issue of susceptibility is important in pain control and should be carefully assessed in studies designed to determine the efficacy of hypnotic procedures in the control of labor pain. Except for the cases reported by August (1961), these studies do not provide sufficient details to adequately evaluate certain aspects of the research. In two of the studies, it is difficult to tell whether self-hypnotic procedures were used, or whether the physician actively administered hypnotic procedures to the parturient (Callan, 1961; Gross & Posner, 1963).

The studies cited suffer from a number of methodological problems. These issues are particularly important because many studies assessing the efficacy of various methods (besides, or in addition to, hypnosis) on the experience of childbirth have suffered from these problems (Barber, 1959; 1963; Davenport-Slack, 1975; Hilgard & Hilgard, 1975; Mandy et al., 1952). One major concern is that none of the studies assessed pain directly. Reductions in pain were inferred from two sources: (1) when the parturient appeared calmer or more relaxed; and/ or (2) when there was less medication used, or fewer obstetrical procedures conducted with or without medication.

The problems inherent in evaluating the experience of pain based solely on external expression have already been addressed. Using the quantity of medication administered to infer the experience of pain is difficult precisely because the medication is "administered." Not only do hospitals differ in their prescription and proscription of medication, but so do individual physicians and childbirth trainers (Richard, 1982; Baruffi et al., 1984). Thus, one may be assessing a hospital or a physician bias rather than pain perception. Not all parturients who request medication are given medication, while others may sometimes be administered medication even when they do not request or want it (August, 1961). A parturient's refusal of analgesics may be based on a number of factors other than pain, such as religion or a concern for potential danger to the fetus. In addition, the parturient may try to live up to either her own expectations or those of her physician or childbirth training regarding the use of medication. Since most births are medicated, studies are often comparing relative differences between groups which, in addition to the problems already noted, is further confounded by individual differences in response to and tolerance of these drugs.

These methodological issues are especially salient in studies which drew their samples at different times. In these instances, the administration of medication is potentially confounded by the phyician's attitude toward and willingness to administer drugs. For example, the comparison group used by Callan (1961) consisted of maternity cases delivered three years prior to the delivery time of the hypnosis group. Gross and Posner (1963) made similar kinds of comparisons. In these studies, the investigator was also the physician who hypnotized and administered treatments to patients. Both the studies by Callan (1961) and by Gross and Posner (1963) were undertaken because the researchers became interested in the use of hypnosis in obstetrics.

The performance of obstetrical procedures (such as episiotomies) without the use of medication is often cited as evidence to support the contention that these parturients were anesthetized. For example, while local medications were administered to all parturients receiving episiotomies in the study reported by Schibly and Aanonsen (1966), seven women were not given this medication in order to "satisfy the curiosity of the operator" (p. 341). No mention is made as to whether or not these episiotomies were rated as painful by the women involved; however, since no apparent objection was made, the authors inferred that the procedure was entirely painless. In fact, as was pointed out earlier, episiotomies themselves and the repair of an episiotomy is not always painful, especially if it is done quickly after delivery (August, 1961). Nevertheless, August (1961) states that it is impressive that more women in his hypnosis group underwent the episiotomy without medication as compared to the group that did not receive hypnosis. Conclusions regarding the success of hypnosis and the experience of pain from these findings suffer from the same logical problems as does drawing conclusions from the administration of analgesics. Since it is the physician who determines whether or not an episiotomy is to be performed, and whether or not it will be done with or without medication, results may simply reflect the physician's willingness to use these procedures.

Four studies reported that labor length was shortened for women who had been trained with hypnosis (Abramson & Heron, 1950; Callan, 1961; Gross & Posner, 1963; Michael, 1952). Two studies found a reduced first stage labor (Abramson & Heron, 1950; Gross & Posner, 1963) one reported a reduced second-stage labor (Michael, 1950) and one found a reduced total time in labor (Callan, 1961) as compared to their respective comparison groups. In addition to the problems regarding the assessment of pain, comparing different groups of parturients on the length of labor can also be problematic. It is difficult to determine when, in fact, labor begins. In the studies presented, Callan (1961) considered labor to have started when the parturient entered hospital. Gross and Posner (1963) appeared to have assessed labor according to cervical dilation (although this is not clear). In one part of their paper, they noted that women in the hypnosis group tended to have more cervical dilation at the time of admission while, in another part of the paper, they state that this difference was not great. Considering that they found a difference only for the first stage of labor and not the second, the operational definition of when labor begins is important. Given that the second stage of labor occurs when dilation is complete it is less difficult to operationalize. However, differences in second stage labor length could be due to differences in the amount of medication administered, as opposed to the technique itself and, as noted, a number of these studies reported differences in the amount of medication administered. The study employing the largest sample did not report differences in labor length (August, 1961).

Verbal reports tend to indicate longer labors than the durations indicated by cervical dilation. Women who have received prepared childbirth training tend to report shorter labors than nontrained women, which is not substantiated by the extent of cervical dilation (Davenport-Slack & Boylan, 1974). These findings have implications for studies reporting that hypnosis and prepared childbirth result in shorter labors. Unless cervical dilation is used in the assessment of labor length, studies must be viewed with caution. Nevertheless, it is interesting to speculate why these verbal reports should underestimate labor. On one hand, it could be the desire of the parturient to appear relaxed and not overly-anxious about reporting "small" contractions. On the other hand, it could be that they are less aware of the contractions. As yet, there are no data to support one hypothesis or the other. Data regarding whether or not hypnotic procedures (or prepared childbirth methods) reduce the length of labor are inconclusive, and the mediating mechanism which would underlie such a finding, is still unclear (Werner, Schauble & Knudson, 1982).

Comparative Studies

In addition to the methodological problems already mentioned, the studies previously cited did not employ adequate control or comparison groups. There are a few studies which, in addition to directly assessing subjective reports of pain, provided more adequate comparisons between nonhypnotic and hypnotic groups. While these studies report on a number of different dependent measures, the data regarding the experience of pain will be the focus of the discussion.

Perchard (1960) compared three groups of primigravidae on a number of variables during childbirth. All women were volunteers and were enrolled by serial rotation into one of the three groups. The first group consisted of 268 parturients who attended three sessions in which information about childbirth was provided and all women visited the labor ward (information-only group). The second group of 126 parturients received the same instruction as the first group but also received three relaxation classes (information-plus-relaxation group). The third group of 986 parturients received the same instruction as the first group, with the addition of three hypnosis sessions (hypnosis group). The hypnotic sessions were conducted by midwives who had no previous training with the technique. A standardized induction was used, followed by suggestions for comfort and relaxation during labor and delivery (i.e., self-hypnosis). It is important to note that the staff on the labor ward were usually unaware of the parturients' group assignment, and the parturients themselves were not aware that there were different methods of preparation.

In the hypnosis group, 547 (55.5 percent) of the parturients were found to be highly susceptible to hypnosis; 257 (26 percent) were rated as moderately susceptible; and 182 (18.5 percent) were rated as not susceptible. The large number of highly susceptible women was attributed to the fact that the criteria employed did not allow for a differentiation between "good" and "somnambule" individuals. The criteria employed for determining responsiveness to hypnosis were based on objective responses to various suggestions, with responsiveness to more difficult items indicating greater susceptibility.

One week after delivery, the mothers' subjective experiences of pain were assessed. Half the women in the information-only group and the information-plus-relaxation group recalled severe pain, compared to 32 percent in the hypnosis group. In addition, 38 percent of the women in the hypnosis group rated the experience as pleasant, compared to 18 percent of women in the information-only group and 25 percent in the information-plus-relaxation group. The majority (78 percent) of all the women felt that the preparation they received had been helpful.

Perchard (1960) concluded that the most impressive result was the confidence and satisfaction shown by the women in the hypnosis group, especially considering the lack of extensive preparation. The reduction in the subjective experiences of pain was rated as limited for the hypnotic group and as not significantly different from the reductions obtained in the information-only and the information-plus-relaxation groups.

In examining the subjective reports of pain in the hypnotic group, there appears to be an effect for susceptibility. For example, while 67 percent of the highly susceptible subjects rated the pain as not severe at any time, nonsusceptible subjects gave this rating 44 percent of the time. The information-only and the information-plus-relaxation groups rated the pain as not severe 44 percent and 42 percent of the time, respectively. In addition, 29 percent of the highly susceptible subjects rated the pain as severe, compared to 54 percent of the information-plus-relaxation group. It is interesting that such large effects were demonstrated considering that the high-susceptible subjects were quite generously classified and a number of medium-high-susceptible individuals would likely have been included in this group.

Davidson (1962) compared hypnotically-trained women with a group of women who received either physiotherapy relaxation (i.e., Read's prepared childbirth techniques) or no special training apart from "mothercraft" information. All three groups comprised 45 primigravidae and 25 multigravidae. The parturients chose the group in which they wanted to participate. The training in self-hypnosis was done in groups of six women each, and all groups received six lessons. A standard induction was administered by the obstetrician-hypnotist, and suggestions were given that the delivery would be comfortable and that they would require fewer chemical analgesics, etc. The prepared childbirth group received six lessons that involved relaxation and controlled breathing as well as pelvic exercises.

Although it is not clearly reported, it appears that pain was assessed after delivery. Parturients in the hypnotic group consistently rated the first and second stages of labor as less painful than did either the prepared group or the control group. The prepared group tended to rate the pain as less severe during the first stage of labor; however, the ratings are quite similar for the second stage. While 46 percent of the parturients in the hypnotic group rated the first stage as painless, only 12 percent of the other two groups (when combined) rated it as painless. The second stage was rated as painless by 24 percent of the hypnotic subjects, but only 3 percent of the other two groups (in total) rated it as such. As had Perchard (1960), Davidson (1962) concluded that the most impressive result was that 70 percent of the parturients in the hypnosis group rated childbirth as pleasant, compared to 23 percent of the prepared group and 33 percent of the controls. Unfortunately, susceptibility was not assessed in this study.

Rock, Shipley and Campbell (1969) randomly assigned 22 parturients to a hypnotic group and 18 to a control group. Full-term parturients, who had not progressed beyond four centimeters of cervical dilation, were assigned to one of the groups. Medical students remained with each parturient throughout most of labor and presented hypnosis to the women. Parturients in the hypnotic group were not formally requested to participate; rather, the student-hypnotist began to talk to the women about making them feel more comfortable, then went into an eye fixation suggestion followed by a typical induction with suggestions for relaxation and comfort. Further suggestions were given when necessary during the balance of the labor period. After delivery, the women rated their amnesia and pain on a five-point scale as follows: (1) complete amnesia; (2) incomplete amnesia; (3) some pain, but satisfied with analgesia; (4) pain, dissatisfied with analgesia (i.e., would have liked more or different medication); (5) failure of method. Parturients in the hypnotic group rated their experiences as significantly less painful than the control group. About half of the women in both groups said they would have liked to have had more medication.

Although hypnotic depth was assessed, it was based on three suggestions and on the impression of the student-hypnotist. This is not as adequate as a standardized procedure, and no mention was made of any relationship between hypnotic depth and the subjective experience of pain. A standardized, less complicated measure of pain should perhaps have been used. The one employed actually assessed amnesia, pain and adequacy of the medication. Another potential problem with this study was that it mentioned a difference between the two groups in parity but failed to specify which group had the larger number of primigravidae.

Of the more recent studies that have been reported, one study did not appear to assess subjective reports of pain (Fuchs, Marcovici, Peretz & Paldi, 1980) and the other did not specify how pain was assessed (Tiba, Balogh, Meszaros, Banyai, Greguss & Jakubecz, 1980). Two other studies were reported adequately enough to be evaluated. Davidson, Garbett and Tozer (1985) randomly divided 50 primigravidae, who had been invited to participate in a study using self-hypnosis into experimental and control groups. The experimental group was offered a training cassette containing a general induction to relaxation and hypnosis and a hypnotic induction followed by specific suggestions for pain relief and positive attitudes toward childbirth. The control group received the same antenatal preparation as the experimental group but were not offered the training cassette. Hypnotic susceptibility was not assessed. Both groups were interviewed after delivery and made global ratings of pain on a visual analogue scale. No differences in length of labor or the amount of medication administered were found. However, women in the self-hypnosis group reported less pain during the first stage of labor, but not the second, and reported more positive attitudes toward labor.

Venn (1987) evaluated parturients who self-selected Lamaze, hypnosis, or Lamaze-plus-hypnosis training. No differences between groups were found on pain ratings taken after delivery, duration of labor, amount of medication taken, or nurses' ratings. One interesting aspect of this study is that of the 122 women approached for this study, only 17 volunteered for hypnosis, and only 8 out of 80 women in the Lamaze group volunteered for a free test of their hypnotizability. The Stanford Hypnotic Clinical Scale for Adults (SHCS; Morgan & Hilgard, 1975) was used to assess the susceptibility of the women in the hypnosis conditions. The author found that the SHCS scores were not highly correlated with outcome measures for Lamaze or hypnosis.

While the multiple case studies presented in the first part of this section are suggestive, they lack the appropriate controls necessary to be conclusive. Some of the comparison studies, however, had large or adequate samples of women. In one of the studies, women were assigned to one of the groups on a volunteer basis, but without awareness of the other groups (Perchard, 1960), and on a nonvolunteer basis in two others (Davidson et al., 1985; Rock et al., 1969). All of the studies employed a control or comparison group that was drawn from the same population of parturients at the same time.

The scales used to assess pain differed from study to study, which makes comparisons difficult. However, the main concern regarding this measurement is that all studies appeared to assess pain after delivery, not during labor and, as has been suggested, women may minimize the negative aspects of their experiences at this time. While caution may be necessary in evaluating the strength of effects within these studies, these data suggest that hypnotic procedures are effective for some women in reducing child birth pain.

DISCUSSION

Hypnotic procedures have failed to meet the grandiose claims that have sometimes been made for them. For example, hypnotic procedures do not generally eliminate reported pain or expressions of suffering, although these procedures have consistently been found to reduce pain, both experimentally and clinically for a number of people (Hilgard & Hilgard, 1975). The proportion of people who can benefit from, or are open to, hypnotic procedures for the control of pain is an issue that has not yet been resolved. The preceding evaluation of hypnotic techniques in childbirth parallels the clinical and experimental findings regarding the use of hypnotic procedures in other settings such as in dentistry. That is, although these procedures are sometimes successful in reducing childbirth pain, they do not generally eliminate it.

The literature indicates that hypnotic procedures are at least as effective as contemporary methods of prepared childbirth or the provision of information in alleviating pain in childbirth. More specifically, hypnotic procedures appeared to be effective in reducing reported pain during at least the first stage of labor, for approximately one-third of women. On the other hand, hypnotic procedures were not at all effective in alleviating pain for at least another third of parturients. However, as noted earlier, anywhere from 9 to 24 percent of women experience relatively painless childbirth, without any intervention. It is important to demonstrate that these procedures reduce pain significantly more than base rates would predict.

The research to date has not determined which components of hypnotic procedures are critical for success. In addition, the effectiveness of various components of prepared childbirth techniques has not, as yet, been evaluated in the clinical setting. Since the components of these techniques overlap, any study seeking to elucidate the critical components of one technique has implications for the others. Methods of prepared childbirth contain four main components: (1) the provision of information about childbirth; (2) breathing exercises; (3) muscle relaxation; and (4) suggestions (either explicit or implicit) that these methods will be effective in controlling or eliminating pain, etc. (Beck & Seigel, 1980; Davenport-Slack, 1975). Historically, these components have almost always been an integral part of hypnotic techniques designed to control pain. As mentioned, it was the close resemblance between the effects and the components of hypnotic and prepared childbirth techniques that led some to conclude that prepared childbirth techniques were "really" hypnosis (e.g., Mandy et al., 1952).

Among the similarities in these procedures are the breathing exercises and muscle relaxation components of prepared childbirth techniques, which are also central to most hypnotic induction techniques. The parturients' concentration on a specific point in the visual field, as part of the Lamaze relaxation procedure, is similar to the eye fixation used in many hypnotic induction techniques. Even the stroking of specific "pain points" advocated by some Lamaze instructors appears to have its historical roots in the "passes" and stroking that Mesmer and his followers often performed near the ovarian area of a woman's body in order to relieve many symptoms, including pain. The one component of the prepared childbirth technique that is often (but not always) included in hypnotic procedures is the provision of information concerning childbirth. However, as has been shown, the provision of information alone is unlikely to result in any significant reduction of labor pain (Davidson, 1962; Perchard, 1960).

The efficacy of prepared childbirth techniques was originally attributed to changes in the physiological processes of childbirth. Now, it is commonly accepted that these techniques, like hypnotic procedures, facilitate pain control through psychological (not physiological) mechanisms. For example, the information component combined with relaxation can often work to reduce anxiety, and thus to reduce the experience of pain. As stressed earlier, this reduction of anxiety does not eliminate pain, and in this setting it is unclear how much effect anxiety reduction has on pain reports. Anxiety management may limit exacerbation of an already-painful experience and reduce the likelihood that the parturient will feel overwhelmed. That is, it may make the experience more positive by allowing a parturient to feel more in control, even if it does not reduce pain. The studies that found that pain and enjoyment or satisfaction with childbirth were relatively independent, support this contention.

Direct suggestion has been found effective in reducing both experimental and clinical pain, with or without a hypnotic induction (Barber, 1970; Spanos, 1986). In part, the efficacy of prepared childbirth techniques has been attributed to distraction (Beck & Seigel, 1980; Davenport-Slack, 1975), through the timing of contractions, trying to breathe "properly," attempting to remain calm and relaxed, and other strategies that give the parturient something to do, other than to focus on the pain. An additional component that has recently become more prevalent is the active participation of the parturient's partner or coach, who often times the contractions, and provides massage, support, and encouragement (Beck & Seigel, 1980; Davenport-Slack & Boylan, 1974; Doering et al., 1980; Norr et al., 1977). This support has consistently been found to increase the probability that a woman will view her childbirth experience as positive. The inclusion of partners in the birth process has increased over the past decade (Baruffi et al., 1984). It could be hypothesized that some unknown portion of the success achieved by August (1961) with parturients unselected for hypnotizability and with no previous training, was due to the support and encouragement he provided, at a time when partners were not encouraged to attend, rather than to the hypnotic techniques per se.

Hypnotic procedures may include additional components that are not always incorporated in prepared childbirth techniques. For example, an examination of the studies reported by August (1961) reveal that, as a hypnotist, in addition to his support, he continually provided parturients with a number of cognitive strategies in an attempt to reduce pain: he sometimes asked parturients to imagine different events or scenes; he distracted them by asking questions; he suggested ways to dissociate from the pain; he asked them to sing, etc. During his interactions with the parturients, he appears to have engaged the women in some activity designed either to minimize the salience of the pain or to emphasize the importance of the "work" in which the women were actively engaged and the results to which it would soon lead. While active manipulation of cognition is less apparent during self-hypnotic procedures the suggestions are similar. It is possible that hypnotic subjects employ imagery to provide comfort or to reduce pain more often than individuals trained in prepared childbirth techniques. Even in the absence of "live" and direct suggestions, the idea of hypnosis has long been associated with fantasy imagery and dreams, rather than with a focus on external reality.

A large number of studies (see reviews by Tan, 1982; Turk, Meichenbaum & Genest, 1983) indicate that various cognitive techniques (such as distraction, imaginal inattention, etc.) are effective in reducing both clinical and experimental pain. In addition, a laboratory study assessing the relative efficacy of the Lamaze focal-point visualization technique compared to an imagery condition that requested the subject to imagine herself relaxed by a lakeside found the latter imagery condition more effective in increasing pain tolerance than the Lamaze technique (Stone, Demchik-Stone & Horan, 1977). While these experimental studies are suggestive, further evaluation of the efficacy of the cognitive components emphasized in hypnosis is necessary. It is interesting that in the attempt to maintain that the techniques were based on physical, as opposed to psychological principles, prepared childbirth proponents may have left behind important components of hypnotic procedures.

It would also be important to examine the types of cognitive and behavioral techniques that are effective at various times during labor. Research from a number of sources tends to point to the idea that pain during the first stage of labor is more variable, and more likely to be affected by various interventions than pain during the second stage (for example, Davenport-Slack, 1975; Davidson et al., 1985). It is possible that the intensity of the pain during the second stage is such that cognitive strategies, such as distraction and imagery, are not feasible. The parturient is often most active during this stage, with little time between contractions. The idea of relaxing with the contractions changes to pushing with them. It is also possible that parturients rate this stage more positively than the first stage (even though it is rated as painful, or more painful, than the first stage) because they are more consumed by the pushing, and because this stage signifies the end of labor and the birth of the child. Thus, it is possible that psychological interventions may be more successful during the first stage of labor than the second. However, it is the first stage that is the longest and the most distressing period for most women.

In addition to pain relief, it is important to note that the majority of parturients using hypnotic and prepared childbirth methods rated the experience of giving birth as satisfying and fulfilling, while only a small minority of women who did not receive these methods rated the experience as such. This finding appears to indicate that these techniques provide something in addition to the potential reduction of pain, because many of the women rating the experience as satisfying must have found the techniques ineffective as a means of pain control. It may be that participating actively in the birth process, and "working" to remain in control and master the pain, are important in leading to a satisfying experience of giving birth (Davenport-Slack, 1975; Melzack, 1984; Oakley, 1983; Richard, 1982).

The most commonly cited disadvantage to the practical use of hypnotic procedures in obstetrics is the large expenditure of time required to train parturients in hypnosis and/or to be present throughout labor (DeLee, 1955; Kroger, 1977; Stone & Burrows, 1980; Wahl, 1962). The studies cited in this chapter do not support this criticism. August (1961) used hypnotic procedures in untrained women in 57 percent of the cases he studied, and found no difference between those trained and untrained in hypnotic procedures on any of the dependent measures. Perchard (1960) used midwives, who had no previous training with hypnosis, to teach self-hypnosis to the parturients in only three sessions. Davidson, Garbett and Tozer (1985) used cassettes with untrained parturients. Thus, there is little support for the contention that excessive amounts of time are required for the use of hypnotic procedures in obstetrics.

Hypnotic procedures are sometimes questioned as impractical in obstetrics because not all individuals are susceptible to hypnosis, and thus many women will not find the technique useful. This criticism makes the implicit assumptions that hypnotic susceptibility is strongly related to the ability to reduce the pain of labor. However, while a moderate relationship between susceptibility and ability to control pain during labor was shown in one study that adequately assessed it (Perchard, 1960), this study also indicated that hypnotic procedures helped to alleviate pain in a substantial number of women who were rated as only moderately susceptible to hypnosis. Moreover, the extent to which relationships between hypnotic susceptibility and suggestion-induced pain reduction are context dependent and mediated by subjects' attitudes and expectations concerning hypnosis, remains controversial (see chapter by Spanos). Clearly, the relationship between hypnotic susceptibility and the control of labor pain requires further investigation. Finally, it is important to emphasize the fact that hypnotic techniques vastly increased most women's enjoyment of the experience of giving birth which, as stated previously, appears to be independent of a woman's ability to reduce childbirth pain.

In conclusion, the research suggests that the relaxation, cognitive strategy, and direct suggestion procedures traditionally associated with hypnosis can play a practical role in helping to make childbirth less distressing. Perhaps the inclusion of procedures such as strategies that involve distraction and imagery for the control of pain could be incorporated into already existing programs. This has the advantage of using the suggestion techniques without involving ideals about control, manipulation, or amnesia, and, as such, these procedures might be more acceptable to more women. Such a combined technique would have most of the components associated with hypnosis except the label. Whether the name, in and of itself, is beneficial because of its historical association with pain control and its license to fantasize and distract oneself from the situation at hand, or harmful because it generates fear about loss of control, requires further research (Hendler & Redd, 1986). Nevertheless, given the evidence, it is unlikely that any psychological techniques, whether labeled hypnosis or prepared childbirth training, will be entirely effective in reducing the pain in childbirth for most women. Perhaps these techniques, when combined with the judicious use of medication, are the most suitable methods of pain control during childbirth for the majority of women. It is hoped that future developments in research will enable women to choose, if perhaps not a painless, then at least a more comfortable and rewarding childbirth experience.

12

Hypnosis, Suggestion, and Dermatological Changes
A Consideration of the Production and Diminution of Dermatological Entities

Richard F. Q. Johnson

Historically, unusual techniques or "home remedies" have been used in attempts to cure common skin ailments. One of the most famous appears in Mark Twain's tale of how Tom Sawyer removed warts by burying a dead cat at midnight under the light of a full moon. Such a "home remedy" is commonly considered to be superstition or nonsense. Nevertheless, (a) by their very nature, such home remedies often suggest to the patient a high expectation for a cure, and (b) a search of the medical and psychological literature shows that there is impressive evidence for cutaneous effects being produced by verbal suggestion. Several types of skin changes that historically have been associated with verbal suggestion will be considered in this chapter. Consideration of selected data is divided into two sections: first, a consideration of some principal phenomena that researchers have investigated that involve the *production* of a dermatological entity, such as a blister formation; and second, a consideration of some phenomena that researchers have investigated that involve the *diminiution or obliteration* of a dermatological entity, such as wart removal. Although the data indicate the possibility of the skin being strongly influenced by thinking and suggestion, the precise relationship between verbal suggestion and changes in the skin has yet to be determined. A set of guiding principles for future research on psychocutaneous effects is outlined.

The views, opinions, and/or findings contained in this report are those of the author and should not be construed as an official Department of the Army position, policy, or decision, unless so designated by other official documentation.

PRODUCTION OF DERMATOLOGICAL ENTITIES

Blisters

At various times, psychologists (Barber, 1961, 1969, 1970; Johnson, 1980; Pattie, 1941; Paul, 1963; Weitzenhoffer, 1953) have critically reviewed more than a dozen studies that ostensibly demonstrated that localized blisters can be produced by suggestions given to hypnotized subjects. In 1974, at the time of my first research study in psychocutaneous medicine, I sent letters to 42 prominent researchers and clinicians who were actively involved in the hypnosis area. I asked them if they had ever tried to produce blisters by means of hypnotic suggestion. Thirty-four of the 42 responded to the survey: of the 34, 22 had never tried, 5 had tried but obtained negative results, and 7 had tried and obtained positive results. The seven who had successfully produced blisters by hypnotic suggestion reported to me anecdotal accounts of their efforts; none had ever published their results. The comments offered by some of the respondents indicated to me that they believed blisters could be produced by hypnotic suggestion, but that they were very skeptical of their findings. That is, they felt that the possibility of being hoodwinked by the subjects was great, since they suspected that highly motivated subjects might purposely and secretly injure themselves to produce the results the hypnotist was suggesting. One of the responders was the late Milton Erickson. He perhaps best summarized the feelings of the seven:

> All the work I have learned about concerning hypnotically induced blisters has made me most dubious about the validity of the reports. My own efforts have taught me that subjects will do things in the ordinary state of awareness that they will not do in a trance state. Any experiment needs constant surveillance for every second of time. [The] human capacity to deceive and to be deceived unintentionally is a serious hazard in hypnotic experimentation where absolute control is not possible. (M. H. Erickson, personal communication, April 23, 1974)

A carefully conducted study by Hadfield (1917) may be considered as the prototype of the published investigations in this area. After the subject was hypnotized, an assistant touched the subject's arm, while Hadfield gave continuous suggestions that a red hot iron was being applied and that a blister would form in the "burned" area. The arm was then bandaged, and the subject was watched continually for 24 hours. After 24 hours, the bandage was removed in the presence of three physicians and the beginning of a blister was noted. During the day, it gradually developed into a large blister surrounded by an area of inflammation.

Some of the problems associated with research on blister formation by hypnotic suggestion was made clear in a study by Ullman (1947). The subject, a soldier with "delicate skin," was hypnotized and asked to recall a battle in which he had participated. He was given the suggestion that a small, molten shell fragment glanced off the back of his hand. At this point, Ullman brushed the subject's hand with a small file to add emphasis. After 20 minutes, a narrow red margin was observed about the specified area. After one hour the beginning of a blister was noticeable. Four hours later, during which time the subject was left unobserved, a full blister had formed. Although this case is a dramatic one, it is open to several interpretations other than that the blister was formed by direct hypnotic suggestion. Since the subject was left unobserved for a considerable period of time before the development of a full blister, the subsequent blister formation may have been due to self-injurious behavior on the part of the subject in order to please the experimenter. Since Ullman actually brushed the subject's hand with a file, the subsequent blister formation may have been due to this extraneous mechanical stimulation by the experimenter himself. Since the subject had "delicate" skin, the subsequent blister formation may have been due to a highly labile skin condition combined with the mechanical stimulation. Since Ullman did not control for the mechanical stimulation of the skin, the possibility of self-injurious behavior on the part of the subject, and the highly labile skin conditions of the subject, the subsequent blister formations following direct hypnotic suggestion for a blister may have been due to any one or a combination of these factors. In addition, since Ullman did not administer the suggestion for blister formation without the prior administration of a hypnotic induction procedure, the role of "hypnosis" in his report remains unclear.

In a study I conducted with T. X. Barber (Johnson & Barber, 1976) on the effects of hypnotic suggestion for blister formation, we attempted to control for the major limitations of past studies in this area. (1) In order to eliminate the possibility of the subject injuring himself (as a means of producing the desired effects), the experimenter carefully observed the subject during the test. (2) In order to control for mechanical stimulation at the test site, an analogous skin area on another part of each subject's body was treated exactly the same as the test site with the exception that the subject was not given a suggestion for blister formation at this control site. (3) In order to control for skin sensitivity, all subjects were assessed on a clinical test for skin sensitivity (dermographia). (4) In order to assess the possible skin changes that might occur as a result of the suggestion, notations were made not only of blisters, but also of erythema, wheals, and changes in skin temperature at both the test and control sites.

During the experiment proper, each of 40 student nurses was asked to read a passage from a book that asserted that indeed blisters could be produced by hypnotic suggestion. Each subject was then administered a formal hypnotic induction procedure and was given the suggestion that she was in her kitchen at home, that it was morning, and that bacon was cooking nearby in a red-hot frying pan. It was then suggested that she was accidentally burned on the back of the hand by the red-hot frying pan, and that a blister was forming there.

In this study, only one subject showed a skin change that could be directly attributed to the suggestion for blister formation. This particular subject showed inflammation at and around the test site during the administration of the suggestion for blister formation. The inflammation formed an irregular pattern that covered approximately 75 percent of the back of the hand including part of the index finger to the first knuckle. The boundary between the inflamed and unin-flamed portions was sharp and easily visible to both the subject and the experi-menter. The inflammation continued during the suggestions for blister formation and subsided within three minutes of completion of the suggestion.

During the postexperimental interview, the subject reported that she had been burned by hot grease on that very spot six years earlier and that the outline of the inflammation coincided with the burned area as she recalled it. Further-more, the subject stated that the accident had occurred six years prior to the experimental session and had occurred in her kitchen, at breakfast time, while she was cooking. Thus, it appears that a previous skin condition was reinstated by using a suggestion that closely resembled what had actually happened to the subject six years earlier. The experimental situation thus led the subject to relive the experience vividly; for example, she stated in the postexperimental interview that she could "feel" the "blister" forming on her hand. The skin change observed was apparently closely related to the fact that she fully accepted the suggestion for blister formation and incorporated it into her thoughts.

The results of the Johnson and Barber (1976) investigation suggest two lines of research be pursued in the future with respect to blister formation by suggestion. First, a study could be conducted comparing the responses of normal subjects with those of subjects with highly sensitive skin. The low response rate (one in 40) to the suggestion for blister formation in the Johnson and Barber study may have been due to the fact that none of the subjects had highly sensitive skin: only one subject displayed a positive response to a clinical test for skin sensitivity (Johnson, 1976), and none had a dermatological history indicating unusual skin sensitivity. Most subjects who were reported to have responded positively in past studies did have such a history (Hadfield, 1917; Kraft-Ebing, 1889; Rybalkin, 1890; Schindler, 1927; Ullman, 1947; Wetterstrand, 1915). Sec-ond, the Johnson and Barber study could be repeated using only subjects who have previously experienced a traumatic experience leading to blister formation, and who report they were able to reexperience that particular traumatic experi-ence vividly during the laboratory suggestion for blister formation. The traumatic experience leading to blister formation could be a natural one in the subject's dermatological history or it may be a laboratory-induced trauma. In either case, the subject would be asked to vividly recall and experience it.

With respect to the second line of possible research, Spanos, McNeil, and Stam (1982) conducted such a study utilizing only subjects who had previously experienced a burn-induced blister in a natural setting (e.g., being burned by hot bacon grease). The effects of hypnotic suggestions for blister formation were assessed in 60 volunteer college students who reported being burned at least six months prior to the study. The subjects were "hypnotically age regressed" and given the suggestion to "relive" the burn experience and suggestions to indi-cate that the blister was forming. Seventeen of the subjects reported vividly imagining the burn events, but not one showed evidence of blister formation or the beginning of a blister (e.g., discoloration of the skin). Like Johnson and Barber (1976) before them, Spanos, McNeil, et al. (1982) also measured skin temperature about the area where the blister was suggested to form; consistent with Johnson and Barber, Spanos, McNeil, et al. did not find any change in skin temperature as a function of suggestions for blister formation.

One of the criteria for inclusion in the Spanos, McNeil, et al. (1982) study was that the burn incident not be associated with severe psychological trauma (e.g., the injury of a parent in a fire). Nevertheless, the emotional atmosphere about the original burn incident that the subject attempts to "relive" may be relevant to the likelihood of a blister being formed in response to hypnotic suggestion. Since anxiety is associated with the production and intensity of other dermatological responses, such as hives (Domonkos, Arnold & Odom, 1982), the presence of anxiety or emotional stress in the subject may be important to the production of blisters by suggestion. Since past research has not evaluated this variable in a rigorous fashion, it remains for future researchers to resolve the issue (cf. Friedman & Booth-Kewley, 1987).

The attempt to produce blisters by suggestion would be of particular value if the original blister-producing injury were experienced in the laboratory under controlled conditions. For example, the blister could be produced by the experimenter with a Hardy-Wolff-Goodell dolorimeter, thereby insuring that the experimenter knows the exact amount of caloric energy used for blister formation, the period of time required for the formation of a blister for each subject, and the specific skin area involved. Although there would be serious ethical problems to be resolved prior to the conduct of such a study, the procedure would insure control over the independent variable and the conditions under which the blister was induced. Future investigations that control the "emotional atmosphere" under which the blister is first produced (e.g., neutral, relaxed, anxious) would be particularly valuable in yielding information relevant to the relationship between blister formation and anxiety or emotional stress. If the formation of blisters were to be observed during one of these suggested studies, parametric studies would then be required in order to determine the necessary and sufficient conditions for blister formation by verbal suggestion. This would include determining the necessity of using hypnotic techniques when administering the suggestion for blister formation; past studies have indicated that the administration of a hypnotic induction procedure prior to the verbal suggestion for blister formation may not be required (Barber, 1969; Kraft-Ebing, 1889; Patite, 1941; Paul, 1963).

Stigmata

Another cutaneous phenomenon associated with verbal suggestion is religious stigmatization. It is likely that the stigmatic's behavior is influenced by suggestions received during religious education. Typically, on Good Friday, the stigmatic will experience pain and bleeding at the backs and palms of the hands, the feet, and the stomach; sometimes bleeding is reported to occur on the forehead (suggestive of the crown of thorns). Nearly all cases of religious stigmatization can be explained in terms of deliberate or "hysterical" self-injury, and therefore stigmata are considered here as a phenomenon associated with the production of a dermatological entity.

The cases of Therese Neumann of the twentieth century and Louise Lateau of the nineteenth century are typcial; both women were carefully studied by serious investigators (Ratnoff, 1969). Each woman was deeply religious, each began experiencing ecstatic paroxysms in their late teens, and each eventually developed painful bleeding on Fridays. Often the bleeding and convulsive attacks ceased either on the same day or by the following Sunday (Easter). Stigmatics (usually adult Roman Catholic women) would receive a great deal of attention and notoriety for their unusual conditions. Since the bleedings are brought to the attention of the investigator only after they have begun, the investigator can never be sure that the initial bleedings were not due to self-injury. Even after the bleedings have begun and show a pattern, it is almost impossible to keep a 24-hour watch on the individual. In the years prior to her stigmatization, Therese Neumann began experiencing convulsive attacks during which her "fingers trembled, and she dug them spasmodically into her hands" (Ratnoff, 1969). In later years, when she became well known for her stigmatization, a noted physician who studied her was "disturbed that under the cover of her bed clothes, she made strange and very intense movements with her arms and legs during the hours before bleeding appeared" (Ratnoff, 1969). While he was in her room, no bleeding occurred; only when he left her room (forced out by her family) did Therese Neumann begin to bleed copiously.

Recently, Early and Lifschutz (1974) reported a case of stigmatization, and their close scrutiny of the case made it unlikely that the lesions were self-inflicted. The case involved a person in Oakland, California, who experienced stigmatic bleeding for the first time during the Easter season of 1972. Unlike most previous cases, she was neither a white adult nor a Roman Catholic. She was a 10.5-year-old black girl of Baptist upbringing. She and her family professed to be religious. Initial bleeding was at school, and she was herself "unaware of its onset." The initial physical exam showed about 1.5 milliliters of dried blood in the patient's left palm, the bleeding having occurred at school about ten minutes earlier. During the initial exam, and on subsequent exams over the next five days, the bleeding sites were examined with a five-and ten-power magnifying lens, revealing no skin abnormality, no skin lesions. Within three hours of the initial examination, she again bled from the right palm. During the following two weeks, she bled from the right palm, the dorsum of the left foot, the dorsum of the right foot, the right thorax, and the middle of her forehead. She bled from the hands more frequently than from the other sites. During her fourth visit to the physician, the physician "observed the blood to increase in volume fourfold, welling up in the center of the [left] palm and spreading over the palmar creases. After wiping the wet blood away, no lesions were present with the exception of a pea-size bluish discoloration remaining in the palm of her left hand for approximately three minutes" (Early & Lifschutz, 1974, p. 199).

This case, as reported by Early and Lifschutz (1947), is striking in the sense that the investigators personally observed the bleeding and found no lesion present after close examination of the skin. They suggest that the girl's stigmata may be related to another phenomenon called psychogenic purpura, or autoerythrocyte sensitization. In psychogenic purpura, strange spontaneous hemorrhages can occur with no current physical trauma. Gardner and Diamond (1956) and Agle and his co-workers (Agle & Ratnoff, 1962; Agle, Ratnoff & Wasman, 1967, 1969) describe psychogenic purpura as consisting of painful spontaneous bleeding following trauma such as an automobile accident, but not occurring until months or even years later during times of emotional stress. Psychogenic purpura occurs in people of a hysterical predisposition and may be reproduced with a hypnotic procedure (Agle, Ratnoff & Wasman, 1967). Early and Lifschutz (1974) felt that since psychogenic purpura is a clinical reality, it may not be so unusual to consider stigmatic bleeding during times of profound, intense religious and emotional conditions as a clinical reality also. Only further serious investigations of both stigmata and psychogenic purpura will shed light on the relationship between cognitive processes and the occurrence of bleeding from skin sites that had been subject to no physical trauma.

Warts

Gravitz (1981) has noted that while suggestion and expectancy for the curing of warts has historically been associated with wart removal (to be considered below), it has also been associated with the production of warts. Gravitz noted that many of the home remedies for wart removal involve the transfer of warts from the person who has them to some unsuspecting bystander. For example, one remedy involves the tying of a ribbon around the affected hand and knotting it as many times as there are warts on the hand; the ribbon is then dropped on a roadway. Whoever picks up the ribbon and unties the knots will get the warts, and the original owner of the warts will lose them. Gravitz reports the little-known fact that in the early twentieth century, the French province of Vaud was noted for its large number of lay wart healers who used such home remedies with their "patients." Apparently, having your warts cured by one of these folk healers was a popular thing to do and gained the "patient" much notoriety and attention. As a result, folk rituals for the production of warts became popular (after all, you could not have your warts removed if you did not have any!). One folk ritual for the production of warts prescribed that the subject go out at night and moisten the tip of the finger with fresh saliva; the wet finger is then applied to the other hand while the subject simultaneously looks at a star. The ritual is repeated while the subject counts "one, two, three . . .," up to the number of warts desired. Wherever the moistened finger has been applied, a wart is supposed to appear.

There have been no serious investigations into the production of warts by suggestion. Nevertheless, Gravitz (1981) suggests that since suggestion and expectancy may be associated with wart removal, then it is not unreasonable to suspect that suggestion and expectancy may be associated with their production as well, especially in light of the reports from the French province of Vaud.

If therapeutic suggestions and illness-producing expectancies are effective in influencing the subject's dermatological response mechanisms, then serious researchers should investigate the possibility of wart production as well as wart removal. Since a virus has been associated with the onset of warts, such research would assist in the understanding of the body's resistance and susceptibility to virus-caused disease.

DIMINUTION OR OBLITERATION OF DERMATOLOGICAL ENTITIES

Of common interest to researchers and clinicians is the attempt by behavioral researchers to diminish or even to obliterate certain dermatological entities by means of verbal or hypnotic suggestion. Case reports abound with attempts to alleviate acne (Hollander, 1958), boils (Jabush, 1969), cold sores (Gould & Tissler, 1984), and the like. Mason (1952) reported dramatic improvement in the skin condition of a young man afflicted with congenital ichthyosiform erythrodermia of Brocq (fish-skin disease) in a matter of weeks as a result of repeated suggestions during "hypnosis" for clearing of the skin condition (Kidd, 1966; Mason, (1955; Schneck, 1966; Wink, 1961). In a now-classic study, Ikema and Nakagawa (1962) have presented data indicating that an allergic skin response to poison ivy-like plants may be reduced if the subjects are first given suggestions that the plant is one that is harmless; conversely, these same investigators presented data that indicated that allergic skin responses can be produced after contact with harmless plants if the subjects are first given suggestions that the plants produce dermatitis. Ikemi and Nakagawa were able to produce these effects regardless of whether or not the subjects received a hypnotic induction procedure prior to the administration of the suggestions. More detailed consideration of these and other skin changes may be found in Barber (1978).

In this section, I will concentrate on two phenomena that have received much attention over the years and that continue to gain the attention of researchers and clinicians alike. These are (1) attempts to remove warts by suggestion, and (2) attempts to diminish the intensity of a burn response and/or accelerate the rate of healing of a burn.

Warts

Whether treated or left untreated, warts often appear to disappear spontaneously and abruptly. In response to direct clinical intervention (e.g., surgical incision, electrical dessication, the application of liquid nitrogen, etc.), warts often reappear within weeks or months (Domonkos, Arnold & Odom, 1982; Fitzpatrick, Arndt, Clark, Eisen, Van Scott & Vaughan, 1971). Left untreated, warts generally remit within two to three years of onset (Rulision, 1942).

With verbal suggestion procedures, such as hypnotherapy, the patient is told that his warts are dying and that they will soon fall off. Since in hypnotherapy no treatment procedure other than words is used, positive results with hypnosis support the notion that warts may be effectively treated with simple direct suggestion. Nevertheless, most investigations of the efficacy of the hypnotic treatment of warts are poorly controlled. When a patient does lose his warts, there are often no control groups with which a comparsion may be made; thus, one cannot eliminate the possibility of the "cure" being due to spontaneous remission, the patient's use of a topical medication at home, or to some other extraneous variable(s).

There have been a few fairly well controlled studies of the hypnotic treatment of warts. Ullman and Dudek (1960), for example, worked with 62 adult patients attending an outpatient clinic. At weekly intervals, each patient was given suggestions of sleep, drowsiness, and hypnosis followed by suggestions that the warts would disappear. Of the 47 patients who were rated as poor hypnotic subjects, only 2 showed wart remission within the 4-week period. However, 8 of the 15 patients rated as good hypnotic subjects were cured of multiple common warts (or, in one case, of a single wart) within a 4-week period. Nevertheless, since Ullman and Dudek did not include a nontreated control group, their study is open to criticism that the warts may have gone into spontaneous remission within the same period of time without the hypnotic suggestive treatment.

A study by Sinclair-Gieben and Chalmers (1959) appeared to control for spontaneous remission. These investigators studied 14 patients with common warts present on both sides of the body. Sinclair-Gieben and Chalmers suggested to each patient during hypnosis that the warts on only one side of the body would disappear. Within 5 weeks to 3 months, 9 of the patients (all of whom were rated as good hypnotic subjects) showed wart involution on the "treated" side while the warts on the control side remained unchanged. No benefit was found in the remaining 5 patients (4 of whom were rated as poor hypnotic subjects). Since Sinclair-Gieben and Chalmers did not employ a nonhypnotic control group, the relative influence of the hypnotic procedures per se is questionable. That is, the suggestions may have been just as effective without the prior administration of a hypnotic induction procedure.

In a study by Surman, Gottlieb, Hackett, and Silverberg (1973), a nonhypnotic control group was used. Their experiment was similar to that of Sinclair-Gieben and Chalmers (1959). Seventeen patients with bilateral common warts or flat warts were administered a hypnotic induction procedure and told that their warts would disappear from one side of their body. Nine, or 53 percent, of the patients showed improvement in 3 months' time. No improvement was found in an untreated control group of 7 patients who were simply told that their "hypnotic" treatment would be postponed for 3 months. In addition, their report stated that the hypnotic treatment did not have a selective effect; i.e., even though the warts were suggested to go away from only one side of the body, when they did go away, they went away from both sides of the body. Similarly, other studies concerned with the removal of warts did not report the suggestion procedure to have selective results (Clark, 1965; Stankler, 1967; Tenzel & Taylor, 1969).

Although the study by Surman et al. (1973) was a carefully conducted investigation utilizing an untreated control group, it lacked a nonhypnotic control group that also received suggestions for wart removal. In a study I conducted with T. X. Barber (1978), an attempt was made to control for this variable. Two groups of subjects, with 11 subjects in each group, received suggestions that the warts were going away. Only one group, however, received a hypnotic induction procedure prior to this suggestion for wart removal. All subjects were asked to return for two follow-up sessions at approximately 2.5 weeks and 6 weeks after the original treatment session. Three of the 22 subjects showed remission of their warts. One subject lost 37 of her 39 warts by the first follow-up session (2.5 weeks); she had had the warts for approximately 3 years. A second subject lost all 5 of his warts by the second follow-up session (4.5 weeks); he had had his warts for 2 years. The third subject lost all of his 13 facial warts within 6 weeks of treatment; he had had his warts for 6 months.

These data support the results of the earlier studies (Sinclair-Gieben & Chalmers, 1959; Surman et al., 1973; Ullman & Dudek, 1960) that found that wart remission is at times closely associated with suggestions for wart disappearance. Of equal importance is the fact that all 3 subjects who showed wart regression were subjects who had been administered the hypnotic induction treatment procedure; none of the subjects in the nonhypnotic condition showed wart regression.

In both the hypnotic treatment and the nonhypnotic treatment, subjects were given identical suggestions for wart removal. The only differences between these two treatments were that in the hypnotic treatment the situation was defined to the subjects as hypnosis and a hypnotic induction procedure was administered, whereas in the nonhypnotic treatment the situation was defined to the subjects as "focused contemplation" and no hypnotic induction procedure was administered. If, as the data suggest, the hypnotic treatment was more effective than the nonhypnotic "focused contemplation" procedure, it may have been due to the greater "believed-in efficacy" of the hypnotic procedure. That is, the hypnotic procedure may have worked better because the hypnotic subjects had heard of the power of hypnosis and had a strong belief that the treatment would work. None of the subjects had ever heard of the term "focused contemplation"—a term that was invented in order to describe the nonhypnotic treatment to the subjects. As stated elsewhere (Barber, 1970, 1978; Johnson & Barber, 1978), other types of suggestive procedures, which subjects apparently believed were effective in curing warts, have been shown to produce just as dramatic results as hypnotic treatments. These other nonhypnotic procedures include, for example, painting the warts with an innocuous dye that the patient was led to believe was a powerful wart remedy (Memmesheimer & Eisenlohr, 1931); placing the patient's hand with warts in an impressive machine that seemed to be "x-raying" the warts—but was actually doing nothing to them (Vollmer, 1946); and placing the subject's hand with warts into an "electric wart curing machine" that seemed to be electrocuting the warts—but was actually doing nothing to them (Bloch, 1927). In each of these reports, the majority of patients "treated" showed wart remission. Since the ostensible treatment procedure varied a great deal (from saline injections to painting warts with innocuous dyes), the only treatment element common to all reports was the strong suggestion by the therapist that the treatment procedure would work; that is, that the treatment procedure was valid and reliable. The fact that remission often occurred soon after "treatment" makes spontaneous remission an unlikely alternative explanation. These studies of nonhypnotic suggestion procedures coupled with those suggestion procedures that did utilize a hypnotic induction procedure support the hypothesis that believed-in efficacy may play an important role in the treatment of warts by psychological techniques.

While the Surman et al. (1973) study lacked a nonhypnotic control group for comparison with hypnotic subjects, and the Johnson and Barber (1978) study lacked an untreated control group for comparison with hypnotic subjects, a recent study by Spanos, Stenstrom, and Johnson (1988) included all three treatment groups. Sixty-four subjects with warts were divided into three groups. Subjects were (a) given a hypnotic induction procedure with suggestions for wart removal, or (b) administered a "cold laser" placebo with suggestions for wart removal, or (c) left untreated for six weeks. Subjects given the hypnotic treatment exhibited more wart regression than did those given either the placebo or no treatment. That subjects given the placebo treatment ("cold laser") did not respond with wart regression is consistent with Johnson and Barber's (1978) findings with a placebo treatment ("focused contemplation"), but it is inconsistent with previous studies using "wart curing machines" (e.g., Bloch, 1927). It may be that the subjects just did not believe that the "cold laser" would work. That is, perhaps they did not believe in the efficacy of the "cold laser" treatment procedure because they had never heard of it before. Further studies focusing on various placebo procedures and the subjects' belief in their efficacy are needed in order to address this important issue.

In the second phase of the Spanos, Stenstrom, et al. (1988) study, an attempt was made to assess the subjects' expectations for the success of the treatment procedure. Seventy-six subjects with warts on either one or both hands were divided into four groups. Subjects were (a) given a hypnotic induction procedure with suggestions for wart removal, or (b) given relaxation suggestions with suggestions for wart removal, or (c) given only suggestions for wart removal, or (d) left untreated. The results of the second phase of the study showed that hypnotic and nonhypnotic subjects given the same suggestions were equally likely to exhibit wart regression and more likely to show this effect than those given no treatment. However, subjects with high expectations for success of the treatment did not lose more warts than did those with low expectations for success. In both phases of the Spanos, Stenstrom, et al. (1988) study, those who lost warts reported experiencing more vivid suggested imagery than those who did not lose warts.

To date, the experimental evidence on the treatment of warts by suggestion supports the hypotheses that (a) with or without the prior administration of a hypnotic induction procedure, suggestions for wart removal are at times effective in the treatment of warts; and (b) that subjects who become vividly involved with the suggestion and the imagery for losing warts are more likely to lose warts than those who do not have vivid imagery.

Since systematic large-scale studies of wart removal by suggestion are difficult to carry out, they appear only rarely in the published literature. In the past ten years, there have been only two (Johnson and Barber, 1978; Spanos, Stenstrom, et al., 1988). Nevertheless, case studies of wart removal by suggestion continue to be reported in the literature. For example, Morris (1985) has reported one case of multiple common warts that had been treated unsuccessfully for over a year by means of standard techniques. Morris treated the patient with hypnotherapy and the Simonton visualization technique, whereby the patient visualizes his own body's defenses attacking the wart. According to Morris, this technique led to successful removal of the warts, which remained in remission at a four-month follow-up. Of course, this was a case study and no controls were used. A formal investigation needs to be carried out to assess the efficacy of Morris's procedure. Morris's report typifies (a) the ongoing efforts on behalf of clinicians to use suggestion and imagery to help rid patients of their warts, and (b) the assumption on behalf of the clinician that the patient needs to "believe in the efficacy" of the procedure in order for it to work.

Burns

The role of verbal suggestion has been implicated in the increased rate of healing of certain wounds. A number of anecdotes and case reports of accelerated healing of burns have been reported. Several experimental investigations of increased rate of healing or diminution of the body's response to a burn stimulus have also been reported. To be considered below are some recent case reports as well as some attempts at experimental investigations in this area.

Ewin (1986) presented a case study of the use of guided imagery in the hospital emergency room for the treatment of the burn patient. A teenage male had accidentally immersed his arm to the elbow in boiling fat. Ewin suggested to the patient that he imagine a pleasant place that was cool and that the injured areas were now cool and comfortable. Ewin did not suggest to the patient that other injured areas were cool and comfortable (the patient had also burned parts of his shoulder with the boiling fat). Those areas that were suggested to be cool and comfortable healed more readily than the burns on the shoulder. It should be noted that although Ewin labeled his technique as "hypnosis," at no time did Ewin define the situation to the patient as "hypnosis," and Ewin does not tell us if the patient construed the situation to be "hypnotic." Since this is a singular case study, it suggests the hypothesis that this type of approach with burn patients may facilitate the rate of healing of burns. This hypothesis should be tested in a more rigorous study with more patients, and with patients who receive a hypnotic induction as well as patients who do not receive a hypnotic induction.

Moore and Kaplan (1983) selected 5 patients on the basis of having symmetrical or bilaterally equivalent burns on some portion of their right and left sides. After the administration of a hypnotic induction, patients were given suggestions that there was increased blood flow to the injury on only one side of the body. Moore and Kaplan reasoned that moderately increased blood flow to a given area would enhance normal healing. The authors rated 4 of the 5 patients as showing accelerated healing on the hypnotically treated side of the body as compared to the nontargeted side of the body. The fifth patient showed rapid healing on both sides.

Margolis, Domangue, Ehleben, and Shrier (1983) conducted a study to assess whether a single hypnotic induction with suggestions for analgesia and coolness in the burned area would facilitate the rate of healing. There were 11 hypnotic subjects and 11 nonhypnotic controls matched for age and percent body-surface area. All subjects were recently hospitalized burn patients. Although there were no differences between the two groups with respect to length of hospitalization, fluid input, or urine output, urine output on the second day (24 to 48 hours postburn) was significantly higher for 6 subjects in the hypnotic group who were rated as at least moderately hypnotized (the other 5 hypnotic subjects were rated as "not hypnotized"). Urine output is a prime indicator in determining the adequacy of resuscitation. The authors concluded that hypnotic suggestion may have been instrumental in reducing urine output on the second day, but they also stated that it could have been an artifact as no other measures evidenced differences between the two groups. Since no subjects were given suggestions for analgesia without the hypnotic induction procedure, no conclusions concerning the necessity of the hypnotic induction are warranted.

Chapman, Goodell, and Wolff (1959a, 1959b) demonstrated that suggestions given after a hypnotic induction procedure may at times influence the amount of inflammation resulting from an experimentally induced burn. These authors induced burns in hypnotic subjects whose one arm had been suggested to be anesthetic and whose other arm had been suggested to be extremely sensitive. In 20 of 27 studies with 13 subjects, there was less inflammation reported on the arms suggested to be anesthetized than on the arms suggested to be sensitive.

Hammond, Keye, and Grant (1983) studied 6 subjects who were given a two-inch-wide burn on both thighs by means of a sun lamp. After the burn, hypnotic suggestions were administered to the subjects that one thigh was analgesic and felt cool. None of the subjects reported pain at the burn area on the analgesic thigh. Compared to the control thigh, the analgesic thigh was rated by a blind evaluator as being less red, and there was a trend for the analgesic thigh to exhibit lower skin temperature. The authors cautiously concluded that hypnotic analgesia may reduce inflammation and aid the healing of burns. They expressed caution because of the small sample size and the need for replication. In addition, because Hammond et al. did not use a nonhypnotic control group, the question whether or not the suggestions for analgesia and coolness require the prior administration of a hypnotic induction procedure to be efficacious remains unanswered. In point of fact, the hypnotic induction procedure may not be necessary for decreased redness, analgesia, and lower skin temperature; it may be that the suggestions for analgesia and coolness in the burned area may be the critical requirement for the diminution of response to the burn stimulus.

The existing studies relevant to increasing the rate of healing of burns in humans by means of verbal suggestion suffer from research design flaws. Principal among the shortcomings is the lack of a large sample size and the lack of controls (mainly, a nonhypnotic control group). However, past studies have also lacked the consistent use of one clearly specified independent variable; studies conducted by different investigators in different laboratories and hospitals have utilized different suggestions for accelerated healing. Some investigators use suggestions of analgesia or coolness or comfort or relaxation or some combination. Some investigators suggest that the control arm remain "normal," while others suggest that it be delicate or sensitive or even painful. If research is to progress rapidly in this important area, interlaboratory reliability based upon standardized techniques is essential.

RECOMMENDATIONS

Future research on the relationship between skin changes and verbal suggestion should be conducted objectively and systematically. In the past, there have been many seminal, yet poorly controlled, case reports on the topic. Future laboratory research should be aimed at eliminating and/or controlling for spurious variables. With more rigorous research methodology, one will be able to determine if the skin changes observed in the clinic are due to verbal suggestion, a hypnotic induction procedure, the lability (stability) of the subject's skin, the personality of the subject, adjunct medication, "believed-in efficacy" of the treatment procedure, vividness of suggested imagery, or a combination of one or more of these and other variables.

It is suggested that future researchers of this topic adhere to the following general principles (Johnson, 1980):

1. Clearly denote the phenomenon of interest. In the study of wart removal by suggestion, too often researchers simply count the number of warts present before and after treatment and use this measure as the index of wart remission. Simply counting warts present on an individual may mislead the researcher as to the precise course of remission, since the subject may gain warts as well as lose them during the course of the investigation. For example, a subject may lose two warts and gain one new wart from one follow-up session to another and thus mislead the researcher into concluding that the subject has lost one wart and gained none. Future researchers should not only count warts, but also note their size, morphology, and precise location on the body. In the study by Johnson and Barber (1978), this was aided by the use of instant color photography; not only did the photographic procedure permit a permanent record, but it also settled any subsequent questions concerning changes in morphology, size, and location from one follow-up session to the next. Similar objective techniques for the denotation and measurement of other skin changes (e.g., blisters, stigmata, ichthyosis) should be used in all future investigations of the relationship between suggestion and skin changes.

2. Clearly specify the independent variable under evaluation. In the past, investigators have carefully reported their observations on the relationship between verbal suggestion and changes in the skin but have often failed to specify clearly the wording of the suggestions administered to the subjects. Mason (1952), for example, simply states that he treated his patient for ichthyosis as follows: "The patient was hypnotized and, under hypnosis, suggestions were made that the left arm would clear" (Mason, 1952, 422). In order for this treatment procedure to be evaluated adequately in future studies, it is essential to know the exact wording of the hypnotic induction procedure, the exact wording of the suggestions that the skin would clear, the type of imagery the subject was asked to employ, the number of times (and length of time) the subject was instructed to practice at home, whether the subject was to continue his normal medication, and so on. Only precise specification of the independent variable employed in a research investigation will permit adequate interpretation of the resultant data.

3. As conditions permit, measure and record as many subject variables as are relevant to the phenomenon under investigation. Characteristics of the subject undergoing evaluation are often relevant to, and necessary for, adequate evaluation of the data. For example, how well a subject responds to suggestions for changes in the skin may be strongly influenced by the lability of the skin, his dermatological history, his anxiety level, his motivation for participation in the study, his personality, his hypnotizability, etc. With respect to blister formation by suggestion, for example, there are indications that responsiveness may be influenced by skin lability (Ullman, 1947), dermatological history (Johnson & Barber, 1976; Ullman, 1947), imaginative ability (Ullman, 1947), hypnotizability (Barber, 1970, 1978), and motivation for self-injury (Johnson, 1980; Johnson & Barber, 1976).

SUMMARY

Studies of several types of skin changes, which historically have been associated with verbal suggestion, indicate that the skin may at times be strongly influenced by thinking and suggestion. Nevertheless, the precise relationship between verbal suggestion and changes in the skin has yet to be determined. The relationship between wart regression and hypnotic suggestion has been studied extensively, but the precise role of the formal hypnotic induction procedure in effecting wart regression is not known. Similarly, research has been directed toward the delineation of the relationship between verbal suggestion and blister formation with the conclusion that verbal suggestion may at times influence blister formation. The objective data on religious stigmatization were reviewed. Although the formation of stigmata remains a mystery, its possible relationship to similar phenomena (e.g., psychogenic purpura or autoerythrocyte sensitization) was pointed out.

It has been shown that there are many skin conditions that may be influenced by verbal suggestion. Although the reasons for these cutaneous phenomena are far from clear, it is proposed that adherence to three principles for research will aid in the determination of the precise relationship between verbal suggestion and changes in the skin: (*a*) clearly denote the cutaneous phenomenon of interest; (*b*) clearly denote the independent variables to be evaluated; and (*c*) measure and record relevant patient/subject variables.

13

From Symptom Relief to Cure
Hypnotic Interventions in Cancer

Henderikus J. Stam

Laboratory psychology has, until very lately, looked askance at hypnosis as a method of psychological investigation; the treatment of suggestion has therefore, to a large degree, been left to the psychopathologists and the psychologists of society, and we have borrowed from them as the occasion arose. Things are changing . . . now that experimental results in general are seen to be functions of the instructions given.

E. B. Titchener (1909)

Historically, the introduction of hypnosis for medical problems has been surrounded by considerable controversy. One or two "pioneering" individuals will intervene with hypnosis for a certain problem and claim varying degrees of success. This is then frequently followed by negative reaction among physicians. As professional medicine finds more appropriate medical or therapeutic means to treat the disorder in question, hypnotic techniques fall out of favor or are relegated to subsidiary roles. The histories of hypnotic treatment for pain, hysteria, "shell shock," and other psychiatric problems satisfy these criteria, at least in broad outline. The treatment of pain, for example, was rapidly taken over by chemical anesthetics in the middle of the nineteenth century and extinguished the furor created by the reports of mesmeric analgesia such as those of James Esdaile ([1846] 1957). Freud himself abandoned hypnosis for free association on the grounds that "a number of his patients could not be hypnotized," and later he found he could "by-pass hypnosis and yet obtain the pathogenic recollections" (Freud, [1895] 1957, 268).[1] Titchener's comment, above, reflects his belief that the proper investigation of hypnosis in psychological laboratories would change the commonly held views of hypnotic phenomena.

CANCER

In this context, what can one make of the treatment of cancer symptomatology, and the disease itself, with hypnotic interventions? In order to examine this question we need to examine the modern context of cancer. First, cancer is a disease for which treatment is only partially effective. When all tumor sites are considered together (excluding non-melanoma skin cancer), the relative five-year survival rate approximates 50 percent (Silverberg & Lubera, 1988). Thus, the disease and its treatment lead to considerable uncertainty about outcome. Secondly, no major discoveries or changes in treatment have been produced in the past decade or more. Although the survival rates for some select tumor sites have improved dramatically over the past two decades (e.g., Hodgkin's disease, testicular cancer), there has been only a gradual overall change. Unless there is a dramatic improvement in survival rates with the recent introduction of biological therapeutics, these rates are unlikely to change dramatically in the near future.

There are several consequences of this. First, physicians and mental health professionals alike have shown increased concerns for the quality of life of cancer patients. Even patients who will succumb to their disease often have their life increased by months or years through varying combinations of existing treatment regimens. Cancer is a chronic illness, that is, a disease of uncertain progression in any individual. Multiple treatments may be given over the course of the disease, and hospitalization is frequently required for acute episodes. Furthermore, both the treatment and the disease may produce multiple symptoms and side effects. Over the past thirty years, hypnosis has been introduced largely as a form of symptom control for cancer patients and as a part of supportive therapies (e.g., Hilgard & Hilgard, 1983; Sacerdote, 1982a, 1982b).

A second consequence of the stabilization of five-year survival rates in cancer has been the renewed search for (a) measures to prevent the disease from occurring in the first instance, and (b) psychological means of influencing the onset and progression of cancer (Stam & Steggles, 1987). It is in this latter area that we find the most controversial claims about hypnosis and cancer.

This chapter will review the literature on hypnosis and cancer from 1959 to the present. Except for isolated reports (e.g., Butler, 1954), there are virtually no papers on the use of hypnosis with cancer patients prior to this date. Butler's (1954) paper is informative, however, in that it already contained all the major themes that would occupy practitioners of hypnosis interested in cancer over the next three-and-a-half decades. Butler presents a theoretical rationale, twelve cases of cancer patients who are treated for pain and other symptoms, and closes with a discussion of the precancerous personality and the possibilities of treating cancer by psychological means. As this review will demonstrate, the literature on hypnosis and cancer has yet to come to terms with the issues raised by Butler: Empirically, it has not solved the most fundamental problems of treatment efficacy, and, theoretically, it languishes in vague generalities about the "essential" nature of hypnosis. The aim of this review is not to solve these problems, but, more simply, to introduce some order where there appears to be none.

This chapter will review the literature on hypnosis and cancer in two sections. The first section will examine the reports of symptom control and supportive therapy using hypnotic techniques. The second section will assess claims made by mental health professionals for the utility of hypnosis in the biological treatment or prevention of cancer. Each section will include a discussion of the theoretical and methodological problems involved in the literature. This will be followed by a discussion that will attempt some concluding statement about the serious limitations of this literature and the conceptions of hypnosis embedded therein.

The dearth of literature on hypnosis and cancer changed, in large measure, with the founding of the *American Journal of Clinical Hypnosis (AJCH)* in 1959. This journal was (and still is) almost exclusively oriented to clinical problems and is much less concerned with research problems than the *International Journal of Clinical and Experimental Hypnosis,* which was first published in 1953. In the first volume of the *AJCH,* Milton Erickson published "Hypnosis in Painful Terminal Illness," which consisted of a description of his use of hypnosis in the treatment of pain in three terminal cancer patients (Erickson, 1959). Thereafter this journal published numerous case studies and commentaries on the use of hypnosis with cancer patients (see, Steggles, Stam, Fehr & Aucoin, 1987).

The Social Context of Health Psychology

The publication of specialty journals was not the only change that could have brought on a greater interest in hypnosis and cancer. The trend that has led to a greater emphasis on viewing cancer as a chronic illness has also led to greater psychological interest in the disease, and psychology has, in general, been much concerned with health issues of late, fostered in part by two major forces. The first is the relative over-production of Ph.D.s in the discipline and the shrinking of traditional job markets (Howard et al., 1986). The second is the change and expansion (in the U.S. at least) of the health care system brought about by an increased supply of physicians and improved insurance coverage (e.g., Ginzberg, 1986; Relman, 1987). The institutional barriers to psychology's involvement in health care settings were thus greatly reduced in the 1970s (Stam, 1988). Health psychology has suddenly risen to prominence in psychology and is claimed to be one of the fastest growing subareas in the discipline (e.g., Stone et al., 1987). At the same time, however, specialties within medicine such as psychiatry, nursing, and family medicine have also been expanding their claims of expertise to cover the psychosocial domain, partially as a function of the same forces noted above (see, Stam, 1988).

How did this lead to increases in the uses of hypnosis with cancer patients? The increases in psychologists in health care settings has led, in general, to a greater push to understand psychological issues in health and illness and the use of a variety of psychological techniques for problems that were, at one time, considered strictly medical. This is reflected in the increased use of hypnosis for a whole range of health care problems. For example, pain emerged as a topic of serious consideration by hypnosis researchers in the late 1960s (e.g., T. X. Barber, 1970; Hilgard, 1969).[2] Thus, cancer as a topic of concern for practioners and researchers of hypnosis has received increased attention as a function of the general push to understand health and illness from psychological perspectives.

HYNOSIS FOR SYMPTON CONTROL AND PATIENT SUPPORT

Hypnosis and Cancer Pain

The most common use of hypnosis in cancer is for symptom control and here the most frequently reported use is the control of pain. It has only been in the past decade that "symptom control" has come to include other symptoms such as nausea, emesis, and anxiety.

Cancer pain. Surveys by the Canadian and American Cancer Societies continue to demonstrate that the general public not only equates cancer with fear and death but also with unmanageable pain (Stam & Scott, 1988). Although the medical establishment is quick to point out that this is an inaccurate perception, a historical view might lead one to the conclusion that the public was, until recently, quite correct. Physicians often viewed pain as exaggerated in cancer patients or as a symptom that had a psychosomatic basis (Pernick, 1985). For example, Butler (1954) concluded his presentation of cases treated with hypnosis for pain with the following:

> One should inquire into the psychodynamic basis for pain, for, of two patients with apparently equal metastatic spread of disease, one will have pain and the other will not. One factor demonstrated in these cases was the influence of a sense of guilt and of a need for punishment. Disease and death were not adequate retribution for the unconscious impulse to kill, to lead an immoral life, or to compensate for the lack of kindness to others. It was necessary to add pain to balance the moral budget. (p. 11)

Such blatant moral reinterpretation of the pain experienced by cancer patients prevented any serious consideration of cancer pain by researchers and clinicians alike. As recently as 1968, Sacerdote claimed that it was important for physicians treating cancer patients to note that "pain may sometimes be nothing more than somatization of a dangerous depression" (1968a, p. 243), and "the need and right that the patient may have to utilize his illness and his pain for the expiation of real or imagined guilt, and in some cases, for the punishment of close members of the family" (1968b, p. 246).

This changed in the 1970s when, for a host of social and medical reasons, chronic pain of malignant origin was finally viewed as a medical problem in its own right and not merely as symptomatic of other, underlying medical problems. Epidemiological data and studies from specialized treatment units now indicate that pain rates vary from 15 percent in patients with early, nonmetastatic disease to 60 to 90 percent in patients with advanced malignant disease (e.g., Bonica, 1979; Foley, 1985). This prevalence is underscored by the fact that cancer patients are still undermedicated for their pain, and that only up to 50 percent of cancer patients with pain report a 70 percent or greater pain relief with analgesics (Foley, 1985; Cleeland, 1984). These figures are, of course, much worse in developing countries where two-thirds of all worldwide cancer deaths occur. Faced with the overwhelming undertreatment of cancer pain and the findings that cancer pain can be controlled in 90 percent of patients, the World Health Organization has begun to conduct worldwide research on cancer pain and to provide guidelines for pain management (Swerdlow & Stjernswärd, 1982; World Health Organization, 1986).

The psychological consequences of this suffering are severe. A number of authors have argued that the psychological impact of cancer pain is frequently much greater than that of nonmalignant chronic pain (e.g., Bond, 1979; Bonica, 1980; Woodforde & Fielding, 1975). A number of studies have also indicated that the intensity of pain experienced by cancer patients was related to the extent to which pain interfered with patients' activities and daily life (Daut & Cleeland, 1982; Stam, Goss, Rosenal, Ewens & Urton, 1985). Stam et al. (1985) also found that reductions in pain in a sample of cancer patients undergoing radiotherapy did not lead to reductions in depression and anxiety following their radiation treatments. Instead, psychological distress continued to be highly related to the extent to which pain interfered in patients' activities of daily life. Thus, it is still not clear what variables account for the increased distress in cancer patients with chronic pain relative to that found in nonmalignant chronic pain patients.

The use of hypnosis for the treatment of cancer pain, like other psychological techniques for the treatment of this problem, has remained largely untested. The bulk of this literature is in the form of case reports. From 1959 to present (1988), I was able to locate 42 published reports of case studies in the periodical literature. Most of these articles reported on more than one case. The large number of books on clinical uses of hypnosis contain numerous other case examples of the use of hypnosis to control pain in cancer patients. All of the usual limitations of case studies apply to this literature (e.g., inability to determine the relative efficacy of the treatment). A second, and perhaps more severe, limitation of this literature in general is that the use of the word "hypnosis" in no way denotes a standard set of procedures. In fact, many of the procedures hardly appear to have more in common than the label.

Despite the dearth of studies there are no lack of prescriptive and "theoretical" treatises on the use of hypnotic techniques with cancer patients. Each of these reviews some selected aspects of the literature on hypnosis and cancer and hypnosis and pain and prescribes some techniques to be used along with a rationale (e.g., Ahles, 1985; Ament, 1982; J. Barber, 1978; 1980; Finer, 1979; Holden, 1977; Sacerdote, 1966, 1968a, 1968b, 1970, 1977; Spiegel, 1985). Disagreements are legion. For example, J. Barber (1978; 1980) claims that hypnosis can be beneficial to "any" patient and that "most" cancer patients can learn hypnotic pain control. Spiegel (1985) claims that "some individuals simply cannot be hypnotized" (p. 223).

Definitions of hypnosis also vary widely but among these there are several recurring themes. They include the definition of hypnosis as "suggestion" and the "establishment of an interpersonal relationship" (Ament, 1982, p. 234), as a "state of intensified attention and receptiveness and an increased responsiveness to an idea or to a set of ideas" (Erickson, 1959, 117), as "self-hypnosis," a "trance state," a "form of aroused concentration coupled with physical relaxation" (Spiegel, 1985, p. 223), as an "altered state of consciousness arising during a specific trusting relationship" (Finer, 1979, p. 225), as a tool "to enable an individual to potentiate inner capacities for self-healing and for creating comfort" (J. Barber, 1978, p. 363), and as a device by which one can elicit mystical states to relieve pain (Sacerdote, 1977). Not only are these claims between authors contradictory but, occasionally, within a single report on hypnotic techniques for cancer pain there are also equally contradictory statements. The problems in defining hypnosis as some special state of the person have long been noted (e.g., Barber, 1969; Spanos, 1986b). This will be discussed further in the conclusion. What is of interest for our current purposes is the efficacy of hypnosis in particular and its comparative efficacy with other psychological methods of pain control. Thus we need to examine what little data is available.

Case studies. The case material, with a few exceptions, follows a very typical pattern (e.g., J. Barber & Gitelson, 1980; Caracappa, 1963; Chong, 1968, 1982; Clawson & Swade, 1975; Cleeland & Tearnan, 1986; Crasilneck & Hall, 1973; Erickson, 1959, 1966; Halpern & White, 1962; Sacerdote, 1962, 1965, 1982a, 1982b; Willard, 1974). Several introductory claims are made about the utility of hypnosis, the need to treat severe pain in cancer patients, and the author's experience in using hypnosis for this problem. What then usually follows is one or more cases wherein hypnosis was successfully used to relieve the pain of the patient and, occasionally, a report of a case where this was not successful. The only exception to this pattern is a report of 10 patients who had received hypnosis for pain control (Crasilneck and Hall, 1962). These authors report that 8 of their 10 patients continued to respond to a hypnotic command despite the fact that they were unconscious and close to death. Like most of the case reports, this report also cannot be evaluated because of the total lack of data and criteria used to determine responsiveness. In general, then, the collection of any form of reliable data in these cases is almost nonexistent.

Several reports of cases of cancer pain treated by hypnosis provide some data about the extent of pain experienced or degree of pain relief obtained (e.g., Cangello, 1961, 1962; Domangue & Margolis, 1983; Kellerman, Zeltzer, Ellenberg & Dash, 1983; Lea, Ware & Monroe, 1960). For example, Lea et al. (1960) treated 20 patients with intractable pain, 10 of whom had pain due to cancer. Their results were defined as "excellent," "good," or a "failure" by the investigators themselves and are thus virtually uninterpretable.

Cangello (1961) provided case material on 22 cancer patients with pain who had been treated with hypnosis. Reductions in narcotic use was the dependent variable. In another report, Cangello (1962) provided data on 81 patients who had a diagnosis of cancer and who were hypnotized for the purposes of anesthesia or for various pain problems. In the latter report, the author made judgments on the "depth of trance" ("light, medium, deep") and determined the degree of pain relief by noting the reduction in narcotic intake on all the patients. Unfortunately, there is no indication of the reliability or validity of these data and it is impossible to determine whether the patient requested reductions in narcotic intake or if this was suggested to the patient by the medical staff following hypnosis.

Domangue and Margolis (1983) compared 12 cancer patients with pain who received hypnosis to 9 patients who did not. Both groups also received analgesics and patients were not randomly assigned to the two groups. There was no difference between the two groups after four months. Although the within-group change in ratings of "worst" pain and "average" pain greater in the hypnosis group, the selective membership of these groups makes this an uninterpretable finding.

It should be noted here that in most reports of the use of hypnosis for cancer pain, there is no exact indication of analgesic use. It is also true that hypnosis, like most psychological techniques, is additional to the analgesics and other medications and pain treatments that patients are already receiving.

Bone marrow aspirations and lumbar punctures. Children with cancer, especially leukemias and lymphomas, frequently are required to undergo aversive medical procedures as part of their treatment. Bone marrow aspirations and lumbar punctures are by far the most painful and traumatic of these (e.g., Katz, Kellerman & Ellenberg, 1987). Kellerman et al. (1983) reported on 16 adolescents who were treated with hypnosis for pain and anxiety associated with either bone marrow aspirations, lumbar punctures, or chemotherapeutic injections. The authors reported that for all 16 patients combined, "discomfort" and "anxiety" were significantly reduced following hypnosis and compared to baseline. The authors pooled their data because "there were no meaningful intergroup differences in response patterns or demographics" (p. 87). The impact of this on their "discomfort" measures is unreported and thus precludes any clear statements about "pain." Bone marrow aspirations and lumbar punctures differ in length and likely impact from each other. Bone marrow aspirations are typically more painful (e.g., Zeltzer & LeBaron, 1982). Both of these are, again, quite different from chemotherapy injections.

J. Hilgard and LeBaron (1982) present a report on the relief of anxiety and pain in children and adolescents with cancer, later expanded into book form (Hilgard & LeBaron, 1984). Although there have been previous case reports of the use of hypnosis for children with cancer (e.g., Gardner & Olness, 1981), these reports—as those of most of the adult cases—have not obtained any quantitative measures of symptomatology, treatment effectiveness, or hypnotic susceptibility. Hilgard and LeBaron measured self-reported and observed pain at baseline and also obtained hypnotic susceptibility scores. On the basis of scores on the Stanford Hypnotic Clinical Scale for Children, 19 of their 24 patients scored in the high-susceptible range. These reported greater reductions in reported pain and anxiety following hypnosis than the 5 low-susceptible subjects. The overall effect of the hypnotic intervention was to reduce pain by approximately 30 percent in these patients.

As with the case studies with adults, however, Hilgard and LeBaron's study still does not indicate the relative efficacy of hypnotic interventions. In fact, very few studies exist that have examined hypnotic interventions with control groups appropriate for testing clinical intervention. For example, in order to make the claims typically made about the utility of hypnosis, not only should such studies include no-treatment controls but they should also at the least, compare hypnotic procedures to some other set of procedures designed to produce the same outcome.

Experimental designs. There are now five recent studies that have attempted to implement at least partial experimental designs and they report mixed results (Katz et al., 1987; Reeves, Redd, Storm & Minagawa, 1983; Spiegel & Bloom, 1983; Syrjala, Cummings, Donaldson & Chapman, 1987; Zeltzer & LeBaron, 1982). Two of these have examined pain in children with cancer and three have examined pain relief in adults with cancer.

Pain control in studies with children. Zeltzer and LeBaron (1982) compared hypnotic techniques to "non-hypnotic behavioral techniques" in children receiving bone marrow aspirations and lumbar punctures. Sixteen patients received hypnosis and seventeen received the nonhypnotic techniques and rated pain and anxiety during lumbar punctures or bone marrow aspirations or both. During bone marrow aspirations, the hypnosis group reported significant reductions in pain and anxiety whereas the nonhypnosis group reported a smaller, but still significant, reduction in pain only. During lumbar punctures, only the hypnotic group reported significantly reduced pain, whereas both groups reported significant reductions in anxiety.

Although the authors claim that "hypnosis is more effective than non-hypnotic techniques" (p. 1035), these results are highly problematic. Zeltzer and LeBaron's hypnotic procedure consisted of guided imagery, the provision of "exciting or funny stories," and other involving imagery. It is not reported whether the situation was even defined as "hypnotic" to either children or parents. In contrast the "nonhypnotic" techniques involved the "use of distraction and encouragement of self-control behaviors; the use of imagery or fantasy was strictly avoided by the therapist" (p. 1033). Not only are the procedures different, but the descriptions alone also make clear that the degree of involvement of the therapists is quite different in each case, with much less involvement in the nonhypnotic group. It is interesting that the authors note this but not its implication when they say that "children have a shorter attention span than adults have, and techniques of nonimagery and cognitive information in the nonhypnotic intervention are less effective in children. After a brief period of counting, breathing, and noticing objects in the room, most children lose interest and refocus their attention on the pain of the procedure(s)" (p. 1034).

In addition to the problem of unequal procedures, it is clear that all changes are minor in absolute terms. The largest mean difference in pre- and post-intervention scores was 1.71 on a 5 point scale. A difference as small as .66 was significant but, it might be argued, perhaps not very meaningful from a treatment perspective.

In the only other report of comparative treatments in the literature, Katz et al. (1987) administered training in "hypnosis and self-hypnosis" to one group of 17 children and compared this with a group of 19 children receiving nondirected play sessions designed to control for the amount of time and attention the child received from a professional. All children had a diagnosis of acute lymphoblastic leukemia, had experienced significant pain and fear during previous bone marrow aspirations, and were scheduled to receive at least three more aspirations. Self-reported pain and fear were significantly reduced by both procedures across the three posttreatment aspirations, Significant interactions indicated that males did somewhat better in the play condition whereas females did better in the hypnosis condition, although the authors qualify these interactions by noting that they are based on very small sample sizes. The main findings of this study clearly indicate no superior effects for hypnotic analgesia in children receiving an aversive medical procedure when compared to a control play condition. Since the Katz et al. (1987) study included a number of controls hitherto not included in reports of hypnotic procedures with children, it places the onus on those claiming that hypnosis is a superior treatment to demonstrate its efficacy in appropriately controlled studies.

Pain control in experimental studies with adults. Only three studies appear to have examined the effects of a hypnotic intervention on cancer pain in adults. One of these was a study in which a "self-hypnosis exercise" of 5-10 minute's duration was added to group therapy for one group of women, but not for another group receiving the same group therapy (Spiegel & Bloom, 1983). The therapy was conducted over a one-year period and all women had metastatic breast cancer. Spiegel and Bloom reported that two of four self-report pain measures were significantly reduced by group therapy in general compared to a no-treatment control group. Only one measure, "pain sensation," was significantly reduced in the hypnosis group compared to the non-hypnosis therapy group.

Spiegel and Bloom claim that this intervention improved patients' experience of pain. Unfortunately, this is impossible to determine from their study. Because of the high dropout rate, data were analyzed using slopes of regression lines obtained from regressing subjects' scores on measurement occasions. It is not clear what effect this had on the data since the untransformed data was not presented. Despite this transformation, the significant effect for hypnosis could only be found on *one* of the four pain self-report measures.

Syrjala et al. (1987) reported a study with leukemia or lymphoma patients who were to receive a bone marrow transplant and were conditioned with supralethal doses of chemotherapy and total body irradiation. This is done to abolish the immune system and rid the body of malignant cells to prepare the marrow of the patient for that of the donor. The side effects of the chemotherapy and irradiation consist of nausea, vomiting, and mouth and throat pain from the breakdown of the oropharyngeal mucosa. Syrjala et al. compared hypnosis (n = 13) with cognitive-behavioral training (n = 12) and two control conditions—a therapist contact group (n = 12) and a no-treatment control group (n = 13)—for the control of pain. The sessions were conducted twice for 90 minutes each prior to the transplantation procedure and ten times after the procedure, for 30 minutes each.

The results were analyzed only for the three treatment groups. The non-treatment control group was dropped from the analysis "since a main effect was found for gender in predicting report of oral pain." A small but significant effect is then reported that indicates that the hypnosis group reported less pain than the combined cognitive-behavioral and therapist contact groups. The authors conclude "as predicted, hypnosis was more effective for pain than was a package of cognitive-behavioral techniques." An examination of a graph of unanalyzed and unadjusted means belies this conclusion. It seems likely that if the no-treatment control group were included, it would have washed out *any* treatment effects. The mean reported pain by the males in this group was *lower* than the mean reported pain by males in any of the other treatment groups. (There were only two females in this group so comparisons are not meaningful, yet even these two patients reported pain at approximately the same level as the females in all other groups.) Finally, there were no group differences in opioid intake or nausea.

The only complete factorial design in this literature that included the division of groups into those scoring high or low in hypnotic susceptibility was a study reported by Reeves et al. (1983). These investigators examined the effects hypnotic analgesia on pain induced by hyperthermia treatments in cancer patients. This consists of heating tumors in excess of 42° C where the heat is produced by a radiofrequency stimulus over periods usually lasting for an hour or longer. Thus, the stimulus conditions are more constant than is typically the case in chronic pain. The twenty-eight patients in this study were assigned to a hypnosis or a control group and each of these was divided into high- and low-susceptible groups on the basis of scores on the Stanford Hypnotic Clinical Scale (Hilgard & Hilgard, 1983). Two sessions of hypnotic training were provided to the hypnosis group and two sessions of hyperthermia were then observed. The hypnotic training was an "indirect" (or "non-authoritarian") version as advocated by investigators influenced by Milton Erickson, who claimed that all subjects are responsive to this techniques regardless of their measured hypnotic susceptibility (e.g., J. Barber, 1980). Patients rated their pain on two baseline trials and again during the two experimental trials.

The results of this study clearly indicated that the only patients to report significant reductions in pain were the high-susceptible subjects receiving hypnosis.

Furthermore, reductions in pain were significantly correlated with measured hypnotic susceptibility in the treatment group, but not in the control group. The authors were able to demonstrate the utility of their procedures for the limited pain of hyperthermia. Further research is still needed, however, to determine whether this hypnotic procedure would be superior to nonhypnotic psychological techniques of pain reduction. The predictability and limited nature of this pain stimulus also makes it unusual among studies of cancer pain. Almost all other studies and reports have been conducted with longer lasting chronic pain due to the disease or one of the treatments of chemotherapy or radiotherapy. Thus the Reeves et al. (1983) study is experimentally more sophisticated yet could have been carried out on any patient population in as much as the pain stimulus was not directly related to cancer but was similar to an experimental pain stimulus of relatively long duration.

Where does this leave the literature on the treatment of cancer pain? More or less where it began, unfortunately. The lack of systematic studies and the continued exaggerated claims made for this technique have left it in scientific and therapeutic limbo. Even if the literature were unequivocal in its evaluation of hypnotic techniques, the reader would still be bewildered by the wide variety of procedures that go by the name "hypnosis." What most of these have in common is (*a*) the definition of the situation as hypnosis, (*b*) the inclusion of some "induction" techniques, which vary from case to case, (*c*) the inclusion of some suggestions for relaxation and focusing on breathing, and (*d*) suggestions for the removal, imaginative transformation, or posthypnotic disappearance of pain. Not all investigators report all of these factors, and some report none, referring instead only to "the fact" that the patient was in a "trance." This problem will be discussed further below. Needless to say, it makes the literature extremely difficult to evaluate.

Treatment failures. If we are to make sense of large numbers of case reports, it might also help if failed cases were occasionally reported. Only three papers have done this with regard to hyponosis and pain. Schon (1960) reports a case of unsuccessful hypnosis for pain in a cancer patient who was not aware of the terminal nature of her disease. Schon attributes failure to her lack of knowledge of impending death and the fact that hypnosis is too frightful because it lays bare the "unconscious knowledge" of impending death. Sacerdote (1965) reports a failed case of hypnosis with an elderly female doctor, also suffering from pain and near death. In this case, the failure is attributed to a number of factors, most notably the patient's "very rigid" personality that could not admit that pain could be controlled by psychological means.

Finally, Hilgard and LeBaron (1982) discuss nine pediatric patients who were unsuccessful in reducing pain below their baseline level. Four of these scored high on their measured hypnotic susceptibility whereas five scored low. In both groups, observer ratings of pain were reduced somewhat while self-reported pain was not. The authors argue that this indicates that the patients now had better control over their pain posttreatment, even though the experience of pain remained constant. An equally persuasive argument could be made from a compliance perspective. After all the efforts of the therapists, the children and adolescents correctly understood the purpose of the treatment and were less active and agitated during treatment but reported their pain as unchanged. Thus, failed cases shed little further light on the utility of hypnotic interventions.

Experimental pain and experiments with other clinical pains. The literature on hypnotic pain control in the cancer patient sheds virtually no light on what mechanisms might be involved in the reduction of pain when such is reported. Although there is no doubt that such ameliorations of pain are genuine in successfully treated cases, there is no evidence that anything particular to hypnosis or hypnotic techniques is responsible for the outcomes. The nature of pain control in the cancer patient is perhaps less difficult to understand when viewed in the light of the research on hypnotic analgesia with experimental pain and other clinical pain conditions. This is not to downplay the significant differences between short-duration, artifically induced experimental pains and long-term chronic pains, and between both of these and chronic pain of malignant origin, but rather to note the clear difficulty in establishing whether there are more straightforward explanations for the reductions in pain obtained following the use of hypnotic techniques.

Experimental research has consistently demonstrated that hypnotic analgesia is equivalent to a variety of psychological strategies in reducing reported pain, including the same suggestions for analgesia presented without hypnotic induction procedures (see, Spanos, 1986b, for a review). Whether hypnotic analgesia is compared to an alternative procedure in a within-subjects design or in a between-subjects design has not altered this conclusion (e.g., Spanos, T. X. Barber & Lang, 1974; Spanos, Kennedy & Gwyn, 1984; Stam & Spanos, 1980). In fact, Stam and Spanos (1980) varied the order of presentation of hypnotic versus "waking" analgesia in high-susceptible subjects in a within-subjects design. Hypnotic analgesia was equally effective, less effective, or more effective than waking analgesia depending upon the order of presentation of these two treatments to the subjects and the expectations conveyed to this subjects. Furthermore, the oft-cited relationship between degree of pain reduction obtained following hypnosis susceptibility appears to hold only if the two measures are obtained in the same context (Spanos, 1986b). The relationship does not appear to hold when subjects are tested for analgesia in contexts that are not obviously related to the hypnotic testing situation.

The clinical efficacy of hypnotic analgesia is more difficult to determine because the investigator has no control over the properties off the painful stimulus. Therefore, hypnotic interventions for clinical pain are rarely subjected to the same scrutiny as the interventions for experimental pain. Even here, however, whenever hypnosis has been tested against comparable interventions, the evidence indicates that hypnosis is not superior to other psychological techniques for controlling pain (e.g., Stam, McGrath & Brooke, 1984). Although equal efficacy does not imply equal processes are at work, efforts to determine the mechanisms of hypnotic analgesia have not uncovered processes that could not be explained by reference to situational and subject variables such as expectancies, imagery, and other cognitions (Spanos, 1986b).

Investigators who do believe that there is something unique and special about hypnotic procedures frequently recognize the dilemma of determining precisely what those effects are in the cancer patient receiving hypnosis for pain relief. For example, Orne (1980a, 1980b) argues that even those who are not capable of "entering profound hypnosis" may obtain some relief from the hypnotic situation. He argues that for the cancer patient "the hypnotic induction procedure and its consequences not related to the presence of hypnosis may serve "an important role" in reversing what had appeared to be a progressive worsening of the patient's overall condition. Thus, the induction of hypnosis and training in self-hypnosis provide the opportunity for someone to offer relief in a manner that involves the patient's active participation" (Orne, 1980a, p. 267). What Orne never specifies is: What is it precisely that remains after one accounts for the situational, person, and imaginal-cognitive variables in hypnotic analgesia? If one concedes the importance of the latter variables, the onus is on the proponent to demonstrate the uniqueness of hypnotic analgesia. While there is no shortage of claims for the uniqueness of hypnotic analgesia, neither the rational analysis nor the empirical demonstration of these claims is forthcoming.

In summary, while hypnotic analgesia may ameliorate cancer pain in at least some individuals and on at least some occasions, there is virtually no indication that hypnosis provides a *unique* analgesic. Furthermore, there is no substantive literature to support the claims made by the proponents of hypnosis for the relief of cancer pain. The techniques used by these therapists may indeed be very effective for controlling pain, but it is important for the reader of this literature to distinguish clearly between what these proponents say they do and what they do. Between these two, the chasm looms large.

Nausea, Anticipatory Nausea, and Vomiting

The proliferation of chemotherapy agents over the past decade, and the increased use of these agents for cancer treatment, has led to a greater concern for the treatment of their side effects. The toxic effects of chemotherapy are not limited to the neoplastic cells but also effect other rapidly dividing cells in the body such as those that line the gastrointestinal tract, the hair follicles, and the bone marrow. One of the most debilitating and frightening problems the cancer patient must face is severe post chemotherapy nausea and vomiting (PCNV). In fact, patients themselves rate this as the most aversive side effect of treatment (Coates et al. 1983).

Not all chemotherapy agents are equally cytotoxic, and their emetic potential varies considerably. Most common chemotherapy regimens can be rated by health care professionals for their expected emetic potential yet even then there are still substantial individual differences in response to the agents by patients (Stam & Challis, in press). This is further compounded by the development, in approximately 20 to 30 percent of patients of an anticipatory nausea and/or vomiting (ANV) response. This may vary from nausea experienced just prior to an injection of chemotherapy, to full-blown emesis occurring the night before treatment. Since ANV appears gradually and does not develop fully until the third or fourth treatment session, it is typically viewed as a respondent learning phenomenon. Most reports indicate that 25 to 35 percent of patients with PCNV also develop ANV (see Andrykowski, Redd & Hatfield, 1985; Challis & Stam, 1988a; Redd & Andrykowski, 1982).

In recent years, a number of authors have argued that hypnosis may be a useful treatment tool to augment the pharmacological treatment of PCNV and may be used as a primary treatment for ANV. The latter has shown itself to be remarkably resistant to treatment by pharmacological means. Most antiemetic medications also have strong sedative effects and most patients find them ineffectual in controlling ANV (e.g., Redd & Andrykowski, 1982; Morrow, 1986). Given the respondent learning view of ANV, most authors argue that the treatment itself ought to be based on psychological principles. Thus, in addition to progressive muscle relaxation, hypnosis is one of the most frequently used treatment approaches for ANV (e.g., Hockenberry & Cotanch, 1985; Kaye, 1984; Redd & Andresen, 1981; Redd & Andrykowski, 1982; Redd, Rosenberger & Hendler, 1983).

Unlike the use of hypnosis for the treatment of cancer pain, its use in treating pre- and post-chemotherapy nausea and vomiting is highly specific. In almost all reports there are indications that the induction and suggestions are meant to enhance relaxation and that suggestions are aimed at distraction (e.g., Kaye, 1984) or used in conjunction with a modified systematic desensitization approach (e.g., Hoffman, 1983).

The efficacy of hypnotic procedures in controlling nausea and vomiting has also been demonstrated in a number of quasi-experimental studies. Redd, Andresen & Minagawa (1982) used a multi-element design across six female patients with anticipatory emesis and an ABAB within-subjects design for three of these patients. In each of these women, the emesis was totally eliminated and nausea significantly reduced. Without hypnosis prior to any treatment the emesis returned and was again eliminated when hypnosis was reinstituted during subsequent treatments. The hypnotic procedures in this study consisted of extensive muscle-relaxation procedures, the provision of pleasant images, and the rehearsal of the treatment procedure in the fashion of systematic desensitization.

Zeltzer, Kellerman, Ellenberg, and Dash (1983) treated nine adolescents with cancer by giving them one to three hypnosis sessions and demonstrated that, compared to baseline recordings, these patients significantly reduced their frequency and intensity of post chemotherapy emesis. In a similar study, Cotanch, Hockenberry, and Herman (1985) demonstrated that, relative to a standard treatment control group, six children who received hypnosis significantly reduced the frequency, severity, and duration of their postchemotherapy emesis.

In a pilot study, Rosberger, Perry, Thirlwell, and Hollingworth (1983) gave twelve cancer patients two hypnotic treatment sessions for nausea and vomiting.

Ten of these patients also experienced ANV. Six of these patients experienced at least some relief of their symptoms and Rosberger et al. indicate that this appeared to be related to measured hypnotic susceptibility on the Stanford Hypnotic Susceptibility Scale, Form C (Weitzenhoffer & Hilgard, 1962). Of the patients who controlled their symptoms, two scored high and four scored in the medium range. There was no relationship however between the development of anticipatory nausea and vomiting and hypnotic susceptibility.

These studies indicate the utility of hypnosis in treating nausea and emesis but do not address the relative efficacy of this procedure compared to other behavioral techniques. In particular, many investigators have used progressive relaxation training (with or without imagery) or systematic desensitization to treat nausea and vomiting (see, Sims, 1987, for a review). The overlap with hypnotic procedures is considerable, and often, aside from their labeling, descriptions of the procedures of progressive muscle relaxation cannot be distinguished from hypnosis. The only study to compare the effects of hypnosis with a treated control group for emesis found no difference between the two procedures. Zeltzer, Le-Baron, and Zeltzer (1984) administered a hypnotic intervention to nine children and supportive counseling to ten other children. All patients had a diagnosis of cancer and had experienced consistent PCNV. Both groups showed significant reductions in nausea and emesis. Patients in the hypnosis group were also tested on the Stanford Hypnotic Clinical Scale for Children (Morgan & Hilgard, 1978-79) and no relationship was found between susceptibility scores and reductions in nausea or emesis following the hypnotic treatment.

As the foregoing makes clear, a definitive study or series of studies has yet to be conducted on the efficacy of hypnotic procedures for the treatment of nausea and emesis. The literature is highly equivocal to this date; no controlled studies have been carried out to compare hypnosis to an appropriate treatment and no-treatment control; measures of nausea and vomiting are inconsistent; few investigators measure hypnotic susceptibility; and investigators need to account for differences in treatment regimens, chemotherapy agents, and pre- and post-chemotherapeutic nausea and emesis.

The available research data have yet to indicate any advantage for hypnosis over standard relaxation or systematic desensitization treatments. These procedures often are more similar than they are different and, as was the case for the treatment of pain, claims about the relative efficacy of hypnosis have yet to be demonstrated. All psychological treatments for ANV have in common (*a*) the use of relaxation procedures (and the concomitant reduction of anxiety), (*b*) distraction, (*c*) the provision of some minimal level of control exercised over treatment by the patient by engaging in such exercises, and (*d*) increased social support gained by the intensive involvement of a therapist in these treatments (Challis & Stam, 1988a).

Some investigators eschew the term "hypnosis" altogether, referring instead to passive or active relaxation training with guided imagery (Redd, 1986). According to Redd, these terms reflect the process presumed to underlie the efficacy of hypnosis and relaxation for treating nausea and emesis. Like a number of psychologists who treat cancer patients, he believes that "the procedures for inducing passive relaxation are identical to those frequently used by many professionals who identify their procedures as hypnosis" (Redd, 1986, p. 21).

In a related study, Hendler and Redd (1986) assigned 105 cancer chemotherapy outpatients to one of three groups. Each group then received an identical brief description of a relaxation/hypnosis session for reducing nausea and vomiting with the exception that the label that was attached to the description was either "relaxation," "hypnosis," or "passive relaxation with guided imagery." Compared to a group of college students, patients held more fearful views about hypnosis. More importantly, compared to patients receiving either of the relaxation labels, patients who received a description labelled "hypnosis" were less likely to state that they would try the procedure if it were offered to them. Hendler and Redd (1986) argue that patients believed hypnosis to be a powerful process that was associated with loss of control and unconscious processes.

None of this is to say that hypnosis is not efficacious, but rather that the mechanisms by which hypnotic procedures reduce nausea and emesis seem to be the same mechanisms operating in relaxation-based procedures. These procedures appear to work best for ANV and only marginally, if at all, for PCNV. In a recent study, Challis and Stam (1988a) found that patients who develop ANV are more likely to score higher on a measure of "absorption" or the proclivity to become involved in imaginative pursuits (Tellegen & Atkinson, 1974). This remained true even when controlling for drug toxicity, state anxiety, the severity of PCNV, and the duration of PCNV. Patients who score high in absorption may ruminate about their upcoming treatment and its side effects and thus maintain the salience of the UCS (treatment) and the UCR (PCNV), facilitating the conditioned anticipatory response. Thus, ANV is likely mediated by psychological mechanisms whereas PCNV is mediated pharmacologically and physiologically. Although these categories are not mutually exclusive, any psychological treatment will be more likely to benefit ANV than PCNV. Hypnotic and relaxation procedures appear to exert their effects in this case through the use of relaxation and imagery procedures imbedded in the technique.

Hypnosis for Support and the Treatment of Problems Secondary to Cancer

Multiple Symptoms. A wide range of case studies have been published over the past three decades dealing with the use of hypnotic techniques to treat other symptoms and problems developed by cancer patients. These included such cases as secondary frigidity after radical surgery for gynecological cancer (Cheek, 1976), other sexual dysfunctions in the cancer patient (Nuland, 1983), and fear of death in a nine-year-old boy (Miller, 1980). Mostly however, these cases report the use of hypnotic techniques to treat or ameliorate multiple physiological and psychological symptoms of the disease and its treatment (e.g., Dempster, Balson & Whalen, 1976; Deyoub, 1980; Ellenberg, Kellerman, Dash, Higgins & Zeltzer, 1980; Kaye, 1987; Milne, 1982; Rosenberg, 1983; Smith & Kamitsuka, 1984). Because symptoms of nausea, vomiting, anxiety, depression, pain, and eating problems often occur together in the cancer patient, these reports detail cases treated with at least two of these present. Only one of these reports presents any quantitative baseline and posttreatment data (Ellenberg et al., 1980), and then only for a single case. The remainder are based wholly on the report of the practitioners involved.

In addition to these case studies there are other claims in the literature about the treatment of multiple symptoms in cancer patients (e.g., Araoz, 1983). These, too, are frequently based on a particular author's experience with patients and are not very useful in elucidating the mechanisms by which hypnotic procedures produce the reported changes or the comparative efficacy of these procedures.

Hypnotherapy. A second group of case studies with cancer patients is even more difficult to evaluate since they are cases of "hypnotherapy" (e.g., Grosz, 1979; LaBaw, 1969; Margolis, 1983; Oliver, 1983; Pettitt, 1979). Most of these are psychodynamic in orientation, and the discussions hinge on the patients' internal dynamics, usually in the terminal phases of the illness. Symptom control is peripheral for these authors, although not ignored. Since hypnotic techniques are included in a package of therapy, there is little that can be said about the efficacy or usefulness of these techniques in this context.

Hypnosis with Children. Although a large number of the studies presented above under the headings of pain and emesis control have been conducted with children, there are also case histories of a general nature that report the use of hypnotic techniques to treat multiple symptoms and help children adjust to the illness in general (Gardner, 1976; Gardner & Lubman, 1983; Gardner & Olness, 1981; LaBaw, Holton, Tewell & Eccles, 1975; Olness, 1981). Despite the presentation of multiple cases (e.g., 27 by LaBaw et al., 1975; and 25 by Olness, 1981) there is little one can conclude from these reports. These authors claim success with hypnotic techniques for symptom control and the development of greater tolerance for diagnostic and therapeutic procedures or they discuss the problems of resistance to hypnosis in children. None of these authors attempts to evaluate these claims with systematic research. And while hypnotic techniques have been enthusiastically endorsed by some practitioners of late for the treatment of problems in childhood cancer (e.g., Hockenberry & Bologna-Vaughan, 1985; Hockenberry & Cotanch, 1985; LaBaw et al., 1975; Lazar, Tellerman, Tylke & Gruenewald, 1983; Olness, 1981; Zeltzer & LeBaron, 1983), these claims are long on promise but short on data. The problems these practitioners are treating are very serious and require immediate attention. Nevertheless, the full range of treatments has not been compared against hypnotic techniques.

HYPNOSIS AS TREATMENT FOR CANCER

The most controversial and, at the same time, least-supported claims made about the utility of hypnotic techniques for cancer are those that suggest that hypnosis can actually aid in the treatment and cure of the disease. In order to understand these claims, we will briefly examine the literature on the spontaneous regression of cancer and unorthodox methods of treatment.

Spontaneous Regression

In cancer treatment, spontaneous regression refers to the partial or complete disappearance of a malignant tumor in the absence of treatment or in the presence of inadequate treatment (Everson & Cole, 1966). Thus, spontaneous regression may be incomplete and may not be permanent. It merely indicates that the tumor growth has been halted or reversed. As Challis and Stam (1988b) indicate, the very term "spontaneous" is a misnomer given that some currently unknown response modifiers are involved in the initiation of the regression. A more appropriate term might be "unidentified regression."

In reporting such regressions, many authors point out the problems in documenting whether a case truly satisfied the criteria for "spontaneous." Others have argued that the rigid criteria have prevented a true understanding of the phenomenon at hand, and that less dramatic occurrences of the regressions are more frequent than often thought by the scientific community (Franklin, 1982). Challis and Stam (1988) also note that practitioners do not often agree on what constitutes adequate treatment for a particular individual and stage of disease. Hence, what some physicians might believe to be adequate treatment may lead to claims of spontaneous regressions by others.

Unorthodox Treatments

A history of the use of unorthodox or unproven treatments for cancer indicates that a wide variety of techniques have been used, typically in opposition to the profession of medicine (Janssen, 1979). These have included mechanical devices, nutritional approaches, and occult techniques (Challis & Stam, 1988b). A technique is defined as unorthodox or unproven if it is "not deemed proven or recommended for current use by scientist and/or clinicians" (American Cancer Society, 1982). Traditionally, psychological methods of treatment have been included under the unorthodox label.

Scientific Literature. This is more than a semantic issue given the continued high rates of use of unorthodox treatments (American Cancer Society, 1975; Faw, Ballentine, Ballentine & van Eys, 1977; Cassileth, Lusk, Strouse & Bodenheimer, 1984). Unorthodox treatments are typically promoted by reference to so-called spontaneous regressions. Challis and Stam (1988b) reviewed the medical and scientific literature on spontaneous regression and included all available cases from 1900 to 1985. In their review they found that reports of the successful treatment of cancer by psychological means or the regression of cancer following psychological changes have appeared in the scientific literature on spontaneous regression in the past two decades (e.g., Lansky, 1982; Meares, 1977, 1980, 1981; Weinstock, 1983; Wooley-Hart, 1979). While these are poorly documented cases often appearing in lesser-known journals, it is a departure from the historical practice of not publishing such cases in the scientific literature. Traditionally, such treatments have been considered unorthodox and inadequate as a form of treatment. The inclusion of such cases in the spontaneous regression literature indicates that this literature sometimes includes as "spontaneous" cases that are treated psychologically (Challis & Stam, 1988b). In fact, psychological mechanisms were the only "unorthodox" mechanisms to appear in the literature on spontaneous regression. Hypnotic techniques fall in this category.

Popular Literature. Despite the appearance of cases of reportedly successful treatment by psychological means in the literature on spontaneous regression, Challis and Stam (1988b) found that only one author presented sufficient information to include actual cases in his reviews (Meares, 1976, 1977, 1979, 1980, 1981). Thus, the documentation for the psychological treatment of cancer is sparse. At the same time there exists a large and popular literature on the healing effects of psychological techniques and therapies (e.g., Achterberg & Lawlis, 1978; Achterberg, Simonton & Matthews-Simonton, 1976; Boyd, 1984; LeShan, 1977; Simonton, Matthews-Simonton & Creighton, 1978). These reports are completely without documentation and evidence and are wholly based on the testimonials of a few individuals who were given short periods of time to live and have outlived their "death sentence" by months or years. Simple mechanisms are then invoked as the cause of these regressions, such as a hormonal imbalance influencing immune functioning (Simonton et al., 1978), resolution of adolescent sexuality conflicts lessening anxiety (Boyd, 1984), and so on. Straddling the popular and scientific literature are reports and claims of the utility of hypnosis in treating cancer.

Hypnosis and Cancer Cures

Reports in the hypnosis literature on the treatment of cancer began to appear at approximately the same time as appeared the popular literature on treating cancer with psychological means, such as the Simonton's imaging techniques. Almost all of this literature dates from the 1970s, although there are foreshadowings in several earlier papers. At this time psychological means of treatment for cancer joined the plethora of mechanical and medicinal unorthodox treatments already available to the cancer patient. Hypnosis was readily included among other techniques such as intensive meditation, imaging, and psychotherapy.

Psychosomatic Medicine. The other major root of the idea that hypnosis may be useful in the treatment of cancer originates with the notion of the cancer-prone personality derived from psychosomatic medicine (see, Stam & Steggles, 1987, for a selective review). While largely spurned by psychiatry, this view generated a tremendous volume of research in the two decades immediately following the Second World War and is making a renewed return in some versions of psychoneuroimmunology. Immune functioning plays an important role in tumorogenesis, but the history of attempts to predict cancer from person variables ought to warn us of the empirical traps in this endeavor (Stam & Steggles, 1987).

A number of early reports of the treatment of cancer with hypnosis were founded on notions derived from psychosomatic medicine (e.g., Butler, 1954; Hedge, 1960; Sacerdote, 1966). Butler (1954), in his classic paper on the use of hypnosis for the cancer patient, concludes his discussion with the claim that, through his intimate association with these patients, he has gained "intuitive knowledge . . . that there is a cancer personality" (p. 11). This is a restatement of the psychosomatic position that the dynamics of the mind could, usually unconsciously, influence health. More importantly, Butler claims that "the future of cancer could lie in the psychological means" (p. 11). Sacerdote supports this same tradition in his proposals for research into the hypothesis that hypnosis may lead to an extension in five- and ten-year cures (Sacerdote, 1966). He believes that hypnotic therapy could lead to objectively measurable changes in cure rates and symptom control if it were inaugurated at the very outset of treatment and became part of the overall strategy of cancer therapy. In fact, he also believed that "hypnosis properly used is a psychotherapeutic means 'par excellence,' and is especially effective when the problem is more specifically a 'psychosomatic' one" (Sacerdote, 1966, p. 105). For Sacerdote, the mechanisms by which hypnosis might be effective for the treatment of cancer would be mediated by cortical, subcortical, hormonal, and biochemical interactions. Unfortunately, Sacerdote never heeded his own call for research.

A more recent version of the psychosomatic statement is provided by Lansky (1982). He argues that cancer itself is either the result of a psychosomatic replacement of a significant loss or the consequence of chronically suppressed anger that is emotional energy turned back upon the self. The therapeutic strategy that leads to cure will come if the patient learns to "love his tumor," an example of paradoxical intention. The patient thus consciously recreates the symptomatology as a means of its elimination. Presumably this must be done under "trance" in order to contact those deep-seated pathologies that cause the tumor growth in the first place. As substantiation of this notion, Lansky relies uncritically on a variety of psychoanalytic and popular notions interwoven with statements about the immune system. The crucial evidence consists largely of a number of theoretical claims made by authors in the psychosomatic medicine tradition.

Visualization. More recent claims about the utility of hypnosis in treating cancer have been heavily influenced by Simonton's techniques and are often variations of this strategy. They rely on the use of imagery (or visualization of the cancer and the body's defenses) and the rhetoric of bolstering immune functioning. For example, Strosberg (1982) uses only the Simonton technique and calls it "auto-hypnosis." Most other authors develop a more complicated rationale and technique. A number of papers on this topic were published in a special issue of the *AJCH* edited by Newton (1983a). These papers, and several others published elsewhere, typically develop a rationale around four popular notions: (*a*) cancer cells develop in most, if not all, people during their lifetime; (*b*) the immune system normally destroys those cells before they develop into detectable cancer; (*c*) the immune system is influenced by many variables, including psychological ones; and (*d*) these psychological variables can be mobilized to strengthen the immune system and hence destroy cancer cells. Hypnosis is then presented as one of these psychological factors capable of influencing the outcome of malignant disease (e.g., Barrios & Kroger, 1975; Finkelstein & Howard, 1983; H. Hall, 1983; M. Hall, 1983; Kroger 1977; Newton, 1983b).

The extent to which such claims have influenced the hypnosis community may be evidenced by the fact that even researchers such as E. and J. Hilgard are willing to consider this as a serious possibility (Hilgard and Hilgard, 1983, p. 219). Although most authors have the good sense to qualify their remarks with the usual calls for more research and by noting the lack of findings supporting these claims, such qualifications are never strong enough to prevent them from making problematic claims in the first place. For example, Bowers (1977; Bowers and Kelly, 1979) has argued that the small number of patients who undergo the Simonton's program may actually be highly hypnotizable. The trait of "high hypnotic ability" is then responsible for the reputed good outcome reported by the Simontons. The implication is that "even if hypnotic procedures proved effective in only a small percentage of (highly hypnotizable?) cancer patients, it would be reason enough to include such a treatment strategy as one line of attack on this dread disease" (Bowers, 1977, p. 234). Given such claims, are there any clinical observations or experimental data to support them? What little there is can be categorized under case reports and research reports.

Case Reports. The most common support for the contention that hypnosis influences disease status in cancer comes from a variety of case reports (August, 1975; Chong, 1979, 1982; Hedge, 1960; Olness, 1981; Shapiro, 1983; Weitz, 1983). These typically include the use of hypnotic procedures in addition to traditional medical treatment. The cases presented by Chong (1979, 1982) and Hedge (1960) will not be discussed here, because of the lack of information provided.

August (1975) reported a case of a thirty-one-year-old woman who received a mastectomy and was then taught (hypnotically) to lower her body temperature in the area of the surgery over a period of four months. Compared to her untreated side, she was able to reduce her body temperature in this area by approximately 4° F and was disease free for over a year. The presumed mechanism of action in this case was that the temperature reduction prevented blood flow and hence restricted cell division. Clawson and Swade (1975) also described this mechanism in detail, without supporting data, as a potential hypnotic treatment for cancer.

The other case reports rely heavily on some form of the Simonton's visualization techniques and refer mostly to the teaching of "self-hypnosis." Olness (1981) reported on twenty-five patients referred for symptom control who were treated with hypnosis. Six of these eventually asked for, and received, imagery exercises aimed at having patients see their immune systems as strong and their cancer as weak. Three of these subsequently died. Although Olness was careful not to make specific claims about this treatment, she did argue that the three who died had difficulty visualizing their disease as weak and their defenses as strong, whereas those who survived had no difficulty with this task.

Two more cases are presented by Shapiro (1983), both of which consist of premenopausal females with breast cancer. These women were taught a form of "auto-hypnosis" with visualization of the immune system fighting cancer. One of these patients died, the other was still alive at time of writing. According to Shapiro, the difference between these patients was not only in the support and attitude of others in the patients' lives, but also in the patients' willingness to fight. The patient who eventually died began to express doubts about her visualizations and her ability to carry them on. According to Shapiro, "once she had accepted its inevitability the disease acted as she stated that it would originally, 'fast and fatal' " (p. 154).

A similar procedure was employed by Weitz (1983) with two women cancer patients, one following mastectomy and one following oophorectomy. Weitz reports both were alive at the time of his writing (with no indication of how long this was from the time of diagnosis), and he implicates his hypnotic treatment in their survival. Furthermore he also reports that he has seen "on the average about two cancer patients a month, specifically referred for hypnotherapy. Some have lived and some have died. In retrospect at this time, there is no question in my mind that those who continue to live have found a reason for living and that those who die quickly do so because they are without purpose" (p. 73).

Research. It is also interesting to note the tangential evidence that is cited and presented in support of the notion that hypnosis can influence immune functioning. Aside from the typical references to Simonton et al. (1978) and Leshan (1977), several authors present qualitative data on the success of treating cancer patients with hypnosis. Gravitz (1985) presents the remission of breast cancer in one case reported in 1846. Needless to say, this is a historically interesting, but wholly unreliable, report. Others have presented cases or a series of cases. For example, Newton (1983b) reports the survival rates of 283 cancer patients who were treated using hypnosis and psychotherapy. These patients were arbitrarily divided into those who were adequately treated and those who were not adquately treated, with the former receiving at least 10 one-hour sessions and the latter receiving from 4 to 9 sessions. The survival rate of the adequately treated (57 percent) was higher than that of the inadequately treated (18 percent). Aside from the obvious lack of a control group and other methodological inadequacies of this conclusion, the result is badly skewed by the inclusion, in the inadequately treated group, of 57 patients who "were very clearly trying to die with a minimum of discomfort" (p. 110). It appears then that palliative cases were placed in the inadequate group and the healthier cases in the adequate group. To claim then, as Newton does, that "this type of intervention can result in lengthening the duration of life and in some instances arrest and reverse the disease process" is misleading at best.

Finkelstein and Howard (1983) make similar claims regarding the efficacy of hypnosis. In their study, however, subjects were instructed to listen to a ten-minute tape recording four times a week. The tape included the suggestion that the listener could take responsibility for his or her own immune system and have it continue functioning. This was interspersed with typical suggestions for relaxation and deep breathing. Forty-three subjects received a follow-up questionnaire after a year of reported use of this tape. These subjects reported increased well-being, both psychologically and physiologically. No verification was provided and no baseline data obtained, yet Finkelstein and Howard (1983) indicate that they are "satisfied that the cassette tape intervention provided psychological and physiological support targeted for participating subjects" (p. 182). Needless to say, this conclusion is wholly unwarranted.

Other data used to support the hypothesis that hypnosis can augment immune functioning are often based on reports that hypnosis can modify allergic responses and treat dermatological conditions such as urticaria, ichthyosiform, and warts (H. Hall, 1983). Whatever the scientific status of these reports, authors cite these findings as evidence for modification of immune functioning by hypnosis. However, such evidence is a long way from showing that immune functions are modified by hypnosis. H. Hall (1983) presented what he believed was more direct evidence in the form of a study wherein twenty subjects had their blood tested for lymphocyte functioning. Following baseline testing, these subjects received hypnotic training in bolstering immune functioning and then were post-tested after hypnotic training and again after one week. Only subjects less than fifty years of age showed improved lymphocyte functioning. Also, high-susceptible subjects (based on a median split on the Stanford Hypnotic Susceptibility Scale, Form C; Weitzenhoffer & Hilgard, 1962) showed greater lymphocyte functioning after their first hypnotic session, but not after one week.

These data are, of course, also difficult to evaluate given the sketchy verbal presentation of the results. In any case, the absence of detailed results makes them preliminary regardless of their manner of presentation. As is typical of such studies, investigators have not included appropriate controls that would unambiguously separate hypnotic effects from others such as relaxation and/or imagination. The base rates of change in physiological measures are also not reported or measured. Whenever appropriate controls have been included in past investigations on the physiological effects of hypnosis, alterations in physiological processes have not been attributable to the specific effects of hypnotic procedures (Frankel, 1987; Sarbin & Slagle, 1979). Furthermore, there are several reports of a failure to affect immune responses with hypnotic suggestions (Beahrs, Harris & Hilgard, 1970; Locke et al., 1987). The data on the immunological effects of hypnosis on cancer onset and progression share the same methodological difficulties as the literature on the physiological effects of hypnosis.

It is obvious even to some proponents of hypnotic treatments for cancer that the research literature rather poorly supports their fond assertion. Replies to this charge have included attacks on the very notion of replicability and a revival of ideas about the relationship between hypnotist and subject. As a case in point, Newton (1983a) introduced the special issue of the *AJCH* on hypnosis and cancer with a direct attack on replication. Failures to replicate should not necessarily cast doubt on the original results. Rather, they illuminate the intensification of the relationship between the hypnotized and the hypnotist. He argues that "the question of who does the study, what his motives are, what his beliefs are, what the structure of personality is, what his expectations are, are to a very great extent as important as the concern over the experimental design, the selection of subjects, the hypnotizability of subjects and the statistical methods used in the analysis of data" (p. 90). Furthermore, the clinical situation merely amplifies this process. For Newton, success comes from the therapist as much as the technique. Failures to replicate cancer cures come not from doubts about the validity of the techniques, but from the failure of the therapist. Newton then gives an example of one "successful" therapist and argues that this therapist's success is due to the fact he is "a most uncommon man who has developed a highly potent therapeutic procedure that is absolutely in tune with himself as a human being and as a therapist" (p. 91).

This defense is often found in writings derived from the Ericksonian tradition. This tradition has, of course, created a double standard. Empirical research is to be lauded for its insights into immune functioning and the findings supporting the connection between the central nervous system and the immune system. On the other hand, empirical analysis is useless in investigating the claims of hypnotists who treat patients for cancer because such is the uniqueness of the psychotherapist-client relationship. Unfortunately, one can't have it both ways. If one is ever to take the hypnotists seriously in their claims for cancer treatment, the burden of proof rests with those making the claims, not with the empirical methods.

The issue of treating cancer with hypnosis parallels a number of hypnotic phenomena that have been investigated over the past half-century. The findings of experimental studies of hypnosis have placed clear limits around these phenomena. For example, in his introductory psychology textbook published in 1935, Gardner Murphy was still able to exclaim that hypnosis can lead to "loss of muscular function . . . loss of a sensory function . . . loss of memories, immediate or remote . . . loss of the capacity to decide or will a course of action" (p. 498), and more. In fact, he also stated that "all the dissociation which occurs spontaneously in hysteria can be made to occur experimentally in hypnosis" (p. 499). That very experimentation would put an end to many of these claims. In the case of phenomena such as hypnotic analgesia or hypnotic amnesia, one rarely sees propositions such as, "hypnosis is capable of total pain relief" or "people are always amnesic after hypnosis." Whatever theoretical perspective one adopts to explain hypnotic analgesia or hypnotic amnesia, one is bounded by the empirical research on these phenomena. The only manner in which one can deny these limiting conditions placed on the phenomena is to deny the validity of empirical research. It is the latter strategy that has been adopted by some practitioners working with hypnotic treatments for cancer. Although the reasons for adopting this strategy may themselves be explainable (e.g., the Ericksonian tradition, the opposition between "hard-nosed" experimentalists and clinicians who must deal with "real problems"), it does not exonerate the proponents from verifying their claims.

THE NATURE OF HYPNOSIS

Essentialists versus Continuous Positions

It does not require a great deal of observation to note the primitive state of the literature on hypnosis and cancer. As already alluded to in places above, perhaps the most puzzling aspect of this literature is determining precisely (*a*) what is meant by hypnosis, and (*b*) what is being done when a patient is "hypnotized." The first question is not unique to the literature on hypnosis and cancer. Widely divergent views of hypnosis can be found throughout the literature on the various hypnotic phenomena. These eventually reduce to two somewhat orthogonal positions, variously called the state/non-state; credulous/skeptical, or special process/social-psychological positions. All of these terms distinguish researchers and practitioners who hold that there is something essential to hypnosis that is fundamentally different from normal psychological activities, from those who hold that hypnotic phenomena are continuous with normal psychological activities. Hence the terms essentialist/continuous might be more appropriate descriptors of these positions.

The literature on hypnosis and cancer is almost wholly written by those who hold essentialist positions. This fact alone accounts for the continued belief that there must be some utility to this powerful technique in alleviating distress, if not in treating cancer. Within this distinction are further divisions—e.g., hypnosis is a psychological lobotomy (Kroger, 1977), hypnosis is a state of intensified attention or receptiveness (Erickson, 1959), hypnosis is a dissociated state of consciousness (Hilgard & Hilgard, 1983), and more. Nevertheless these various definitions do not differ in their emphasis on an essential nature of hypnosis. Of course, if one begins with the premise that hypnotic phenomena are continuous with normal psychological activities, then one is less likely to look for ways to use this "special" tool.

The distinction between essentialist and continuous views is even more apparent if we ask of this literature: What is it that is being done when the patient is being hypnotized? It is obvious that the context is usually clearly defined as one involving "hypnosis." Beyond this distinction, however, very little can be divined that would differentiate it from a host of other procedures typically used with cancer patients (e.g., Redd, 1986; Sims, 1987). These include various forms of progressive or systematic relaxation training, the use of imagery or visualization, meditation, and suggestions for relief of symptoms such as nausea, pain, and anxiety. These then are frequently integrated with other forms of psychotherapy. In cases where hypnosis is *not* explicitly mentioned, such as in the treatment of very young children or adults anxious about "losing control," the hypnotic procedures used are in fact indistinguishable from those called by a procedural name (e.g., Olness, 1981). It is only an author's preference that leads to labeling the procedures "hypnotic" instead of "imagery."

This problem has long been a concern to experimental researchers of hypnosis. As soon as one attempts to determine the necessary and sufficient conditions for the presence of hypnosis, it becomes readily apparent that they can be subsumed under a host of phenomena that do not require esoteric explanations (e.g., T. X. Barber, 1969; Spanos, 1986b). The resistance of clinical researchers and practitioners to such "continuous" explanations is well known and has yet to be explained.

This is not the place to argue for a particular conception of hypnosis. If the reader has come this far, then the author's inclinations should, by now, have become obvious. Surely the more important point is that this large and diverse literature on hypnosis and cancer does not shed much light on our understanding of either hypnosis or cancer. It is crippled by a lack of sophisticated research, weakened by the strongly "essentialist" preconceptions brought to the topic by the authors, and is doomed to obscurity by virtue of its post-hoc conclusion. It appears largely that most of it is written by and for a narrow group of practitioners that share certain preconceptions. This might not matter but for one final point I should like the reader to ponder.

Placing Responsibility on the Patient

Providing psychological interventions for treating cancer raises a moral issue that is not easily ignored. Proponents do not claim theirs is the *sole* treatment, but they often do claim that the effectiveness of any other therapeutic modality relies on the proper psychological state of the patient. Thus. responsibility is placed on the patient for the development and progress of cancer and the outcome of treatment. Psychological methods of cancer treatment are far from benign (Holland, 1982). Patients may already feel guilty and vulnerable and may be placed at risk for greater psychological distress and hopelessness when the disease and its treatment become their personal responsibility. Psychological interventions for psychological problems may be very helpful and even necessary for the cancer patient (e.g., Stam, Bultz & Pitman, 1986). There is no support, however, for the claims that psychological techniques actually reject or contain cancer or otherwise lead to its regression (e.g., American Cancer Society, 1982; Challis & Stam, 1988b). Whatever links exist between immune functioning and distress do not allow one to claim a directional relationship (Stam & Steggles, 1987; Wellisch & Yager, 1981).

Hypnosis practitioners are not immune from these arguments. If they treat the symptoms of cancer and the side effects of its treatment, they may be contributing to the general well-being of their clients. At worst, they are a benign influence. If they are "treating" the cancer itself, they appear to be accepting the premises of other unorthodox medical practitioners, even when they do so at their clients' request. Whether the client is fleeing a hostile, orthodox medical establishment or merely following up on claims made in the popular literature, it makes no difference. At the least, "treating" cancer requires the practitioners to make unsubstantiated claims. At worst, they create an illusion that may lead to greater client hopelessness as an outcome. Perhaps the usual qualifying remark—further research is needed—is appropriate as a conclusion, if only as an understatement to highlight the long labor that remains to be done if we are to demythologize hypnotic therapies for cancer.

NOTES

1. Freud was quite emphatic about his changed attitude on hypnosis, which followed directly from his experiences. While he first treated hypnosis as a highly useful tool for the treatment of hysteria, he later argued, "I soon dropped the practice of making tests to show the degree of hypnosis reached, since in quite a number of cases this roused the patients' resistance and shook their confidence in me, which I needed for carrying out the more important psychical work. Furthermore, I soon began to tire of issuing assurances and commands such as: 'You are going to sleep! . . . sleep!' and of hearing the patient, as so often happened when the degree of hypnosis was light, remonstrate with me: 'But, doctor, I'm *not* asleep' " (Freud, [1895]/1957, p 108).

2. It is interesting to note in this context that T. X. Barber had already reviewed the pain literature in 1959 (T. X. Barber, 1959) and begun experimental research in hypnosis and pain in the early 1960s (e.g., T. X. Barber & Hahn, 1962). Hilgard and others began their research on hypnosis and pain much later in the context of the general push for psychological approaches to pain management (e.g., Melzack, 1973).

14

Forensic Aspects of Hypnosis

Graham F. Wagstaff

As hypnosis has often been construed historically as a trance state or special process, it is perhaps inevitable that it should come in contact with the legal system. The main alleged feature of hypnosis, which has led many to advocate its use in forensic contexts, is its ability to enhance memory (Reiser, 1980; Haward and Ashworth, 1980; Hibbard and Worring, 1981). Thus Haward and Ashworth (1980) argue that hypnosis can "induce a mental state which facilitates recall and enables the subject to produce more information than he would be able to provide in the so-called waking state" (p. 471). However, hypnosis has also been advocated as a truth-seeking device, a technique to evaluate a defendant's sanity, an aid in the preparation of witnesses or parties for trial, a means of detecting malingering, an aid in obtaining admissions and confessions, and as a defense in criminal cases (Kline, 1983; Udolf, 1983). Nevertheless, the traditional state or special process view of hypnosis might also lead us to suspect that there may be special dangers attached to hypnosis that have legal implications. The most obvious dangers arise from the possibility of hypnotizing individuals into a somnambulistic state of hypersuggestibility; a state in which they may have little or no knowledge of their actions, in which they may be induced to do things against their wills, or in which they are unusually prone to accepting false information.

THE HYPNOTIC STATE AND CRIMINAL LIABILITY

Haward and Ashworth (1980) argue that in the hypnotic state "the good hypnotic subject loses the power to monitor sensation from the outside world or to engage in any mental processes until so directed by the hypnotist" (p. 470). Hilgard (1986) also comments that one of the characteristics of the hypnotic state is "The hypnotized subject loses initiative and lacks the desire to make and carry out plans of his own; he appears to have turned over much of this to the hypnotist" (p. 164).

According to some state theorists, the obvious dangers accompanying the achievement of such a state are magnified by the fact that it is possible to "hypnotize" unwilling victims without their knowledge. Thus Marcuse (1976) argues that providing subjects are hypnotically susceptible, they can be hypnotized, even if unwilling, by some devious techniques. According to Marcuse a most useful technique for "hypnotizing" the unwilling person is the "disguise method" in which "one takes a person from sleep into hypnosis, and at the termination of hypnosis returns the subject to sleep again without the subject's ever being aware of the fact that he has been hypnotized" (p. 58). Udolf (1983) argues that "it is not possible to hypnotize a person who actively resists hypnosis," but "it is possible to hypnotize persons without their awareness by using a variety of techniques." Such techniques allegedly include avoiding the use of the terms "sleep" or "hypnosis," or by using the "chaperone" technique, whereby the subject undergoes hypnosis "by watching a confederate ostensibly being hypnotized" (p. 7).

Given this potential for abuse, cases in which hypnosis has allegedly been used for criminal purposes are remarkably rare (Barber, 1969; Udolf, 1983). In the few cases that have arisen in which defendants have claimed they were unwittingly "hypnotized" into committing a crime and were therefore not responsible for their actions, the courts have generally treated such claims with skepticism (Udolf, 1983). Some victims, usually of seduction, have claimed they were victimized through hypnosis; though once again courts have tended to doubt the role of "hypnosis" in such cases (Udolf, 1983). Hypnosis has even been employed as an argument for both prosecution and defense simultaneously. In a case reported by Perry (1979) a lay hypnotist freely admitted that he had "hypnotized" two female subjects for sexual purposes. His defense was that since it is impossible to coerce people under hypnosis into committing acts that they believe to be immoral, the women must have been willing. The women claimed they did not want to have sex but could not resist because of the hypnosis. The man was first convicted but found innocent on appeal.

While the dangers of "hypnotizing" people into doing acts against their wills seem, in general, to have been treated with skepticism by the courts, nevertheless, in Canadian law, hypnotic suggestion, along with other external influences such as drugs and alcohol is allowed as a basis for the defense of "automatism" (Udolf, 1983). In one case the Supreme Court of Canada held that a confession should be excluded as involuntary because the defendant "had been induced into a state of hypnosis during an interview with a skilled police interrogator, whose voice had a hypnotic quality" (Haward and Ashworth, 1980, p. 477). Similarly, the American Law Institute's Model Penal Code (ALIMPC) requires that an act must be voluntary or an omission in order to render the perpetrator criminally liable and states that conduct during hypnosis or resulting from hypnotic suggestion is *not* voluntary within the meaning of the proposed statute (Udolf, 1983).

HYPNOSIS AS AN INVESTIGATIVE PROCEDURE

As has been mentioned, hypnosis has most often been advocated as a memory enhancement procedure. This has given rise to a debate with regard to the problems that may arise from "hypnotizing" witnesses who may subsequently be asked to give evidence in court. According to the state approach to hypnosis, problems arise because the hypnotic state renders the "hypnotized" individual particularly susceptible to cognitive distortion. The reasons for this are apparent in Hilgard's (1986) description of the defining features of the "hypnotic state": (1) increased suggestibility, (2) enhanced imagery and imagination, (3) the subsidence of the planning function, and (4) the reduction in reality testing. The fourth feature seems particularly pertinent to the present discussion. Hilgard argues that in the hypnotic state, the subject becomes susceptible to reality distortions including "falsified memories," and the "absence of heads or feet of people observed to be walking around the room." Hilgard remarks that "these and many other distortions of reality that would normally be readily detected and corrected can be accepted without criticism in the hypnotic state" (p. 165). This means, in the forensic context, that "hypnotized" witnesses may be particularly susceptible to confabulations (the filling in of memory gaps with spurious detail), hallucinations, suggestive questioning, and nonverbal cueing. They may be more confident in evaluating the veridicality of memory and actually believe that their falsified memories are true (Udolf, 1983; Orne et al., 1984). The problem emerges, therefore, that even if no attempt is made deliberately to distort or shape the testimony of a witness, or extract a confession from a suspect (confessions produced by hypnosis are "involuntary" according to Udolf, 1983), the very production of a hypnotic state may lead to memory distortion and an irretrievably contaminated witness. According to Diamond (1980), the problem of contamination is so great that a hypnotized witness "has been rendered incompetent to testify" (p. 349).

There has also been some controversy over who should and who should not be allowed to conduct hypnotic interviews and whether suspects should be "hypnotized." For example, Orne et al. (1984) argue that hypnotic interviews can be entrusted only to qualified psychologists and clinicians with experience of hypnosis. The researchers also argue that because individuals can successfully simulate hypnosis, and "hypnotized" individuals are capable of willfully lying, "There is no justification for the authorities to hypnotize suspects in a case" (p. 209). However, Hibbard and Worring (1981) claim that hypnotic interviews can be safely conducted by trained police officers, and that hypnosis can be used successfully on defendants as "an operator can easily reliably test for both simulation and lying given he knows the proper techniques" (p. 282). Haward and Ashworth (1980) also argue that hypnosis can be used to good effect on suspects, and remark that "statements under hypnosis are likely to be closer to objective truth than ordinary statements made in the waking state" (p. 478).

The state position would thus lead us to accept that hypnosis has both unique advantages and disadvantages in the forensic arena. The main alleged advantage is its ability to enhance memory; its main disadvantages are that victims and witnesses may be encouraged to do or say things unknowingly or against their wills, and that memory distortions are more likely in the hypnotic state. According to Perry and Lawrence (1983), different emphases on the advantages and disadvantages have led to three main positions on the use of hypnosis for investigative forensic work. In France hypnotically elicited testimony is banned by the courts. This extreme position has been advocated in the United States by Diamond (1980) and in Britain by Morton (1984). Others have concluded that hypnosis does have some value as an investigative procedure, but it should only be used with strict guidelines. Thus, for example, it should be induced only by professionally trained personnel such as physicians, psychiatrists, and psychologists who have previous training in hypnosis. Furthermore, all interviews should be videotaped, and hypnosis should not be used on witnesses who are subsequently to appear in court (Orne, 1979; Orne et al., 1984). Others propose that hypnosis is essentially safe and an effective way of recovering material for use in court (Reiser, 1980; Hibbard and Worring, 1981; Haward and Ashworth, 1980). Most learned societies based in the United States have tended to support the second position, i.e., hypnosis may have some use as an investigative tool, but it must be applied only with strict safeguards (see reports of the Society for Clinical and Experimental Hypnosis, 1979; the International Society of Hypnosis, 1979; and the American Medical Association, 1986). In Britain the British Society of Experimental and Clinical Hypnosis has adopted a cautious view on the use of hypnosis (see BSECH report, 1983), and the British Home Office has recently issued some guidelines to police that recommend procedures similar to those laid down by the AMA (Serly, 1987).

A wide range of opinion is also evident in Supreme Court decisions in the United States. Thus, New Jersey, North Carolina, Wyoming, and Wisconsin have admitted hypnotically elicited testimony (in Wisconsin, regardless of whether safeguards have been adhered to), whereas California, Florida, Georgia, Indiana, Nebraska, Pennsylvania, Virginia, Maryland, Arizona, and Michigan have excluded previously hypnotized witnesses from appearing in court (Perry and Laurence, 1983; Anderton, 1986; Serly, 1987). In a recent test case in England, at Maidstone, the judge ruled that the testimony of four witnesses who had been previously "hypnotized" was not admissible in court (Serly, 1987).

HYPNOSIS, THE LAW AND THE EXPERTS

Legal case reports indicate that courts are becoming increasingly reliant on the testimony of "experts" on hypnosis before deciding whether to proceed with or how to judge a particular case. One of the possible reasons for this is that hypnosis has been shrouded in the mystique that attaches to the concept of a hypnotic state. This places hypnosis outside the range of normal experience and understanding. However, confusion has been created because supporters of the state approach have been vocal in proclaiming both the advantages and disadvantages of forensic hypnosis, often taking up somewhat different positions (see, for example, Haward and Ashworth 1980; Reiser, 1980; Waxman, 1983; Orne et al., 1984; Perry and Nogrady, 1985). Often the terms used to explain the alleged positive and negative effects seem to perpetuate the mystique of the hypnotic process. Hibbard and Worring (1981), for example, argue that the enhancement of memory under hypnosis comes about through a "dissociative mechanism" that allows direct access to the subconscious. They say, "Hypnosis is a controlled dissociated state in which the conscious, critical, intellectual and logical portion of one's mind is dissociated, inhibited, misdirected, or distracted, allowing for direct access to one's subconscious" (p. 32). Emphasizing the dangers, Kline (1983) argues that confabulation and distortion occur through a "regression in ego functioning." The mystique is perhaps also perpetuated by the tendency of those who have more skeptical attitudes about the memory enhancement properties of hypnosis to propose, nevertheless, that it should only be carried out by trained psychiatrists and psychologists with experience in hypnosis (see the 1986 AMA report).

However, in the remainder of this chapter it will be argued that there is an alternative way of viewing hypnosis that may help considerably in bringing legal cases that have involved hypnosis within the area of expertise of the layperson, and out of the sole domain of psychiatric and psychological experts on the characteristics of the "hypnotic state."

THE STATE-NONSTATE DEBATE

One of the most significant aspects of the debate of issues relating to hypnosis in the legal context has been a tendency to avoid a fundamental theoretical issue on which interpretations of different findings are based. The issue that still appears to dominate contemporary theorizing in hypnosis is the "state-nonstate" debate, which more recently has been presented as a distinction between special process and social psychological approaches to hypnosis (Spanos, 1986b).

One of the important characteristics of nonstate approaches to hypnosis, as typified in works by Barber (1969), Barber, Spanos & Chaves (1974), Sarbin and Coe, (1972), Spanos (1982, 1986b) and Wagstaff (1981a), is that hypnotic phenomena are interpreted in terms of "normal" psychological processes, such as attitudes, expectancies, conformity, imagination, and relaxation. In particular, they lay strong emphasis on the hypnotic situation as a *social interaction*. As Barber et al. say: "The area subsumed under the term "hypnotism" is a social psychological phenomenon *par excellence* in that one individual exerts a potent influence on the behavior and experience of another individual" (1974, p. 144). According to the cognitive-behavioral approach of Barber and his associates, subjects carry out so-called "hypnotic" behaviors when they have positive attitudes, motivations, and expectations toward the test situation that lead to a willingness to think and imagine with the themes suggested (Barber et al., 1974). More recently, Spanos (1986b) has defined hypnotic behavior similarly as a "purposeful, goal-directed action that can be understood in terms of how the subjects interpret their situation and how they attempt to present themselves through their actions" (p. 449). Wagstaff (1986) has construed hypnotic behavior as resulting from a "willingness and/or response to pressure, to play the role of a "hypnotized" person. The role is determined by personal preconceptions and the social context, as defined by the hypnotist and the hypnotic situation" (p. 69). Thus while the state view of hypnosis construes "genuine" hypnotic phenomena to be involuntary rather than deliberate, the nonstate cognitive-behavioral/social psychological view takes the position that while good hypnotic subjects may act *as if* they have lost control of their actions, the actions are, nevertheless, voluntary. Spanos (1986b), for example, argues that "responsive hypnotic subjects behave as if their responses were involuntary because their preconceptions about hypnosis and the persuasive communications they receive in the hypnotic test situation define acting that way as central to the role of being hypnotized" (p. 449). It should be noted that "voluntary" in this context refers to the opposite of "automatic," rather than the opposite of "coerced" (as through external pressure). The legal distinction will be elucidated shortly. One implication of these nonstate views is that any hypnotic situation can be reevaluated in a way that is meaningful in terms of everyday language and understanding. The hypnotic situation is one in which subjects are invited, or even pressured in some cases, to enact the role of a "hypnotized" person as defined by their own expectations and the instructions and cues given by the hypnotist and the situation. The subject may refuse to do this or engage in various activities designed to convince the hypnotist, and often him- or herself, that he or she is experiencing the suggested effects. If subjects' experiences coincide with expectations, they may actually *believe* they are "hypnotized" (Sarbin and Coe, 1972; Wagstaff, 1981a, 1986). Barber et al. (1974) have suggested that the example of a shaman may serve as a useful analogy. A shaman may behave in unusual ways, frothing at the mouth and talking in a strange voice. The shaman's explanation of his behavior may be that he is possessed by a spirit, yet few anthropologists would agree with this as an explanation. Nevertheless, few would argue that he is faking. The most parsimonious interpretation would be that he behaves in this manner because he *believes* he is possessed by a spirit, i.e., he enacts the role of someone possessed by a spirit. According to Barber et al. (1974) it is no more meaningful to explain the shaman's behavior in terms of spirit possession than it is to explain the hypnotic subject's behavior in terms of a trance or state.

At first the distinction between *being* "hypnotized" (i.e., in a hypnotic state) and *believing* one is "hypnotized" may seem pedantic. However, let us consider some possible implications of such an analysis for the defense of "automatism" in a forensic situation.

ROLE-ENACTMENT AND HYPNOTIC AUTOMATISM

Suppose a man appears in court on a charge of murder. The defendant claims he did not act voluntarily but was taken over by the devil. Who would be called as an expert witness, a clergyman or a psychiatrist? In most courts in the Western world there would be little doubt that a man who confessed to a murder with the sole defense that he was "possessed by the devil" would be judged either culpable or insane. Most jurors and jurists would be unlikely to pay much attention to experts purporting to describe the "characteristics and powers of the devil" or to claim the defendant's testimony was "contaminated by the devil." If the behavior of a man who claims he has been "hypnotized" into committing murder is interpreted in an equivalent way, then the evidence necessary for the court to make a decision might be rather different from that implied by a "state" view of hypnosis. If it is established that the man murdered under the delusion that he was "hypnotized" and with no other motive, then that might be sufficient to pronounce him deluded and insane. If he was coerced by another who pressured him to murder and required him to enact the role of a hypnotized person as he did it, then the jury could decide how to weigh this coercive factor in coming to a decision. If he would probably have murdered the person anyway, regardless of whether he was enacting the hypnotic role, then presumably he would be found culpable. In such a case, the court might deem it useful to call a psychiatrist to adjudge the man's sanity, but it would be of little value calling experts on the "powers of the hypnotic state." It would be as irrelevant to ask whether the man was "hypnotized" with or without his knowledge as it would be to ask whether a person can "willingly" agree to be possessed by the devil.

If the nonstate position is valid, then it is perhaps fortunate that the courts have tended to be skeptical about claims that crimes have been committed due to the influence of "hypnosis." However, strong doubt should perhaps be cast on the grouping in Canadian law of hypnotic suggestion along with other external influences such as drugs and alcohol as a basis for the defense of automatism, or the proposal in the ALIMPC that conduct during hypnosis or resulting from hypnotic suggestion is *not* voluntary.

This is not to say, however, that the only circumstances under which a plea of involuntary conduct because of hypnosis would be allowed from a nonstate perspective would be on grounds of insanity. Hypnotic situations from a nonstate view are social situations like any others and are susceptible to the same coercive influences such as threats, loss of face or status, fear of embarrassment, and so on (Wagstaff, 1981a). In English law a distinction is made between the defense of *compulsion*, an act performed involuntarily as the result of another's actions, and *automatism*, which is an act performed involuntarily as the result of a spasm or convulsion, or by a person not conscious of what he or she is doing, as when concussed or sleepwalking or insane (Curzon, 1980). The defense of compulsion covers duress by threats, necessity (to avert a greater evil), obedience to orders, and marital coercion. Thus, unless some extra pathological condition is evident, the most viable defense on grounds of involuntariness for a person who commits a criminal act while enacting the role of a "hypnotized" person would be on grounds of *compulsion*, that is, through duress or obedience to orders as might occur in other social situations. However, importantly, from this perspective laypersons would presumably be held no less fit to judge whether a "hypnotized" person acted involuntarily out of "compulsion" than they would be able to judge, for instance, whether a patient acting under the orders of a doctor; or a soldier acting under the orders of an officer; or a suspect bullied, tricked, or brow-beaten by a police interrogator acted "involuntarily."

Nevertheless, in order to maintain that a cognitive-behavioral/social psychological approach is a more useful and parsimonious way of approaching forensic aspects of hypnosis, it is necessary to examine the credibility of claims that might appear to favor a state interpretation of relevant phenomena.

HYPNOSIS AND ANTISOCIAL ACTS

The debate whether "hypnotized" individuals can be induced to commit immoral or criminal acts of which they would be incapable in a waking "state" is an old one (Barber, 1969). Actual criminal case histories provide no definitive answer as such cases are comparatively rare, and the role that hypnosis played in such cases seems mainly confined to providing a rationale for justifying behavior (Barber, 1969; Wolberg, 1972; Udolf, 1983). However, some experimental studies seem to confirm that "hypnotized" persons can be made to perform acts that are immoral or harmful, either to themselves or others. The acts include indecent exposure (Kline, 1958), picking up a dangerous snake and throwing acid at people (Rowland, 1939; Young, 1952), minor thefts, verbal attacks on people and verbalizing secrets (Brenman, 1942), and calling people obscene names (Parrish, 1974). However, a number of reviewers of these studies have concluded that the concept of a hypnotic state is not necessary to explain the results (Barber, 1961, 1965; Coe, Kobayashi & Howard, 1972a, 1972b; Orne, 1962; 1965; Udolf, 1981). Instead, they can be explained primarily in terms of subjects being willing to carry out the actions because they (a) wanted to help the hypnotist/experimenter, (b) thought their actions would really be safe, and/or (c) assumed the experimenter would take responsibility for the consequences of the acts he instructed them to perform. For example, in one experiment (Young, 1952) "deeply hypnotized" subjects were asked to throw acid at an experimenter and also to pick up a dangerous snake (both the experimenter and the snake were behind an "invisible" plate of glass). The majority of subjects attempted to throw acid at the experimenter and reached for the snake when "hypnotized" but refused to perform these actions when not "hypnotized." However, Orne and Evans (1965) found that both hypnotic subjects *and* nonhypnotic subjects simulating hypnosis carried out the same tasks when given emphatic suggestions to do so. Postexperimental interviews revealed that all subjects admitted that they were convinced that no one would really be harmed because the context was an experimental one. Of importance in this study was the finding that whereas five out of six subjects carried out the acts when "hypnotized," only two of the same subjects carried out the acts when "unhypnotized." However, *all* six "unhypnotized" simulators carried out the tasks. These results are strongly supportive of the social psychological view that subjects in hypnosis experiments modify their behaviors to comply with experimental demands (Wagstaff, 1981a; Spanos, 1986b).

In another experiment Coe, Kobayashi, and Howard (1973) found that hypnotic procedures made no difference to whether subjects could be induced to sell heroin. In fact there was a trend for those *without* "hypnosis" to be more likely to commit the act. Coe et al. found that the subject's moral stance on the issue was more important than either hypnotic induction or whether subjects believed the requests for antisocial conduct were part of an experiment. Similarly, Levitt et al. (1975) found that hypnotic procedures made no difference to whether subjects would cut up the American flag or mutilate the Bible; overall only 3 subjects out of 23 refused to cut the flag, and 4 out of 13 refused to mutilate the Bible. While some have argued that most subjects are only likely to commit such acts if the situation is perceived as "safe" (Orne and Holland, 1968; Mixon, 1974), other research indicates that a large proportion of subjects will also commit harmful acts even if the situation is not actually safe or innocuous. For example, Calverley and Barber (1965) found that almost all of a group of nursing students would sign derogatory-slanderous statements about a nursing superintendent if emphatically directed to do so. However, while some nurses subsequently stated they believed no harm would come from signing the statement, others said that they really believed that the statements would be harmful. Almost all of those in the latter category nevertheless signed the statements when the directions were sufficiently emphatic. Most significantly, like other experimenters, Calverley and Barber found that hypnotic induction made no difference to whether or not the subjects carried out the acts.

To summarize, there is no definitive evidence, either anecdotal or experimental, that indicates a necessity to postulate any special hypnotic process or hypnotic state to explain claims that people have committed antisocial acts while "hypnotized." As Wagstaff (1981a) has pointed out, while the concept of the hypnotic automaton is a useful "cover-up" for denying responsibility for actions, it is conceivable that a person might commit a crime and honestly believe that a special state of "hypnosis" was responsible. However, such self-persuasion would usually be confined to someone suffering with delusions, who, if unable to use "hypnosis" to justify criminal actions, would probably choose something else.

HYPNOSIS, TRUTH TELLING, CONFESSION, AND SIMULATION

Contrary to the claims of writers such as Haward and Ashworth (1980), it is the opinion of most contemporary reviewers (see, for example, Udolf, 1983; Orne et al. 1984; AMA report, 1986; Anderton, 1986) that there is no conclusive evidence, either anecdotal or experimental, to indicate that hypnosis can act as a "truth serum." On the contrary, according to Wagstaff (1981a; 1986) there are elements in the hypnotic situation that may pressure subjects to actually falsify accounts, and Anderton (1986) argues that the possibility of hypnotic subjects lying is particularly high in a forensic setting. Even one of the most ardent proponents of the forensic use of hypnosis, Reiser, has argued that "If a subject is motivated to lie, it would be as easy to do under hypnosis as it would be for that person in a nonhypnotic state" (1980, p. xvii). While this position may seem somewhat paradoxical for state theorists wishing to propose that hypnotic behavior is, at least partly, involuntary or automatic, the conclusion that a person, if so motivated, can and will lie in hypnotic situations accords well with a nonstate perspective.

There are a few anecdotal cases in which suspects in criminal cases have confessed during a hypnosis session but subsequently denied their confessions (Udolf, 1983). However, in these cases it is not necessary to postulate a hypnotic state to explain the confessions. For example, in one case an appeals court ruled against the claim that a confession made by a particular suspect was involuntary simply because hypnosis had been used; however, they ruled that the confession was still involuntary because the hypnotist had used deception, physical pressure, persistent and unceasing questions, and false offers of friendship and help—all of which added up to the equivalent of mental coercion (Udolf, 1983). This case illustrates well the fact that hypnotic situations, like other situations, can be judged sufficiently coercive to extract "involuntary" confessions; however, the grounds do not have to be those of "automatism." Kline (1983) has also pointed to a number of factors that might account for a confession, none of which would require the induction of a hypnotic state. For example, he argues that the suspect's perception of an interrogating officer as a friendly figure may create extreme pressure to confess, and because of "compelling psychodynamic needs" (presumably these include guilt), the suspect may "try with pathetic eagerness to confess to those details which he senses the police were seeking" (pp. 136–37).

While there seems to be some disagreement among state theorists whether the simulation of hypnosis can be detected (see Hibbard and Worring, 1981; Orne et al., 1984), from a nonstate perspective the question itself begs a question and is too simplistic. From the view of a state theorist, an individual who role-acts hypnosis, and even believes he or she is "hypnotized," but does not fall into the prerequisite dissociated, altered state of consciousness, could be considered to be "simulating." However, a person who deliberately claims to be "hypnotized" when not is also simulating. The assumption that "genuine" hypnosis involves the achievement of a dissociated altered state of consciousness thus leads to the odd conclusion that it is possible to "simulate hypnosis" without actually exercising any form of deliberate deceit. This problem does not occur for nonstate theorists who have tended to use "simulation" purely in an operational sense, to denote an experimental instruction. Thus a "simulator" is someone who has been instructed to imitate the role behavior of a "hypnotized" person as it is construed by him or her. Wagstaff (1981a, 1986) has argued that the distinction between acts with and without private acceptance or belief is the most appropriate one for dealing with deliberate deceit from a nonstate perspective.

Nevertheless, contrary to the claims of writers such as Hibbard and Worring (1981), there appears to be no way of detecting "the simulation of hypnosis" even if a hypnotic state is accepted. Hibbard and Worring (1981) claim that the double-hallucination test of trance logic is the most reliable indicator of the "simulation of hypnosis." It is claimed that when asked to hallucinate a person actually before them in another place, "hypnotized" subjects see both the hallucinated person *and* the actual person, whereas "unhypnotized" simulators claim to see only *one* recognizable person. However, this claim seems based solely on invalid anecdotal evidence, as a number of experimental studies have failed to find significant differences on the double-hallucination response between "real" hypnotic subjects and subjects required to simulate hypnosis (Spanos, 1986b). Moreover, there appears to be no other response that can reliably distinguish between subjects in hypnotic and nonhypnotic conditions (Wagstaff, 1981a, 1986; Spanos, 1982, 1986b).

The difference in emphasis between state and social psychological views of hypnotic phenomena can be illustrated by an analysis of the notorious "Hillside Strangler Case." In 1979, Kenneth Bianchi was arrested and charged for the rapes and murders of a number of women. Bianchi said he was innocent, but during a pretrial examination in which a hypnotic interview was used, a "hidden" personality who claimed to have committed the murders emerged. According to Hilgard's (1986) neo-dissociation theory, it is perfectly feasible that preexisting multiple personalities should emerge in the hypnotic state, as hypnotic procedures allegedly facilitate the process of dissociation and allow contact with "hidden" subsystems normally dissociated from consciousness. The defense maintained that Bianchi had been suffering from multiple-personality syndrome at the time he committed the murders. However, the prosecution maintained that Bianchi's multiple-personality syndrome was a role enactment conveyed using background information available in our culture and cued by information given during the hypnotic interview. This latter interpretation coincides with a social-psychological, role-enactment view of multiple personality (Sarbin and Coe, 1979; Spanos, Weekes & Bertrand, 1985). Support for the social psychological interpretation of this case comes from a study by Spanos, Weekes, et al. (1985) that showed that most subjects who were instructed to role play a defendant undergoing hypnosis displayed the main signs of multiple personality even though they were given no previous information about multiple personality or specific symptoms. According to Spanos, Weekes, et al. (1985), it is unlikely that anyone in Bianchi's situation would really believe in his or her role enactments; however, in some clinical situations it is possible that some patients may come to believe they have multiple personalities. According to a nonstate social psychological perspective, the credibility of hypnotically elicited multiple personalities as a defense cannot rest on objective tests of whether the defendant is "simulating hypnosis" or whether he or she *has* multiple personalities. No such tests exist, and any claim that they do is likely to mislead the courts. Instead, the important issues concern whether the court decides the defendant *believes* he or she has multiple personalities, and the implications of this for a defense of insanity on the grounds of a defect of reason or insane delusion. (One is perhaps tempted to ask how a man who deliberately committed brutal rapes and murders could be considered "sane" regardless of whether he "faked" multiple personalities or not; however, the law in Western countries seems prepared to make this kind of distinction.)

HYPNOSIS AND MEMORY ENHANCEMENT

Of the issues in the area of forensic hypnosis, the pros and cons of using hypnotic procedures as a memory enhancement procedure remain the primary source of debate. Advocates of the use of hypnosis for this purpose (for example, Kleinhauz, Horowitz & Tobin, 1977; Haward and Ashworth, 1980; Reiser, 1980; Hibbard and Worring, 1981) have tended to base their arguments on three sources of evidence: anecdotal case-histories, results of general experiments on hypnotic hyperamnesia and age regression, and experimental analogues of the forensic context. However, although some experimental studies of hypnotic hyperamnesia appear to show that hypnotic procedures have a special capacity to improve memory, reviewers such as Barber (1965), Wagstaff (1981b, 1982b, 1984) and Orne et al. (1984) have drawn attention to some major methodological shortcomings in these studies. These include:

1. The use of within-subjects that allow for subjects to "hold-back" in the waking control condition in response to the demand characteristics of the situation.

2. The failure to counterbalance designs to allow for order effects.

3. The failure to equate hypnotic and waking control groups in terms of motivating suggestions.

4. The failure to use adequate controls for experimenter and subject bias effects.

5. The failure to measure the proportion of errors (i.e., false alarms) to correct responses.

If these criteria are applied, then a number of older studies are methodologically unsatisfactory: for example, Stalnaker and Riddle (1932), Illovsky (1963), Eisele and Higgins (1963), Sears (1955, 1956), Krippner (1963), McCord (1956), Lodato (1964), Rosenthal (1944), McCord and Sherrill (1961), Hammer (1954), Rosenhan and London (1963), White, Fox, and Harris (1940). Some more recent studies are also subject to methodological criticism. Dhanens and Lundy (1975) claimed to have demonstrated superior recall with hypnotic procedures, but this study has been criticized by Smith (1983) for anomalies in the data, and Orne (1979) points out that if the appropriate comparison is made the study does not indicate a greater increase in recall with hypnosis. De Piano and Salzberg (1981) purported to find evidence for hypnotic hyperamnesia. However, no attempt was made to measure error rates or accuracy in this study.

In contrast, a number of better-controlled studies have failed to find any superiority for hypnotic over nonhypnotic memory facilitation procedures, regardless of whether the material is abstract or meaningful, tested by free recall or by recognition, or emotional or neutral (Parker and Barber, 1964; Cooper and London, 1973; Wagstaff and Ovenden, 1979; Wagstaff and Sykes, 1983). The present state of the literature in this area seems well summarized by Smith (1983): "In the presence of the appropriate controls . . . the absence of any hypnotic memory enhancement becomes clear" (p. 393).

Studies of hypnotic age regression have been deemed relevant by some proponents of hypnosis for memory enhancement, because regression techniques are sometimes advocated as a way of facilitating the memories of witnesses (Hibbard and Worring, 1981). Some early studies purported to demonstrate that hypnotic subjects can give more convincing and accurate performances of age regression (for example, Reiff and Sheerer, 1959; True, 1949; Gidro-Frank and Bowersbuch, 1949). However, these studies have been extensively criticized (Barber, 1962, 1969; Yates, 1961; O'Connell, Shor & Orne, 1970). More recently, claims have been made that hypnotic age-regression procedures can facilitate the production of developmental trends in visual illusions and reinstate child-like eidetic imagery and other behaviors of young children (Parrish, Lundy & Leibowitz, 1969; Walker, Garratt & Wallace, 1976; Fellows and Creamer, 1978; Nash, Johnson & Tipton, 1979; Riakov, 1982). However, these studies either have not been replicated by other researchers, or have been subject to methodological criticism or reinterpretation (Wagstaff, 1984).

As a defense against the negative view, it could be argued that these studies are too artificial to yield results comparable to those found in forensic investigations. If this were the case, then presumably the more analogous studies become to real-life forensic investigations, the more likely a superiority for hypnotic procedure will be demonstrated. However, the contrary appears to be the case. When the *accuracy* of recall (both errors as well as correct answers) is determined, the vast majority of studies that have attempted to reproduce more lifelike situations indicate that hypnotic procedures do *not* have any special capacity to enhance memory to a level above that achievable by nonhypnotic procedures. The absence of any superiority for hypnotic procedures is evident regardless of the nature of the stimulus materials (objects, people, faces, words), the way they are presented (incidently, intentionally, on slides, films, or "real-life" staged events), or the method of recall (forced choice recognition or free recall, immediate or delayed) (Buckhout et al., 1981; Baker, Haynes and Patrick, 1983; Dywan and Bowers, 1983; Gregg and Mingay, 1987; Mingay, 1985; Sanders and Simmons, 1983; Sheehan, Grigg and McCann, 1984; Sheehan and Tilden, 1983, 1986; Putnam, 1979; Nogrady, McConkey & Perry, 1985; Geiselman, Fisher & Holland, 1985; Timm, 1981; Wagstaff, 1982a; Wagstaff, Traverse & Milner, 1982; Wagstaff and Maguire, 1982; Yuille and McEwan, 1985; Zelig and Beidleman, 1981). The main apparent exception to this overwhelming evidence is a study by Griffin (1980) who reported superior recall for hypnotic procedures. However, this study was methodologically confounded, the hypnotic groups received more testing, the statistical analysis is incorrectly interpreted, and recall errors were not determined.

While conceding that hypnotic procedures have no special capacity to enhance accurate memory, some have argued that, nevertheless, hypnosis may have special advantages in applied contexts where a guilt-stricken witness may feel reluctant to disclose details, (Perry and Nogrady, 1985). However, as Wagstaff (1984) has pointed out, there are a number of techniques that hypnotists have employed in forensic investigations that could conceivably produce better results than *routine* police interrogation, but none of which requires the introduction of a hypnotic induction procedure. These include systematic relaxation to reduce anxiety and trauma; sympathetic unauthoritarian interrogators who establish rapport; reminscence and repeated testing; ingenuity in providing associative cues such as guided memory procedures; role playing and picture drawing; and, if appropriate, the adoption of a more lax criterion for report. There is no evidence to suggest that hypnotic procedures would be any more effective than a sympathetic counsellor or clinician in extracting details from a guilt-stricken witness, though *both* might be better than a routine police interview.

Although the vast majority of studies show that hypnotic procedures do not facilitate accurate memory, there are some inconsistencies with regard to other variables. For example, Geiselman et al. (1985) report that although a hypnosis group did no better than a group given a "cognitive interview" designed to facilitate memory, *both* groups did better than a group given a standard interview. However, other studies have failed to find a significant memory improvement for subjects given either hypnotic or nonhypnotic memory facilitation instructions over untreated control subjects (Wagstaff, Traverse, & Milner, 1982; Wagstaff and Maguire, 1982; Nogrady, McConkey & Perry, 1985; Timm, 1981). However, probably the most controversial issue concerns the extent to which hypnotic procedures produce errors in memory. Putnam (1979), Sanders and Simons (1983), and Zelig and Beidleman (1981) found that hypnotic subjects made more errors on leading questions than nonhypnotic control subjects; however, Sheehan and Tilden (1983) and Yuille and McEwan (1985) did not find that hypnotic subjects were more susceptible to misleading information. A number of writers (Orne, 1979; Laurence and Perry, 1983) have argued that one way hypnotic procedures may appear to enhance memory is by encouraging the subject to increase the amount of information generated, both correct and incorrect (i.e., the subject adopts a more lax criterion for report). An early study by Stalnaker and Riddle (1932) is frequently cited as supporting this view, but more recent support has come from an experiment by Dywan and Bowers (1983). They found that hypnotic subjects reported over twice as many items as, but three times the errors of, nonhypnotic control subjects. However, Wagstaff and Sykes (1983), Sheehan and Tilden (1983), and Sanders and Simmons (1983) did not find that hypnotic subjects generated more information. One of the more consistent findings concerns the certainty that hypnotic subjects express in their responses. A number of studies have shown that hypnotic procedures either make subjects more confident in their answers when they are only as accurate as controls, or they are as confident as controls when they are actually *less* accurate. In both cases the implication is the same: hypnotic subjects tend to express greater confidence in inaccurate responses or produce more false positive responses (Buckhout et al., 1981; Nogrady et al., 1982; Putnam, 1979; Sanders and Simons, 1983; Sheehan and Tilden, 1983; Wagstaff, 1982a; Wagstaff et al., 1982). Nevertheless, Timm (1985) found this effect only when subjects of high-hypnotic susceptibility in a hypnotic condition were compared with subjects of low susceptibility in a nonhypnotic condition, and Gregg and Mingay (1987) found no evidence that hypnotic procedures increased false positive responding.

The variability in these results would suggest it is different expectations generated by different experimental situations that account for the reporting errors shown by hypnotic subjects, rather than some feature of a "hypnotic state." In line with this interpretation, Sheehan and Tilden (1984) suggest that the confident reporting of inaccurate information may be associated with the "social psychological pressures generally existing in the situation that then motivate subjects to report with certainty that something is true when it is not" (p. 203). If this is the case, then it might be predicted that if subjects were not given instructions that conveyed either implicitly or explicitly that they should remember better, then errors would be less likely. Some indirect support for this view comes from the study by Gregg and Mingay (1987). In this experiment subjects were given either a hypnotic induction or a relaxation procedure, but very limited suggestions for memory enhancement were given. As mentioned previously, they found no differences between the hypnotic and nonhypnotic groups for the number of accurate items recalled or the number of false positive errors.

In spite of inconsistencies there seems to be sufficient evidence to warrant the conclusion that when memory facilitation procedures are placed within the context of "hypnosis," more false or inaccurate reports are evoked (Wagstaff, 1985). This in itself is not surprising from either a state or nonstate perspective. Simply labeling a situation as "hypnosis" is in itself sufficient to increase responsiveness to test suggestions due to additional task demands (Barber, 1969). It should perhaps be emphasized that the issue here concerns what happens if hypnotic induction is *added* to an existing procedure. It would obviously not be difficult to devise a procedure in which nonhypnotic subjects would produce more errors than hypnotic subjects. Simply give the nonhypnotic subjects a reward for every detail produced, either correct or incrorrect, and punish the hypnotic subjects for every error. However, what seems more at issue is how any additional errors produced by hypnotic subjects are to be interpreted. In particular, do hypnotic subjects *really* believe that they saw or heard the extra inaccurate details that they report? It is commonly accepted by state theorists that the uncritical acceptance of distortions of reality is a defining feature of the hypnotic state (Hilgard, 1986); therefore, in all likelihood the distortions of memory that are manifested by hypnotic subjects are irreversible. Thus Orne et al.

(1984) remark, "the problem is not merely the inaccuracy of the confabulations (i.e., the 'filling in' of gaps with spurious detail), but the fact that these are likely to be accepted as accurate by the hypnotized individual" (pp. 186–87). The classic demonstration that has been alleged to show the irreversibility of hypnotically distorted memory concerns the hypnotic creation of pseudomemories (Laurence and Perry, 1983). Using a procedure described by Orne (1979), 27 subjects were age regressed and instructed to "relive" a night they had previously described. They were then asked whether they had heard loud noises that awakened them. Since none had actually described a loud noise, this question acted as a subtle suggestion that loud noises had actually been heard. After the termination of the hypnotic session, 13 subjects not only claimed that they had actually heard the noises on the night in question but also continued to maintain this even when told that the noises had only been suggested to them. While some have assumed that this demonstrates the capacity of hypnosis to distort memory permanently, it should be noted that no control group was used to test whether the responses were simply the result of compliance (Wagstaff, 1981a), i.e., subjects *say* they heard the noises to comply with experimental demands, when privately they know they did not. To test this alternative hypothesis, however, Spanos and McLean (1986) repeated the experiment with an additional instruction to subjects that each had a "hidden part" that can always distinguish what was suggested from what really happened. When this "hidden part" was contacted, only 2 of 11 subjects who had reported that they heard the noises continued to maintain that they were not imaginary. Spanos and McLean conclude that so-called pseudomemories of this kind may reflect reporting biases in response to contextual demands rather than actual permanent memory distortions. A further study by McCann and Sheehan (1987) indicated that pseudomemories could be "breached" by giving subjects incontrovertible evidence relating to original events. This result can also be interpreted in terms of Spanos and McLean's analysis (Gregg, 1987). These results cast doubt on the view that hypnotic procedures have some special capacity to produce permanent, irreversible memory distortions.

To summarize, in accordance with a nonstate view, the bulk of the experimental evidence suggests that hypnotic procedures do not facilitate accurate memory to a degree greater than that achievable in motivated nonhypnotic conductions. Because of the contextual demands of situations, hypnotic procedures may lead subjects to offer more false reports, but there is as yet little experimental evidence to support the view that such reports reflect greater *actual* memory distortion than that which might occur in comparable situations where hypnotic procedures have not been employed.

CONCLUSION

In this chapter it has been argued that much is to be gained from approaching forensic aspects of hypnosis from nonstate cognitive-behavioral or social psychological approaches. One important advantage is they can help to bring hypnotic phenomena within the range of understanding of laypersons and, while not eliminating the need for experts in psychology and psychiatry, reduce the reliance on the conflicting accounts by experts of the nature and characteristics of the "hypnotic state." However, what are the implications for practice? Clearly, it would make sense from a nonstate view to remove hypnotic phenomena from the domain of "automatism," however, the issue of whether hypnotic procedures should be banned or witnesses subjected to them disqualified from giving evidence in court is too complex to warrant a simple answer.

It could be argued that if hypnotic phenomena are not "unusual" in any way, why should the use of hypnotic techniques be legally curtailed? However, the problem with this argument as it confuses the nature of the procedure (which may; be innocuous or harmful, usual or unusual) with the nature of the explanation (which may be mundane or extraordinary). The fact that the effects of a procedure may have a mundane explanation does not necessarily make that procedure acceptable. One does not need to posit a special process to explain why a suspect might give a confession after having been subjected to electric shocks; however, such a mechanism would not be allowed as an interrogation device by most Western courts. But, one could still argue that if hypnotic procedures have no special capacity to actually alter memory irretrievably, then the risks attached to using them would appear to be minimal. Moreover, it presumably matters not whether the hypnotist is a consultant psychiatrist, university professor, police cadet, or unqualified stage hypnotist. The worst that can happen is the police will be wasting their time. Unfortunately, the issues are not that simple. Although the evidence is not totally consistent, it does seem to be the case that when hypnotic induction procedures are added to other treatments, subjects are more likely to proffer false information (Wagstaff, 1985). The problem then arises that even if additional false reports given by witnesses following hypnotic procedures are not actually memory distortions, witnesses may, nevertheless, be extremely reluctant to retract them, just as Laurence and Perry's (1983) subjects were reluctant to retract their pseudomemories of noises. This problem is compounded by the fact that it is popularly believed that hypnosis is a reliable memory enhancement procedure (Wagstaff, 1988). Jurors and jurists may thus place a spurious credibility in these inaccurate reports. As for the use of "lay-hypnotists," there is much evidence that people tend to underestimate the situational pressures that exist in social situations (Milgram, 1974; Wagstaff, 1981a). At least a qualified psychologist or psychiatrist is more likely to be aware that an apparently innocuous situation may give rise to inaccurate reports when it is defined by its participants as "hypnosis" or a "memory enhancement" procedure.

From a nonstate perspective, the practical problem is not should the police use a procedure that uniquely enables them to implant pseudomemories and false confidence in witnesses, but should one allow a procedure that encourages or pressures a witness to role play a person with "super-memory," that is (incorrectly) publicly accepted as a reliable memory enhancement procedure?

Though the questions are different, the answers could reasonably be the same. Given that hypnotic procedures do not enhance memory to a level above that achievable in comparable nonhypnotic situations, and given that they can sometimes induce additional false reports (even if reporting biases), there seems little point in using them; one would be better off attempting some other nonhypnotic memory facilitation procedure such as a cognitive interview, guided memory, or relaxation. Even if these nonhypnotic procedures should prove ineffective and also plagued by the production of false reports, why risk making the situation worse by adding to them the additional task demands of hypnotic induction? Furthermore, although it may seem presumptuous to limit the use of "hypnotic procedures" when they vary so much, the courts have a number of practical and legal issues to consider, such as the implications of their decisions for other cases, how the jury is to be instructed, and how experts are to be used. Such issues are particularly complex in the case of "hypnosis" as so many exaggerated and misleading cultural conceptions exist. Given these problems, then even if the case concerning the dangers of hypnotic procedures has been overstated, from a legal point of view, it may still be more expedient to limit their use.

Part Four

Theoretical Overviews and Emerging Paradigms

15

Response Expectancy as a Determinant of Hypnotic Behavior

Irving Kirsch and James R. Council

The idea of a link between expectancy and hypnosis can be traced to the experiments conducted in 1784 by the French Royal Commission appointed to investigate claims made by Mesmer and his followers regarding animal magnetism (Franklin, Majault, LeRoy, Sallin, Bailly, D'Arcet, De Borie, Guillotin & Lavoisier, [1785] 1970; Pattie, 1967). The commissioners demonstrated that the occurrence of a magnetic crisis or other mesmeric phenomenon was determined by a "sensitive" subject's belief or expectation that he or she was being magnetized or in contact with a magnetized object. For example, crises could be elicited by falsely informing subjects that they were being magnetized through a closed door or by having them touch a tree that they were led to believe had been magnetized. Because they were investigating Mesmer's hypothesis of a universal magnetic fluid, the conclusion that mesmeric effects were due to imagination and belief was tantamount to concluding that they were not real. Thus from the first, expectancy was viewed as an unwanted artifact in hypnosis research, an unfortunate status that it retained when the concept of magnetism was replaced with that of trance (cf. Orne, 1959).

In the nineteenth century, there was one hypnosis theorist who saw expectancy as the primary determinant of many hypnotic responses, and who did so without simultaneously dismissing those responses as artifactual. That theorist was Albert Moll (1897). Anticipating the response expectancy hypothesis (Kirsch, 1985a), Moll maintained that two fundamental principles determine hypnotic behavior: "(1) men have a certain proneness to allow themselves to be influenced by others through their ideas, and in particular to believe much without making conscious logical deductions; (2) a psychological effect tends to appear in a man if he is expecting it" (Moss, 1897, p. 241).

Moll recounted a number of anecdotes and experiments demonstrating the role of belief and expectancy in producing perceptual, motoric, and physiological alterations in hypnotic and nonhypnotic contexts and concluded that these phenomena stemmed from the subject's focusing attention on the desired effect and firmly believing the effect would occur. For example, he elicited hallucinations by leading blindfolded subjects to believe they were being mesmerized, replicating the findings of the French Royal Commission of 1784.

An undeservedly neglected figure in the history of hypnosis, Moll anticipated other important points made in this chapter. For example, he noted the effects of watching a responsive subject model hypnotic behavior in enhancing the observer's hypnotic response expectancies. In addition, he stressed the importance of situational perceptions, credibility of procedures, and the utilization by the hypnotist of naturally occurring physical symptoms (e.g., eye fatigue) during induction procedures to heighten expectancy.

As did other nineteenth-century theorists, Moll believed that a special altered state of consciousness was necessary for the occurrence of some hypnotic phenomena. However, unlike other state theorists, Moll afforded equal status to expectancy as an explanatory construct and believed that some genuine hypnotic effects did not require a trance state. His general emphasis was on the continuity, rather than the discontinuity, between hypnotic and nonhypnotic phenomena. Where possible, his inclination was to explain behavior occurring in hypnotic contexts and similar behavior occurring in nonhypnotic contexts as due to a single set of psychological mechanisms. Thus, Moll's theory can be considered a transitional approach between state and nonstate conceptions of hypnosis.

RESPONSE EXPECTANCY AS A UNIFYING CONSTRUCT

Unlike special state theorists, cognitive-behavioral and social psychological theorists view expectancy as an essential part of the process by which hypnotic behavior is generated. Sarbin's (1950) role-theoretical analysis of hypnotic behavior emphasizes the subject's perceptions of the role of hypnotized subject. In addition to role expectations, Barber (1969, 1970, 1972) has stressed the importance of subjects' perceptions of the degree to which the situation is appropriate for the occurrence of hypnotic behavior, the perceived difficulty of particular suggestions, and people's beliefs about their ability to experience hypnotic phenomena. These may be termed, respectively, situational perceptions, perceived task difficulty, and expected hypnotizability.

How do these expectancy-related cognitions affect hypnotic response? Expanding on Moll's (1897) hypothesis, we suggest that response expectancies are the final common path through which hypnotic responses are generated. Response expectancies are subjective probabilities of the occurrence of nonvolitional responses, that is, responses experienced as occurring automatically, without conscious effort. In an extension of cognitive-learning theories, Kirsch (1985a) hypothesized that response expectancies generate corresponding subjective experiences and their behavioral and physiological correlates, a phenomenon that is particularly apparent when changes in response are produced by placebos.

From this perspective, the occurrence of a particular hypnotic response is a function of the subject's expectancy (subjective probability) that it will occur. Various expectancy-related cognitions (e.g., role perceptions, situational perceptions, perceived task difficulty, and expected hypnotizability) affect hypnotic response via their effect on response expectancies. Specifically, people expect to experience particular suggested effects to the extent that they perceive the response as consistent with the role of hypnotic subject, perceive the situation as hypnotic, judge the response to be "easy," and judge themselves to be good subjects.

In the next section of this chapter, we summarize data demonstrating that nonvolitional responses can be generated by expectancy in nonhypnotic contexts. In subsequent sections, we review data bearing on the influence of role perceptions, situational perceptions, perceived difficulty of response, and hypnotic response expectancies on subsequent experiential and behavioral responses to hypnosis. In the final section, we return to a consideration of our hypothesis that response expectancies are *immediate* causes of responses to hypnotic suggestion.

RESPONSE EXPECTANCY IN NONHYPNOTIC CONTEXTS

A considerable body of data demonstrates that nonvolitional responses can be elicited by the expectancy of their occurrence (Kirsch, 1985a). For example, nonhypnotic manipulations designed to alter response expectancies have been found to produce significant changes in phobic anxiety, generalized anxiety and depression, pain perception, sexual arousal, nausea, alertness, tension, relaxation, and drowsiness. In many cases, the genuineness of these response changes has been substantiated by the observation of corresponding changes in physiological function. For example, self-reported changes in subjective experience have been accompanied by corresponding changes in pulse rate, blood pressure, galvanic skin response, gastric function, and penile tumescence. These data demonstrate that response expectancy effects can be genuine rather than artifactual.

Many placebo-generated responses are similar or identical to hypnotic effects. For example, both hypnosis and placebos are effective in treating skin conditions, pain, and asthma (Barber, 1978; Evans, 1985; Wadden & Anderton, 1982). Because these response changes can be produced in nonhypnotic as well as hypnotic situations, uniquely hypnotic mechanisms (e.g., trance) are not needed to explain their occurrence. A more parsimonious explanation is that the same mechanism (i.e., response expectancy) produces these responses in both hypnotic and nonhypnotic situations.[1]

Many hypnotic suggestions ask subjects to temporarily exhibit symptoms of conversion disorders. For example, subjects may be asked to experience partial paralysis or selective loss of sensation. Conversion symptoms appear to go in and out of style and tend to be consistent with patients' perceptions of physiology. In addition, they appear to be responsive to convincing, nonhypnotic expectancy-modification procedures, as indicated by the following report:

We use a form of indirect suggestion psychotherapy to remove the fixated symptoms of hysteria, otherwise unyielding to ordinary methods.

A week before treatment starts, the patient is informed at considerable length that his illness is functional in character, distinguished by conversion phenomena. The patient is assured, however, that he is to be treated in a manner that will be of considerable help. After spending several days in expectation of the "medication" intended to remove the symptoms of his ailment, the patient is conducted to the treatment room and invited to lie down on a couch. He is then informed that the "medicine" will be poured slowly on a special mask and assimilated by his organism by means of breathing in the evaporated drug. He is furthermore assured that the substance brings no unpleasant reactions whatsoever, such as nausea or headache. These remarks help considerably to avoid any possible complications arising in auto-suggestion. The patient is then told, in a manner well adjusted to the level of his education, that he will feel much better, that the symptoms of his disease are a product of cortical inhibition and that the drug, being a powerful stimulating substance, is intended to remove the inhibition. It is explained, for instance, that the patient's hyperkinesia is determined by excitation of brain cells, and that the drug, by calming the nervous system, puts them back into a normal state.

Immediately after this, a registered nurse begins to pour, drop by drop, some aromatic liquid, such as menthol dissolved in alcohol, on the mask already on the patient's face. The whole procedure of treatment takes no more than ten minutes. In the meantime, a discussion is conducted with some other physician concerning the effectiveness of the treatment, with which the latter concurs. They point out that the drug has an excellent effect upon the nervous system and is capable of removing many pathological manifestations. No remarks are addressed directly to the patient; from the very beginning of the treatment he remains a passive listener to the conversation conducted only between the two physicians; the conversation is actually a question of indirect suggestions.

This method of treatment has been used by us for a great variety of symptoms, including hysterical contracture, hyperkinesis, partial paralysis, astasia-abasia [inability to stand or walk without legs wobbling or collapsing, although the patient has normal control while sitting or lying down], mutism, and persistent vomiting. (Schreiber, 1961, pp. 85-86)

The production of perceptual alterations, including imaginings that are reported to occur at quasi-hallucinatory levels of vividness, is a hypnotic phenomenon frequently reported for highly suggestible subjects. In the nonhypnotic context of an experiment in psychophysics, Juhasz and Sarbin (1966) induced gustatory hallucinations via a manipulation designed to produce a strong expectation that plain water would be tasted as salty. Subjects were shown a series of bottles labeled "1" through "10" and received instructions that implied that these bottles went in order from lowest to highest concentration of salt. In reality, all of the bottles contained plain distilled water. Subjects administered samples to themselves, starting with the bottle marked "1" and proceeding in order through the series of bottles. Thirteen out of 14 subjects who had the stimuli visible to them reported tasting salt. The other half of the subjects had their backs turned to the bottles, and seven of these subjects reported tasting salt. Of the 20 subjects from both groups who reported tasting salt, 12 maintained that they would testify at a murder trial to the reality of their perceptions.

Heaton (1975) induced substantial alterations in subjective experience, including reports of hallucinations by about 50 percent of his subjects, by false-ly informing them that they were ingesting a drug that produced psychedelic flashbacks. It is interesting to note that some of the specific characteristics of these expectancy-induced experiences are similar to frequently reported characteristics of hypnotic trance. For example, in addition to experiencing hallucinations, most subjects reported perceptual distortions, numbness or tingling sensations, a dreamlike feeling, and changes in time perception.

The data reviewed above indicate that the kinds of experiences and behaviors that are elicited by hypnotic procedures can also be produced by placebos and other expectancy-modification procedures. It is possible, though not parsimonious, to hypothesize that different mechanisms are operative in different contexts—that these responses are due to expectancy in nonhypnotic contexts but are due to other factors when elicited by means of a hypnotic induction. For that reason, we turn to data about the role of expectancy-related cognitions in hypnotic situations.

ROLE PERCEPTIONS

In the late eighteenth and early nineteenth centuries, when hypnosis was called mesmerism and was believed to be due to the action of a universal magnetic fluid, the defining symptom of the "magnetized" subject was the *crisis,* a violent convulsive seizure that could persist for several hours and was seen as instrumental in effecting a patient's cure. Spanos and Gottlieb (1979) have argued that the mesmeric crisis paralleled the convulsions associated with the ritual of demonic exorcism, and that the behaviors associated with the roles of the mesmerist and magnetized subject evolved from existing reciprocal behaviors enacted by the exorcist and victim of demonic possession. Another reason for the frequency of convulsions in response to early inductions is that the first patient that Mesmer treated by means of "magnetism" happened to be suffering from a hysterical disorder, the most prominent symptom of which was convulsions. This historical coincidence led to a popular association between mesmerism and convulsions and to an expectancy that convulsive spasms followed successful magnetization.

Accounts of the ensuing history of mesmerism/hypnotism (e.g., Pattie, 1967; Sarbin, 1962) clearly demonstrate that the behaviors associated with the roles of hypnotist and subject varied considerably as a function of general standards for social behavior and theoretical construals of hypnotic phenomena. As an example, one can contrast the histrionic and violent behavior associated with mesmerism to the restraint and tranquillity typical of Braid's neurohypnology. Sarbin (1962) has suggested that the difference was due to cultural differences between France and England during that era with respect to violence and sensationalism, differences in patient characteristics (Mesmer worked primarily with female hysterics), and Braid's belief that the patient, not the hypnotist, was ultimately in control of hypnotic experiences.

Contemporary Data on Hypnotic Role Perceptions

Just as hypnotic procedures have become standardized over the course of time, so too has the role of the hypnotic subject. Currently, the hypnotized person typically sits passively with eyes closed, shows little or no spontaneous speech or movement, and speaks slowly and softly in response to questions. Role-theoretical analyses view the behavior of hypnotized subjects as a function in part of their expectations of how a good subject ought to behave, and considerable data support this hypothesis. For example, people who are informed that hypnotized subjects display catalepsy of the dominant arm are likely to experience this effect when hypnotized (Orne, 1959; Sheehan, 1971), and being informed that spontaneous amnesia is characteristic of hypnosis significantly increase the likelihood of its occurrence (Young & Cooper, 1972).

Popular fiction has portrayed the deeply hypnotized subject as one who is unable to resist the hypnotist's suggestions, and highly suggestible subjects frequently behave as if this were so. However, two recent studies have convincingly demonstrated that the inability of highly hypnotizable subjects to resist suggestions is functionally related to their perceptions of the role of a hypnotized subject (Lynn, Nash, Rhue, Frauman & Sweeney, 1984; Spanos, Cobb & Gorassini, 1985). In these studies, subjects were instructed to resist responding overtly to suggestions and were informed that either the ability or the inability to resist was characteristic of deep hypnosis. In both studies, subjects who were informed that successful resistance was an indication of deep hypnosis successfully resisted test suggestions, whereas those who were not so informed did not.

Role-expectancy manipulations can also produce a complete reversal of hypnotic amnesia. Silva and Kirsch (1987) told one group of highly hypnotizable subjects that the purpose of their research was to study hypnotic amnesia, and that deeply hypnotized subjects are unable to recall forgotten information no matter how hard they tried. A second group was told that the purpose of the experiment was to study the memory enhancement effects of hypnosis, and that deep hypnosis enabled subjects to breach hypnotic barriers. After hearing one of these conflicting rationales, subjects were exposed to a tape-recorded hypnotic induction that included an amnesia suggestion, a challenge to remember, a "trance-deepening" procedure, and a second challenge to remember. Subjects in both groups showed high levels of amnesia following the first challenge. On the second challenge, subjects in the amnesia-expectancy condition displayed even more amnesia than they had following the first challenge. In contrast, all but one of the subjects in the memory enhancement condition displayed full recall following the second challenge.

Role Perceptions and Altered States of Consciousness

Besides affecting overt responses, role perceptions are important determinants of self-reported experiences of altered states of consciousness. In a nonhypnotic context, this has been convincingly demonstrated in a series of studies designed by Plotkin and his colleagues (reviewed in Plotkin, 1979). In the most compelling of these studies (Plotkin, 1976), subjects receiving veridical alpha-wave biofeedback were given intermittent verbal feedback indicating either success or failure. They were also given varying information about the characteristics of the state of consciousness that they would experience if they were successful. For half of the subjects, these characteristics were those that are typically reported as the "alpha experience." The others received descriptions that in most respects were the opposite of the usual alpha experience.

Although there were no significant differences among the four groups in the degree of alpha enhancement achieved, there were dramatic differences in the reports of their subjective experiences. Whereas most subjects in the "failure" conditions reported "nothing unusual," almost all persons in the "success" groups reported experiences that corresponded to the information they received. These data suggest that the nature of the state of consciousness experienced during alpha biofeedback training is dependent upon subjects' role expectations and that the degree to which changes are experienced varies as a function of the strength of their response expectancies.

Henry (1984) demonstrated a similar correspondence between expected and experienced alterations in conscious state in a hypnotic context. Instead of manipulating role expectancies, Henry assessed individual differences in hypnotically naive subjects' beliefs about the experiential characteristics of a hypnotic "trance" state. This was accomplished by means of a questionnaire consisting of opposing subjective experiences that might be associated with hypnosis.

In order to test the hypothesis that role perceptions influence the subjective experience of trance, it was necessary to find a set of subjective experiences that were not associated with hypnosis in a uniform direction by inexperienced subjects. A large pool of potential bipolar items were assembled, and subjects were asked to indicate the direction of change that they thought would be experienced by a hypnotized subject. In other words, they were asked to indicate whether hypnosis would produce more or less relaxation, more or less control of movement, and so forth. The criterion for retaining an item in the final version of the scale was an endorsement rate of not more than 60 percent in either direction. Subjects were then asked to predict whether they would personally experience each of those changes in consciousness when they were subsequently hypnotized.

The degree of change in state of consciousness that subjects expected to experience significantly predicted the number of unsuggested alterations in experience that they subsequently reported. In turn, changes in experience predicted responsiveness to test suggestions. However, the nature of those changes in experience was largely determined by subjects' preconceptions. Depending on their expectancies, hypnotic subjects described "trance" as a state in which time either passed more slowly or more quickly than usual, logical thought was either more or less difficult than normal, the hypnotist's voice sounded closer or farther away than before, sounds were experienced as more muffled or more clear than usual, the subject felt more of less involved than usual, and so on.

Henry's data suggest that there is no particular state of consciousness that can be labeled "hypnotic trance." Rather, there are a variety of changes in experience that are interpreted as evidence of "trance" when they are experienced in a hypnotic context. Some of these are directly suggested in typical inductions (e.g., relaxation), others occur as a function of subjects' preconceptions. To the degree that changes in conscious state are experienced and are interpreted as evidence that a hypnotic trance has been achieved, subjects come to believe that they will be able to experience suggested effects, an expectation that is capable of generating those effects (Council, Kirsch & Hafner, 1986).

PERCEPTIONS OF THE SITUATION

In the eighteenth century, mesmerists used a variety of procedures to induce "crisis." These included stoking or making "passes" over the patient bare-handed or with a magnet, having patients sit around a bucket containing iron filings, having the subject stand by a "magnetized" tree or drink "magnetized" water, and having the person sit with his or (more frequently) her knees pressed between the thighs of the mesmerist who applied pressure to the hypochondria (the area between the rib cage and navel) or the ovarium. In modern placebo terminology, eighteenth-century induction procedures were nonspecific in the sense that no particular components were necessary for successful induction of a crisis. Experiments conducted by the French Royal Commission established to investigate mesmerism concluded that belief in the appropriateness of the situation was sufficient to elicit crises in susceptible subjects.

Although there is still variety in induction procedures, most hypnotic inductions involve suggestions for deep relaxation. However, equivalent degrees of response enhancement have been produced by "alert" inductions in which relaxation is inhibited (Edmonston, 1981) by task motivational instructions (Barber, 1969), by brief training in the use of imaginative strategies (Council et al., 1983; Katz, 1978, 1979; Vickery, Kirsch, Council & Sirkin, 1985), and by a variety of expectancy modification procedures. For example, subjects have been hypnotized by ingesting placebos (Glass & Barber, 1961), gazing at a flashing light (Kroger & Schneider, 1959), and listening to false "brainwave" biofeedback (Council et al, 1983). Techniques for successfully inducing hypnosis appear to be limited only by the creativity and credibility of the hypnotist. As had the French Royal Commission two centuries earlier, Sheehan and Perry (1976) have concluded that "it is not the procedural conditions per se that are important but whether or not the subject perceives them as part of a context that is 'appropriate' for displaying hypnotic behavior" (p. 723).

The level of expectancy generated by a particular induction is likely to be mediated by the congruence between a subject's preexisting beliefs about hypnosis and the implicitly or explicitly stated rationale for that induction. Council, Kirsch, Vickery, and Carlson (1983) presented rationales for hypnotic inductions to subjects who rated them for credibility (cf. Borkovec & Nau, 1972) before the inductions were administered. An overall correlation of .70 between expectancy and credibility was found for data collapsed across rationales for traditional trance inductions, cognitive-behavioral skill training, and a high-credibility placebo induction. Within-cell correlations ranged from .59 to .79, indicating that this relation held for traditional as well as nontraditional inductions.

"You are becoming very, very relaxed." Just hearing those words evokes the idea of hypnosis to most people in our culture (Edmonston, 1984). For that reason, relaxation procedures can effectively increase responsiveness independently of an explicit label indicating that it is a hypnotic procedure. Less traditional procedures require explicit labeling. For example, Barber and Calverley (1964, 1965a) have shown that simply defining the administration of test suggestions as hypnosis has significant effects on suggestibility. In another study, these authors told subjects that a tape-recorded hypnotic induction was either very effective or very ineffective in producing hypnosis (Barber & Calverley, 1965b). Those who were told that the induction was effective were subsequently more responsive to test suggestions than those who were told that it was not effective.

At the beginning of this chapter, we described the experiments conducted by the French Royal Commission appointed to investigate mesmerism in the eighteenth century. The first contemporary replication of those experiments were reported by Glass and Barber (1961). They devised a highly credible rationale and setting, including medical props and procedures, to convince subjects that an inert pill described as a "powerful hypnotic drug" would produce a state of hypnosis. With this set and setting, the placebo pill was as effective as a standard hypnotic induction in raising levels of response to suggestion.

In a conceptually similar treatment, Council et al. (1983) used the setting of a psychophysiological laboratory to lend credibility to an expectancy-modification procedure involving "biofeedback." Subjects were presented with the rationale that a hypnotic state could be generated through amplification of particular brainwaves. They were then wired to a polygraph, viewed their "brainwaves" on an oscilloscope, and heard a false feedback tone through headphones. This procedure was equivalent to standard trance-induction procedures on most measures of hypnotic response.

One early demonstration of the use of an expectancy-modification procedure as a hypnotic induction was unintentional. Kroger and Schneider (1959) presented their "Brain Wave Synchronizer" as a bona fide scientific tool for inducing hypnosis. The synchronizer, a variable stroboscopic light at which subjects stared, was said to alter alpha rhythms through photic driving to produce a trance state. Kroger and Schneider claimed to induce deep hypnosis in 50 percent of their subjects, and light hypnosis in 30 percent with five minutes of exposure. Hammer and Arkins (1964) examined whether the synchronizer alone was sufficient to induce hypnosis or whether it had to be supplemented with verbal suggestion in order to be effective. It was found that while a verbal induction combined with the synchronizer was effective in increasing suggestibility, exposure to the synchronizer alone with no expectation of hypnosis had no such effect.

PERCEIVED TASK DEDUCTION

One way to alter people's beliefs about the difficulty of particular suggestions is by providing verbal information. Barber and Calverley (1964) varied statements by the experimenter regarding the level of difficulty of suggestions. They reported that subjects who were told that responding to suggestions would be easy scored significantly higher on a test of suggestibility than subjects who were told that the suggestions would be difficult.

Modeling is a second way in which subjects might learn about the relative difficulty of suggestions. In two studies on the effects of modeling (Botto, Fisher & Soucy, 1977; Klinger, 1970), experimenters had subjects view a model who passed either all or none of the suggestions on standard measures of hypnotic responsiveness. Subjects exposed to a responsive model subsequently achieved significantly higher hypnotic response scores than those who had seen an unresponsive model.

In a later study (Botto and Fisher, 1978), relatively unresponsive subjects saw a model pass hypnotic suggestions and relatively responsive subjects saw a model fail to respond completely to test suggestions. When they were subsequently tested on the complete scale, subjects who had been exposed to the successful model were more responsive than they had previously been. Conversely, subjects who had been exposed to an unsuccessful model were less responsive than they had been. Unfortunately, the subject assignment procedure makes it impossible to rule out the possibility that these results were due to a statistical regression to the mean.

In a particularly well-designed study, Coe and Steen (1981) independently assessed the effects of modeling on expectancy and on hypnotic response. Subjects were exposed to one of two videotapes on which they observed a model being tested on a standard measure of hypnotic responsiveness. Both videotapes showed the model passing half of the suggestions and failing the other half, but the items that were passed on one tape were failed on the other and vice versa. One group of subjects was then tested for hypnotic response. Another group was not tested, but was asked to predict how they would respond to each suggestion if they were tested. Modeling produced parallel effects on expectancy and on actual response. Subjects expected to be more responsive to positively modeled suggestions than to negatively modeled suggestions, and subjects were more responsive to positively modeled than to negatively modeled suggestions. Thus, in addition to demonstrating a modeling effect on hypnotic response, Coe and Steen (1981) provided evidence that the effect was mediated by response expectancy. This data also provide evidence of the specificity of response expectancies.

SELF-PERCEPTIONS OF HYPNOTIC RESPONSIVENESS

Self-reported expectancies of subjects with no previous experience of hypnosis have typically accounted for about 10 percent of the variance in measures of hypnotic responding after traditional trance inductions (Barber & Calverley, 1969; Melei & Hilgard, 1964; Saavedra & Miller, 1983; Shor, 1971). Shor (1971) noted the paradox of such weak research findings in view of the universal clinical observation that expectancy and belief play vital roles in hypnotic behavior. The response expectancy hypothesis also suggests a substantially stronger relation than has typically been reported.

Substantially higher correlations between self-predictions and subsequent response, accounting for about 25 to 40 percent of the variance, have been reported in some studies (Barber & Calverley, 1964; Council, Kirsch, Vickery & Carlson, 1983). Unlike studies in which smaller correlations were reported, these studies included groups of subjects that did not experience traditional trance inductions. Instead, they were asked to place themselves in hypnosis or were given brief training in using goal-directed fantasy to generate response to suggestions. Combining data from two different studies, Kirsch, Council, and Vickery (1985) demonstrated that there was a significantly stronger relation between expectancy and response when a traditional induction was not part of the experimental procedure than when it was. Thus, the imposition of a trance induction procedure attenuates the relation between measures of expectancy and hypnotic response.

How do trance inductions attenuate correlations between expectancy and response? Part of the answer can be found by considering the parallels between the construct of response expectancy and that of intention. Except for the volitional quality of the response, the definition of response expectancy is identical to the definition of intention proposed by Fishbein and Ajzen (1975). These authors define an intention as a person's subjective probability that he or she will perform a voluntary behavior and propose that intentions are "immediate determinants of the corresponding overt behaviors" (p. 372), a relation that is virtually identical to the expectancy-response relation hypothesized by Kirsch (1985a) for nonvolitional response.

Just as correlations between response expectancy and subsequent response are often weaker than one might expect them to be, measured intentions are rarely as predictive of behavior as they ought to be. Fishbein and Ajzen (1975) have suggested that correlations between intentions and behavior are often attenuated because there is generally a period of time intervening between the measurement of the intention and the observation of the intended behavior. Intentions are not stable over time. Rather, they are often contingent on the occurrence of certain events, and when those contingencies are not met, one's intentions are likely to change. For example, we intend to travel to Europe next summer if we have sufficient funds. However, if our funds prove insufficient, our intention is likely to change.

Response expectancies are like intentions in that they are often contingent on particular criteria being met and are subject to change if those criteria are not met. For example, people may believe that their excessive fear of snakes can be alleviated by treatment. But if the treatment is not sufficiently credible, that belief is likely to change (Kirsch, 1978). In a similar manner, the common belief that hypnosis involves a special state of consciousness imposes contingencies on expected responsiveness. Many people have preconceptions about hypnosis that link it with very pronounced alterations in experience. They may not know the exact nature of this "trance" state, but their criteria for concluding that they are in fact hypnotized includes having experiences that are extremely different from those of normal waking consciousness. They may also believe that when people are hypnotized their responses to suggestions occur without any cooperation on their part, perhaps even with continual active resistance.

According to response expectancy theory, "the probability of occurrence of a nonvolitional response varies directly with the strength of the expectancy of its occurrence and inversely with the magnitude or difficulty of the expected response. Therefore, a weak expectancy for a large change in subjective response is likely to be disconfirmed, whereas a strong expectancy for a small change is likely to be confirmed, thereby strengthening the expectancy and initiating a cycle for continued change" (Kirsch, 1985, p. 1199). Prior to experiencing hypnosis for the first time, people are likely to have weakly held expectancies about their own responsiveness. They may expect to be very responsive, but they do not hold that expectancy with very much conviction. If, in addition, their subjective criteria for concluding that they are hypnotized include very profound changes in conscious experience, their expectations of experiencing a "trance" are likely to be disconfirmed. When these weakly held expectancies are disconfirmed, their expectancies for response to suggestions are lowered, which in turn reduces their responsiveness. Others who hold less extreme expectancies about the nature of hypnosis are more likely to have their hypnotic response expectancies confirmed and thereby strengthened.

Trance Inductions as Expectancy-Modification Procedures

Trance induction procedures are typically designed so as to increase subjects' expectancies for responding to suggestions. In clinical practice, hypnotists tailor inductions to the characteristics and ongoing behavior of individual subjects (Erickson, 1980). Subjects' spontaneous behaviors are observed and commented on as evidence that trance is occurring, naturally occurring phenomena (e.g., eye strain following eye fixation) are suggested so that they might be similarly interpreted, failure to comply with suggestions is prevented by using quasi challenges, and failures that do occur are reinterpreted as successes. Some of these techniques have been incorporated into standardized induction procedures (e.g., Weitzenhoffer & Hilgard, 1962). As Barber et al. (1974) have noted, "the major purpose of these techniques appears to be to lead the subject to believe that he is responding well to suggestions and thus may expect that he will continue to respond well" (p. 29). Hypnotic inductions can thus be interpreted as expectancy-modification procedures (Kirsch, 1985a).

The implication of this analysis is that trance induction procedures are effective to the degree that they lead subjects to believe that their state of consciousness has been sufficiently altered to permit the occurrence of hypnotic phenomena. Experiences of relaxation and disorientation confirm the belief that one is in a "hypnotic trance" and thereby generate positive expectancies for subsequent confirmatory experiences (i.e., positive responses to hypnotic test suggestions). Conversely, insufficient changes in conscious state lower hypnotic response expectancies. Thus, response expectancies can change dramatically between the beginning and end of a traditional trance induction. The degree and direction of expectancy change depends on subjects' implicit criteria for concluding that hypnosis has occurred and, to a lesser extent, on the skill of the hypnotist.

The hypotheses that trance inductions alter response expectancies and that responsiveness is due to these alterations in expectancy were tested by Council et al. (1986). Hypnotic response expectancies were assessed prior to administering a traditional trance induction and again after the induction, but prior to the administration of test suggestions. In addition, subjective reports of trance depth were obtained immediately after the induction procedure. Although preinduction expectancies were only moderately correlated with hypnotic responsiveness, the correlations between postinduction expectancies and responsiveness were substantially higher, approximately equaling the test-retest reliability coefficient of the expectancy measure.

Because these data are correlational, it is possible to interpret the relation between expectancy and response as epiphenomenal rather than causal. That is, it is possible that hypnotic inductions produce a hypnotic trance state that has parallel effects on expectancy and suggestibility. In order to test the hypothesis that responsiveness was due to expectancy, rather than to an altered state of consciousness, trance depth was assessed on the Long Stanford Scale (Tart, 1979), and the results were analyzed by means of causal modeling. This analysis revealed that when hypnotic response scores were simultaneously regressed on expectancy and trance depth, only expectancy uniquely predicted responsiveness. In other words, although expectancy significantly predicted responsiveness even when variance associated with trance depth was statistically controlled, the reverse was not true. Reported trance depth was not significantly related to responsiveness when variance associated with expectancy was statistically controlled.

Altering Expected Responsiveness

Hypnotic response expectancies are easily manipulated by verbal information. For example, Gandolfo (1971) asked subjects to try to resist complying with a posthypnotic suggestion. One group of subjects was led to expect that they probably would be able to resist the suggestion, a second group was led to believe that they probably would not be able to resist, and neutral expectations were imparted to a third group. Those given positive expectancies about their ability to resist showed greater resistance than subjects in the other two groups.

Vickery and Kirsch (1985) manipulated subjects' expectancies about the effects of repeated testing of response levels. One group of subjects was told that repeated testing led to an increase in responsiveness, a second group was told that it decreased responsiveness, a third group was informed that hypnotizability was a stable trait, and a fourth group was not given any information at all about the effects of repeated testing. Response to suggestions was then assessed in two separate sessions. Although subjects in all four groups were equally responsive in the first session, positive expectancy information significantly enhanced second-session responding and negative expectancy information significantly decreased second session-responding. The hypnotic behavior of the stable expectancy and no-information groups did not change from one session to the next.

Two studies have used feedback from bogus personality tests as an expectancy manipulation. After an initial test of hypnotizability and administration of a "personality" scale composed of randomly selected items from the MMPI, Gregory and Diamond (1973) provided experimental subjects with bogus feedback to the effect that the personality test indicated that they ought to be responsive to hypnosis. Upon retesting, subjects in whom positive expectancies had been induced were significantly more responsive than control subjects and were also more responsive than they had been during the initial testing session.

Saavedra and Miller (1983) manipulated expectancy by using false feedback from a battery of tests. After completing the test battery, subjects were instructed to return for a second experimental session, during which they received "feedback" in the form of a "hypnotizability coefficient" indicating low, medium, or high hypnotizability. Hypnotic responsiveness was then assessed. Subjects in the low-expectation group were significantly less responsive than those in other groups. However, in contrast to the data reported by Gregory and Diamond (1973), high-expectancy subjects in Saavedra and Miller's study were not more responsive than control subjects who had received no feedback or subjects who had been told they would be moderately hypnotizable.

If the relation of test items to hypnotizability is logically clear, personality assessment can affect hypnotic response expectancy even without experimenter feedback. Tellegen and Atkinson's (1974) Absorption Scale, for example, consists of items that, when read in a hypnotic context, might easily be recognized as related to hypnotic responsiveness (e.g., "If I wish, I can imagine that my body is so heavy that I could not move it if I wanted to"). Because the meaning of its items are clear, Council et al. (1986) hypothesized that administering the absorption scale in a hypnotic context might be a way of indirectly providing subjects with bogus feedback about their hypnotizability. We reasoned that subjects who completed the scale in a hypnotic context and found themselves answering "true" to many items like this one might conclude that they were good hypnotic subjects. Conversely, subjects responding "false" to many items might conclude that they would not be very good at hypnosis.

In order to test this hypothesis, we administered the absorption scale to 64 subjects in the context of a hypnosis experiment, and to an additional 64 subjects in a context unrelated to hypnosis (Council et al., 1986). Regression analyses revealed a significant interaction between the absorption scale and its context of administration, affecting its relation to hypnotic behavior. As predicted, absorption was significantly correlated with responsiveness and expectancy only when the scale was administered in a context that was clearly associated with a subsequent hypnotic experience. When the apparent relation between the scale and hypnosis was disguised, absorption was unrelated to any measure of hypnotizability. These data suggest that the frequently reported association between absorption and responsiveness is an artifact of the scale's effect on response expectancies.

There Are No Low-Hypnotizable Subjects

Wilson (1967) devised an especially persuasive expectancy manipulation, by means of which he was able to demonstrate a powerful effect on hypnotic response. Wilson suggested a variety of perceptual effects to experimental subjects and then produced those effects via hidden lights, tape recordings, and fans. For example, following the suggestion that subjects would see the color red, a red tinge was surreptitiously imparted to the room. Similarly, a suggestion to hear music was accompanied by tape-recorded music played at a very low volume. Following the example of Perky (1910), who had demonstrated that at near-threshold levels subjects are unable to discriminate between real and imagined stimuli, Wilson presented these stimuli intensely enough to be perceived, but not in sufficient intensity to arouse suspicion.

Wilson's study was designed to maximize subjects' response expectancies, while minimizing effects due to other variables. For example, subjects were informed that the study was an investigation of imagination, rather than of hypnosis, and no formal hypnotic induction was used. Relatively neutral experimental demand was imparted by telling subjects that "because little is known about this area, we have few expectations about what behavior should occur; our interest is in what behavior does occur" (Wilson, 1967, p. 54). Finally, in order to minimize the influence of rapport and other interpersonal factors, subjects were left alone in the room during the experimental manipulation and subsequent testing of hypnotic response levels. All instructions were presented via audiotape, and subjects' responses were unobtrusively observed through peepholes.

Wilson found generally low levels of response to the Barber suggestibility scale among control subjects. This is not surprising given the various procedures by which hypnotic role demands were minimized. In contrast, response levels of *all* experimental subjects were at or above the midpoint of the scale and above the mean response level of control subjects. In fact, none of the experimental subjects responded at levels that would typically lead to a classification of low hypnotizability.

RESPONSE EXPECTANCY AND OTHER NONSTATE THEORIES

The response expectancy hypothesis is generally consistent with earlier nonstate theories (Barber, 1969; Barber et al., 1974; Sarbin, 1950, Sarbin & Coe, 1972; Spanos, 1982, 1986b; Wilson & Barber, 1983). All are in agreement that hypnotic responses can be conceptualized as believed-in imaginings and that these experiences occur when people voluntarily take on the role of hypnotic subject. Nevertheless, subtle differences in emphasis between these theories are worth noting. Unlike previous theories, response expectancy theory hypothesizes that expectancies are *immediate*, rather than mediating, causes of hypnotic response.

Imagery and Expectancy

Barber and his colleagues have emphasized the importance of imagining events that are consistent with suggested effects. From this perspective, positive expectancies enhance hypnotic response because they "give rise to a willingness to think and imagine with the themes that are suggested" (Barber et al., 1974, p. 19). Extending Arnold's (1946) ideomotor action hypothesis, Barber et al. (1974) maintained that thinking about and imagining an event produce corresponding overt behaviors, subjective experiences, and physiological changes. Thus, subjects who pass particular test suggestions are likely to have engaged in goal-directed fantasies, that is, they are likely to have imagined events that, were they to actually occur, would produce the suggested response (Spanos, 1971; Spanos & Barber, 1972; Spanos & Ham, 1973). Also, teaching subjects to engage in goal-directed fantasies tends to enhance responsiveness to suggestions (Council et al., 1983; Katz, 1978, 1979; Vickery et al., 1985). In agreement with Sarbin and Coe (1972), Barber et al. (1974) conceptualized good hypnotic subjects as people who were skilled at becoming involved in imaginary events (also see, Hilgard, 1979; Wilson & Barber, 1983).

Although involvement in goal-directed imagery generally enhances hypnotic response, we believe that the causal link between imagery and expectancy is contrary to that proposed by Barber. From a response expectancy perspective, goal-directed imagery enhances responsiveness by virtue of its effects on expectancy.

Evidence that the effects of imagery on hypnotic response are mediated by response expectancy is provided by a number of studies (Council et al., 1983; Council et al., 1986; Kirsch et al., 1984; Vickery & Kirsch, 1985). However, the clearest evidence about the relation between imagery and expectancy as determinants of hypnotic response can be found in a series of five studies in which these variables were pitted against each other. Lynn et al. (1984) and Spanos, Cobb, et al. (1985) found that when provided with information leading them to believe that they would be able to do so, highly hypnotizable subjects resisted complying with suggested effects while simultaneously becoming absorbed in imaging those effects. Conversely, Zamansky (1977) and Spanos, Weekes, and de Groh (1984) reported that when given appropriate instructions, highly hypnotizable subjects could experience a suggested effect while actively imagining conflicting events.

Finally, Kirsch, Council, and Mobayed (1987) demonstrated that these effects are generalizable to moderately hypnotizable subjects as well. Following a no-imagery, baseline assessment of responsiveness, test suggestions were repeated along with instructions to imagine either compatible or incompatible events. Regardless of type of imagery, half of the subjects were told that the imagery would enhance responsiveness and half were told that it would inhibit responding. Goal-directed imagery enhanced responding when subjects were led to believe that that would be its effect and inhibited responding when subjects were provided with contrary information. Conversely, counterimagery inhibited responding only when subjects expected it to do so.

Honesty and Impression Management

In his most recent theoretical work, Spanos (1986b) has stressed the role of impression management as the primary motivator of hypnotic behavior. According to Spanos, the behavior of hypnotic subjects is completely under voluntary control. Highly responsive subjects act as if they were experiencing nonvolitional responding and other hypnotic effects in order to convey the impression that they are deeply hypnotized. Spanos notes in passing that many of these subjects appear to convince themselves that they are experiencing these effects, but this belief is treated as a form of self-deception that is incidental, rather than essential, to his conception of hypnotic behavior.

In contrast, we believe that most subjects are motivated more by a desire to experience hypnotic effects than by a wish to convey the impression that they are experiencing those effects. Although some people might be motivated by a desire to fool a hypnotist or experimenter, unless given explicit instructions to simulate, most subjects respond overtly to suggestions only to the degree that they honestly experience the suggested effects. State theorists maintain that genuine hypnotic responses can be distinguished from faked responses in that they are consistent with alterations in subjective experience. Without adopting the view that hypnotic responses are produced by some special state of consciousness, we nevertheless maintain that this distinction between genuine and faked responses is valid. Faked responses are easy to explain. The more interesting and difficult problem is to account for the changes in subjective experience that are the defining characteristics of genuine hypnotic responses.

Considerable research effort has been devoted to the behavior of a small minority of highly responsive subjects. However, the genuineness of hypnotic behavior is most clearly evident in the responses of the vast majority of people who are only moderately successful in responding to suggestions. Although there are some exceptions (e.g., wart removal), most hypnotic responses are easy to fake, as demonstrated by the frequent failure to find differences between the behavior of simulators and that of nonsimulating, highly responsive subjects. The failure of most subjects to respond to many suggestions indicates that they are not merely faking the responses that they do emit. It is very unlikely that people voluntarily select particular levels of hypnotizability and then play a role that is consistent with their selected response level (Kirsch, 1986).

Although genuineness in responding is most easily demonstrated in moderately hypnotizable subjects, it can also be confirmed among more responsive subjects. Kirsch, Carone, and Johnston (1985) played a tape-recorded induction and test suggestions twice to a group of simulators and a group of nonsimulating subjects who had been selected for high levels of responsiveness. During the first administration, subjects were led to believe that they were alone. Unbeknown to them, their behavior was surreptitiously observed via a hidden camera attached to a video monitor in an adjacent room. They were then observed again, listening to the same recording with an experimenter present in the room. Simulating subjects were twice as responsive when the experimenter was present as they had been when they were alone. In contrast, the presence of an experimenter had no effect on the behavior of subjects who had not been instructed to simulate. Because no one was present for them to impress during the first trial, their responses to suggestions cannot be explained as voluntary behaviors aimed at conveying the impression that they are hypnotized.

Hypnosis and Volition

People voluntarily take on (rather than "play") the role of hypnotic subject, just as they voluntarily—and sometimes involuntarily—take on other social roles (e.g., psychologist, parent, student, patient). The role of hypnotic subject typically includes implicit or explicit demands to cooperate in imagining suggested effects and to report honestly one's experience of those effects (Spanos, 1986b). Although imagining and reporting are voluntary behaviors, the experience of suggested effects is not fully controllable by most people. If hypnotic experiences were completely under voluntary control, we would all be capable of genuinely full hypnotic responding.

Hypnotic subjects are generally assured that their willingness to experience hypnotic responses is a necessary precondition for the occurrence of those responses, and that information is also widely available in the popular media. Furthermore, because they regard hypnosis as intrinsically interesting, many subjects actively attempt to experience suggested effects. Some are quite ingenious in devising cognitive strategies that help them to experience suggestions, and the responsiveness of others can be dramatically increased by teaching them similar strategies (Gorassini & Spanos, 1986; Spanos, de Groh & de Groot, 1987). However, even when engendered by intentional cognitive strategies, genuine hypnotic responses are experienced as occurring nonvolitionally. More importantly, the same responses can be occasioned in situations that discourage active compliance.

The study by Juhasz and Sarbin (1966) is an example of the elicitation of a hypnotic-like response in a situation that does not encourage active compliance. In the presumed context of an experiment in psychophysics, subjects were asked to indicate when they experienced water tasting salty. Because the water was not in fact salty, subjects can be said to have imagined the salty taste. However, the experimental context was not one that suggested voluntary imagining. Instead, the context implied that honest reporting of sensory, rather than imaginary, experience was called for. For that reason, the experienced salty taste can best be understood as an automatic consequence of subjects' expectations, rather than as a voluntarily imagined response.

Because it ensured that suggested effects were experienced regardless of volitional effort, Wilson's (1967) expectancy manipulation procedure, which was described above, reinforced a passive response to suggestions. Nevertheless it resulted in substantial enhancement of hypnotic responsiveness. Similarly, placebo administration, which produces many of the same effects that can be brought about by hypnosis, reinforces passivity rather than an active attempt to bring about change. In placebo contexts, the implication is that the "drug" will produce an effect regardless of the subject's intentional efforts.

Perhaps the most conclusive evidence that hypnotic phenomena cannot be fully accounted for as volitional behavior is the fact that hypnosis (and placebos) can produce changes in warts and other skin conditions (Barber, 1978). Changes in skin condition are not under voluntary control. One could offer subjects a substantial sum of money to make their warts disappear; but it is unlikely that many would be able to do so. The effect of hypnosis on skin conditions is a particularly puzzling phenomenon. It is also one that clearly demonstrates the commonality between hypnotic phenomena and placebo effects. Both are examples of the nonvolitional nature of response expectancy effects.

CONCLUSIONS

In nonhypnotic contexts, nonvolitional responses, many of which are similar or identical to hypnotic responses, can be generated by the expectancy of their occurrence. One could hypothesize that the occurrence of these responses in hypnotic contexts and their occurrence in nonhypnotic contexts are due to different mechanisms. However, it is more parsimonious to explain these occurrences in terms of a common underlying mechanism. Neither trance nor intentional cognitive strategies can account for the occurrence of these effects in nonhypnotic situations. In contrast, the activation of response expectancies appears to be a common factor in all of them.

Variables other than response expectancy—imaginative involvement, role perceptions, and rapport, for example—also influence hypnotic behavior. However, the effects of these variables are mediated by response expectancy. Goal-directed fantasies enhance response only to the degree that subjects expect them to have that effect. Subjects' perceptions of the hypnotic role lead them to expect to experience particular responses as a function of being hypnotized. Rapport enhances responsiveness because it is associated with increased trust in the hypnotist's statements. Unlike imagery, role perceptions, and rapport, the effect of response expectancy is immediate. Just as intention is the immediate determinant of voluntary behavior, response expectancies are immediate determinants of hypnotic and other nonvolitional responses.

A variety of strategies can be used to convince subjects that suggested effects will occur. In hypnotic contexts, these include hypnotic inductions that produce minor sensory alterations and suggestions for active involvement in goal-directed imaginings. In other contexts—for example, psychophysical experiments and placebo administration contexts—trance inductions are not used and response expectancies are activated by procedures that imply a more passive role for subjects. Nevertheless, these contexts generate response changes that are similar to those observed in hypnosis. The most parsimonious explanation of these data is that nonvolitional responses are generated by the expectancy of their occurrence in both hypnotic and nonhypnotic contexts. Trance inductions and goal-directed strategic cognitions are not necessary precursors of these responses. Rather, they facilitate hypnotic experiences via their effects on expectancy.

NOTE

1. It has been suggested that expectancy accounts for only part of the pain-reducing effects of hypnotic suggestions. Among highly hypnotizable subjects, McGlashan, Evans, and Orne (1969) reported significantly greater pain reduction following hypnosis than following administration of a placebo presented in a Darvon capsule as an experimental pain-relieving drug. However, two features of the experimental design render the experimenters' conclusion arguable, at best. First, the magnitude of a placebo effect depends on the perceived strength of the drug for which the placebo is substituted. Thus, placebo morphine is more effective than placebo codeine, which in turn is more effective than placebo Darvon or placebo aspirin (Evans, 1985). It is likely that a sample of subjects selected for extremely high responsiveness to hypnosis would have greater faith in the effects of hypnosis than in the effects of an experimental analgesic resembling Darvon. Second, the use of an ischemic muscle task as the means of producing pain introduces an unfortunate artifact. Stam and Spanos (1987) demonstrated that a hypnotic induction reduced the rate of "work" at the pain-inducing task used by McGlashan et al., an effect that would artificially reduce the degree of experienced pain.

16

The Cognitive Skills Model

An Emerging Paradigm for Investigating Hypnotic Phenomena[1]

Michael Jay Diamond

This article represents the early stages of what might be considered a "working model" of clinical hypnosis. Its thrust is exploratory, speculative, and descriptive. The ideas presented are intended to generate further research and clinical application in hopes of providing a better understanding of hypnotic phenomena. Practically all parameters of the model are now considered by most sophisticated workers to be part of modern hypnosis. However, it is the gestalt emerging from the integration of these separate elements that renders the model paradigmatic and of particular heuristic value. It is believed that a more complete understanding and effective application of hypnotic phenomena require the development of a metatheoretical position encompassing both the phenomenological and behavioral perspectives to hypnosis (cf. Fromm & Shor, 1979).

This alternative model is termed the *Cognitive Skills* approach to hypnosis (Diamond, 1977a, 1977b; Katz, 1978, 1980) and has elsewhere been discussed in terms of the so-called "new hypnosis" (Araoz, 1985). Following an introduction to this new paradigm, the data supporting the model are briefly examined. The key parameters and controversial issues surrounding the model are then discussed, while its clinical implications are highlighted throughout.

INTRODUCTION: WHY A NEW MODEL?

An alternative approach to hypnosis is stressing the unique cognitive, and yet frequently unconscious,[2] processes of the hypnotized individual largely stems from a growing dissatisfaction with the more traditional trance model that is dependent on classical, ritualistic hypnotic inductions. Barber, Spanos, and Chaves

(1974); Gibbons (1979); Sarbin and Coe (1972); Spanos (1982a, 1986b); and Bandler and Grinder (1975); among others, have questioned the usefulness of the trance paradigm and have promoted the investigation of hypnosis from a more varied perspective. The cognitive-behavior theory of Barber et al. (1974), the social-psychological or contextualist positions of Coe and Sarbin (1977; Sarbin & Coe, 1972) and Spanos (1982a, 1982b), the phenomenological and ego-psychological inquiries of Fromm (1977) and Shor (1979), the unique clinical contributions of Milton Erickson (Erickson, 1980; Erickson & Rossi, 1979; Erickson, Rossi & Rossi, 1976; Haley, 1967), the research on modifying hypnotic responsivity (Diamond, 1974, 1977a, 1977b; 1982; Gorassini & Spanos, 1986; Kinney & Sachs, 1974; Sachs & Anderson, 1967; Spanos, 1986a; Stolar, 1979), the newer generation of interpersonal theorists (e.g., Bányai, 1985; Diamond, 1987; Nash, 1984; Sheehan, 1980; Sheehan & McConkey, 1982), and the studies of cognitively oriented experimentalists (e,.g., Crawford, 1982; Crawford & Allen, 1983; DeStefano, 1977; Karlin, 1979; Katz, 1978, 1979; Nogrady, McConkey, Laurence & Perry, 1983; Sheehan & McConkey, 1982; Spanos, 1971, 1982b; Spanos & Barber, 1972; Wallace & Patterson, 1984) have all contributed to the development of this approach.

The traditional trance paradigm or trait-state position has been useful for both experimentalists and clinicians in enabling molar, global descriptions of the central dimensions of hypnotic trance, for example, trait reliability and stability over time. In contrast, the cognitive skills model assumes a more molecular, contextual-bound set of constructions and focuses more directly on the cognitive-behavioral, within-person variance during hypnosis. The newer model is distinguished by its attempt to investigate and utilize the internal, *cognitive* processes initiated and/or evoked by a subject during the hypnotic experience. Moreover, the *skill* metaphor is used to emphasize the fact that cognitive processes within the hypnotic domain may be learned or acquired. Thus, hypnosis is viewed as a process rather than structure or thing, and the word "hypnosis" is regarded as a verb rather than noun.

It is well accepted that the essence of good clinical hypnosis is the ability to understand and make use of the unique needs and characteristics of the client. A hallmark of the cognitive skills approach is an appreciation for the client's unique phenomenological world and a methodology to affect that world. Careful attention is placed on *discovering, understanding,* and *utilizing* the hypnotized individual's unique cognitive abilities and skills and, subsequently, *collaborating* with the S to utilize his/her talents in ego-syntonic ways.

The clinical methods of the cognitive skills model are drawn from such diversified sources as modern psychoanalytic practice, humanistic-existential psychology, strategic therapy, systems theory, and contemporary cognitive behaviorism. More specifically, the goals of *discovering* and understanding the client's internal processes, representational systems, and unique needs are most typically achieved by active and empathic listening skills (Kohut, 1977; Langs, 1976). The cognitive skills approach also uses the intuitive and empathic methods that Erickson and his colleagues designed to delineate and alter the client's frame of reference (Erickson et al., 1967; Haley, 1967, 1973; Watzlawick, 1978).

Cognitive skills methodology relies on advances in modern cognitive behavioral psychology and hypnotherapy in order to achieve the goal of *utilization* (i.e., evoking and making use of the client's mental processes in ways that are outside his/her usual range of intentional or voluntary control), and subsequently, modification of problematic cognitive processes. Cognitively oriented therapies (Beck, 1976; Horowitz, 1978; Mahoney & Thoresen, 1974; Meichenbaum, 1977; Singer, 1974) have been integrated with developments in experimental and clinical hypnosis to produce a different approach to hypnotic intervention. This approach stresses the role of cognitive strategies in affecting imagery and thought processes, dissociation, experienced involuntariness of responding, self-observation, attribution, and self-control of these processes.

COGNITIVE PROCESSES, SKILLS, AND HYPNOSIS

The cognitive skills model posits that internal cognitive processes under the S's voluntary or involuntary direction (and oftentimes, quite independent of conscious awareness) are the critical ingredients in the experience of hypnosis. Thus, the focus is more upon the process of "what" the hypnotized S is doing (or might do) than upon the "why" it is being done. The emphasis on cognitive processes and skills is a considered strategem geared to avoid the more global language and the psychodynamically dominated metaphors of the classical trait-state theory. Nevertheless, this alternative cognitive model is in no way antithetical to the notion of trance and/or altered state(s) of consciousness. The concern rather is upon *what* the trance experience represents for the *unique* individual being hypnotized.

The cognitive skills model seems to have naturally developed from the current resurgence of interest in cognition and internal experience (e.g., Hilgard, 1977; Kihlstrom, 1985; Sheehan & McConkey, 1982). This contemporary Zeitgeist encourages a more intensive focus on the specifics of the cognitive skills used in hypnosis.[3] As suggested elsewhere (Diamond, 1973, 1977a, 1977b, 1980; Gibbons, 1979; Katz, 1980; McConkey & Cottee, 1985; Perry, Gelfand & Marcovitch, 1979; Shor & Easton, 1973; Spanos, 1982a, 1982b), it may be most fruitful to think of hypnotizability as a set of cognitive skills rather than as a stable trait. Thus, it is conceivable that the so-called "insusceptible" or refractory S is simply less adept at creating, implementing, or utilizing the requisite cognitive skills in hypnotic test situations. Similarly, what makes for a highly responsive or "virtuoso" S may very well be precisely the ability or skill to generate those cognitive processes within the context of a unique relationship with a hypnotist (Diamond, 1977a, 1984, 1987). Moreover, hypnotic suggestions differ in the nature of the cognitive processes necessary to experience as well as enact the suggestion (Tellegen, 1978-79). Some suggestions implicitly contain requisite strategies for the hypnotic response (e.g., arm immobilization to suggested imaginal rigidity), while as Barber et al. (1974) noted, other suggestions require that the S create a strategy in order to devise and implement an internal representation of a suggestion. Moreover, certain suggestions are worded in a "hypnotist-centered" way in which the hypnotist declares the effects to be occurring, whereas other suggestions are worded in a more "subject-centered" way wherein the *S* is encouraged to use his/her own skills to create the effect (Barber et al., 1980; Spanos, 1982b). Coe (1978; Schuyler & Coe, 1981) differentiated those hypnotic responses where the subject is a *passive* participant to whom things happen (i.e., "happenings") from those where one *actively* makes things happen (i.e., "doings"). Both "subject-centered" suggestions and active "doings" are directly addressed in the cognitive skills model by the explicit attention paid to creating *appropriate hypnotic cognitive strategies.*

One of the inherent consequences in using the social learning-based metaphors of "skill" and "strategy" is that some of the "magic" surrounding the experience of hypnosis may be lost. Scientific materialism can be as limiting in understanding human experience as the concept of "animal magnetism" was in inhibiting the development of scientific hypnosis. One of the most appealing facets of hypnosis is the opportunity it affords both the clinician and scientist to study and utilize elements of consciousness outside the range of everyday awareness. It is from this region of the so-called unconscious that most creative work and discovery stems. Thus, it is important to alert ourselves to the human tendency to reify constructs and make "explanatory fictions" into tiny homunculi. Processes labeled "cognitive," "skills," and "strategies" are no more immune from this fact of cognition than are constructs like "id," "atavism," and even "trance." It will continue to be a most difficult task to utilize the new model's constructs in a flexible, empirical, and open-ended manner.

To set the stage for a presentation of the cognitive skills approach, I would like to consider an analogy from sexual behavior. In the "fantasy model of sex," one merely does "what comes naturally" and doesn't need to learn to do anything because satisfying sex occurs spontaneously if the "conditions" are right (Zilbergeld, 1978). As the author argued, this analysis was fine and good for many, but what about those with sexual dysfunctions? More recently, developments in sexual therapy have focused on the importance of choice and the role of learning in the development of appropriate skills (Araoz, 1982). As these sexual skills become well learned, either in the course of normal development or as a result of sex therapy, spontaneity becomes possible and sexual responses seem to become "second nature" as one learns to simply "let things happen."

In hypnosis, as in sexual behavior, changes occur in many response systems (for example, physiological, emotional, and cognitive functioning) and alterations in consciousness apparently occur in both endeavors. Hypnotic learning too involves at least those three levels of functioning. The data appear the least equivocal in the cognitive sphere (Hilgard, 1977; Kihlstrom, 1985). However, the nature of the cognitive skills involved has been, heretofore, left rather vague. Researchers have nevertheless attempted to speculate; thus, Barber et al. (1974), J. Hilgard (1970), and Sarbin & Coe (1972) have likened the hypnotic skills to those required for involvement and absorption in books, movies, and dramatic role enactment, labeling these skills "thinking and imagining with," "imaginative involvement," and "role enactment." Other constructs include "absorption" (Tellegen & Atkinson, 1974) and "utilization of sense memories" (Erickson & Rossi, 1977). Sheehan and McConkey (1982; McConkey & Cottee, 1985) discussed the specific cognitive skills involved in hypnosis in terms of *absorption, attention, imagery, and dissociation.* I would add to this list a capacity for *enactment or involuntary responding* (cf. Spanos, Rivers & Ross, 1977) *synthetic-holistic or primary process thinking* (Crawford 1982; Fromm, 1977), and a cognitive-affective skill pertaining to one's *readiness for a (positive) transference* to the hynotist. These terms remain imprecise and rather speculative; nonetheless, they do suggest the importance of relevant learning and developmental experience in hypnotic skill development. Moreover, as McConkey and Cottee (1985) put it: "we do not yet know the relative importance of each of these cognitive skills to hypnotizability, and we do not yet know the particular configuration of these skills that is essential for high hypnotizability to occur" (p. 7).

Although our understanding of the cognitive processes involved is rudimentary, we do have evidence to indicate that developing skills of a cognitive nature can considerably enhance the experience of hypnosis. What data there are will be briefly considered next.

EVIDENCE LEADING TO THE COGNITIVE SKILLS MODEL

Two types of studies have provided the empirical foundation for the development of the cognitive skills model: (1) those training *S*s in cognitive skills and then comparing their hynotic experiences with the experience of *S*s exposed only to more traditional trance inductions; and, (2) those increasing hypnotic responsiveness by using cognitively oriented training programs. These two sets of studies overlap in some ways and extensive reviews have been provided by Barber et al. (1974), Diamond (1974, 1977a, 1977b, 1982), and Smyth (1981). In these studies, cognitive skill training took varied forms and employed numerous terminologies including "goal-directed fantasy" (Spanos, 1971; Spanos & Barber, 1972), "think-with suggestions" (Barber et al. 1974; Barber & Wilson, 1977; DeStefano, 1977), and "social-learning or skill training" (Council, Kirsch, Vickery & Carlson, 1983; Gorassini & Spanos, 1986; Katz, 1978, 1979). The last set of studies, for example generally demonstrated enhanced responsivity as well as greater generalization and feelings of self-control as a result of cognitively oriented training as compared to traditional trance methods. Other modification studies have successfully employed some or all of the following cognitively oriented training approaches: facilitative information about hypnosis; disinhibitory information designed to correct misconceptions; operant learning procedures; modeling; practice; and cognitive self-control strategy instruction (Diamond, 1974).

Overall, studies employing variables focused on cognitive strategies have undoubtedly provided the strongest support for the cognitive skills model (Diamond, 1972; Gorassini & Spanos, 1986; Spanos, Robertson, Menary & Brett, 1986; Kinney & Sachs, 1974). These strategies seem to include: (1) suspension of reality-orientation; (2) facilitation of imagination and imagery control; (3) focused thinking with; and (4) encouragement of specific covert self-control skills (i.e., information concerning how to interpret specific types of suggestions). The meaningfulness of the changes produced in these studies remains controversial however (Hilgard, 1977; Kihlstrom, 1985; Perry, 1977), and while the data appear clinically significant (Diamond, 1977a; Gorassini & Spanos, 1986; Spanos, 1986c), the limits of change remain to be established empirically. The basic parameters and key issues of the model are discussed next.

PARAMETERS AND KEY ISSUES

A more extensive perusal of table 1 suggests some areas of contrast between the basic parameters of the cognitive skills model and the more traditional trance model with its emphasis on trance capacity, passivity, involuntary processes, formalized ritual, and the hypnotist's control. Naturally, distinctions made between the two paradigms are established for heuristic purposes, differences are purposefully highlighted, and oversimplification are likely. Nonetheless, rapprochement seems premature and the establishment of reasonable boundaries should further facilitate open and informed inquiry. Distinguishing the models in this way should be seen as an effort towards enhancing clarity and clinical application, rather than another foray into polemics.[4]

TABLE 1
DISTINGUISHING CHARACTERISTICS OF THE TRADITIONAL TRANCE
AND COGNITIVE SKILLS PARADIGMS OF HYPNOSIS

FEATURE	TRADITIONAL PARADIGM	COGNITIVE SKILLS PARADIGM
General Background Features		
1. Descriptive characteristics.	Trance metaphors—e.g., sleep; manhole entering; deepening; entering trance—hypnosis as a *noun*.	Skill-learning and cognitive metaphors—e.g., cognition-strategy; experience; absorption; involvement; choice; practice—hypnosis as a *verb*.
2. Theoretical influences.	Psychodynamic theory; psychoanalytical research—topographical model of consciousness.	Social-learning theory; ego psychological and cognitive theory; existential-humanistic psychology; field systems, and strategic psychotherapy; cognitive-behavioral

FEATURE	TRADITIONAL PARADIGM	COGNITIVE SKILLS PARADIGM
		research—*horizontal* model of consciousness.
3. Methodology.	Introspection; theoretical speculation.	Participant observation; behavior-observation skill; empathic listening.

Phenomenological Experience and Cognitive Processes

4. Alteration of consciousness.	Trance state typically characterized by undimensional *explanatory* construct discussed according to regressive, dissociative, atavistic, and more primitive processes.	Emphasis upon the search for multidimensional *descriptive* constructs describing our varied cognitive perceptual alterations as imaginal, involvement, active imagination, goal-directed fantasy, absorption, dissociation, role enactment, yielding, hemispherical activation, and depotentiating the generalized reality orientation.
5. Mediational processes.	Regressive mechanisms including dissociation.	Cognitive skills and strategies (either within or outside *S*'s awareness) including imagination, enactment, dissociation, distraction, and yielding.
6. Conscious-unconscious distinction.	Unconscious particularly important; conscious emphasis limited to willingness to be hypnotized (otherwise often characterized as stimulation or compliances.)	Conscious choice (to utilize hypnotic skills) emphasized; unconscious refers to processes outside of *S*'s immediate awareness or verbal-labeling mechanisms that contribute to hypnotic experience.

FEATURE	TRADITIONAL PARADIGM	COGNITIVE SKILLS PARADIGM
7. Activity level of *S*.	Passivity (particularly cognitive passivity) encouraged.	More active, creative cognitive processes emphasized (frequently concomitant with bodily relaxation and nonlinear informational processing).
8. Voluntary-involuntary distinction.	Involuntary processes and experiences (i.e., automatisms) are stressed.	Interplay stressed between voluntary activation (of hypnotic skills) and experienced involuntariness (i.e., automatisms).
9. Role of choice.	Not necessarily important except to commence hypnosis.	Extremely important throughout hypnotic experiences.
10. Role of cognitive strategies.	Only occasionally employed, e.g., in hypnotic pain control (with only minimal interest in *how* they are generated and *what* they are).	Considered as either devised or implemented (e.g., when provided by the hypnotist) for each hypnotic suggestion (much attention paid to *how* and *what* of them); regarded important to be made explicit.
11. Locus of control.	External, e.g., hypnotist or *S*'s "unconscious"; occasionally internal.	Internal (i.e., *S*'s utilization of hypnotic skills) with or without conscious awareness.
12. Attribution as to agent of change.	Hypnotist to large extent (who hypnotizes *S* for change solutions); self to less consistent extent.	Self (generates change strategies and solutions).
13. Power source for effective hypnosis.	Power more often than not to hypnotist, by virtue of his/her skill as hypnotist or clinical acumen and strategy.	Explicit "power-to-the-person"; person (subject)-centered inasmuch as *S*s actively devise or implement hypnotic skill-based solutions.

FEATURE	TRADITIONAL PARADIGM	COGNITIVE SKILLS PARADIGM

Hypnotic Interactional Processes

14. Role of hypnotic induction.	Formal ritualized induction necessary.	Induction unnecessary; setting events for skills utilization necessary.
15. Role of hypnotist.	Passive, clinical observer and skilled technician.	Active participant observer, employing modeling feedback, shaping, and participation (e.g., mutual hypnosis); creates a "holding environment" for client hypnotic processes.
16. Administration of suggestions.	More authoritative (sometimes permissive).	Permissive (*S* often actively cooperates).
17. Method of suggestion.	Indirect or direct, individualized or nomethetic.	Direct and individualized (idiographic) albeit indirect suggestions used to disinhibit skills.
18. Role of attitude, expectation, and motivation.	Important but regarded as separate from trance ability (and thus, to some extent, artifactual).	Strongly emphasized (and interdependent with cognitive skills).
19. Conceptualizing individual differences in hypnotic responding.	Relatively stable trait of hypnotizability posited (with genetic factor likely).	Social learning history and environment interacting with person (n.b.: reciprocal determinism) to produce complex response system and individual differences in requisite skills.
20. Issue of modification of hypnotizability.	Only minor, more situational variations considered possible (inasmuch as trait is quite stable).	Significant modifications can occur as a result of training and reinforcement in cognitive skills.

FEATURE	TRADITIONAL PARADIGM	COGNITIVE SKILLS PARADIGM
21. Differentiating refractory from more responsive and "virtuoso" *S*s.	Qualitative differences posited, "virtuosos" often regarded as unique (and possessing extraordinary abilities).	Differences conceptualized according to developmental deficits or enrichment in requisite cognitive skills—deficit amelioration possible with appropriate (and sometimes extensive) training; "virtuosos" regarded as developed primarily by identical processes of learning.

Application

FEATURE	TRADITIONAL PARADIGM	COGNITIVE SKILLS PARADIGM
22. Goals.	Varied depending upon the clinician's theoretical orientation, but essentially oriented toward eliciting particular experiences in response to suggestion.	Varied according to clinician's theoretical orientation, albeit distinguished by emphasis on learning to develop cognitive strategies useful outside the therapeutic context.
23. Type of learning.	Generally, stimulus specific within therapeutic context.	Emphasis on "learning to learn"; creating of client as self-therapist.
24. Type of client-therapist relationship.	Traditional, more authoritative based upon therapist orientation.	Interactive, more cooperative according to client needs and frame of reference.
25. Role of diagnosis.	Utilized in gross fashion with some contraindictions for more extreme psychopathology; motivation and hypnotizability assessed initially and thereafter assumed relatively stable.	Extremely important in terms of nature of pathology, motivation, and hypnotic skills, all of which may vary during treatment and which dictate differential hypnotic intervention strategies.

FEATURE	TRADITIONAL PARADIGM	COGNITIVE SKILLS PARADIGM
26. Clinical interventions.	Varied with no particular emphasis on client's subsequent understanding or utilization of therapist's technique; influence may be direct or indirect.	Broad-based approach emphasizing client understanding and utilization of therapist technique, albeit according to client's frame of reference; influence either direct or indirect but latter procedures are to be brought under client self-control.

Treatment and Long-term effects

27. Role of generalization, transference, and maintenance.	Not necessarily focused upon; self-hypnosis occasionally taught in order to facilitate these effects.	Made explicit and strongly emphasized in conjunction with practice in requisite cognitive skills.
28. Relationship to self-hypnosis.	Indirect relationship—self-hypnosis typically taught after hetero-hypnosis.	Directly linked as self-hypnosis trained as cognitive skills are facilitated; self-hypnosis frequently taught prior to heterohypnosis.

Self-Cognition

29. Relationship to self-control.	No necessary relationhip (and can indirectly foster dependency).	Directly linked—parameters are of a self-control nature (and thus clear-cut implications for the development of self-control, mastery, and competence).
30. Relationship to self-esteem.	No necessary relationship (albeit most hypnotists attempt to increase S's sense of well-being).	Direct in that it provides a basis for S's experiences of mastery, competence, and creativity in the psychological domain.

The table attempts to differentiate the cognitive skills paradigm, from the more traditional model across a number of features in hypnosis. The reader will notice that the first two features highlighting *descriptive metaphors* and *major theoretical influences* were briefly mentioned in the introductory section. The third feature concerning *investigative methodology* stresses the role of empathic listening and participant as well as behavioral observation skills in the emerging paradigm. There are five additional dimensions of the model that will be discussed more thoroughly and considered according to the parameters presented in table 1. These are (1) *phenomenological experience and cognitive processes;* (2) *hypnotic interactional processes;* (3) *applications;* (4) *treatment and long-term effects;* and (5) *self-cognition.*

PHENOMENOLOGICAL EXPERIENCE AND COGNITIVE PROCESSES

The key to understanding both hypnosis, and the basis of the proposed model, is an appreciation for the subjective experience of the hypnotized person. The level of abstraction and inference here is somewhat more molecular and thus oriented toward discovering the specific cognitive processes used to experience hypnosis. Thus, in contrast to the more Aristotelian-dominated logic of intro-spective, analytic psychology, the emerging paradigm is characterized by a more process-oriented phenomenological orientation to the hypnotic experience. The key phenomenological and cognitive features can be seen in table 1 by reference to points 4-13. Hypnosis is characterized as an experience associated with specific cognitive and behavioral patterns primarily under the S's volitional control rather than as a "place" (the trance) that S enters. It is not a matter of the hypnotist's creativity and artistry except in the sense that the hypnotist creates the appropriate conditions for the S to utilize his/her own skills. Nor is it the result of mysterious, unknown, unconscious, or even "mystical" powers lying somewhere within the S. Consistent with an existential position, choice lies with the S to the extent that (s)he is willing to accept that assumption. Of course, psychodynamic fac-tors may reduce the likelihood of such acceptance among certain individuals. There is, however, considerable freedom to modify internal as well as external behavior, and the locus of control is posited to rest with the S. The experience is primarily self-produced within the limits of what Bandura (1978) calls naturally occurring reciprocal determinism.

The skillful hypnotist can no longer assume the S to be a passive, receptive organism during the hypnotic trance, prepared to imagine and enact suggestions in an automatic fashion. In contrast, the model focuses on what the S does internally in response to a suggestion, with a particular emphasis on the kinds of translations and embellishments that occur (cf. Sheehan & McConkey, 1982). The S is viewed as cognitively active, even though his or her phenomenological experience may be one of tranquillity and passivity. Moreover, at any given moment the S may or may not be aware of the internal activities (s)he is invok-ing. Splitting and/or other dissociative processes may occur throughout hyp-notic experiencing, albeit such activity can be partly available in a conscious fashion (Beahrs, 1982; Hilgard, 1977; Watkins & Watkins, 1979). Such cognitive activity is believed to occur irrespective of the direct or indirect nature of the suggestion and whether or not the suggestion explicitly delineates a strategy for responding (e.g., Barber et al., 1980; Spanos et al., 1977).

The existence of perceptual alterations in hypnosis representing varied states of consciousness is no longer an issue. A more difficult matter is generating some sort of descriptive analysis of what is involved in this alteration of consciousness. The experience is certainly multidimensional (Hilgard, 1965; Weitzenhoffer, 1963), and yet some continue to search for a unidimensional explanatory mechanism. There are however some very useful metaphors employed to describe the alternate states of consciousness that are congruent with cognitive skill theory. They include Shor's (1959) notion of fading or depotentiation of the "generalized reality orientation, "Hilgard's (1977) neo-dissociation, Miller, Galanter, and Pribram's (1960) activation of more receptive or passive modes of information processing (e.g., releasing the "planning function"), Fromm's (1977) utilization of primary processes, Deikman's (1966) deautomization of ordinary cognitive processes, and Reyher's (1977) disengaging or suspending left-hemispherical information processing or, alternatively, engaging the analogic-synthetic mode of the right hemisphere. Nevertheless, these concepts remain global and, at best, characteristic of the "map" rather than the "territory."

In the cognitive skills model, the emphasis remains on what the S actually does experientially to alter consciousness. Thus, starting from the individual's *choice* to alter perceptual experience, the investigator must follow the S's experience in an ideographic fashion in order to determine precisely what cognitive skills need to be employed. Attention may then be paid to such cognitive processes as imagination, enactment, dissociation, distraction, and yielding to determine their role in producing the experience of trance.

Traditionally, the cognitive processes involved in hypnosis have been characterized according to the psychoanalytic construct of regression. Others have argued that these mechanisms are more transpersonal or transcendental than regressive (Welwood, 1979). Perhaps the difference is more one of language than experience and reflects separate biases of Western- and Eastern-oriented psychologies. At any rate, the cognitive skills involved in hypnosis do seem to be characterized primarily by the experience of "allowing," "yielding," or "letting go" (cf. Fromm, Brown, Hurt, Oberlander, Boxer & Pfeifer, 1981) and may be more congruent with triphasic rather than bimodal models of consciousness (Wilber, 1980).[5]

Though it may seem paradoxical, choice (i.e., self-control) and cognitive skills appear necessary to produce alterations in consciousness that are experienced as more flowing, spontaneous, receptive, yielding, and/or unconscious. As the gestalt therapists remind us, changes occur in a paradoxical fashion (Beisser, 1970). Thus, it is not surprising that the sense of "letting go" in hypnosis follows the S's choice to abandon efforts to experience what he or she would like to experience and simply to attempt to experience what (s)he is experiencing. An analogy might be drawn to the Eastern-dominated disciplines of aikido, jujitsu, meditation, yoga, and tantric sex in which focused concentration precedes or is associated with letting go. Related self-initiated altered states of consciousness apparently occur in our Western approach to jogging, "inner" tennis, sensate focusing, and the forementioned activities of reading, movie viewing, and dramatic acting. Shapiro (1978) has attempted to integrate the techniques of Eastern spiritual disciplines with Western psychotherapy and behavior modification. He regards the skill of *letting go* as frequently being "a conscious choice" and, paradoxically, "the ultimate in self-control."

The issue of the voluntary-involuntary nature of hypnotic experience remains a controversial one and plays a crucial role in the cognitive skills approach. The latter model is characterized by an emphasis on the continual and frequently quite subtle interplay between voluntary and involuntary behavior. Thus, hypnosis is viewed as neither a passive, involuntary experience (e.g., in the early traditional trance notions), nor simply as a consciously directed set of imaginings (e.g., Barber, 1969). Thus, consistent with writers from Bernheim (1889) and White (1941) to Coe (1978), Weitzenhoffer (1980), and Sheehan and McConkey (1982), hypnosis is viewed as a mixture of conscious voluntary elaborations (i.e., "doings") and automatisms, "happenings" or acts that do not involve higher cortical processes, volition, and/or the so-called "executive apparatus of the ego" (Weitzenhoffer, 1963). However, earlier writers have invariably adopted a topographical model (witness terms like "higher," "executive," etc.) to convey the nature of the distinction. The cognitive skills approach is based largely on a more horizontal view of such processes and is most consistent with Hilgard's (1977) experimental data and Watkins & Watkins's (1980) as well as Beahrs's (1982) clinical observations of partial dissociations in consciousness. Thus for example, even a profound experience of hypnotic amnesia involves some voluntary activity on the part of the *S* (Hilgard, 1977). The degree of experienced voluntariness varies considerably between and within *S*s according to the type of suggestion (cf. Spanos et al., 1977). The evidence indicates that even the most hypnotizable *S*s (experiencing hypnotic analgesia) "implemented in their own ways the suggestions given by the hypnotist" (Hilgard, 1977). The *S*'s inability to tell us how (s)he accomplished a particular hypnotic suggestion can no longer be accepted as "prima facie" evidence that (s)he is inactive in the process. Thus *S*s are both *active* and *passive-receptive, voluntary* and *involuntary* during hypnosis.

It is also the case that an experienced involuntariness is a frequent concomitant of much self-generated activity. It may be that *S*s differ considerably in the extent to which they experience (and/or label) their hypnotic responses as voluntary. Researchers operating from quite varied theoretical sets (e.g., Coe, 1978; Hilgard & Hilgard, 1975) have independently suggested that even highly hynotizable *S*s may describe their experiences primarily from a voluntary perspective (i.e., hypnosis as a "doing") or, alternatively, describe them according to more involuntary processes (i.e., as a "happening"). Radtke & Spanos (1981) have offered an attributional account of hypnotic experiences as influenced by contextual factors. The cognitive skills approach offers a congruent method for discerning the basis of these subjective experiences. It may well be that while the phenomenologically occurring events are essentially similar, *S*s may differ in the ability to *observe* their cognitive processes and, in turn, to *discriminate*, *utilize,* and *report* such activities. The cognitive skills model suggests that individuals particularly skilled in these self-control, introspective abilities are more likely to report hypnosis as a series of "doings." Thus, individuals evidencing hysteric symptomatology and who are more likely to show up in psychiatric settings as high hypnotizables (cf. Frankel, 1976; Spiegel & Spiegel, 1978) may skew the distribution toward "involuntariness" by virtue of their lack of well-developed introspective abilities across a wide range of their functioning. The growing psychological sophistication of our society at large may be consistent with the increasing tendency to respond favorably to the self-generated, subject-centered approach to hypnosis and even, perhaps, to consider self-hypnosis as the basis for all hypnosis (Barber, 1985; Ruch, 1975). It remains an important empirical matter, however, to determine the precise extent to which one experiences hypnosis as involuntary.

In addition, it is clinically useful to determine the implications of the skills model for more dependent, passive *S*s expecting to be "put into a trance." In practice, consistent with an ideographic approach, my own inclination with such clients is to employ more traditional interventions in order to maximize short-term beneficial effects of hypnosis. However, the procedures of the skills model have not been demonstrated to detract from the qualitative experience of "involuntariness." It may be that the mediational skills and strategies that are employed become more automatic and spontaneous (and thus apparently involuntary) as they are well learned and established.[6] In addition, for reasons still unclear, some *S*s do require ritualistic trance induction in order to utilize the necessary skills, and there is evidence that traditional inductions facilitate responding to hypnotist-centered test suggestions (Barber et al., 1980; Katz & Crawford, 1978). The skills model predicts that the relaxation accompanying traditional trance-induction facilitates cognitive skill usage for certain *S*s, which then enhances subsequent responsivity. Thus, the importance of mediational skills is emphasized in contrast to traditional explanations that emphasize the activation of primary process.

THE INTERACTIONAL PROCESS IN HYPNOSIS

The cognitive skills model is distinguished by its emphasis on the lack of a formalized *hypnotic induction* ritual, the more *permissive,* cooperative, and nonauthoritarian orientation, and the *individualized,* idiographic, and *actively participatory* approach to induction, suggestion, and training in cooperation with the *S*. These features are highlighted in points 14-16 of table 1. The therapeutic alliance between the subject and hypnotist is considered a critical variable in maximizing responsivity by lessening the potentially threatening nature of hypnotic experiences. Thus, trust and rapport are essential, and the technological approach to hypnosis is specifically disavowed (cf. Diamond, 1984, 1987). The induction within the skills model is construed as "setting the stage" for *S*'s utilization of the requisite cognitive skills and thus need not contain the more ritualistic and formalized behaviors of traditional "trancing." An experientially rich description, and yet more parsimonious metaphor, derives from the British Object Relations School of psychoanalysis and is termed "the holding environment" (Winnicott, 1965). This is most applicable to the hypnotic environment wherein the patient/subject can feel sufficiently safe (i.e., "held") to allow the requisite therapeutic regression (i.e., internal processes) to occur. Permissive or naturalistic hypnotic inductions appear particularly effective with so-called "resistant" subjects unresponsive to more authoritarian suggestions (J. Barber, 1980). Thus, useful inductions frequently require no more than an invitation by the trusted hypnotist that the S give him or herself "permission" to utilize hypnotic skills in combination with, for example, eye closure or bodily relaxation. Traditionally, the hypnotist was viewed as doing something to the S (i.e., "entrancing"). This influence of the authoritarian and more Mesmeric-like conception continued to plague hypnosis until more recently when the pendulum swung in the opposite direction, perhaps to an extreme as witnessed in Barber's early work (1969; Barber et al., 1974). Today we see that both the S and the hypnotist are viewed as playing a major role in the interactive hypnotic experience (Diamond, 1984, 1987).

The cognitive skills approach is unique however in its emphasis on the role played by the hypnotist as model for the requisite hypnotic skills. The role of client feedback here thus becomes pivotal. An innovative clinical application deriving from this model may be seen in the use of a variant of "mutual hypnosis" in the form of the "client-as-hypnotist" (Diamond, 1980, 1983). Additional interesting experimental uses of the hypnotist-as-a-model have been reported elsewhere (Diamond, 1972, 1974; DeStefano, 1977; Katz, 1979), while Diamond (1980, 1983) reviewed its clinical uses.

A number of requisite social psychological factors, including the S's *attitudes, expectations,* and *motivation* as well as environmental and ecological variables, are construed as strongly related to the hypnotic experience by virtue of the reciprocal, interactive nature of cognition, personality, and situation (see point 17; cf. Barber et al., 1974; Coe & Sarbin, 1977; Sarbin & Coe, 1972; Spanos, 1982a). In addition *individual differences* in hypnotizability, differentiating the so-called *"refractory" from the "virtuoso,"* and the *issue of modifying* hypnotizability also relate to the interactional framework of the model (see points 18-21). Individual differences are seen as essentially a matter of varied learning experiences leading to differential cognitive skill development so that refractory Ss are differentiated from virtuosos by developmental learning deficits rather than postulated traits. Thus, modification of hypnotizability is conceptualized as real (rather than spurious) and as meaningful in that training facilitates the development of the necessary cognitive abilities.[7] The upper limits of such training are unknown and do require investigation (Diamond, 1977a, 1977b). The role of "critical periods" and cognitive maturational factors would seem important in understanding the limits that might emerge. Nonetheless, trait conceptualizations appear less useful than social learning principles within the skills model.

APPLICATIONS

It is in the area of applications that the unique features of the cognitive skills approach, as depicted in points 22-26, are most likely to stand out. Traditionally, hypnotic suggestions are administered in a more authoritative fashion to a *S* said to be in a trance. The *S* then either does or does not respond experientially and/or behaviorally to the suggestion and is regarded to be hypnotized based on some sort of estimation of his/her response. (See, Tellegen, 1978-79, for an excellent discussion of the variety of methods for assessing hypnotizability.)

These trance-based approaches are typically characterized by a lack of attention paid to devising strategies geared toward enhancing the *S*'s experience of the suggestion. It is the cognitive skills model, used in a "naturalistic" fashion, that is unique in its emphasis on explicit strategy formation in the clinical hypnotic context (cf. Araoz, 1985; J. Barber, 1980; Barber, 1985). Moreover, consistent with the person-centered approach, the model typically relies on permissive suggestions describing alternative response possibilities. The client is encouraged to give as much feedback as possible to the hypnotist about the hypnotic experience in order that ego-syntonic cognitive strategies may be devised and used in treatment. The emphasis herein then is more on learning to *respond in hypnotic ways* than on generating *particular responses* to hypnotic suggestions.

The clinician using hypnosis within this new framework must establish an atmosphere where the client can learn how to utilize his/her cognitive skills toward the realization of everyday goals. As in all hypnotherapy, the goals may range from the most circumscribed behavioral or symptomatic to more global, open-ended ones. Irrespective of the clinical goal, the therapist will be concerned with helping the client use cognitive strategies and skills to reach his/her destination (cf. Barber, 1985). Depending on the goal, the hypnotherapist may utilize *direct instruction of a verbal-explanatory sort* (e.g., "In order to experience yourself at that party of fifteen years ago, you may start by picturing your girlfriend, then smelling the burning wood of Vermont, and next, letting yourself imagine that a part of you can travel backwards in time while the critical part of your mind simply watches the experience without needing to interfere for now . . .") *modeling* (e.g., "Watch how I allow myself now to just close my eyes, relax my body, pretend I'm going to pump warm air into my right arm with each breath, and just allow my thoughts to drift by without holding on to any one in particular as I . . ."); *encouragement of client cognitive strategizing* (e.g., "How might you experience yourself as partly in this chair and partly outside jogging?" with the hypnotherapist then using the client's response to further develop the appropriate hypnotic strategy); and; more *indirect strategic interventions* that may evoke useful cognitive skills that otherwise might be inhibited by more direct, verbal, and consciously oriented methods. In this last approach, in addition to the use of such indirect strategic methods (perhaps best represented in the work of Erickson), the cognitive skills-oriented clinician will attempt to facilitate the client's bringing the skill under volitional control. For example, the cognitive skills clinician may use an Ericksonian method such as confusion or the "My friend John" technique (Haley, 1967) to first evoke the skill of "trusting the unconscious," but unlike, certain non-skill-oriented applications of these procedures (e.g., Bandler & Grinder, 1975; Grinder et al., 1977), would then work to insure that the client had learned to use this cognitive skill independent of any charismatic teacher or creative heterohypnotic intervention. Practically speaking then, the *S* might be invited to reexperience the "confusion" state (or whatever the *S* may identify it as) using his/her own strategies and may subsequently utilize these cognitive processes (which may be experienced as "a certain kind of trance," "a letting go," or perhaps "when I trust my unconsious") as befits his/her needs.

The key is for the client and hypnotist to work together in order to best restructure the situation, using the appropriate cognitive skills, in order to optimally fit the client's needs. The role of diagnosis in terms of psychopathology and particular cognitive defensive style, motivation to use hypnotic skills, and hypnotic skill abilities is thus essential to appropriate hypnotic intervention. A variety of cognitive strategies may then be utilized (i.e., following diagnosis), including focused imagining, distraction, thinking with, displacement, dissociation, yielding, and reframing. Clinical techniques borrowed from imaginally oriented therapies (e.g., guided fantasy, focusing, gestalt procedures, active imagination), from cognitive behavioral (e.g., covert conditioning, thought-stopping, stress inoculation, cognitive restructuring) and from traditional hypnotherapy (e.g., Erickson-like indirect procedures, affect bridges, direct suggestions, hyperempiria) are all useful when integrated in this fashion. In addition, the work of the cognitive behavior modifiers, including Bandura (1977), Beck (1976), Lazarus (1971), Mahoney & Thoresen (1974), Meichbaum (1977), and Mischel (1968), has been useful in translating principles of learning and motivation into the cognitive experiential domain. Finally, innovations offered by the cognitive training strategies of Barber (Barber et al., 1974; Barber & Wilson, 1977; Wilson & Barber, 1978), Spanos (1971; Gorassini & Spanos, 1986; Spanos & Barber, 1972), Katz (1979), Diamond (1972, 1977a, 1977b), and Sachs (Sachs & Anderson, 1967; Kinney & Sachs, 1974), as well as the clinical procedures of Araoz (1982; 1985) and Barber (1985), suggest further applied interventions.

TREATMENT AND LONG-TERM EFFECTS

Additional key features within the proposed model (see points 27-28) pertain to the more explicit role of *generalization, transference,* and *maintenance* effects of treatment. The emphasis placed upon the self-generated and, subsequently, self-controllable aspects of hypnotic experiences, as well as the direct link with self-hypnosis, implies an increase in the likelihood for maintenance and ultimately internalization of the therapeutic learnings. This is suggested by the fact that the client is taught to recognize, develop, and utilize the necessary cognitive skills, with emphasis placed on employing them outside the formally defined hypnotic setting. Thus, for example, a client trained in migraine control might employ similar cognitive skills in the dentist's chair or at a tense family gathering. The *S* is encouraged to practice these skills that become defined as self-hypnotic skills. In effect, self-control is what the *S* learns, developing his or her own ability to experience hypnosis by choice, initiative, and skill. Empirical data are necessary, however, to substantiate these speculations.

SELF-COGNITION

Finally, the cognitive skills model has direct implications for various cognitions concerning one's *self* (see points 29-30). It would seem that the *S*'s feelings of positive *self-esteem* are directly encouraged because the cognitive skill utilization provides experiences in creativity, self-efficacy. mastery, and competence. As Frank and his colleagues (Frank, Hoehn-Saric, Imber, Liberman & Stone, 1978) pointed out, experiences of competence are crucial in any successful psychotherapeutic or change process. Others have stressed the value of personal mastery in hypnotherapy (Barber, 1985; Frankel, 1976; Gardner, 1976; Kir-Stimon, 1978). Katz (1978: Katz & Crawford, 1978) indeed demonstrated increases in perceived *self-control* when the model is applied, while Diamond (1980) presented several case studies employing the client-as-hypnotist method and suggesting that heightened feelings of *self-worth* and esteem followed its use. It is quite likely that a therapeutic framework encouraging autonomy, competence, internal locus of control and self-determination will prove particularly valuable in a contemporary Western culture so characterized by self-disorders (cf. Kohut, 1977).

CONCLUSION

A cognitive-based model of clinical hypnosis, termed the cognitive skills model, has been presented as an alternative to the more traditional trance model. Learned, cognitive behavior and modifiable skills have been stressed in a discussion of the key parameters of the model. The importance of a *S*'s cognitive skills are differentially emphasized by various practitioners and researchers, and in turn, hypnotic suggestions and techniques are frequently *not* matched to the *S*'s specific cognitive strengths. It is the author's hope that this chapter will contribute to a more precise assessment of cognitive hypnotic skills and, concomitantly, a more collaborative and systematic effort to employ hypnosis in ways that are sensitive to the unique hypnotic talents of both our experimental subjects and clinical patients.

NOTES

1. The author wishes to thank Daniel Araoz, Michael Bond, Jean Holroyd, Norman Katz, Jerrold Shapiro, and Donald Stolar for their constructive comments on an earlier version of this article. In addition, I am grateful for the collaborative efforts of Norman Katz, with whom I have

developed the clinical foundation of this model in an ongoing series of clinically oriented workshops. A portion of this paper was presented at the Annual Meeting of the American Psychological Association, Toronto, 1978.

2. For our purposes the term "unconscious" is used descriptively to refer to processes going on outside conscious awareness; there is no implied psychoanalytic connotation (cf. Shevrin & Dickman, 1980; also, Hilgard, 1977).

3. Studies of hemispheric specialization indicate shifts in cortical activation from the left to the right hemisphere when hypnotizable individuals enter hypnosis (Graham & Pernicano, 1979; MacLeod-Morgan & Lack, 1982).

4. It may be noted that an alternative approach that is beyond the purview of this paper is represented in the work of Milton H. Erickson (e.g., Bandler & Grinder, 1975; Erickson, 1980; Erickson & Rossi, 1977; Erickson et al., 1976; Grinder, DeLozier & Bandler, 1977; Haley, 1967). However, the distinguishing features of this latter approach are not readily classified in either paradigm and, in fact frequently represent a compromise between the two. In my view, familiarity with the parameters of both the traditional and cognitive skills model enhances the understanding and utilization of Erickson's so-called "strategic model" (Haley, 1973).

5. Bimodal models differentiate egoic from nonegoic modes of experiencing whereas triphasic model distinguish between pre-egoic, egoic, and transegoic experiencing modes.

6. The specific cognitive skills and strategies will not be discussed here. The interested reader is referred to Barber & Wilson (1977), Barber et al. (1974), Diamond (1977a), Gorassini & Spanos (1986), Katz (1979a), and Spanos & Barber (1972) for a perusal of several specific strategies proven effective. In addition, Shapiro (1978) presents a series of innovative strategies combining cognitive dimensions of both Eastern spiritual disciplines and Western psychotherapy.

7. Katz (1978) has suggested that the use of the term susceptibility might be replaced by discussing "hypnotic skills."

17

The Construction and Reconstruction of Hypnosis*

Theodore R. Sarbin

The contributors to this book share a common metapsychology. Unlike the heirs of Mesmer and Charcot, they take as their point of departure the axiom that human beings are intentional, goal-seeking agents. This axiom includes persons who serve as subjects in hypnosis experiments and persons who are clients in psychotherapeutic encounters.

The adoption of this metapsychology has opened the door to skepticism about traditional theories of hypnosis that postulate a special state of mind—a postulate that in earlier times satisfied the mystery requirements of romantic descriptions of human conduct. The history of hypnosis is replete with theories that regard the person as an inert organism, passively and mechanically exhibiting behavior that is qualitatively discontinuous from everyday behavior. The claim that hypnosis is a special state of the organism has had popular ratification in imaginative novels and films, comic cartoons, the media attention given to reports from police interrogators, the case reports of clinical practitioners, and by *ex cathedra* pronouncements from respectable scientists. If ever there were an entrenched paradigm in the human sciences, hypnosis as a special state of the organism would qualify as a prime exemplar.

The long-lasting debate about the nature of hypnosis is informed by the arguments made by Thomas Kuhn in his seminal book, *The Structure of Scientific Revolutions* (1962). His thesis that science is a social enterprise that follows normative rules has been widely adopted. From an axiomatic framework, scientists—often unwittingly—follow a pattern, both in their theory construction and in their experiments. The pattern of scientific activities takes on the characteristics of a set of rules. Over time, to accommodate findings that are contrary to existing

*This chapter is an updated and extended version of an invited address delivered to Division 30, American Psychological Association, Los Angeles, California, August 1981.

theories, scientists are compelled to add categories to the framework. At some point, critical scientists recognize that the paradigm has become too cumbersome, has lost its elegance, and fails to provide interesting hypotheses. When a paradigm no longer stimulates convincing explanations, a new paradigm takes over. Introducing fresh metaphors, nonconforming scientists carry on their experiments and observations without depending on the traditional categories.

Some writers challenged Kuhn's use of the metaphor of revolution, and in a later edition of his book, Kuhn assented to the evolutionary nature of some scientific enterprises. Whether paradigms shift suddenly or slowly, it is clear that the beliefs that guide the work of scientists are resistant to change. Even when faced with acceptably valid observatons that challenge conventional theory, scientists have been creative in inventing explanations to sustain the life of the paradigm to which they owe allegiance.

Born during the historical period when the rationality rules of science were gradually displacing theological explanations, the study of hypnosis became the province of healers, primarily physicians. Influenced by the causality requirements of science, physicians of the eighteenth and nineteenth centuries subscribed to the prevailing ideology that the universe was a giant clockwork machine. A corollary to the ideology was reflected in the slogan that "man is a machine," a corollary that directed physicians to look for cause-and-effect sequences within the body.

Even a casual acquaintance with the history of hypnosis theories would demonstrate the overriding presence of the mechanistic conception of life. Because of the uncritical assumption of the equivalence of brain and mind, nineteenth-century physicians employed mechanistic conceptions in their efforts to uncover cause-and-effect sequences within the immaterial mind. Although the search for causes within the body has not been entirely abandoned (see, for example, Spiegel and Spiegel 1978), the search for connections within the mental apparatus is still with us (see, for example, Hilgard, 1977).

We must not lose sight of the fact that the prevailing theories in the discipline of psychology have not rejected the category of mentalistic determinants. Although psychologists are now the most visible theorists, many of them continue to be influenced by the paradigm laid down by their medical forerunners. In this respect, the traditional study of hypnosis shares the mentalistic paradigm of a large majority of contemporary psychologists—that human conduct is a function of internal forces.

Restricting our discussion now to hypnosis theories, what are the observations and arguments that challenge the conventional paradigm?

The answer to this question requires that we turn out attention to the first series of controlled experiments in the study of hypnosis. In the 1920s and early 1930s, Clark Hull and his graduate students carried out a series of laboratory experiments designed to uncover the mysteries of hypnosis. Unlike most of the prior literature that was anecdotal, Hull's research made use of control subjects, using the stimulus response format in designing the experiments. He reported the research in a now-seldom-cited book, *Hypnosis and Suggestibility* (1933).

In his conclusion, perhaps unwittingly, he shifted from explaining hypnosis as habit phenomena to prestige suggestion as the focal variable. Although prestige suggestion was not defined nor further developed as an explanatory concept, it is patently a concept drawn from observations of social life. Although Hull's work in no way sounded the death knell of the mechanistic search for causes, his ultimate use of a social psychological explanation departed radically from the behaviorist orientation of his work and helped open the way for a new framework.

Although not without precedent, in my early writings I pointed to the well-known observation of individual differences in responsiveness to standard induction procedures as a source of skepticism about the prevailing mechanics of mentalism (Friedlander and Sarbin, 1938; Sarbin 1943, 1950). I rejected the categories of the mechanistic perspective—a perspective that sometimes formed an uneasy alliance with the alien metaphysic of formism. I questioned the reliance on the ill-defined trance concept as a way of explaining the individual differences that could not be accounted for by mechanistic theories. Rejecting the mechanistic framework, I opted for a social psychological perspective. I saw the actions of the participants in the hypnosis dialogue as a miniature drama, and I presented a preface to a theory that leaned heavily on the concept of social interaction, communication, and role taking. With this orientation, the focus of study changed radically. Instead of searching for the assumed cause-and-effect relations in the mental apparatus, the focus was the social encounter. Locating hypnosis in the domain of social encounters was a corrective to the decontextualized view of human action so dear to practitioners of the normal science of psychology. Clearly, the observer of social encounters would have a different research agenda from that of an observer trying to uncover forces operating within the psyche. For example, the observer would be guided by such questions as "What is the subject trying to do?" "What is the hypnotist trying to do?" "How do the interactants define their roles?" "What strategies of impression-formation are employed by each interactant?" and so on. The observer of the social encounter is especially sensitive to the premise that people are capable of dramaturgical solutions to ambiguous situations, among them acting "as if," deception, secrets, masking, disattending, and even self-deception (Scheibe, 1979).

The most important conceptual shift centered on the fundamental definition of the person. In traditional mechanistic theorizing, the person is an object or an organism acted upon by forces of various kinds. The responses to these forces are perceived as *happenings*. Such a perception enables the scientist to frame experiments on the model of those conducted in physiological laboratories, such as measuring reaction times in the muscle fibers of decerebrate frogs. In the social psychological perspective, the person is an agent, a doer, a performer. The person does not emit a mechanical set of movements to a given stimulus but engages in intentional acts. Such actions are performed within the constraints imposed by contexts, such as time, place, person, institutional pressures, normative expectations, audience effects, etc. The recognition of such contextual constraints was greatly facilitated by the appearance of Martin Orne's paper on the social psychology of the psychological experiment (1962c). The happening-versus-doing dichotomy is central to the paradigm clash in the study of hypnosis as it is in the study of other forms of human conduct. The history of hypnosis contains repeated references to the so-called classic suggestion effect, the apparent absence of volition in the performances of hypnosis subjects. This apparent lack of agency was not problematic to those scientists and practitioners who subscribed to the mental state theory. Given that the person was regarded as an object or organism, the scientific observer would merely record evidence of purported *happenings* within the organism. It was thus irrelevant to raise the question whether the subject willfully performed a particular action. In the social psychological framework, the interest is in the *doings* of the participants. The classic suggestion effect poses a question: What epistemic, linguistic, or expressive actions does the subject perform to convince the observer (or self) that his/her actions were performed nonvolitionally? Contained in the question is a parallel question: What are the credibility rules of the observer that would lead to the acceptance of the subject's declaration of nonvolition as a valid self-description? A careful reading of published reports makes clear that skeptical observers adopt different credibility rules from credulous observers.

A paradigm shift is accompanied by changes in the language employed to describe phenomena. It has been customary to speak of *susceptibility* to hypnosis—a metaphor consistent with the mental state doctrine. With the recognition that the participants in a hypnosis episode engage in a dialogue, *responsiveness* became the preferred descriptor. Another metaphor, the *depth of hypnosis,* made sense during the period when the older paradigm was unchallenged. Depth as a descriptive metaphor was probably borrowed from the language of anesthesia. Deep anesthesia can be differentiated from superficial anesthesia by appropriate standard tests. The depth of hypnosis metaphor influenced psychologists and their subjects to assimilate hypnosis to anesthesia in the operating room. Under the guidance of the competing social perspective, some of the observations that had been connoted as degrees of depth are more transparently described as *degrees of involvement* in the role of hypnotic subject. The social encounter paradigm calls for assimilating the hypnotizable subject to a dramatic actor highly involved in portraying a particular role.

Our chosen metaphors guide our observations and the structure of our experiments. During the heyday of mentalism, when psychologists tried to emulate the work patterns of physicists and chemists, pivotal metaphors were drawn from telephone and telegraph technology and from the physics of energy. Again, this made sense to mechanistically committed scientists. Nerve trunks were like wires, carrying messages from one place to another. With the recognition of the failure of the mechanistic perspective in the human sciences, metaphors were borrowed from such nontraditional sources as rhetoric, game playing, drama, and textual criticism (Geertz, 1980). These sources have traditionally given privileged status to human beings as doers, as actors intentionally trying to meet their obligations and make good their claims to identity.

One of the ironies of the traditional paradigm with its roots in mechanism and mentalism is the source of a central metaphor, trance. The label "trance" has been employed to identify a purported mental state that is different from other purported mental states. Although widely used to support the doctrine that the subject is the carrier of a happening, "trance" is not drawn from the same sources as other terms in the mechanistic or mentalistic paradigm. The source is romantic poetry, such as when the hero is en*tranced* by the beauty of a fair maiden. The remote etymology of trance is movement from one status to another, as from life to death. It is instructive to note that one of the most significant events that challenged the older paradigm was the recognition of the circularity of the trance concept. Trance was defined as the counterexpectational conduct of the person who responded to the hypnotic induction. When asked how one could account for the counterexpectational conduct, the proponents of the mental state theory would point to the trance as the casual agency. The absurdity of the formula trance = trance was not noticed until critics of the old paradigm called attention to the circularity of employing the same term on both sides of the causality equation.

The traditional mental-state paradigm is in crisis when experimenters unequivocally demonstrate that acts supposedly under control of the hypnotic trance can be performed by unhypnotized, properly motivated subjects; that a special kind of logic—trance logic—is ephemeral; that so-called dissociative phenomena are dramaturgic acts; that manipulated expectations can produce hypnotic-like behavior; that the actions of the subject (and the experimenter) may be felicitously described in the language of strategic interaction, game playing, and dramatism (Spanos & Coe, 1972; Spanos, 1986b).

A discussion of contemporary views of hypnosis as a clash of paradigms leads to the inference that the direction taken by scientists (and others) is influenced by the particular metaphor employed to account for problematic conduct. The obvious historical example is Mesmer, whose theory reflected the then-current interest in magnets. The observation that a magnet could attract iron filings served Mesmer as the ground for a grand metaphor: it is as if human influence is brought about by an invisible force, like mineral magnetism. The "as if" quality of the metaphor was submerged after he and fellow mesmerists asserted that animal magnetism was a unique force, and further, that such a force could be manipulated to influence the status of medical patients.

From Mesmer to the present, observations that today go under the heading "hypnosis" have been the subject of construction and reconstruction. Theorists of all kinds have rendered explanations that centered on the primary observation: the apparent influence of the verbal and gestural behavior of one person on the behavior of another. These theorists tried to make sense out of apparent nonsense, and clarity out of apparent contradiction. As I noted before, under the impetus of the mechanistic metaphysic, statements made in the vocabulary of science displaced earlier statements couched in vocabularies more suited to occult mysteries.

Whether framed by scientists or by ordinary people, explanations are conceptual constructions, the products of problem-solving activities. The form of the construction varies with the information available to the theorist, the prevailing scientific and political climate, and, not least, the pool of potential metaphors available as aids for describing perplexing and counterexpectational conduct. Strands in the texture of explanation are interrelated: for example, if the information available to the scientist included measures of reaction time, the conceptual construction would probably be communicated in the language of neurology, especially if the theorist found the telephone system useful as a model.

The history of hypnosis has been a history of attempts to fashion explanations that made sense of the salient fact: the hypnosis subject or patient engages in public conduct that is *contrary to expectations*. The theorist is not interested in conduct that conforms to expectations. Theories are not created to explain the compliance of the subject to a simple request, such as, "come in and be seated." It is only when the subject performs in counterexpectational ways that the need to explain is activated. The constructional efforts of a theorist are challenged when a person does not recall his or her name, is apparently unable to perform simple motoric acts, or reports being in another place at another time. These are examples of conduct that violate ordinary expectations. We expect as a matter of course that a person will remember his or her name.

The present discussion follows from my earlier efforts to penetrate the vagaries of past and present theories (Sarbin, 1943, 1950, 1962, 1972, 1979, 1984). Parenthetically, since theories of hypnosis and theories of general psychology flow from the same cultural sources, an exploration into the interior of the history of ideas relating to hypnosis may illuminate the history of psychology.

As I mentioned earlier, the machine has been the prevailing metaphor for theorists of hypnosis. At least that part of the history of hypnosis that has been preserved in our libraries shows unmistakably that the root metaphor of the machine generated various clinical and investigative models. The world is a machine and so is man—this was the metaphor that had its modern rebirth in the seventeenth century and reached maturity in the latter half of the nineteenth century. It has served the scientific community in many ways and has been responsible for impressive achievements in the physical and biological sciences. The central category—the transmission of force—was explicit in Mesmer's thesis, in Braid's early physiological theories, and in Charcot's neuropathological formulation. It was implicit in Bernheim's employment of the vaguely defined concept of suggestion.

It is worthy of note that few, if any, psychological constructions based on the principle of mechanistic causality have been self-sustaining. Human beings, whether in the hypnosis experiment or in everyday life, refuse to act exclusively as if they were machines. The record of the past two hundred years makes clear that transmission-of-force theories have failed to account for individual differences in the performance of counterexpectational conduct. When the transmission-of-force theories proved insufficient to account for observations, some theorists borrowed categories from an alternate root metaphor—the root metaphor most often associated with Platonic forms (Pepper, 1942). Trance, hypnotic state, odylic force, and *elan vital* are conceptions that do not accommodate to the requirements of mechanistic science. They belong to the metaphysics of forms, of abstractions, and are not subject to the pulls and pushes that characterize the actions of levers, clocks, engines, nerve fibers, or computers.

Having been nurtured on the ideology of mechanistic science, members of the disciplines that have adopted hypnosis—psychology and medicine—have traveled along a familiar path. They have focused on the subject or patient who has been the target of the hypnotist's attention. Actions of the subject not accounted for by concurrent theory or common sense are singled out for special attention and explanation. Myopically focusing on the subject, in modern times the all-pervasive question has been: What property of the individual was the cause of the counterexpectational behavior? The causality requirement—the quintessential feature of mechanistic science—is taken for granted, and the bounded individual is the locus of interest. Through experiment or other systematic observation, antecedent events (including the hypnotic induction) are partitioned from consequent events, the actions and verbalizations of the subject. When systematic covariation occurs between antecedent and consequent, causality is inferred.

The traditions of the scientific enterprise call for explanations where the antecedent condition, e.g., the induction, does not lead to hypnosis behaviors. In reviewing the history of hypnosis, it is plain that mechanistic theories have been kept alive by invoking categories outside the rules of the transmission-of-force doctrine. Nondemonstrable entities are introduced to mediate between the induction and the performance. As I have already indicated, these entities are illicitly incorporated into theory from the metaphysic of Platonic forms, the most famous of these forms is "trance." It is an embarrassment to trance theorists that the abstraction can be employed only through circular reasoning.

CONTEMPORARY RECONSTRUCTIONS

I have intended the foregoing pages as a framework, a setting to serve as background for contemporary constructions of hypnosis. The recorded history shows that hypnosis has been reconstructed over and over again. This history shows that most of the constructions have leaned on metaphors that served the causality requirement of mechanistic science. In this connection I need but mention the numerous attempts to establish hypnosis as a neurological entity residing within the organism. The imagery stimulated by such metaphors as special nervous pathways, electrochemical forces, vapors, and magnetic fluids helped to place the causal agency inside the person. The actions of the hypnotized person— in these constructions—are *happenings* presumably caused by the electrochemical or electromechanical forces in the nervous system. Illustrative of this type of construction is a report by a prominent team of investigators. On the basis of tenuous relationships between scores on hypnosis scales and preinduction EEG profiles, they concluded that "hypnotic susceptibility is a function of brain physiology" (London, Hart & Leibovitz, 1968). In a replication of the study, Miller (1973) was unable to confirm even the tenuous relationship that served as the basis for the mechanistic construction. Another team of investigators made a similar claim. On the basis of a borderline significant correlation ($r = .27$) between fast EEG waves and a suggestibility scale, Ulett, Akpinar, and Itil (1972) concluded that "hypnosis . . . exists in reality as a phenomenon demonstrable in the physiology . . . of the nervous system." Flaws in experimental design and data interpretation made the conclusion unacceptable (Sarbin, 1973).

During the half-century that I have been working in the field of hypnosis, I have been able to increase my understanding through the employment of metaphors that are remote from neurology and other traditional scientific disciplines. I have turned to the humanities for guiding metaphors. Early I raided the humanistic discipline of theater arts to introduce *role* as the central metaphor.

Prior to my reconstruction of hypnosis as role enactment, I had assimilated from my teachers and from recognized authorities the prevailing notion that hypnosis was a personality trait, possibly related to suggestibility. The locus of causality was inside the subject's head, personality, psyche, or nervous system. The refiguration of the events of the hypnotic scene as role enactment demanded some marked alterations in interpretation. It was but a short step from regarding hypnotic conduct as the performance of a special role to the overarching conception that life is theater. If "all the world's a stage" then auxiliary concepts of the drama could be enlisted to help explain the counterexpectational conduct of hypnosis. Among such concepts are role preparation, rehearsal, acting skill, scripts, audiences, and so on. It is important to note that the same conceptions were fruitfully employed to describe social behavior of all kinds, not only hypnosis (Sarbin, 1954; Sarbin and Allen, 1968). Of central importance, both for social actions generally and for hypnosis particularly, is that the human being is regarded as a doer, a performer, an actor, an agent, not an inert object that passively processes information. This is not the place to spell out the specifics of the role-theoretical constructions of hypnosis or the research that has provided the empirical supports (Sarbin and Lim, 1963; Sarbin and Coe, 1972, 1979). Suffice it to say that the central variable is role enactment. The focus is on what the subject does and how he or she does it, taking into account the context in which the performance occurs.

The dramaturgical perspective has been widely used by literary critics and by sociologists identified as symbolic interactionists. In this perspective, actors not only responded to situations, but also mold and create them. So-called mental processes have no place in the construction of the situation. The actions of the participants define the situation. To the theorist who employs dramaturgical metaphors, the units of interest are not organisms, not individuals, not trait assemblies, but interacting persons in identifiable social contexts. The role theorist, then, is interested in the participation of both the subject and the hypnotist. The interactants are inseparable parts of a dramatic episode, the meaning of the subject's role enactment cannot be studied apart from the meanings the subjects assign to the hypnotist's role enactments. As in any dramatic encounter, the performances of any actor may influence the performances of co-actors as well as audiences.

The development of the role-theoretical conception of hypnosis has been influenced by a readiness to depart from the formist and mechanist metaphysics and, instead, to regard human action as dependent on context. I have written elsewhere of the advantages to human science of adopting the contextualist world view, the root metaphor of which is the historic act in all its complexity. Unlike mechanistic and formist metaphors that emphasize the search for invariant truth, the historic event is subject to change, novelty, and negotiation (Sarbin, 1977).

The initial statement of a construction is hardly ever a complete theory. Clinical observations and empirical findings raise questions not directly considered in the first approximation to theory. For example, in the absence of data to support the notion of a special trait of personality, how should one account for individual differences in hypnotic performance? How should theory deal with the widely recognized observation that the performance of one subject is more convincing than the performance of another? Consider the frequently used finger-interlock test of responsiveness. The responses of subjects to the finger-interlock test may be sorted into three classes: (1) non-compliance, that is, the subject separates the finger; (2) compliance, the subject passively keeps the fingers interlocked; and (3) vigorous effort, the subject tries to unlock the grip without success. From the dramaturgical standpoint, the third is a more *convincing* enactment.

To help understand observations of this kind, I turned to another humanistic discipline, rhetoric. The purpose of rhetoric is to persuade, to convince, to influence belief and action. Although rhetoric is most often defined as the art of using spoken or written language to influence others, it is also employed to denote expressive movements of the body as an accompaniment of speech. Glances, shrugs, gestures, facial movements, jerks, and other bodily actions fall under the rubric of rhetoric—they are involved in persuasive communication. The subject who vigorously tries to separate the interlocked fingers makes the performance more convincing.

Whether the actor is on the professional stage or in the hypnosis laboratory, the rhetoric of role enactment is employed to enhance the actor's credibility. The actor, upon commitment to the performance of a role, engages in expressive conduct to demonstrate that he or she is legitimately entitled to enact the role. This description applies equally to the hypnotist and to the subject. Both engage in rhetorical acts. The task of credibility enhancement falls upon the hypnotist no less than on the subject. Since Mesmer's time, hypnotists have employed linguistic devices, gestures, "passes," costumes, white coats, bedside manners, and even stage props in the service of the rhetoric of role enactment. A moment's reflection on the typical induction procedure makes clear that it is loaded with verbal and phonic rhetoric. The content may be directed to reassurance and rapport building, but the rhetorical style is different from ordinary conversation. The hypnotist may lower the pitch of the voice, speak in a slower tempo than is customary, repeat key words and phrases, and otherwise communicate that his or her occupancy of the status of experimenter or healer is legitimate.

In most theories of hypnosis, the hypnotist's rhetoric of role enactment is given little attention. The rhetorical devices in the induction are more than embellishments, they have communicative goals. Hardly anyone would subscribe to the proposition that oral delivery of certain strings of words as auditory stimuli would have the power to create so-called hallucinations, amnesias, analgesias, and so on. Clearly the strings of words must be assigned meaning before they can function as guides to action. Not to penetrate the meanings of the induction is to treat it as something of a mystery.

To take some of the mystery out of the induction, I borrowed from other humanistic sources, religion and ethnology, the concepts of ritual and ceremony. The structural similarities of the hypnotic induction and the healing rituals of shamans and witch doctors are immediatedly apparent. Both the hypnotist and the shaman apparently follow a prepared script, with only minor deviations from one time to the next. The content and style of ritual performances and ceremonial utterances facilitate the passage from one social status to another and ratify entrances into, and exits from, certain social roles. The hypnotic induction is the formal ceremony that facilitates the entrance of the person into the role of hypnotized subject or patient.

As in all rituals, there are theatrical elements. The induction emphasizes cooperation, and specially chosen words and phrases instruct the subject in bodily relaxation and the promise of a rewarding experience. The ritual behavior of the hypnotist provides the setting for the entrance of the subject into a dramatic encounter, the outcome of which is uncertain but potentially rewarding. It is important to underscore the fact that the induction ceremony emphasizes sleep and relaxation. Edmonston (1981) has argued convincingly that the typical induction is designed to encourage the subject to relax. He claims that the phenomenon of hypnosis would be nonexistent if the subject failed to take the attitude conducive to relaxation. In his extensive review of the literature, Edmonston shows that some minimal, but predictable, physiological changes are to be expected when a person performs the relaxation response (Benson, 1975).

Included in the relaxation response are proprioceptive changes. The subject may monitor these changes and assign meanings to them, meanings that become part of the context when he or she renders a self-report. To be sure, the meanings assigned vary from person to person, depending in part on the subject's concurrent interpretation of the ambiguities in the induction ritual. The interpretation of proprioceptive cues has been shown to be an important element in certain religious rituals of conduct reorganization (Sarbin and Adler, 1971). A sympathetic belief system is a prerequisite for attributing magical implications to proprioceptive cues generated by the relaxation response.

To penetrate further into the communicative aspects of the induction ritual, I turned for help to another humanistic discipline, semiotics. This discipline is ideally suited as a source of hypotheses about the meaning of messages contained in the hypnotic induction. The question to be addressed is: What are the textual features of the induction that influence a subject to engage in conduct that is contrary to expectation? Earlier investigators, unfamiliar with the power of semiotic analysis, cavalierly answered the question by relying on mental state concepts, especially trance.

Semiotics, among other things, is concerned with metaphoric analysis. It is not enough, however, to look for poetic metaphors of the simple kind so often used to illustrate figurative language. For our purposes, we point to the fact that a metaphor has two terms, the figurative and the literal. Further, each term can be expressed or implied. Thus, four classes of metaphor are generated. In the first class, the figurative and the literal are both expressed, e.g., the poet is a nightingale, Richard has the heart of a lion, Jefferson was a giant. In the second class, the literal term is expressed and figurative term is suppressed, as in religious rituals. In the third class, the figurative term is expressed and the literal term is silent, as in proverbs. In the fourth type, neither term is expressed, both must be inferred from the context. Deciphering any metaphor requires cognitive work, and the work increases with the suppression or silencing of the terms. Metaphoric encounters of the fourth kind require the most cognitive work. The listener works to make sense of the intentions of the speaker by entertaining such questions as: Does the speaker mean such-and-such a statement to be taken literally or figuratively? What meanings should I assign to the speaker's utterance? etc.

The hypnosis encounter may be construed as a metaphor of the fourth kind (Sarbin, 1980). The actions of both participants, including their speech acts, follow from the mutual intentions of both parties, and these mutual intentions are tacitly held together in a grand extended metaphor. Both the literal and figurative components of the metaphor are implied and the listener must construct an interpretation. Beginning from the most obvious and unchallenged observation, we recognize that the hypnotist *talks* to the subject. The talk is modulated by rhetorical devices, as mentioned before. In addition to the stylistic shifts, the hypnotist utters declarative sentences. To organize the subject's expectations, he or she makes use of similes and marked metaphors such as "hypnosis is a state of absorbed attention somewhat like that experienced when reading a novel or seeing a movie." More significant is the fact that the hypnotist utters fictional, counterfactual statements such as "your legs are getting heavier," "you are becoming drowsy," "you are drifting away," "you are surrendering your normal state of consciousness." Some inductions even provide epistemological frameworks for the subject such as "your subconscious mind is being activated."

It must be emphasized that the content of the entrance ritual—the induction—includes fictional, contrafactual, and problematic statements such as "your legs are getting heavy" and "you are drifting away." Clearly, the subject is placed in a problematic situation. How does one make sense of these fictional, contrafactual utterances? The subject may engage in an internal dialogue somewhat as follows: "The hypnotist says my legs are getting heavy. My life experiences tell me that body parts don't increase in weight merely because someone says so. Drifting is something that happens in a canoe on the lake, not in a laboratory or clinic." Sense making is called for. If the subject joins his observation that the hypnotist is uttering fictional, contrafactual statements with the observation that the hypnotist has shifted his style of talking, the next step in the silent dialogue would be the semiotic question: "What is the *meaning* of these strange utterances?"

Two possible answers are immediately forthcoming. The first is "the utterances are nonsense, my legs are not getting heavier and I am not drifting." In this case, the interactants have no basis for continuing the encounter. The second answer to the semiotic question might be formulated as follows: "Since the hypnotist is dramatizing his talk to me in telling me things that both of us know are fictional, perhaps he is inviting me to participate in a game of 'let's pretend' and also to pretend that it is serious business." The subject might conclude his silent dialogue with a self-directed statement: "By dramatizing his actions and by uttering fictional, contrary-to-fact statements, the hypnotist is casting me in a role for a theatrical enterprise, a role that calls for *as if* behavior, for actions that help created illusions." Such a conclusion follows from construing the hypnotist's utterances as an extended metaphor of the fourth kind. That is, the subject rejects the literal interpretation of the fictional utterances and instead constructs the figurative interpretation. Having concluded that the messages are not to be taken literally, the subject now has the task of supplying the tacit terms. The hypnotist's talk does not openly direct the subject to enter a metaphorical transaction—the subject must establish the metaphoric meaning from the total context. Another way of describing this sequence is that the participants communicate by indirection. The intent of the grand metaphor is that the two interactants will engage in a miniature drama, each employing his or her skills to follow an unvoiced script.

I want to stress that the overall metaphor contained in the problematic, fictional utterances of the induction invites the subject to participate in a dramaturgical enterprise. If the subject accepts the implied invitation, both interactants will perform to the limit of their skills, neither overtly expressing the literal and figurative terms that make the enterprise a theatrical one. The suppressed metaphor is the same as that contained in much of Shakespeare's work, namely, "all the world's a stage."

Closely related to dramaturgical and semiotic conceptions are those drawn from strategic interaction and game playing. My understanding of hypnosis has been enlarged as a result of employing conceptions enunciated by the late Erving Goffman (1959, 1969) and Karl Scheibe (1979). When the self-reports of hypnosis subjects are taken as data reflecting phenomenal experience, it is in order to consider the possible strategic elements in the form and quality of the reports. Because we now recognize that hypnosis subjects are still social beings capable of managing impressions, it is necessary to examine self-reports contextually.

The self-report is necessarily the datum from which the theorist constructs inferences about the private experience of the subject. Examples of phenomena that depend upon self-report are so-called hallucinations, amnesia, and analgesia. What makes self-report interesting to students of hypnosis is the obvious contrafactual nature of the report. No theory is complete if it cannot account for convincing reports of a nonexistent but bothersome insect, for claims of amnesia for an event that occurred only a minute ago, or assertions of analgesia under ischemia or cold-pressor conditions. To claim that the nonexistent insect is "phenomenally real" to the subject only puts an end to inquiry on how a person can convince self or other of a contrafactual event.

The phenomenal veridicality of contrafactual reports has been a pivotal topic in theoretical debates. Theorists who hold the belief that hypnosis is accompanied by neurological changes or modification in the "psychic apparatus" are comfortable in assuming that the self-report is a veridical reflection of experience. Theorists who are guided by the paradigm that hypnosis is a social encounter look for the influence of social contexts on the self-report. They are sensitive to the possibilities that self-reports that deform consensual or empirical validity may serve strategic goals.

To serve his or her manifold purposes, a person may engage in a variety of strategies, among them masks, mirrors, lies, and secrets (Scheibe, 1979). Aware of these commonplace strategies, the contemporary student of hypnosis will examine the self-report from a perspective that is different from earlier students who had not been exposed to the literature on strategic interaction.

One of the categories of strategic interaction is deception. It is proper for an investigator to entertain the hypothesis that a contrafactual self-report may be a deceptive maneuver. In employing strategic interaction as a framework for reconstructing hypnosis, we begin from the postulate that the subject is not a passive object manipulated by environmental forces but is an active, problem-solving, sense-making, social creature. When the subject utters a self-report, the contemporary investigator asks: "What is the subject doing?" The question is framed in the context of a parallel question: "What is the hypnotist doing?" These questions lead to more detailed queries such as "What are the interactants trying to achieve?" and, narrowing our focus on the subject who utters contra-factual statements, "What strategies of social action and rhetorical communication does the subject employ?"

The posture of asking what the subject is *doing* directs us to the intentions of the subject. If we can infer the subject's intentions, then we can search for the strategies that he or she employs to realize the intentions. In those cases where the subject is trying to ratify his or her role, we can posit the use of various game-playing strategies. We now know that one class of subjects holds the intent to pretend, to create an illusion, to make believe, to deceive. These are subjects who, e.g. first claim amnesia and, later, under pressure for veridicality, breach the amnesia.

Given the clinical or research purposes of most hypnosis settings and the expectation of truth telling, an apparent moral element is introduced when we attribute to subjects the use of deception as a strategy for realizing his or her intentions. However, it is unlikely that either the hypnotist or the subject would employ the attribution "deception" without qualification. The problem for both participants is to neutralize the moral component of deception. Moral neutralization is commonplace in such settings as the theater, stage magic, warfare; competitive sports such as boxing, fencing, and football; in poker and chess;

in practical joking; in fairy tales; and in the exercise of rules of politeness. Deceptions in these contexts are free of moral judgment. It requires no superior epistemic skill to assign the acts of the hypnosis subject to the same class of actions. The neurtralization is enhanced by the hypnotist's assertions of unlabeled fictions, as I discussed earlier. The subject's conferral of legitimate authority on the scientific investigator or the clinical healer facilitates the removal of any moral taint from the intention to deceive.

The person who employs the impression-management strategies to realize his intentions (e.g., to be regarded as a good-natured, cooperative scientific collaborator), then, is like a professional stage actor. The goal is to convince the audience that one is enacting the role sincerely. The impression-management strategy is supported by the rhetoric of role enactment, discussed before. The task of rendering a contrafactual self-report as if it were a true report requires subtle histrionic skills.

The self-reports of all subjects cannot readily be assimilated to the use of strategies of deception. Using amnesia as an example, not all subjects breach when pressured to remember. That is, they claim amnesia and maintain the amnesia. When the conduct of the subjects convinces the experimenter that they *believe* that the self-report "I don't remember" is genuine (not a deception), the strategic game-playing explanation requires supplementation.

The contemporary reconstruction of hypnosis must explain the phenomenon where the subject says "I believe" or otherwise communicates that the contrafactual report reflects a veridical state of affairs, not a fictional one. It has proven unproductive to look for imaginary psychic structures or hypothetical dissociation mechanisms. More continuous with observations is locating the self-report of the subject within the context of his or her metaphysical assumptions. The actions antecedent to a person saying "I believe" involve more than a theatrical performance. Believing is a complex act and involves at least the placing of a value on a proposition. In the case of amnesia, for example, subjects must resolve a paradox. They must confront the fact of two contrary knowings: (1) the recognition that they are engaged in a theatrical enterprise in which the strategy of deception is fostered; (2) holding the belief that deception is an inappropriate or improper strategy. The paradox is resolved through the adoption of an unconventional metaphysical assumption: the suspension of the law of non-contradiction, the rule that something cannot be both *A* and *not-A* at the same time. Although unconventional in most mundane problem-solving situations, the suspension of this rule is not unique to hypnosis. It occurs in other settings, for example, in the creating and telling of fairy tales, in the practice of magic, and in certain theological doctrines.

An apt label for this state of affairs is self-deception. The subject "believes" under belief-adverse circumstances. In order to deceive himself or herself, the actor must be proficient in two epistemic skills, the skill to spell out certain of his engagements with the world, and the skill to not–spell out certain engagements. (For a more detailed account of self-deception see, Sarbin, 1981.)

The incursion into the field of strategic interaction has directed me to employ yet another set of metaphors derived from humanistic sources. It has proven useful to look upon the actions of human beings as conforming to the requirements of self-narratives. The idea of a self-narrative as providing guidelines for action flows from everyday observations. We dream in narrative, our fantasies and daydreams are untold stories, our career plans are stories, we interpret the random movements of geometric figures according to conventional plots (Michotte, [1946] 1963), the sources of meaning for interpreting our lives are stories—myths, parables, morality tales, epics, etc.

When subjects in a hypnosis experiment enter the laboratory they do not deposit their life stories in the vestibule along with their raincoats and hats. One's self-narrative continues to serve as background for interpreting the requirements of the experiment. Individual differences in how persons employ their self-narratives will be reflected in the degree and style of responsiveness to the induction and to subsequent suggestions and commands.

To tell a story or to employ a narrative is to organize the elements of unorganized experience into a coherent account. Our interest is in exploring how a person creates a coherent self-narrative when he or she must assimilate contradictory bits of knowledge such as in the "classic suggestion effect," i.e., the self-report of nonvolition. In the self-report, the subject claims that he or she is not the agent of an action, say, arm levitation. From the perspective of a jury of observers, the disclaimer is false. The contradiction is striking: "I claim not to be the agent of my act" versus "No other person or force moved my arm, therefore I am the agent of my act."

To maintain a coherent self-narrative requires strategic and epistemic skills already identified as deception and self-deception. About half the subjects elect the strategy of deception to maintain a coherent story. These are the subjects who claim nonvolition and under prodding, demands for honesty, and other pressures repudiate the claim to nonvolition. Those subjects who insist on maintaining the contradiction, as I have already indicated, adopt an unconventional metaphysic to keep the story whole. It is as if they say "Although I appear to be the agent, I am not."

Both kinds of subjects construct self-narratives, taking into account the behavior of the experimenter, the setting, the audience, etc. Their self-narratives are different, however, and depend on the differential use of grammatical forms. At one time, the self can be the *author* of action, represented by the pronoun "I," at another time, the self can be the *object* of happenings, represented by the pronoun "me." The focus of an episode in a self-narrative, then, may be on the "I" (author) or on the "me" (the narrative figure, the role being played). The subjects who employ the strategy of deception tell their stories from the perspective of the self-as-author. The self-deception subjects employ their stories differently. The covert story focuses on the "me," the object of action, the narrative figure imaginatively created by the self-as-author. The subject must be skillful in *not spelling out* those engagements that would challenge plausibility and coherence.

In the same way that a person can become deeply involved in the lives of characters in fictional or biographical narratives, so can self-deceptive subjects become deeply involved in the role of narrative figure in their own life stories. In uttering the contrafactual "I did not raise my arm, it just happened to me," the person elides the ongoing social encounter into the plot of his or her self-narrative—the plot in which he or she is the central character. The self-report and the publicly performed actions are directed to the hypnotist or other spectators as audience. The contrafactual self-reports, convincingly given, charter the actor as someone special, as the star of the show, at least as a potential fifteen-minute celebrity. The self-report of nonvolition validates a story in which the subject has entered a magical kingdom of enchantment. (For more elaborated accounts see, Sarbin, 1984, 1986.)

CODA

In the preceding pages, I have tried to show that the field of hypnosis may be described in terms of a paradigm clash. The older theories for the most part have been shown to be inadequate to explain counterexpectational conduct, mainly because the subject or patient had been regarded as a passive entity, mechanistically processing stimulus inputs. The competing viewpoints, well represented in this volume, begin from the postulate that human beings are agents, and that the conduct of hypnosis subjects requires no explanatory categories other than those employed to explain any social encounter

Free from the restrictions of mechanistic models, a sizable body of scholars has been able to engage in the refiguration of the human sciences. We no longer find it necessary to borrow our metaphors from the physical sciences. To help understand hypnosis, I have presented a series of metaphors drawn from humanistic sources that have proven useful in reconstructing hypnosis. The theater, religion and ethnology, rhetoric, semiotics, and narrative have provided metaphors to give body to the observations that make up the corpus of observations that are subsumed under the rubric "hypnosis."

Will the paradigm clash be resolved by the wide acceptance of the social encounter metaphor and the submerging of the special state doctrine? On logical and scientific grounds, one would reply in the affirmative. The chapters in this book would support this affirmation. However, there is more to the social enterprise of science than logic and scientific method. There are political, economic, and institutional factors to consider (Coe, 1987). In some clinical settings and in forensic investigations, practitioners continue to present hypnosis as a special mental state, albeit with a large mystery component. The mass media in general report hypnosis from the standpoint of the conventional paradigm, usually supported by quotations from medical experts. Professional workshops provide training to would-be hypnotists and, for the most part, support the mental state doctrine. These factors, I believe, will continue to reinforce belief in hypnosis as a special mental state and will do little toward changing the public image of hypnosis—an image that has remained fairly constant since Svengali was presented to the book-reading public. For the academic community, on the other hand, the older paradigm has outlived its usefulness. Psychologists and other observers of human action are developing sophisticated methods for understanding counterexpectational conduct. They begin their work from the uncomplicated fact that the hypnotic situation is a social encounter. The paradigm shift, as I indicated before, is not restricted to hypnosis. In the human sciences, the world view that nurtured special state theories—man is a machine—is being displaced by the world view of contextualism, the root metaphor of which is the historic act in all its complexities.

Looking upon hypnosis as a social encounter is but one derivation of the contextualist world view. At the same time that we adopt the social encounter framework to study how persons influence each other (historic acts in miniature), we must be content with pursuing the goal of historians and other humanists, i.e., *understanding*. The twin goals of mechanistic science, prediction and control, are bound to be frustrated when we remind ourselves that the subjects in our experiments are active agents who (like the rest of us) can employ strategic skills to invalidate predictions generated either from fallible theories or from probabilistic outcomes of laboratory studies.

Part Five

Politics and Prospects

18

Hypnosis

The Role of Sociopolitical Factors
in a Paradigm Clash

William C. Coe

Hypnosis has characteristically been associated with the mystical, the strange, the unusual and the dramatic. The mass media and popular literature nearly always report hypnotic experiences as the ultimate of wonderment—the dramatic cure, the multiple personality, or the powerful influence of the hypnotist. From the mesmerizer of the eighteenth century to the stage hypnotist of the present, the lay public has been exposed to hypnosis as a phenomenon of power and influence. The more conservative views of hypnosis, although present since its beginnings, have been given scant attention. In recent times hypnosis is being viewed increasingly as a legitimate therapeutic tool in medicine, dentistry, and psychotherapy. Less dramatic expectations are replacing the overstated ones, but an aura of mystery and sensationalism often remains. Unfortunately, the image of hypnosis as mysterious has caused some practitioners to avoid its use, and persons who might benefit from it to shy away. This same aura, on the other hand, opens the practice of hypnotism to otherwise unqualified persons who take advantage of people looking for an instant cure.[1]

From Kuhn's framework of the evolution of science, the special process view of hypnosis holds the position of the "traditional paradigm" (Kuhn, 1962, 1970). Normal science concerns itself with the elaboration and extension of traditional paradigms. As science continues, a second phase of activity emerges with the appearance of a "new paradigm." The new paradigm requires a reconstruction of traditional theory, a reevaluation of empirical findings, and a redefinition of admissible problems.

Viewing hypnosis with the same social psychological theories as those employed to understand other kinds of "nonspecial" conduct represents the "new paradigm" for hypnosis.

The scientific controversy over the nature of hypnosis, earlier called the state/nonstate issue, had its beginnings at least as far back as Mesmer's claims of animal magnetism in the late 1700s (see e.g., Sarbin & Coe, 1972; Sheehan & Perry, 1976). The more recent antecedents of the alternative conceptualization are found in the works of Hull (1933), Dorcus (1937), Pattie (1935, 1941, 1950), White (1941), and Sarbin (1950). While these investigators challenged some of the exaggerated claims made for hypnosis, they did not criticize the fundamental assumptions of hypnotic state theory, except for Sarbin, who attacked the special state as a mentalistic concept.

Sutcliffe's (1960) article on the "skeptical" and "credulous" views of hypnosis appeared to set the stage for experimental investigators to move in the direction of using more naturalistic metaphors in examining the hypnotic context. A good deal of support for the nonstate paradigm was generated in the 1960s through the theoretical and empirical efforts of Theodore Barber and his colleagues (e.g., Barber, 1969; Barber, Spanos & Chaves, 1974) and Theodore Sarbin and his colleagues (e.g., Sarbin & Coe, 1972, 1979). Also, during this period both Chaves (1968) and Spanos and Chaves (1970) pointed out the relevance that the state/nonstate debate held for Kuhn's views of paradigm clashes in the evolution of science.

In the late 1970s, Hilgard and his colleagues reintroduced Janet's (1901) earlier discarded concept of dissociation as "neodissociation" (Hilgard, 1973, 1974, 1977a, 1977b, 1979; Hilgard, Morgan & McDonald, 1975). The neodissociation position offered new life to the failing special state paradigm. It postulated involuntary, cognitive processes as the basis for hypnotic responsiveness. Clinical hypnotists, who generally support a special state position, found the new dissociation postulate compatible with the notion of an altered state explanation. Hilgard's prestige as a scientist and experimenter undoubtedly helped in acceptance of the theory and provided authoritative support for the clinical orientation. The research orientation in the 1980s again returned to the question of whether or not hypnosis is best viewed as the result of special processes in the form of dissociated cognitive subsystems, or as the result of social psychological interactions of the context with the person.

At present, the issue is seen most clearly in the published exchanges between Spanos and his colleagues and Hilgard and his colleagues. The results of carefully worked out studies and articles have led Spanos to conclude that neodissociation theory is unnecessary and probably misleading (e.g., Spanos, 1982a, 1983, 1986b; Spanos & Hewitt, 1980). In response, Hilgard's supporters and coworkers rally to the defense of the "hidden observer" and neodissociation theory (e.g., Laurence & Perry, 1981; Laurence, Perry & Kihlstrom, 1983; Nogrady, McConkey, Laurence & Perry, 1983).

I was puzzled over the liveliness of the debate on an issue that had seemed to be resolving itself rather easily as the data were gathered. In conversations with colleagues on both sides of the neodissociation issue, it seemed that there was a great deal of agreement that the experimental findings indicated nothing very "special" about hypnosis. Still, some of my colleagues seemed rather uncomfortable in applying the same social psychological metaphors to hypnosis as they might easily do to other types of conduct. A "feeling" remained that hypnosis should somehow retain its "specialness." Because the research findings did not appear to be having as significant an impact as I thought they should on theorizing, I wondered if *non*scientific issues were involved.

SURVEY OF RECENT JOURNAL ARTICLES

My first data'were derived from an evaluation of all the hypnosis articles published in three recent years (1981-83) in four journals where hypnosis articles are commonly published: the *American Journal of Clinical Hypnosis (AJCH)*, the *International Journal of Clinical and Experimental Hypnosis (IJCEH)*, the *Journal of Abnormal Psychology (JAP)*, and the *Journal of Personality and Social Psychology (JPSP)*.

Each article was evaluated on two criteria. First, I recorded whether or not the term "hypnotic state" was used as an explanatory concept, or in a way that did not seem to question the concept's validity. Second, each article was classified as either an *experimental* study based on the use of systematically collected data, comparison groups and methodology, or as a *clinical* study, including case reports, theory with case examples, or reviews of clinical topics.

The results are presented in table 1. The number of clinical articles versus the number of experimental articles in each journal is essentially what would have been expected from the title of the journal and a knowledge of the professional association by which it is published. Approximately 78 percent of the articles in the *American Journal of Clinical Hypnosis* are clinical articles and 22 percent experimental papers. There is somewhat of a reversal in the *International Journal of Clinical and Experimental Hypnosis* with approximately 63 percent of its articles being experimental and only 37 percent clinical. Both of the *American Psychological Association* publications contained all experimental articles (100 percent). Thus, a substantial majority of the clinical studies are found in the *American Journal of Clinical Hypnosis* and a smaller number in the *International Journal of Clinical and Experimental Hypnosis*.

The percentage of articles employing the term "state" as it relates to the experimental/clinical dichotomy is of interest. Authors of experimental articles favor the use of *nonstate* language about 90 percent of the time in the hypnosis journals and closer to 100 percent of the time in the APA journals. (Two of the experimental articles were classified as state articles in the *Journal of Abnormal Psychology*, however, the question mark in table 1 indicates that the choice was unclear even in those two instances.) Almost the reverse percentages are found for clinical articles. About 85 percent mention the state concept in a way that could lead one to believe that *there is*, without question, a palpable, but mysterious trance or hypnotic state.

TABLE 1.

THE USE OF THE "STATE" CONCEPT IN FOUR JOURNALS
OVER THE LAST THREE YEARS (1981–83) IN ARTICLES
JUDGED AS EXPERIMENTAL OR CLINICAL

	American Journal of Clinical Hypnosis (AJCH)			International Journal of Clinical & Experimental Hypnosis (IJCEH)		
	State	Nonstate	Total	State	Nonstate	Total
Experimental	1	16	17	6	36	42
Articles	(5.9%)	(94.1%)	(22.1%)	(14.3%)	(85.7%)	(62.7%)
Clinical	52	8	60	21	4	25
Articles	(86.7%)	(13.3%)	(77.9%)	(84.0%)	(16.0%)	37.3%)

	Journal of Abnormal Psychology (JAP)			Journal of Personality & Social Psychology (JPSP)		
	State	Nonstate	Total	State	Nonstate	Total
Experimental	2 (?)	14	16	0	8	8
Articles	(0–12.5%)	(87.5–100%)	(100%)	(0%)	(100%)	(100%)
Clinical	0	0	0	0	0	0
Articles						

Special state concepts seemed to me to be used primarily in one of two ways. The more frequent use was most often seen in clinical case reports. The author would simply mention the fact that trance was involved, with no further explanation. For example, "I put the patient in trance," "Trance was induced," "While in the hypnotic state the patient . . ." etc. However, the mention of a special state was almost always only a very minor part of the article's content. Most of the information had to do with the client's history, a description of the clinical problem, and a description of the intervention techniques. Nearly all of these cases could have been read with little or no loss of meaning if terms like "hypnotic state" or "trance" had not been mentioned. State terms seemed to have been employed solely for the purpose of showing that the authors believed that their procedures were really different from relaxation, guided imagery, or other common therapeutic techniques that are applied without hypnosis (see, Mott, 1985; Spinhoven, 1987; and Wadden & Anderton, 1982, for similar conclusions).

The second use of the state concept, where it appeared at all, was confined to a relatively few experimental articles. The authors seemed to be using it out of habit and as a procedural shorthand to indicate subjects had been hypnotized. For example, there might be a brief mention that the subjects were placed in hypnosis or hypnotized. However, the notions of "trance" or "state" were used quite sparingly and without indications that they were considered causal or explanatory concepts. Experimental investigators who have been characteristically associated with the special state position in the past now seemed to favor a skills metaphor over a state metaphor. Terms such as "hypnotic ability," "hypnotic talent," "hypnotic virtuosos," even "dissociative skills" appeared frequently (e.g., Hilgard, 1982). The shift in emphasis to a "skills" metaphor is especially interesting because it is the same emphasis that the social psychological theorists have proposed for at least the past thirty-five years (e.g., Sarbin, 1950).

What can the results tell us about the use of state metaphors? It seems clear that the vast majority of clinicians prefer using special state concepts in vague ways, perhaps naively, or perhaps to mystify purposely. It seems equally clear that the vast majority of experimental investigators avoid using special state concepts, and even when they do, they appear to stand for a procedural shortcut. The evidence therefore appears, at least on the face of it, to indicate that the special state position has won the day with clinical hypnotists and that the social psychological position has won the day with experimental hypnotists.

However, the interesting challenge of understanding the differences in the use of special state concepts between clinicians and researchers is raised. A logical analysis of the rewards that each group may attain from support of a special state position may help to understand their choice more clearly.

First, we can attempt to outline the primary goals and aims of clinical practitioners. Most clinical hypnotists participate in a private practice and/or clinic and hospital work. (They may combine several endeavors, of course.) They are applied scientists in the helping professions who apply their knowledge as a service to the public and, in turn, receive remuneration for their services. It is obviously important that they have a clientele for their services.

What advantages might occur for clinicians if an altered state metaphor for hypnosis is accepted? Viewing hypnosis as a special state separates out hypnotic techniques and hypnotherapists as being unique and different from other therapists. Once such a separation is accomplished, clinical hypnotists may be viewed as possessing special training and special skills, which in turn, creates a special demand for their services. Also, the opaqueness and vagueness of special state concepts allows the aura of mystery and power long associated with hypnosis and hypnotists to remain alive. Such beliefs may lead clients to seek out hypnotic practitioners on their own or encourage other professionals to refer clients for the "magic" of hypnosis.[2]

The major goal of experimental scientists, on the other hand, is to discover new knowledge and an objective understanding of the world. Metaphors are useful insofar as they lead to theories that can account for empirical observations and guide research into fertile domains. The apparent overwhelming choice of researchers to avoid the use of vague, special state concepts suggests that the metaphors of social psychology rather than those of special processes best fulfill their goals.

As Spanos (1982a, 1986b) has recently pointed out, fewer and fewer items of behavior are regarded as specific to hypnosis. The controlled experiments over the past twenty-five years have yielded objective data demonstrating that behaviors like catalepsies, posthypnotic conduct, memory changes, and so on, are not necessarily specific to the induction of hypnosis. Even the conduct so frequently quoted as representing unique, subjective experiences in hypnosis, like, "trance logic," a "tolerance for logical ambiguity" (Evans, 1968; Orne, 1959, 1966; Perry & Walsh, 1978), or "source amnesia" (Coe, 1978; 1988; Evans, 1979) are not withstanding the empirical or logical tests of time (see Spanos, 1986b for a review and my chapter on Posthypnotic Amnesia in this volume). The behaviors once believed to be the products of a special state can be brought about through a variety of instructions, e.g., exhortation, instructions to imagine, instructions to concentrate, or instructions to simulate. In short, shifts in theoretical emphases and advances in experimental designs have reduced the number of so-called hypnotic-specific behaviors to none, or practically none, at all.

The central issues in the modern-day analysis of hypnotic phenomena are focused on those portions of the hypnotic performance that have been refractory to a social psychological analysis or to a common sense analysis (e.g., Allen & Scheibe, 1982; Coe, 1978, 1980; Coe & Sarbin, 1977; Sarbin & Coe, 1979; Sarbin, 1984). Because most subjects do not enact the behaviors that have been historically associated with deeply hypnotized subjects, special state or trance concepts are usually not adopted to explain their actions. Most investigators would agree with the statement that the conduct of 90 percent to 95 percent of the people who submit to hypnotic induction procedures can be accounted for adequately by social-psychological concepts. The notion of special states is not necessary for understanding their actions.

Even for the 5 to 10 percent of subjects who respond dramatically to hypnotic techniques, the "somnabulists" or "hypnotic virtuosos," the major research focus is on their subjective experiences as they report them, rather than the fact that they overtly respond to suggestions in unique ways. The self-reports that are of interest are those that are counterfactual and claim that the hypnotic experiences were "real." Even though such reports are infrequent, they have taken on a major role in the special state controversy. Because such reports are not easily accounted for by *any* current theoretical concepts, the door remains open for special process propositions. Social psychological constructs such as situational demands, skills, expectations, self-congruence, self-desception, beliefs, and attributions do not quite satisfy theorists who view hypnotic behavior as discontinuous from other everyday conduct.[3]

Current state propositions may also be criticized on logical grounds. One sort or another of an altered state theory has been postulated for hypnosis dating back at least as far as Mesmer's "Animal Magnetism." All special state views tend to focus on the internal workings of the subjects, and to postulate differences between the physiological or psychological conditions of the subjects while in the "hypnotic state" compared to the normal "waking state." Such views nearly always stipulate, or at least strongly imply, that the special state underlies, and accounts for in a causal sense, the subjects's conduct during hypnosis.

To remain viable for scientific purposes, special state concepts must provide independent, empirical referents of the state. It is not acceptable to define the special state by the observations that it is postulated to explain, the tautological use of state concepts so forcefully exposed by Ted Barber a number of years ago (Barber, 1969). Current, experimental state theorists, but not some clinical state theorists, are careful to avoid the pitfall of tautology. However, they have not been so successful in providing satisfactory referents for their concepts (Coe, 1980).

Even though there appears to be little empirical or logical support for a special state, a sizeable group of experimental investigators are quite tolerant, if not strongly supportive, of that position. Thus, it seems appropriate to inquire whether or not there are benefits within the hypnosis community, other than the scientists' goals, that are contingent upon supporting a state position.

THE SECOND SURVEY

The idea for another survey grew from the hypothesis that there are some not-so-obvious personal, political, and professional benefits associated with being friendly to the special state position. To test such a hypothesis it was necessary to locate benefits that are both desirable and available for empirical evaluation. Several prestigious, scientific-related activities seemed possibilities: (1) editorships on journals, (2) awards from scientific hypnosis societies, and (3) positions of leadership in these societies.[4] Each activity is made public, otherwise they would carry little prestige. Each activity is therefore amenable to empirical evaluation.

A questionnaire was mailed to all of the members of the editorial boards (as of January 1984) of the *American Journal of Clinical Hypnosis (AJCH)* and the *International Journal of Clinical and Experimental Hypnosis (IJCEH)* (N = 42 total). Fifty-nine and one-half (59.5) percent returned the questionnaire and made up the "Editorial" sample. Questionnaires were also sent to five investigators who are widely known as supporters and primary contributors to the social psychological view of hypnosis. These five made up the "Socialpsych" sample. One member of this sample was on the editorial board of *IJCEH*. His responses were not included in the Editorial sample's data. All respondents in both samples held the Ph.D. degree.

Three subsamples were also selected from the Editorial sample for comparisons with the Socialpsych sample. One subsample, the "IJCEH," was composed of the 19 members of the *IJCEH* editorial board who returned their questionnaires. Another subsample was composed of the six members of the *AJCH* editorial board who returned their questionnaires, the "AJCH" sample. A third subsample of eleven (11), the "Select" sample, was selected from the 19 *IJCEH* subsample for being more similar in years of involvement in hypnosis research (mean = 22.64 yrs., sd = 7.97) to that of the Socialpsych sample (mean = 25.20 yrs., sd = 12.62; $t < 1.0$, df = 14), than either the total Editorial sample (mean = 16.08 yrs., sd = 9.54) or the other two subsamples (*IJCEH*: mean = 16.00 yrs., sd = 9.96; *AJCH*: mean = 16.33 yrs., sd = 8.64). The purpose of the Select sample was to have a comparison group who had approximately the same amount of time as the Socialpsych subjects to be productive and to receive awards, honors, etc.

The questionnaire asked for various information about publications and professional contributions, memberships in societies, editorial activities, positions of leadership in societies, and awards from hypnosis groups. Information was also obtained from two, seven-point rating scales. One asked respondents to rate their theoretical preference for understanding hypnosis (1 = definitely a nonstate view; 7 = definitely a state view). The other asked them to rate the degree to which their contributions to hypnosis had been Experimental/ Theoretical versus Clinical (1 = 95%-100% Experimental/Theoretical; 7 = 95%-100% Clinical).

Scientific Contributions

Table 2 shows the results of the four samples' data on publishing and professional contributions and the results of the two rating scales.

Socialpsych Sample versus Select Sample

The nature of the questionnaire return created an unexpected bias in the samples. Four of the older and most published of the Editorial sample, who are very well-known for their special process positions, refused to respond to the questionnaire. As a consequence, the Socialpsych sample tended to have higher levels of scientific productivity than the other samples, and, by those criteria, would be expected to have received more awards and honors than the total Editorial sample or its subsamples.

The first five items compare various publishing and professional contributions to hypnosis. The Socialpsych sample had published significantly more total articles than the Editorial sample (mean = 60.8 vs. mean = 18.5). (Column 2 of the table 2 reports the relevant t-test results.) A breakdown of the total articles into specific journals showed that the Socialpsych sample had published significantly more articles than the editorial sample in each journal, with the exception of the *International Journal of Clinical and Experimental Hypnosis,* where they were about equal. The Socialpsych sample had also presented significantly more papers at hypnosis meetings than the Editorial sample (mean = 40.00 versus mean = 21.29). There were no significant differences between the two samples in number of "book chapters" published, the number of "books published," or the number of "workshops presented." The Socialpsych sample was nevertheless numerically higher in each category.

The next five items in table 2 show contributions similar to the first five except that they are in areas other than hypnosis. None of the comparisons between the Socialpsych sample and the Editorial sample reached acceptable levels of statistical significance. However, the Socialpsych sample was again numerically higher in each instance.

The last two items in table 2 show the ratings of theoretical preference for hypnosis and the type of personal contributions to hypnosis. As expected, the Socialpsych sample favored completely and unanimously a nonstate position while the Editorial sample leaned significantly more toward a state position (mean =

TABLE 2
COMPARISON OF PUBLISHING AND PROFESSIONAL CONTRIBUTIONS

Contributions in Hypnosis	Total Editorial Sample (N=25)	t	Socialpsych Sample #1 (N=5)	t	Select Sample (N=11)	IJCEH Sample #2 (N=19)	AJCH Sample #3 (N=6)	F	ANOVA (#1,#2,#3) Newman-Keuls Post-Hoc
1. Total # journal articles published in hypnosis. Of these:	18.5† (13.7)+	3.49**	60.8 (56.2)	1.89 <.10 >.05	28.27 (11.24)	20.53 (13.42)	12.17 (13.96)	6.25**	1>2,1>3
a) # in IJCEH	5.84 (4.44)	<1.0	6.80 (5.63)	<1.0	8.72 (4.02)	6.95 (4.08)	2.33 (3.93)	2.71 p=.08	
b) # in AJCH	2.28 (4.02)	2.25*	7.20 (6.54)	2.97**	1.45 (0.93)	1.16 (1.17)	5.83 (7.25)	5.91**	1>2,1>3,3>2
c) # in JAP	2.24 (3.44)	3.46**	10.20 (9.12)	1.91 <.10 >.05	3.91 (4.37)	2.74 (3.78)	0.67 (1.21)	6.40**	1>2,1>3
d) # in JPSP	0.48 (0.87)	2.42*	2.60 (4.22)	1.29	0.91 (1.04)	0.63 (0.96)	0.00 (0.00)	3.17*	1>2,1>3
2. # Book chapters published in hypnosis.	3.92 (4.58)	<1.0	5.80 (3.35)	<1.0	6.00 (6.12)	4.32 (5.15)	2.67 (1.63)	0.68	–
3. # Books published in hypnosis, author or editor.	1.12 (1.74)	<1.0	1.60 (1.34)	<1.0	1.27 (1.10)	0.84 (1.01)	2.00 (3.10)	1.30	–
4. # Papers presented on hypnosis at meetings.	21.29 (16.28)	2.15*	40.00 (24.15)	1.14	27.10 (19.46)	22.83 (17.08)	16.83 (13.95)	2.56	–
5. # Workshops presented on hypnosis.	17.83 (20.79)	1.19	33.20 (46.68)	<1.0	17.20 (17.43)	15.44 (18.12)	25.00 (28.11)	0.99	–

Contributions to Other Areas	Total Editorial Sample (N=25)	t	Socialpsych Sample #1 (N=5)	t	Select Sample (N=11)	IJCEH Sample #2 (N=19)	AJCH Sample #3 (N=6)	ANOVA (#1, #2, #3) F	Newman-Keuls Post-hoc
1. # Journal articles.	25.28 (37.02)	<1.0	29.40 (41.10)	<1.0	35.27 (40.21)	24.05 (33.26)	27.50 (46.54)	0.05	-
2. # Book chapters.	2.52 (3.81)	1.88 <.10 > .05	8.80 (15.39)	<1.0	4.00 (4.45)	2.63 (3.76)	2.67 (4.32)	1.72	-
3. # Books, author or editor.	1.04 (1.95)	1.51	2.60 (2.88)	<1.0	1.73 (2.57)	1.21 (2.20)	0.50 (0.55)	1.38	-
4. # Papers presented at meetings.	10.58 (13.16)	1.22	18.60 (14.67)	<1.0	14.60 (17.14)	11.72 (13.49)	7.17 (12.62)	0.98	-
5. # Workshops	4.25 (8.32)	<1.0	4.80 (6.57)	<1.0	7.40 (10.99)	4.72 (8.86)	2.83 (6.94)	0.13	-
Rating Scales (seven points)									
1. Theoretical preference for hypnosis 1 = nonstate 7 = state	5.16 (1.60)	-5.74**	1.00 (0.0)	-7.18**	5.27 (1.19)	4.95 (1.62)	5.83 (1.47)	17.68**	3>1,3>2,2>1
2. Type of contribution to hypnosis 1 = Experimental/Theoretical 7 = Clinical	3.24 (1.94)	-1.83 <.10 > .05	1.60 (0.89)	-1.56	2.59 (1.28)	3.18 (1.76)	3.17 (2.14)	1.70	-

† = mean   + ( ) = sd   *p< .05   **p< .01

1.00 vs. mean = 5.16). The type of contributions to hypnosis did not differ significantly between the Socialpsych sample although the tendency was for the Socialpsych subjects to view their contributions as more "experimental/theoretical" than did the Editorial sample (mean = 1.60 vs. mean = 3.24, p = .08).

Table 2 reflects the clear theoretical differences between the Socialpsych sample and the Editorial sample and also demonstrates that the Socialpsych subjects have contributed as much or more to the literature of psychology, especially to hypnosis, than the Editorial sample. The Socialpsych sample appears to represent a highly productive group of investigators who have contributed to the knowledge of hypnosis over a considerable number of years (24.40 years on average). Further, even a casual examination of the special state theorists who hold editorships on the hypnosis journals quickly dispels the possibility that they are more qualified individually than the members of the Socialpsych sample. They range from well-known scientists through recent Ph.D.s, many of whom have only begun to contribute to the literature on hypnosis. This is not to say that the editorial members are poorly qualified, but only that the five Socialpsych investigators are better qualified than many of them in terms of quantity and quality of their scientific contributions.

Socialpsych Sample versus Select Sample

Column 4 of table 2 shows the t-test results for each variable between the Socialpsych and Select sample. Only one significant difference was found between these two samples on their contributions to hypnosis. The Socialpsych subjects had published significantly more articles in the *American Journal of Clinical Hypnosis* than the Select subjects (mean 7.20 vs. 1.45), although the Socialpsych sample had published marginally more total articles in hypnosis (mean 60.8 vs. 28.27) and in the *Journal of Abnormal Psychology* (mean 10.30 vs. 3.91). None of their contributions to other areas differentiated the two samples significantly. There was, however, a clear difference between the samples on their preferred theoretical interpretation of hypnosis, with the Socialpsych sample preferring nonstate interpretations completely (mean = 1.0, sd = 0.0) versus a much stronger preference for state interpretations in the Select sample (mean = 5.27, sd = 1.19). The samples did not differ in their type of contribution; both rated themselves toward the experimental/theoretical direction rather than the clinical. In sum, these two samples were minimally different in terms of their years and types of productivity.

Socialpsych, IJECH, and AJCH Samples

The last column of table 2 shows the results of 1 × 3 ANOVAs across the three independent samples along with the direction of significant differences (where appropriate) on post-hoc tests. As regards contributions to hypnosis, the Socialpsych sample had published significantly more (1) total articles on hypnosis, (2) articles in *AJCH*, (3) articles in *JAP*, and (4) articles in *JPSP* than both of the other two samples. The AJCH sample had published more articles in the *AJCH* than had the IJCEH sample. A marginal difference is suggested for articles published in the *IJCEH* where it appears that both the Socialpsych and IJCEH samples published more articles than the AJCH sample.

The three samples did not differ on any of their contributions to areas other than hypnosis. There was also no significant difference in the way they rated their type of contributions to hypnosis. However, there were clear differences among the samples in the preferred theories for hypnosis with the AJCH favoring a state position more than both of the other samples and the IJCEH sample favoring a state position more than the Socialpsych sample.

In sum, the Socialpsych sample showed at least equal productivity across a broad range of contributions as either the IJCEH or the AJCH sample, and more productivity in selected areas of hypnosis contributions than both of the other samples.

Editorial Positions and Awards

I hypothesized that the membership structure of an organization was important. If the membership is made up largely of clinicians, then experimentalists who are friendly to the special state position, would be more likely to receive the awards, honors, etc. that the organization controls than would experimentalists supporting a social psychological position.

The American Society of Clinical Hypnosis (ASCH), composed almost entirely of clinicians, publishes the *American Journal of Clinical Hypnosis (AJCH)*. The Society for Clinical and Experimental Hypnosis (SCEH), which publishes the *International Journal for Clinical and Experimental Hypnosis (IJCEH)*, has a large majority of clinician members (approximately 94 percent estimated from the July 1984 directory). (Many members of these hypnosis societies hold medical or dental degrees.) The American Psychological Association's Division 30, Psychological Hypnosis, is composed entirely of psychologists, therefore, the proportion of clinicians to researchers is substantially lower than it is in the other two societies. A recent survey found that over 50 percent of Division 30's members have conducted research on hypnosis (Kraft & Rodolfa, 1982).

Editorial Positions

The questionnaire asked subjects if they had ever been on the editorial board, or if they had ever reviewed articles, for the four journals surveyed earlier. The responses of the Socialpsych sample are shown in the top half of table 3 and those of the Select Editorial sample in the bottom half.

TABLE 3

EDITORIAL AND REVIEWING ACTIVITIES

	American Journal of Clinical Hypnosis (AJCH)		International Journal of Clinical & Experimental Hypnosis (IJCEH)		Journal of Abnormal Psychology (JAP)		Journal of Personality & Social Psychology (JPSP)	
	Ever on Editorial Board?	Ever Reviewer?	Ever on Editorial Board?	Ever Reviewer?	Ever on Editorial Board?	Ever Reviewer?	Ever on Editorial Board?	Ever Reviewer?
Socialpsych Sample (N = 5)								
Yes	0 (0%)	0 (0%)	1 (20%)	3 (60%)	2 (40%)	5 (100%)	0 (0%)	4 (80%)
No	5	5	4	2	3	0	5	1
Select Editorial Sample (N = 11)								
Yes	1 (9%)	1 (9%)	11 (100%)	-	2 (18%)	4 (36%)	0 (0%)	4 (36%)
No	10	10	0	-	9	7	11	7

As the journals' emphases move toward a higher percentage of experimental publications and a lower percentage of using state concepts (toward the right in table 3), the Socialpsych nonstate investigators are more likely to be included in their editorial and reviewing processes.

At the time of the survey there were 11 editorial positions available on the *American Journal of Clinical Hypnosis* and at the time of this writing there are 22 positions available. However, none of the Socialpsych sample has ever been asked to serve as an editor or as a reviewer for the journal despite their generally higher level of productivity in hypnosis compared to the editors on the *AJCH* who responded to the questionnaire (table 2). But, the Select Editorial subjects are also not well represented in the editorial or reviewing processes of the *AJCH*.

The *International Journal of Clinical and Experimental Hypnosis* has only one of the five Socialpsych persons on its 44 member editorial board despite the fact that they have contributed as much or more to the hypnosis literature compared to the *IJCEH* editors who responded to the questionnaire (table 2). However, three of the five Socialpsych subjects have served as ad hoc reviewers for *IJCEH*.[6]

As would be expected from the variety of topics published in the two APA journals, the number of specialists in hypnosis who serve on their editorial boards is relatively small. Nevertheless, two persons in the Socialpsych sample have served on the *Journal of Abnormal Psychology*'s editorial board, and all five of them have reviewed papers for the journal. Table 3 shows that the percentage of persons from the Select Editorial sample compared to that from the Social-psych sample does not differ significantly on *JAP*'s editorial board (Fishers exact p = .30). However, the Socialpsych investigators have been represented more often than the Select Editorial investigators as reviewers for *JAP* (Fishers exact p = .03).

The *Journal of Personality and Social Psychology* follows a similar pattern in that four of the five Socialpsych sample have reviewed for the journal although none of them have been on its editorial board. (The editorial board contained no specialist in hypnosis.) The Select Editorial sample's representation in *JPSP*'s editorial and reviewing processes does not differ significantly from that of the Socialpsych sample (Fisher's exact p = 1.0 and 0.13 respectively).

The results generally support the hypothesis that a positive association with the special state position increases the chances of becoming a member of the editorial boards of the two journals published by the hypnosis societies. It is not obvious for the two journals published by the American Psychological Association.

A possible explanation for the low representation of the Socialpsych investigators on the hypnosis journals' editorial boards is that these individuals do not meet the levels of scientific productivity necessary for inclusion. However, the results of table 2 have already strongly contraindicated such a hypothesis. It would appear that were the invitations to editorial boards and reviewing for hypnosis journals based on past contributions to hypnosis, the five Socialpsych subjects would have been well represented in the editorial activities of the hypnosis journals. Since they were not, the hypothesis that they have not been asked because of their nonstate, theoretical preferences remains viable.

Officerships

Subjects were asked (1) if they were, or ever had been, a member of three hypnosis societies; (2) if they had ever been an officer of each society; and (3) if they had ever received an award from each society. Table 4 shows the results of the distribution of officerships from each society. The pattern of officerships is similar to that of editorial positions in table 3. As a society's membership has more experimentally oriented members, the chances that the Socialpsych investigators will have held positions of leadership increases.

ASCH: None of the Socialpsych sample have been officers in the ASCH; however, only two of them have been members. In fact, only one person from the entire sample who belonged to ASCH claimed to have been an officer. The data cannot determine whether theoretical preference is related to becoming an officer in the society.

TABLE 4

DISTRIBUTION OF OFFICERSHIPS TO
SOCIETY MEMBERS BY SUBSAMPLE

	(ASCH) American Society for Clinical Hypnosis (8 officers)			(SCEH) Society for Clinical and Experimental Hypnosis (4 officers)			Division 30 Psychological Hypnosis (5 officers)		
	Number of members who have been officers	# fellow	# member	Number of members who have been officers	# fellow	# member	Number of members who have been officers	# fellow	# member
Socialpsych Sample (N = 5)	0/2 (0.0%)	1	1	0/4 (0.0%)	3	1	3/4 (75.0%)	3	1
Select Sample (N = 11)	0/7 (0.0%)	4	3	7/11 (63.0%)	8	3	4/9 (44.4%)	8	1
IJCEH Sample (N = 19)	0/12 (0.0%)	4	8	8/19 (42.1%)	13	6	7/16 (43.8%)	10	6
AJCH Sample (N = 6)	1/5 (20.0%)	1	4	1/3 (33.3%)	1	2	1/4 (25.0%)	1	3

SCEH. Four of the Socialpsych investigators are, or have been, members (two are Fellows) of the SCEH. Nevertheless, none of them have ever held an official position.

The Select sample held significantly more officerships in SCEH than the Socialpsych sample (63.6% versus 0%, Fishers exact $p = .05$). None of the other subsample comparisons reached statistically significant differences.

Division 30: None of the subsamples differed significantly in the percentage of officerships held in Division 30 of APA. However, three of the four Socialpsych investigators who are members of Division 30 have been officers (the three had each been president) where none of them had ever been officers in either SCEH or ASCH.

Awards

Table 5 shows the distribution of awards across the subsamples for the ASCH and the SCEH.

TABLE 5

DISTRIBUTION OF AWARDS FROM HYPNOSIS SOCIETIES BY SUBSAMPLE

	(ASCH) American Society of Clinical Hypnosis (8 per year)		
	Number of recipients	Total number of awards	Mean number of awards (sd)
Socialpsych Sample #1 (N = 5)	1 (20.0%)	1	0.20 (0.45)
Select Sample (N = 11)	1 (9.1%)	1	0.09 (0.30)
IJCEH Sample #2 (N = 19)	2 (10.5%)	2	0.11 (0.32)
AJCH Sample #3 (N = 6)	3 (50.0%)	4	0.67 (0.82)

	(SCEH) Society for Clinical and Experimental Hypnosis (6 per year)		
	Number of recipients	Total number of awards	Mean number of awards (sd)
Socialpsych Sample #1 (N = 5)	2 (40.0%)	2	0.40 (0.55)
Select Sample (N = 11)	9 (81.8%)	27	2.45 (1.86)
IJCEH Sample #2 (N = 19)	14 (73.7%)	36	1.89 (1.73)
AJCH Sample #3 (N = 6)	1 (16.7%)	6	1.00 (2.45)

ASCH: The number of recipients of awards across the four samples does not reach significance by Fisher's exact test. However, the AJCH sample tended to receive a higher percentage of awards than both the IJCEH Total sample (50% vs. 10.5%, Fisher's exact p = .06) and the Select sample (50.0% vs. 9.1%, Fisher's exact p = .09). Comparing the mean number of awards across the three independent samples, the AJCH sample received significantly more awards than either the Socialpsych sample or the IJCEH sample who did not differ from each other (F = 3.29, $p < .05$; Newman Kuel's post hocs, 3 >1, 3 >2).

SCEH: The number of recipients of awards across the four samples shows significant differences between the Select sample and the AJCH sample (81.8%

vs. 16.7%, Fisher's exact p = .02) and between the IJCEH sample and the AJCH sample (73.7% vs. 16.7%, Fisher's exact p = .02). The Socialpsych sample did not differ significantly from the other samples in regard to the number of award recipients.

Comparison of the three independent samples on the *number of awards* received did not reach significance (F = 1.19, p< .05). However, the comparison of the Socialpsych sample with the Select sample showed a significant difference in favor of the Select sample (mean = 0.40 vs. mean = 2.45, t = 2.38, p< .05).

SUMMARY OF OVERALL FINDINGS

The Socialpsych investigators had contributed more to the hypnosis literature than the editorial investigators as a whole. They also differed from the editorial sample in preferring a nonstate view of hypnosis, but did not differ in the type of contribution (experimental/clinical) of their works. Nevertheless, none of them has been asked to serve on the editorial board of the *American Journal of Clinical Hypnosis* or to review for that journal. Only one of them has served on the editorial board of the *International Journal of Experimental and Clinical Hypnosis,* although the service of three of the five as ad hoc reviewers has been requested. The APA publications (*JAP* and *JPSP*) do not reflect such differences using the Select sample for comparison, except that the Socialpsych investigators have been used as reviewers on *JPSP more often* than the Select sample investigators.

Awarding officerships in the American Society of Clinical Hypnosis showed no clear patterns. In fact, only one person from all the samples claimed to have been an officer for this organization. In the Society for Clinical and Experimental Hypnosis, however, the Select sample had held significantly more officerships than the Socialpsych sample. The samples did not differ in officerships held in APA Division 30 although three of the Socialpsych persons had been president of the Division whereas none of them had ever held an office in the two hypnosis societies.

The number of persons receiving awards from the American Society for Clinical Hypnosis tended to favor the *American Journal of Clinical Hypnosis* (*AJCH*) subsample over the *International Journal of Clinical and Experimental Hypnosis* (*IJCEH*) subsample but not the Socialpsych sample. The AJCH subsample received more awards on the average, however, than the Socialpsych subjects and the IJCEH subjects. The number of persons receiving awards from SCEH showed the Select and IJCEH samples receiving higher percentages than the AJCH sample but not the Socialpsych sample. However, the Select sample received more awards on average than the Socialpsych sample.

CONCLUSION

The combined results suggest that important sociopolitical variables are operating which may affect the choice of theoretical metaphors for investigators of hypnosis. For clinical practitioners, the special state interpretation acts to set hypnosis apart as a special technique that requires unique skills and training. As a consequence, possibilities for hypnotic practitioners to attain practical, personal, and political goals related to their occupational pursuits are enhanced. Since clinical practitioners make up a large majority of the memberships in the two hypnosis societies investigated, they are likely to hold the power for determining status-enhancing positions in these societies. Clearly, these two societies have not recognized the five leading social psychological investigators sampled in this report to the degree that their scientific contributions would seem to warrant.

The results were not as clear for the American Society of Clinical Hypnosis as they were for the Society of Clinical and Experimental Hypnosis, but there seems little doubt that the social psychological theorists tended to be excluded from these societies' editorships, officerships, and awards, especially compared to a select sample of investigators who have been involved in hypnosis research for a similar number of years but espouse a special state interpretation of hypnosis rather than a social psychological interpretation.

The third hypnosis group studied, Division 30 of the American Psychological Association, with a much larger percentage of experimentally oriented members, did not appear to discriminate against the social psychological theorists. In fact, they were at least equally represented as officers, and the APA journals (*JAP* and *JPSP*) used them equally, or more than, state oriented investigators for editorial assignments.

In general, this investigation suggests that being friendly to the special state view of hypnosis enhances a researcher's chances of attaining high status accoutrements from the hypnosis community. Even though the scientific purpose of theories is to help guide research and to enhance the understanding of hypnosis, and social psychological concepts seem to best fill such a purpose, the sociopolitical climate of the larger hypnosis community makes supporting special state concepts more attractive. The data also suggest that younger investigators are likely to be influenced toward a special process (or state) position because of the accoutrements controlled by their more clinically oriented colleagues. Thus, values other than those presumably espoused by scientists appear to have a significant effect on the direction of theorizing and research taken by research oriented investigators.

NOTES

This chapter is based in part on the author's invited address to Division 30, Psychological Hypnosis, at the APA Annual Meeting in Los Angeles, August 29, 1983, titled "Trance: A Problematic Metaphor for Hypnosis." I am grateful to Theodore R. Sarbin and Richard L. St. Jean for their thoughtful and helpful suggestions on the final manuscript.
    1. See Meeker and Barber (1971) for a critical accounting of stage hypnosis "feats." See Coe and Ryken (1979) for a discussion on the *lack* of dangers from being hypnotized.

2. I am not suggesting that clinical hypnotists are out to dupe the public (or their fellow professionals), or that they are any less adequate as helpers than therapists who employ other methods. Many of them truly believe that hypnosis creates special, unique changes in their clients.

Hypnosis as a special state, however, raises some problems for licensed clinicians as well. First, lay hypnotists (almost without exception in my experience) use the definition of hypnosis as special in order to support legislation that will legitimize them as state sanctioned practitioners without the need for training in one of the mental health professions. At the same time, they employ its uniqueness to block legislation that would limit the practice of hypnosis to licensed health professionals.

The aura of mystery surrounding hypnosis as a special state may also create difficulties in practice. Clients who expect "magic" may be easily disappointed with the progress of therapy. Alternatively, the magical connotations of hypnosis may keep potential clients from trying it, or from showing up at all. Nevertheless, the present data suggests that the positive benefits from the special state metaphor appear to outweigh any negative consequences.

3. See Wagstaff (1981) for logic and data that argue against the special state metaphor in accounting for even the most dramatic examples of hypnotic conduct.

4. I am grateful to my deceased colleague, Mitri Shanab, for suggesting some possibilities.

5. It is appropriate to point out that some of the socialpsych theorists are members of both the American Society of Clinical Hypnosis and the Society for Clinical and Experimental Hypnosis. Their lack of editorial positions cannot be explained by their lack of membership. Further, phone conversations with the respective association offices who publish the journals confirmed that membership in the society was not a requirement for appointment to their editorial board or a requirement for receiving most of the awards each grants yearly.

19

The Cognitive-Behavioral Perspective

Synopsis and Suggestions for Research

Nicholas P. Spanos and John F. Chaves

The cognitive-behavioral perspective begins with the hypothesis that hypnotic behavior is historically rooted social action that is fundamentally similar to other, more mundane forms of social behavior. From this perspective the concept of hypnosis as an altered state of consciousness that is induced by certain rituals (hypnotic induction procedures) and that, in turn, produces unusual behavior is highly misleading. Instead, hypnotic induction rituals are viewed as historical curiosities that reflect outmoded nineteenth-century attempts to conceptualize the behaviors associated with this topic as linked in some way to sleep. Relatedly, the suggested behaviors that have figured most prominently in the history of hypnosis (e.g., limb catalepsies, amnesia, analgesia, hallucinations) coalesced into a coherent social role (the role of hypnotic subject) not because of any intrinsic correlations among these different behaviors, but instead, because they were conceptualized as being related in eighteenth-and nineteenth-century special process theories of mesmerism and hypnosis (Spanos & Gottlieb, 1979).

As theories of mesmerism and hypnosis evolved, components of the hypnotic role that were once considered central dropped away. For example, as the theoretical connection between hypnosis and hysteria became increasingly tenuous and difficult to maintain in the late nineteenth century, convulsions became an increasingly less common "symptom" of the "hypnotic state." Similarly, attempts to make hypnosis scientifically respectable and nonmystical led investigators to deemphasize displays of clairvoyance and other seemingly occult manifestations that, at one time, had been among the most prominent characteristics of mesmerism and hypnosis (Dingwall, 1968). In short, viewed from a cognitive-behavioral perspective, hypnotic behaviors are, in Radtke's terminology, social artifacts. The patterns of behavior carried out by "hypnotized" subjects do not reflect the essential characteristics of an invariant psychological state. Instead, these behaviors are rule-governed social actions that are determined by the conceptions of hypnosis shared by subjects and hypnotists in particular sociohistorical circumstances. As conceptions of hypnosis change, so do the behaviors that constitute the hallmarks of "being hypnotized."

Alternatively, special process theories are based on the assumption that hypnotic behavior does involve invariant psychological processes that are independent of social context and that constitute the "essence" of hypnosis (Orne, 1959). Consequently, research generated from this perspective has been aimed at identifying that "essence" and separating it from the artifact of social context. However, the search for an hypnotic essence had by and large been fruitless. Candidates for essential characteristics of hypnosis have, at one time or another, included heightened suggestibility, trance logic responding, hidden observer responding, source amnesia, disorganized recall during hypnotic amnesia, and context-independent posthypnotic responding. As the research reviewed in the various chapters of this volume makes clear, whenever these patterns of response have been subjected to careful empirical scrutiny, their status as context-dependent and their relation to subjects' goal-directed strivings have been clearly revealed.

From cognitive-behavioral perspectives, the goal of research is not to isolate an hypnotic essence but, on the contrary, to demystify hypnotic responding and to engage in empirical work and theory construction that will serve to integrate hypnotic responding into a more general theory of social behavior.

Taken together, the chapters in this volume testify to the vitality of cognitive-behavioral perspectives. The work conducted in this tradition has very clearly demonstrated the utility of viewing hypnotic responding as the context-generated, goal-directed enactments of sentient agents. A wealth of information has been amassed concerning the roles of social psychological antecedents and cognitive mediators in the genesis of the behavioral and subjective components of hypnotic responding, and in determining the ways that subjects come to define and interpret their responding. This tradition has also provided the conceptual tools that enabled the seemingly esoteric phenomena that constituted the empirical mainstays of special process approaches to be more parsimoniously reinterpreted in terms of social action. For example, Coe's chapter on amnesia makes it clear that the varied phenomena associated with posthypnotic amnesia (e.g., breaching of amnesia, disorganized recall, source amnesia, instruction-induced enhancements and decrements in amnesia) cannot be accounted for by viewing amnesia as a "passive happening." On the other hand, these phenomena can be integrated into a coherent theory when hypnotic amnesia is conceptualized as reflecting an "active doing," the attempts of subjects to self-present as unable to remember. Relatedly, the chapter by Spanos suggests that a similar conceptualization is required to adequately account for hidden observer responding, the equivalence of hypnotic and nonhypnotic suggestions for pain reduction, the context-dependent relationship between hypnotizability and suggestion-induced pain reduction, and other aspects of hypnotic analgesia. De Groot and Gwynn's chapter enumerates the inadequacies and inconsistencies that result from attempting to explain so-called "trance logic" responding in terms of a hypnosis-specific "tolerance for logical incongruity." These investigators also provide a more parsimonious account that revolves around the active, but less than completely successful, attempts of motivated subjects to meet the task demands associated with difficult suggestions.

The chapters by Flynn and Jones and by St. Jean also document the failures of special process formulations. In these cases it is the failures of such formulations to provide adequate accounts for the reports of sensory and perceptual alterations associated with hypnotic procedures and suggestions that are discussed. Relatedly, the chapter by Lynn, Rhue, and Weekes documents the failure of special process formulations to provide an adequate account for those responses to suggestion that are defined by subjects as involuntary occurrences. Misled by their own tacit assumption that hypnotic responses are automatic "happenings," special process theorists took reports of involuntariness at face value. Consequently, they were unable to account for the strategic nature of responses to suggestion. By conceptualizing reports of involuntariness as reflecting schema-based interpretations that are activated by the communications transmitted in the hypnotic context, Lynn, Rhue, and Weekes provide a formulation that can account for the strategic nature of hypnotic responding as well as for the involuntariness reports of the responding subjects.

The chapter by Radtke demonstrates the inadequacies involved in conceptualizing reports of hypnotic depth as reflecting the degree to which subjects have entered an altered (hypnotic) state of consciousness. By drawing on contemporary attribution theory she provides a more coherent and parsimonious cognitive-behavioral account for such reports. Rather than positing unusual "states," her account emphasizes the interacting roles of context, preconceptions, and self-observations in shaping subjects' interpretations of themselves as more or less "hypnotized."

While the chapters in this volume clearly document the increases in knowledge gained by conceptualizing hypnotic phenomena from cognitive-behavioral perspectives, it is equally clear that our understanding of hypnotic behavior and its antecedents remains incomplete. A good deal of research remains to be done before hypnotic phenomena can be fully integrated into a comprehensive account of human social behavior. Below we will examine several of the issues that, in our opinion, deserve more extensive research consideration.

THE PROBLEM OF HYPNOTIZABILITY

In the last thirty years, hypnotizability has emerged as a pivotal construct in theories of hypnosis, and people who attain high scores on hypnotizability scales have been lauded as "hypnotic virtuosos" who purportedly possess extraordinary but little understood cognitive talents (Register & Kihlstrom, 1986). As Bertrand indicates, hypnotizability scores remain relatively stable over even long intervals, and different hypnotizability scales intercorrelate to a substantial degree. The usual approach to these findings is to attribute them to stable psychological dispositions (Hilgard, 1977). Thus, from this perspective the temporal stability and high interest correlations obtained with hypnotizability measures reflect a stable capacity for dissociation, imagery vividness, absorption, fantasy proneness, or whatever. This approach has fostered the kinds of correlational studies reviewed by de Groh. Dispositional measures, usually in the form of questionnaires, have been correlated with measures of hypnotizability. As de Groh indicates, the findings in this area have frequently been contradictory or negative. Even consistent correlations between attribute measures and hypnotizability have rarely exceeded $r = .30$, and recent work suggests that even the most consistent relationships—such as that between absorption and hypnotizability—may be expectancy-mediated artifacts (Council, Kirsch & Hafner, 1986).

In the last decade, the stable capacity hypothesis has been challenged with increasing frequency by studies demonstrating that hypnotizability can be modified to a very substantial degree (Diamond, 1977; Spanos, 1986a). As Bertrand's chapter indicates, a substantial proportion of the low hypnotizables who are exposed to brief training regimens aimed at altering their attitudes, expectations, and interpretational sets score in the high-hypnotizability range on posttest measures.

Related to modification studies are those demonstrating a context-dependent relationship between hypnotizability and subjects' responsiveness to nonhypnotic suggestions for analgesia (e.g., Spanos, Kennedy & Gwynn, 1984). These studies indicate that low hypnotizables given instructions for analgesia in nonhypnotic contexts report as much pain reduction as high hypnotizables given hypnotic analgesia, and more pain reduction than low hypnotizables given hypnotic analgesia. Studies of this kind indicate that degree of hypnotic analgesia may have less to do with a stable cognitive capacity assessed by hypnotizability scales than with the situation-specific attitudes, expectations, and preconceptions concerning hypnosis that influence the interpretations subjects develop of the pain-reduction test situation and their likelihood of employing pain-reducing strategies in the situation.

Finally, several recent studies (Katsanis, Barnard & Spanos, 1988; Spanos, Gwynn, Gabora & Jarrett, 1988) indicate directly that hypnotizability scores are related to subjects' tacit interpretations of suggested demands. Even among subjects with positive expectations for hypnotic performance and high imagery-vividness scores, those who interpreted suggestions as requests to wait passively for suggested effects to "happen" attained significantly lower hypnotizability scores than those who interpreted the same suggestions as tacit requests to generate the subjective and behavioral effects called for.

Taken together, the above findings suggest that the usual stability in responsiveness associated with measures of hypnotizability may have to do at least as much with stable elements what are intrinsic to the definition of the situation as a test of hypnotizability, as with stable cognitive capacities. For example, all modern tests of hypnotizability begin with a hypnotic induction procedure that consists of interrelated suggestions for relaxation and that explicitly defines the situation as hypnosis. Furthermore, the test suggestions administered on all of these scales are worded passively to imply that hypnotic responses just happen by themselves (e.g., your arm is rising higher and higher), and these suggestions usually instruct subjects to imagine events that are consistent with the subjective effects called for (e.g., imagine that your arm is pumped up with helium, making it feel lighter and lighter). Many of these scales (e.g., Weitzenhoffer & Hilgard, 1959) also include repeated suggestions for relaxation and sleep interspersed between the test suggestions, and these serve to continually reinforce the definition of the situation as hypnosis.

In short, all modern hypnotizability scales share important and highly salient common elements, and these common elements are likely to call up the same situation-specific attitudes, interpretations, and expectations regardless of the specific hypnotizability scale in which they are embedded. For example, subjects with strong negative attitudes toward hypnosis are likely to translate those attitudes into noncooperativeness with suggested demands regardless of the specific hypnotizability scales they are administered, and those who tacitly interpret passively worded suggestions as requests to wait for effects to happen automatically are likely to develop this interpretation regardless of the particular scale on which the passive suggestions appear.

Thus, elements common and specific to hypnotizability scales may elicit situation-specific attitudes, interpretations, and expectations that play a major role in mediating the cross-test and test-retest stabilities that characterize performance on these scales. Moreover, because the attitudes and interpretations called up by these common elements are, by and large, specific to *hypnotic* situations, they will tend to reduce the likelihood of finding strong or consistent correlations between context-free measures of cognitive ability (e.g., trait measures of imagery vividness) and hypnotizability scores.

These ideas suggest that future studies might manipulate the elements common to hypnotizability scales and examine the effects of such manipulation on the magnitude of cross-test correlations. For example, one recent study (Spanos, Gabora, Jarrett & Gwynn, experiment 1, 1988) administered subjects the Carleton University Responsiveness to Suggestion Scale (CURSS; Spanos, Radtke, Hodgins, Stam & Bertrand, 1983) in one session and the Creative Imagination Scale (CIS; Barber & Wilson, 1979) in a second session. The CURSS was always defined as a test of hypnotizability. For half of the subjects the CIS was also defined as a test of hypnotizability, while for the remaining half it was defined as a test of creative imagination. The correlations between CURSS and CIS scores were significantly and substantially higher when both tests were defined in terms of hypnotizability than when one was defined in terms of hypnotizability and the other in terms of creative imagination.

A second study (Spanos, Gabora, et al., experiment 2, 1988) employed subjects who had previously scored either high or low on the CURSS. In a latter session these subjects were administered the CIS in nonhypnotic contexts that indicated either that CIS performance would resemble earlier CURSS performance or that it would be highly discrepant from earlier CURSS performance. Correlations between CURSS and CIS scores were high and significant when subjects expected similar performance in the two test situations, but very low and nonsignificant when subjects expected discrepancies in performance on the two scales.

The notion that hypnotizability reflects a stable cognitive capacity has dominated research in this area for the last thirty years. Nevertheless, consistent correlations of even a modest magnitude between cognitive attribute variables and hypnotizability have proven difficult to demonstrate. Moreover, the cognitive capacity hypothesis, with its emphasis on the assessment of intrasubject attributes, has deflected attention away from a detailed analysis of the situational components that make up the hypnotizability test situation. Recent evidence appears to be converging on the importance of situation-specific attitudes, interpretations, and expectations in determining performance in the hypnotizability test situation and in influencing the magnitudes of cross-test and test-retest hypnotizability correlations. A broadening of research along these general lines might lead to a viable, contextually based cognitive-behavioral alternative to the stable capacity hypothesis of hypnotizability. Moreover, if stable cognitive abilities are related to responsiveness to suggestion, these abilities are likely to be uncovered only after important situational influences can be specified and controlled.

CLINICAL HYPONOSIS RESEARCH

Mesmerism and hypnosis began as clinical endeavors and, as the chapters in the applied section of this volume make clear, hypnotic procedures continue to be employed on a regular basis for treating a wide range of clinical problems. For example, the chapters by Chaves, D'Eon, and Stam review a large number of reports that have assessed the efficacy of hypnotic procedures for reducing the pain associated with a wide range of medical and dental disorders and procedures. Reviewed in those chapters are studies that dealt with the effects of hypnotic interventions on childbirth pain, surgical and postsurgical pain, and other uncomfortable medical procedures, as well as the effects of these interventions in reducing the pain associated with such disorders as cancer and headache. Relatedly, the chapters by Stam and Johnson describe a wide variety of nonpain disorders and other problems in living that have been treated with procedures labeled as hypnotic. These problems include sexual dysfunction; difficulties in habit control; anticipatory nausea and vomiting in chemotherapy patients; warts and other dermatological disorders; and a wide range of other personal, interpersonal, and marital problems.

Perhaps the most obvious aspect of the work reviewed in all of these chapters is its overall lack of methodological rigor. For the most part, research in clinical hypnosis consists of anecdotal reports and uncontrolled clinical studies. Frequently these studies do an inadequate job of specifying the characteristics of the treatments that are labeled "hypnotic" and an equally inadequate job of specifying the criteria used to infer therapeutic change. Moreover, in many studies that do compare hypnotic and nonhypnotic treatments the independent variables are confounded so that meaningful interpretation of the findings is impossible. Stam, for example, noted how Zeltzer and Le Baron (1984) (*a*) failed to specify how their so-called "hypnotic" treatment was different from nonhypnotic guided imagery procedures, (*b*) failed to specify whether this treatment was even defined as "hypnosis" to the patients, and (*c*) confounded rather than independently assessed the effects of the independent variables in their study. In short, in 1988, clinical hypnosis as a research area appears to be at roughly the same point as experimental hypnosis research before Barber began his systematic controlled experimentation in the late 1950s.

What needs to be done in this area is, of course, easier to specify than to implement. Nevertheless, even investigators who conduct uncontrolled clinical outcome studies can (and should be required by journal editors to) clearly define the components of the various treatments that they label as hypnotic, operationally define the criteria used to assess therapeutic change, assess the reliability and validity of those criteria, and, where feasible, use multiple, converging dependent variables.

With pain phenomena that are relatively well circumscribed and relatively common (e.g., childbirth pain, migraine, chronic tension headache), controlled comparison studies can and should be carried out. The study by Stam, McGrath and Brooke (1984) on hypnotic intervention for temporomandibular joint pain can serve as a useful model. In that study subjects were randomly assigned to a no-treatment control group and two treatment conditions. Subjects in both treatments were provided with the same cognitive strategy procedures. However, those in one treatment were also administered an hypnotic induction procedure while those in the other treatment were not. Three important characteristics in this study deserve emphasis: (*a*) Subjects were drawn from a common population and assigned randomly to treatments. (*b*) A no-treatment group controlled for the effects of spontaneous remission and repeated assessments. (*c*) The two treatments differed with respect to only a single variable: the presence or absence of an hypnotic induction procedure. Stam et al. (1984) found that subjects in the two cognitive strategy treatments showed equivalent levels of improvement on all dependent measures and more improvement than no-treatment controls. In other words, the hypnotic procedure added nothing to the benefits produced by the cognitive treatment alone.

Studies modeled after that of Stam et al. (1984) are sorely needed to evaluate the effects of hypnotic procedures on a wide range of clinical phenomena. In fact, given subject availability such studies would do well to include placebo control groups as well as no-treatment control groups. The placebo groups would, of course, provide some estimate of the effects of expectancies and beliefs in treatment efficacy in patients who were not provided with cognitive strategies, hypnotic inductions, or other specific treatment procedures. For example, several recent studies (Spanos, Stenstrom & Johnston, 1988; Spanos, Williams & Gwynn, 1988) indicated that hypnotic and nonhypnotic imagery-based suggestions were equally effective at inducing wart regression, but that the imagery-based suggestions were more effective in this regard than placebo treatments.

Stam et al. (1984) found that improvement in both the hypnotic and cognitive treatments correlated significantly with pretested hypnotizability, and related findings have also been reported in other studies (see the chapter by Chaves for a review). On the other hand, a number of studies have reported no significant correlation between hypnotizability and outcome when using hypnotic interventions in the treatment of dental pain (J. Barber, 1977; Gillett & Coe, 1984), smoking (Perry, Gelfand & Marcovitch, 1979), warts (Spanos, Stenstrom & Johnston, 1988; Surman, Gottlieb, Hackett & Silverberg, 1973), and the control of hemophilic bleeding (Swirsky-Sacchetti & Margolis, 1986). As described in several chapters, the relationship between hypnotizability and suggestion-induced reductions in laboratory pain appears to be more context dependent and expectancy mediated than was once supposed. Similar variables may be determining whether or not significant correlations emerge between hypnotizability and treatment outcome in clinical settings. Clinical studies that assess patients' hypnotizability both within the treatment context and outside of the treatment context are required to resolve this issue.

Since the time of Mesmer, procedures that are now labeled as hypnotic have been lauded by some clinicians as highly effective for a wide range of psychological and physiological problems. In fact, in the case of most clinical problems there is very little evidence to indicate that hypnotic interventions are effective at all, and no good evidence to indicate that such interventions are any more effective than other forms of treatment (Wagstaff, 1987). This, of course, does not mean that hypnotic treatments are *ineffective*. It simply means that the effectiveness or ineffectiveness of most of the treatments labeled as hypnotic has yet to be adequately evaluated. One important priority for hypnosis research in the next decade should involve carefully controlled clinical studies that begin to delineate the effective components in hypnotic treatment packages.

HYPNOSIS AND HAPPENINGS

The chapters in this volume have emphasized that hypnotic responses can be viewed more fruitfully as actions or enactments than as automatic occurrences or "happenings." Moreover, the research conducted on the suggested phenomena considered most central to the topic of hypnosis (e.g., age regression, amnesia, analgesia, hallucination, limb catalepsies) has clearly borne out the utility of this view. However, some of the phemonena linked historically with the topic hypnosis are very clearly happenings rather than actions, and these phenomena require careful consideration by any comprehensive approach to this topic.

Some of the "happenings" associated with hypnotic performance can be conceptualized rather easily as indirect and unintended consequences of subjects' goal-directed strivings. For example, "trance logic" responses such as transparent hallucinations and duality responding during age regression are not, in themselves, goal-directed or strategic actions. Subjects do not intend to generate transparent hallucinations or to feel adultlike during age regression. Instead, such patterns of responding appear to reflect the failures of subjects to generate in complete form the goal-directed responses called for by the test suggestions (cf. the chapter by de Groot & Gwynn). Relatedly, the body image changes sometimes associated with hypnotic induction procedures (e.g., I felt as if I was floating; I couldn't feel my legs) can be understood rather easily as unintended consequences of enhanced relaxation (Edmonston, 1980), and the changes in time perception that occur during hypnotic enactments can be conceptualized as unintended consequences of the information processing actively engaged in by hypnotic subjects (cf. the chapter by St. Jean).

Other "happenings," however, cannot be conceptualized as unintended consequences of goal-directed activity. These are events that are very clearly intended and, what's more, that appear to result at least indirectly from some aspect of subjects' goal-directed activity. Nevertheless, their occurrence is not itself an action that subjects directly generate. A prime example of this kind of happening is the suggestion-induced disappearance of warts that, Johnson's chapter makes clear, cannot be explained away in terms of spontaneous remission.

Some of the important antecedents of suggestion-induced wart regression are goal-directed actions. For instance, subjects' imagining their warts shrinking and disappearing is obviously goal-directed activity. Just as obviously, however, such imagery doess not in any direct way produce wart regression. For instance, both suggestion-induced wart regression and suggestion-induced arm rising involve goal-directed cognitve activity. Nonetheless, arm rising is itself an action that can be accounted for in terms of subjects' motivations, plans, intentions, and the like. Wart regression is *not* an action at all, it is an event, something that happens as opposed to something that is done. Consequently, an account of wart regression in terms of variables like motivations and intentions must necessarily remain incomplete. The same is, of course, true for other suggestion-induced happenings such as the remission of ichthyosis (e.g., Mason, 1952), the control of bleeding in hemophilics (e.g., Swirsky-Sacchetti & Margolis, 1986), the production and suppression of alergic responses (e.g., Ikemi & Nakagawa, 1962), and the control of lesion outbreaks in patients with genital herpes (Longo, Clum & Yaeger, 1988).

Understanding suggestion-induced happenings of these kinds remains an important and fascinating challenge to the cognitive-behavioral perspective. Perhaps the first step toward meeting this challenge should involve attempting to delineate which aspects of the hypnotic/suggestion situation are important in eliciting these effects. For example, with respect to warts, recent work indicates that neither an hypnotic induction nor preliminary instructions for relaxation add to the effectiveness of imagery-based suggestions in producing wart regression (Spanos, Stenstrom et al., 1988). Moreover, the effects of suggestions cannot be accounted for simply in terms of enhanced expectancies. Subjects given placebos and those given suggestions reported equivalent expectations of treatment success, but suggestions were more effective than placebos at producing wart regression (Spanos, Williams et al., 1988). Suggestions, however, were not effective with all subjects. Interestingly, they were most effective for subjects who possessed multiple warts as opposed to a single wart, and for those who rated their suggested imagery of wart regression as relatively vivid. On the other hand, wart regression was unrelated to hypnotizability or to attribute measures of imagery vividness or absorption (Spanos, Stenstrom et al., 1988). Early work by Sinclair-Gieben and Chalmers (1959) indicated that suggestions could produce remission that was limited to specific bodily regions (e.g., the warts on one hand and not the other). As Johnson's chapter points out, however, more recent work has consistently failed to replicate these findings.

Taken together, all of this seems to imply tentatively that subjects' active involvement in suggestion-related thinking and/or imagery activates or strengthens systemic (as opposed to region-specific) physiological processes that can lead to eventual wart remission. The more vivid subjects' suggestion-related imagery (which perhaps in part reflects their degree of absorption in or commitment to the suggested task), the greater likelihood that the relevant physiological processes will become strengthened or activated. Also, the greater the amount of wart virus in the system (as reflected by multiple as opposed to a single wart), the greater the likelihood that the strengthened or activated physiological processes will make contact with and kill the virus.

Obviously, these tentative ideas will require modification and refinement as more information about the antecedents of suggestion-induced wart regression become available. For example, it remains unclear whether active cognitive involvement in some nonimaginal activity that subjects believe will "work" would be equally effective.

The antecedent variables that are important in eliciting other suggestion-induced happenings may well be different from the variables that are important in wart regression. For example, relaxation, which appears to be relatively unimportant in wart regression, may be extremely important in the control of hemophilic bleeding. The important point is that each of the different suggestion-induced happenings requires systematic and individualized investigation. Little is likely to be gained by attempting to conceptualize suggestion-induced happenings in terms of vaguely defined special processes such as "dissociation" or "trance states." A theoretical and methodological framework that emphasizes the delineation, systematic assessment, and manipulation of the contextual components associated with each suggestion-induced phenomenon is likely to yield important returns on research investments.

References

Aaronson, B. (1973). ASCID trance, hypnotic trance, just trance. *American Journal of Clinical Hypnosis, 16,* 110-117.

Abelson, R. P. (1981). Script as a psychological concept. American Psychologist, *36,* 715-729.

Abramson, M., & Heron, W. T. (1950). An objective of hypnosis in obstetrics. *American Journal of Obstetrics,* May, 1969-1974.

Achterberg, J., & Lawlis, G. F. (1978). *Imagery of cancer.* Champaign, Ill.: Institute for Personality and Ability Testing.

Achterberg, J., Simonton, O. C., & Matthews-Simonton, S. (1976). *Stress psychological factors and cancer.* Dallas: New Medical Press.

Agle, D. P. & Ratnoff, O. D. (1962). Purpura as a psychogenic entity: A psychiatric study of autoerythrocyte sensitization. *Archives of Internal Medicine, 109,* 685-694.

Agle, D. P., Ratnoff, O. D., & Wasman, M. (1967). Studies in autoerythrocyte sensitization: the induction of purpuric lesions by hypnotic suggestion. *Psychosomatic Medicine, 29,* 491-503.

Agle, D. P. Ratnoff, O. D., & Wasman, M. (1969). Conversion reactions in autoerythrocyte sensitization. *Archives of General Psychiatry, 20,* 438-477.

Ahles, T. A. (1985). Psychological approaches to the management of cancer-related pain. *Seminars in Oncology Nursing, 1,* 141-146.

Allen, V. L., and Schieb, K. E. (1982). *The social context of conduct: Psychological writings of Theordore Sarbin.* New York: Praeger Publications.

Alman, G. M., & Carney, R. E. (1980). Consequences of direct and indirect suggestions on success of posthypnotic behavior. *American Journal of Clinical Hypnosis, 23,* 112-118.

Ament, P. (1982). Concepts in the use of hypnosis for pain relief in cancer. *Journal of Medicine, 13,* 233-240.

American Cancer Society (1975). Unproven methods of cancer management: Cancer quackery. *Ca—A Cancer Journal for Clinicians, 25,* 66-71.

———. (1982). Unproven methods of cancer management: O. Carl Simonton. *Ca—A Cancer Journal for Clinicians, 32,* 58-61.

American Journal of Clinical Hypnosis. (1983). Special issue: *Hypnosis and Cancer* (Vol. 25, Nos. 2-3).

American Medical Association (1986). Council Report: Scientific status of refreshing recollection by the use of hypnosis (August, 1985). *International Journal of Clinical and Experimental Hypnosis, 34,* 1-12.

Amman, B. M., & Carney, R. E. (1981). Consequences of direct and indirect suggestions on success of post-hypnotic behavior. *American Journal of Clinical Hypnosis, 23,* 112-118.

Anderson, J. A. D., Basker, M. A., & Dalton, R. (1975). Migraine and hypnotherapy. *International Journal of Clinical and Experimental Hypnosis, 23,* 48-58.

Anderson, M. N. (1957). Hypnosis in Anesthesia. *Journal of the Medical Association of Alabama, 27,* 121-125.

Anderson, N. H. (1974). Algebraic models in perception. In E. C. Carterette and M. P. Friedman (Eds.), *Handbook of Perception* (Vol. 2). New York: Academic Press.

Anderson, N. H.. (1975). On the role of context effects in psychophysical judgement. *Psychological Review, 82,* 462-482.

——. (1982). Cognitive algebra and social psychology. In B. Wegener (Ed.), *Social attitudes and psychophysical measurement.* Hillsdale, N. J.: Erlbaum.

Anderton, C. H. (1986). The forensic use of hypnosis. In F. A. De Piano & H. C. Salzberg (Eds.), *Clinical applications of hypnosis.* Norwood, N.J.: Ablex.

Andreychuk, T., & Skriver, C. (1975). Hypnosis and biofeedback in the treatment of migraine headache. *International Journal of Clinical and Experimental Hypnosis, 23,* 172-173.

Andrykowski, M. A., Redd, W. H., & Hatfield, A. K. (1985). Development of anticipatory nausea: A prospective analysis. *Journal of Consulting and Clinical Psychology, 53,* 447-454.

Angelini, R. F., & Stanford, R. G. (1987). *Perceived involuntariness: The interaction of incongruent proprioception and supplied imagery.* Paper presented at the meeting of the American Psychological Association, New York.

Anonymous. (1905). A new anesthetic. *British Journal of Dental Science, 48,* 544-545.

Araoz, D. L. (1981). Negative self-hypnosis. *Journal of Contemporary Psychotherapy, 12,* 1, pp. 45-51.

Araoz, D. L. (1982). *Hypnosis and sex therapy.* New York: Brunner/Mazel.

——. (1983). Use of hypnotic techniques with oncology patients. *Journal of Psychosocial Oncology, 1,* (4), 47-54.

——. (1983a). Transformation techniques of the new hypnosis. *Medical Hypnoanalysis, 4,* (3), 114-124.

——. (1983b). *Ericksonian hypnosis: The quintessence of client-centeredness.* Paper presented at the 2nd International Congress of Ericksonian Psychotherapy, Phoenix, Ariz.

——. (1985). *The new hypnosis.* New York: Brunner/Mazel.

Arnold, M. B. (1946). On the mechanism of suggestion and hypnosis. *Journal of Abnormal and Social Psychology, 41,* 107-128.

As, A. (1962). Non-hypnotic experiences related to hypnotizability in male and female college students. *Scandinavian Journal of Psychology, 3,* 112-121.

——. (1963). Hypnotizability as a function of non-hypnotic experiences, *Journal of Abnormal and Social Psychology, 66,* 142-150.

As, A. & Lauer, L. (1962). A factor analytic study of hypnotizability and related personal experiences. *Journal of Abnormal Social Psychology, 10,* 81-89.

As, A., O'Hara, J. W. & Munger, M. P. (1962). The measurement of subjective experiences presumably related to hypnotic susceptibility. *Scandinavian Journal of Psychology, 3,* 47-64.

As, A., & Ostvold, S. (1968). Hypnosis as subjective experience. *Scandinavian Journal of Psychology, 9,* 33-38.

As, A., Hilgard, E. R., & Weitzenhoffer, A. M. (1963). An attempt at experimental modification of hypnotizability through repeated individualized hypnotic experiences. *Scandinavian Journal of Psychology, 4,* 81-89.

Asch, S. E. (1958). Effects of group pressure upon modification and distortion of judgements. In E. E. Maccoby, T. M. Newcomb & E. L. Hartley (Eds.), *Readings in social psychology,* (3rd ed., pp. 174-183). New York: Holt.

Astbury, J. (1980). Labor Pain: The role of childbirth education, information and expectation. In C. Peck & M. Wallace (Eds.), *Problems in pain.* London: Pergamon.

August, R. V. (1961). *Hypnosis in obstetrics.* New York: McGraw Hill Book Company Inc.

——. (1975). Hypnotic induction of hypothermia: An additional approach to postoperative control of cancer recurrence. *American Journal of Clinical Hypnosis, 18,* 52-55.

Austrin, H. R., & Pereira, M. J. (1978). Locus of control as a predictor of hypnotic susceptibility. *The American Journal of Clinical Hypnosis, 20* 199-202.

Avard, D. M., & Nimrod, C. M. (1985). Risks and benefits of obstetric epidural analgesia: A review. *Birth, 12,* 215-225.

Averill, J. R. (1982). *Anger and aggression: An essay on emotion.* New York: Springer-Verlag.

Avia, M. D., & Kanfer, F. H. (1980). Coping with aversive stimulation: The effects of training in a self-management context. *Cognitive Therapy and Research, 4,* 73-81.

Baker, E. L. (1986). Hypnosis with psychotic and borderline patients. In B. Zilbergeld, M. G. Edelstein & D. L. Araoz (Eds.), *Hypnosis: Questions and answers.* New York: Norton.

Baker, E. L., & Levitt, E. E. (in press, 1988). The hypnotic relationship: An investigation of compliance and resistance. *International Journal of Clinical and Experimental Hypnosis.*

Baker, R. A., Haynes, B., & Patrick, B. S. (1983). Hypnosis, memory and incidental memory. *American Journal of Clinical Hypnosis, 25,* 253-262.

Balthazard, C. G. & Woody, E. Z. (1985). The "stuff" of hypnotic performance: A review of psychometric approaches. *Psychological Bulletin, 98,* 283-296.

Bandler, R., & Grinder, J. (1975). *Patterns of the hypnotic techniques of Milton H. Erickson, M.D. Volume 1.* Cupertino, Calif.: Meta Publishers.

Bandler, R. J., Madaras, G. R., & Bem, D. J. (1968). Self-observation as a source of pain perception. *Journal of Personality and Social Psychology, 9,* 205-209.

Bandura, A. (1977a). Self-efficacy: Toward a unifying theory of behavioral change. *Psychological Review, 84,* 191-215.

——. (1977b). *Social learning theory.* Englewood Cliffs, N.J.: Prentice-Hall.

——. (1978). The self system in reciprocal determinism. *American Psychologist, 33,* 344-358.

Bandura, A., O'Leary, A., Taylor, C. B., Gauthier, J., & Gossard, D. (1987). Perceived self-efficacy and pain control: opioid and nonopioid mechanisms. *Journal of Personality and Social Psychology, 53,* 563-571.

Bányai, E. I. (1985). On the interactional nature of hypnosis: A social psycho-physiological approach. Paper presented at the International Congress of Hypnosis and Psychosomatic Medicine, Toronto, Canada.

Bányai, E., & Hilgard, E. R. (1976). A comparison of an active alert hypnotic induction with traditional relaxation induction. *Journal of Abnormal Psychology, 85,* 218-224.

Barbasz, A. E., & Lonsdale, C. (1983). Effects of hypnosis on P300 of olfactory-evoked potential amplitudes. *Journal of Abnormal Psychology, 92,* 520-523.

Barber, J. (1976). Effectiveness of hypnotic analgesia in the reduction of experimental dental pain in individuals of both high and low hypnotic susceptiblity. Unpublished doctoral dissertation, University of Southern California.

——. (1977). Rapid induction analgesia: A clinical report. *American Journal of Clinical Hypnosis, 19,* 138-149.

——. (1978). Hypnosis as a psychological technique in the management of cancer pain. *Cancer Nursing, 1,* 361-363.

——. (1980). Hypnosis and the unhypnotizable. *American Journal of Clinical Hypnosis, 23,* 4-9.

——. (1982). Incorporating hypnosis in the management of chronic pain. In J. Barber & C. Adrian (Eds.), *Psychological approaches to the management of pain.* New York: Brunner/Mazel.

Barber, J., & Gitelson, J. (1980). Cancer pain: Psychological management using hypnosis. *Ca—A Cancer Journal for Clinicians, 30,* 130-136.

Barber, J., & Mayer, D. (1977). Evaluation of the efficacy and neural mechanism of a hypnotic analgesia procedure in experimental and clinical dental pain. *Pain, 4,* 41-48.

Barber, T. X. (1956). A note on hypnotizability and personality traits. *Journal of Clinical and Experimental Hypnosis, 4,* 109-114.

——. (1959). Toward a theory of pain: Relief of chronic pain by prefrontal leucotomy, opiates, placebos, and hypnosis. *Psychological Bulletin, 56,* 430-460.

——. (1960). The necessary and sufficient conditions for hypnotic behavior. *The American Journal of Clinical Hypnosis, 3,* 31-42.

——. (1961). Antisocial and criminal acts induced by 'hypnosis': A review of clinical and experimental findings. *Archives of General Psychiatry, 5,* 301-312.

——. (1962). Hypnotic age regression: A critical review. *Psychosomatic Medicine, 24,* ; 286-299.

Barber, T. X. (1963). The effects of "hypnosis" on pain: A critical review of experimental and clinical findings. *Psychosomatic Medicine, 25,* 303-333.

——. (1964). Hypnotizability, suggestibility and personality: V. A critical review of research findings. *Psychological Reports, 14* (Monograph Supplement 3).

——. (1965). The effects of "hypnosis" on learning and recall: A methodological critique. *Journal of Abnormal Psychology, 21,* 19-25.

——. (1969). *Hypnosis: A scientific approach.* New York: Van Nostrand Reinhold.

——. (1970). *LSD, marijuana, yoga and hypnosis.* Chicago: Aldine.

——. (1972). Suggested ("hypnotic") behavior: The trance paradigm versus an alternative paradigm. In E. Fromm & R. E. Shor (Eds.), *Hypnosis: Research developments and perspectives.* New York: Aldine-Atherton.

——. (1976). *Hypnosis: A scientific approach.* New York: Psychological Dimensions.

——. (1978). Hypnosis, suggestions, and psychosomatic phenomena: A new look from the standpoint of recent experimental studies. *American Journal of Clinical Hypnosis, 21,* 13-27.

——. (1979a). Training students to use self-suggestions for personal growth, *Journal of Suggestive Accelerative Learning and Teaching, 4* (2).

——. (1979b). Suggested ("hypnotic") behavior: The trance paradigm versus an alternative paradigm. In E. Fromm & R. E. Shor (Eds.), *Hypnosis: Developments in research and new perspectives.* (2nd ed.). Chicago: Aldine, 217-271.

——. (1981). Medicine, suggestive therapy and healing. In R. J. Kastenbaum, T. X. Barber, S. C. Wilson, B. L. Ryder, & L. B. Hathaway. *Old, sick and helpless: Where therapy begins.* Cambridge, Mass.: Ballinger Publishing Company.

——. (1982). Hypnosuggestive procedures in the treatment of clinical pain. In T. Milton, C. J. Greene, & R. B. Meagher, Jr., (Eds.), *Handbook of health care clinical psychology.* New York: Plenum.

——. (1983a). Changing "unchangeable" bodily processes by (hypnotic) suggestions: A new look at hypnosis, cognitions, imaginings and the mind-body problem. In A. A. Sheikh (Ed.), *Imagination and healing.* Farmingdale, N.Y.: Baywood Publishing Company.

——. (1985). Hypnosuggestive procedures as catalysts for psychotherapies. In S. J. Lynn & J. P. Garske (Eds.), *Contemporary psychotherapies. Models and methods* (pp. 333-375). Columbus, OH: Charles E. Merrill.

Barber, T. X., & Calverley, D. S. (1963). "Hypnotic-like" suggestibility in children and adults. *Journal of Abnormal and Social Psychology, 66,* 363-389.

——. (1964a). The definition of the situation as a variable affecting "hypnotic-like" suggestibility. *Journal of Clinical Psychology, 20,* 438-440.

——. (1964b). Experimental studies in hypnotic behavior. Suggested deafness evaluated by delayed auditory feedback. *British Journal of Psychology, 55,* 439-446.

——. (1964c). Toward a theory of "hypnotic" behavior: An experimental study of "hypnotic time-distortion." *Archives of General Psychiatry, 10,* 209-216.

——. (1964d). Toward a theory of hypnotic behavior: Effects on suggestibility of defining the situation as hypnosis and defining the response as easy. *Journal of Abnormal and Social Psychology, 68,* 585-592.

——. (1965a). Hypnotizability, suggestibility, and personality: II. Assessment of previous imaginative-fantasy experiences by As, Barber-Glass and Shor questionnaires. *Journal of Clinical Psychology, 21,* 57-58.

——. (1965b). Empirical evidence for a theory of hypnotic behavior: Effects on suggestibility of five variables typically included in hypnotic induction procedures. *Journal of Consulting Psychology, 29,* 98-107.

——. (1965c). Empirical evidence for a theory of "hypnotic" behavior: The suggestibility-enhancing effects of motivational suggestions, relaxation-sleep suggestions, and suggestions that the S will be effectively hypnotized. *Journal of Personality, 33,* 256-270.

——. (1966). Toward a theory of hypnotic behavior. Experimental evaluation of Hull's postulate that hypnotic susceptibility is a habit phenomenon. *Journal of Personality, 34,* 416-433.

Barber, T. X. & Calverley, D. S. (1969). Multidimensional analysis of "hypnotic" behavior. *Journal of Abnormal Psychology, 74,* 209-220.

Barber, T. X., & Cooper, B. J. (1972). Effects on pain of experimentally-induced and spontaneous distribution. *Psychological Reports, 31,* 647-651.

Barber, T. X., Dalal, A. S., & Calverley, D. S. (1968). The subjective reports of hypnotic subjects. *American Journal of Clinical Hypnosis, 11,* 74-88.

Barber, T. X., & Glass, L. B. (1962). Significant factors in hypnotic behavior. *Journal of Abnormal and Social Psychology, 64,* 222-228.

Barber, T. X., & Hahn, K. W. Jr. (1962). Physiological and subjective responses to pain-producing stimulation under hypnotically-suggested and waking-imagined "analgesia." *Journal of Abnormal and Social Psychology, 65,* 411-418.

——. (1964). Experimental studies in "hypnotic" behavior: Physiological and subjective effects of imagined pain. *Journal of Nervous and Mental Disease, 139,* 416-425.

Barber, T. X., Spanos, N. P., & Chaves, J. F. (1974). *Hypnosis, imagination, and human potentialities.* Elmsford, N.Y.: Pergamon Press.

Barber, T. X., & Wilson, S. C. (1977). Hypnosis, suggestions, and altered states of consciousness: Experimental evaluation of the new cognitive-behavioral theory and the traditional trance-state theory of "hypnosis." In W. E. Edmonston (Ed.), *Conceptual and investigative approaches to hypnosis and hypnotic phenomena* (pp. 34-74). New York: New York Academy of Sciences.

——. (1979). The Barber Suggestibility Scale and the Creative Imagination Scale: Experimental and clinical applications. *American Journal of Clinical Hypnosis, 21,* 84-108.

Barber, T. X., Wilson, S. C., & Scott, D. S. (1980). Effects of a traditional trance induction on response to "hypnotist-centered" versus "subject-centered" test suggestions. *International Journal of Clinical and Experimental Hypnosis, 28,* 114-126.

Bargh, J. A. (1984). Automatic and conscious processing of social information. In R. S. Wyer and T. K. Srull (Eds.), *Handbook of social cognition* (Vol. 3, pp. 1-43). Hillsdale, N.J.: Erlbaum.

Barrios, A. A., & Kroger, W. W. (1975). Hypnosis as a tool in the fight against cancer. *Journal of Holistic Health, 1,* 71-80.

Baruffi, G., Dellinger, W. S., Stobino, D. M., Rudolph, A., Timmons, R. G., and Ross, A. (1984). Patterns of obstetrics procedures used in maternity care. *Obstetrics and Gynecology, 64,* 493-498.

Baum, D. & Lynn, S. J. (1981). Hypnotic susceptibility level and reading involvement. *International Journal of Clinical and Experimental Hypnosis, 29,* 366-374.

Baumeister, R. (1982). A self-presentational view of social phenomena. *Psychological Bulletin, 91,* 3-26.

Beahrs, J. O. (1982). *Unity and multiplicity: Multilevel consciousness of self in hypnosis, psychiatric disorder, and mental health.* New York: Brunner/Mazel.

Beahrs, J. O., Harris, D. R., & Hilgard, E. R. (1970). Failure to alter skin inflammation by hypnotic suggestion in 5 subjects with normal skin reactivity. *Psychosomatic Medicine, 32,* 627-631.

Beck, A. J. (1976). *Cognitive therapy and the emotional disorders.* New York: International Universities Press.

Beck, N. C., Geden, E. A., & Brouder, G. T. (1979). Preparation for labor: A historical perspective. *Psychosomatic Medicine, 41,* 243-258.

Beck, N. D. & Hall, D. (1978). Natural childbirth: A review and analysis. *Obstetrics and Gynecology, 52,* 371-379.

Beck, N. D., Siegel, L. J., Davidson, N. P., Kormeier, S., Breitenstein, A., & Hall, D. G. (1980). The prediction of pregnancy outcome: Maternal preparation, anxiety and attitudinal sets. *Journal of Psychosomatic Research, 4,* 343-351.

Beecher, H. K. (1946). Pain in men wounded in battle. *Annals of Surgery, 123,* 96-105.

——. (1959). *Measurement of subjective responses.* New York: Oxford University Press.

Beers, T. M., & Karoly, P. (1979). Cognitive strategies, expectancy, and coping in the control of pain. *Journal of Consulting and Clinical Psychology, 47,* 179-180.

Bem, D. J. (1965). An experimental analysis of self-persuasion. *Journal of Experimental and Social Psychology, 1*, 199-218.

———. (1967). Self-perception: An alternative interpretation of cognitive dissonance phenomena. *Psychological Review, 74*, 183-200.

———. (1972). Self-perception theory. In L. Berkowitz (Ed.), *Advances in experimental social psychology* (Vol. 6). New York: Academic Press.

Bennett, A. (1985). The birth of a first child: Do women's reports change over time? *Birth, 12*, 153-158.

Bensen, V. B. (1971). One hundred cases of post anesthetic suggestion in the recovery room. *American Journal of Clinical Hypnosis, 14*, 9-15.

Bensen, H. (1975). *The relaxation response.* New York: William Morrow & Company.

Berger, P. L., & Luckman, T. (1966). *The social construction of reality.* New York: Anchor.

Berk, S. N., Moore, M. E., & Resnick, J. H. (1977). Psychosocial factors as mediators of acupuncture therapy. *Journal of Consulting and Clinical Psychology, 45*, 612-619.

Bernheim, H. (1880/1906). *Suggestive therapeutics.* New York: G. P. Putnam's Sons.

———. *Suggestive therapeutics: A treatise on the nature and use of hypnotism.* (2nd ed., C. A. Herter, Trans.). New York: Putnam.

Bernheim, H. M. (1891). *New Studies in Hypnostism.* (R. S. Sandor, Translator). New York: International Universities Press.

Bernstein, M. R. (1963). Management of burned children with the aid of hypnosis. *Journal of Child Psychology, 7*, 93-98.

———. (1965). Significant values of hypnoanesthesia: Three clinical examples. *American Journal of Clinical Hypnosis, 7*, 259-260.

Bertrand, L. D., Spanos, N. P., & Parkinson, B. (1983). Test of the dissipation hypothesis of hypnotic amnesia. *Psychological Reports, 52*, 667-671.

Bertrand, L. D., & Spanos, N. P. (1985). The organization of recall during hypnotic suggestions for complete and selective amnesia. *Imagination, Cognition & Personality, 4*, 249-261.

———. (in press, 1988). Hypnosis: Historical and social psychological aspects. In A. A. Sheikh & K. S. Sheikh (Eds.), *Eastern and western approaches to healing.* New York: Wiley and Sons.

Besser, A. R. (1970). The paradoxical theory of change. In J. Fagan & I. L. Shepherd (Eds.), *Gestalt therapy now* (pp. 77-80). Palo Alto, Calif.: Science and Behavior Books.

Betts, G. S. (1909). The distribution and functions of mental imagery. *Teachers College—Contributions to Education* (No. 26).

Birnbaum, M. H. (1974). Using contextual effects to derive psychophysical scales. *Perception & Psychophysics, 15*, 89-96.

———. (1982). Controversies in psychological measurement. In B. Wegener (Ed.), *Social Attitudes and Psychophysical Measurement.* Hillsdale, N.J.: Erlbaum.

Bitterman, M. E., & Marcuse, F. L. (1945). Autonomic response in posthypnotic amnesia. *Journal of Experimental Psychology, 35*, 248-252.

Bjork, R. A. (1972). Theoretical implications of directed forgetting. In A. W. Melton & E. Martin (Eds.), *Coding processes in human memory.* Washington, D.C.: Winston & Sons.

Bjork, R. A., & Geiselman, R. E. (1978). Constituent processes in the differentiation of items in memory. *Journal of Experimental Psychology: Human Learning & Memory, 4*, 347-361.

Black, S., & Wigan, E. R. (1961). An investigation of selective deafness produced by direct suggestions under hypnosis. *British Medical Journal, 2*, 736-741.

Blum, G. S. (1975). A case of hypnotically induced tubular vision. *International Journal of Clinical and Experimental Hypnosis, 23*, 111-119.

Blum, G. S., & Graef, J. R. (1971). The detection over time of subjects simulating hypnosis. *International Journal of Clinical and Experimental Hypnosis, 19*, 211-224.

Bodorik, H. L., & Spanos, N. P. (1977). Suggested amnesia of semantic components of memory in hypnotic and task-motivated subjects. Unpublished manuscript, Carleton University, Ottawa, Canada.

Bond, M. R. (1979). Psychologic and emotional aspects of cancer pain. In J. J. Bonica & V. Ventafridda (Eds.), *Advances in pain research and therapy* (Vol. 2, pp. 81-88). New York: Raven Press.

Bonica, J. J. (1979). Importance of the problem. In J. J. Bonica & V. Ventafridda (Eds.), *Advances in pain research and therapy* (Vol. 2, pp. 1-12). New York: Raven Press.

———. (1980). Cancer pain. In J. J. Bonica (Ed.). *Pain* (pp. 335-362). New York:Raven Press.

Bonilla, K. B., Quigley, W. F., & Bowers, W. F. 1961. Experience with hypnosis on a surgical service. *Military Medicine, 126,* 364-366.

Bonnell, A. M., & Bourreau, F. (1985). Labor pain assessment: Validity of a behavioral index. *Pain, 22,* 81-90.

Borkovec, T. D., & Nau, S. D. (1972). Credibility of analogue therapy rationales. *Journal of Behavior Therapy and Experimental Psychiatry, 3,* 257-260.

Botto, R. W., & Fisher, S. (1978). A preliminary report on social learning behavior in the hypnotic situation: Modeling or mimicry. In F. H. Frankel & H. S. Zamansky (Eds.), *Hypnosis at its bicentennial.* New York: Plenum.

Botto, R. W., Fisher, S., & Soucy, G. P. (1977). The effect of a good and a poor model on hypnotic susceptibility in a low demand situation. *International Journal of Clinical and Experimental Hypnosis, 25,* 175-183.

Bowers, K. S. (1966). Hypnotic behavior: The differentiation of trance and demand characteristic variables. *Journal of Abnormal Psychology, 71,* 42-51.

———. (1971). Sex and susceptibility as moderator variables in the relationship of creativity and hypnotic susceptibility. *Journal of Abnormal Psychology, 78,* 93-100.

———. (1975). The psychology of subtle control: An attributional analysis of behavioral persistence. *Canadian Journal of Behavioral Science, 7,* 78-95.

———. (1976). Hypnosis for the seriously curious (pp. 41-52). Monterey, Calif.: Brooks-Cole.

———. (1977). Hypnosis: An informational approach. *Annals of the New York Academy of Sciences, 296,* 227-237.

———. (1979). Time distortion and hypnotic ability: Underestimating the duration of hypnosis. *Journal of Abnormal Psychology, 88,* 435-439.

———. (1981). Do the Stanford scales tap the classic suggestion effect? *International Journal of Clinical and Experimental Hypnosis, 31,* 293-308

Bowers, K. S., & Brenneman, H. A. (1979). Hypnosis and the perception of time. *International Journal of Clinical and Experimental Hypnosis, 27,* 29-41.

Bowers, K. S., & Kelly, P. (1979). Stress, disease, psychotherapy and hypnosis. *Journal of Abnormal Psychology, 88,* 490-505.

Bowers, K. S., & Quan, A. (1978). Imaginative absorption, time distortion, and hypnotic ability. Unpublished manuscript, Waterloo University.

Bowers, P. (1978). Hypnotizability, creativity and the role of effortless experiencing. *The International Journal of Clinical and Experimental Hypnosis, 26,* 184-202.

———. (1982). The classic suggestion effect: Relationships with scales of hypnotizability, effortless experiencing, and imagery vividness. *International Journal of Clinical and Experimental Hypnosis, 3,* 270-279.

Bowers, P., Laurence, J-R., & Hart, D. (in press, 1988). The experience of hypnotic suggestions. *International Journal of Clinical and Experimental Hypnosis.*

Bowers, W. F. (1966). Hypnosis: Useful adjunct in surgery. *Surgical Bulletin, 46,* 8-10.

Boyd, P. (1984). *The silent wound: A startling report on breast cancer and sexuality.* Reading, Mass.: Addison-Wesley.

Brady, J. P., Levitt, E. E., & Lubin, B. (1961). Expressed fear of hypnosis and volunteering behavior. *Journal of Nervous Mental Diseases, 133,* 216-217.

Braid, J. (1846/1976). *Neurypnology, or the rationale of nervous sleep, considered in relation with animal magnetism.* New York: Arno Press. (Original work published in London by J. Churchill, 1946).

Braid, J. (1846/1970). The power of the mind over the body. In M. M. Tinterow, *Foundations of hypnosis: From Mesmer to Freud.* Springfield, Ill.: Thomas. (Original work published in London by J. Churchill, 1846).

Bramwell, J. M. (1903). *Hypnotism: Its history, practice and theory.* London: Grant Richards. Reissued with new introduction. New York: Julian Press, 1956.

Braun, B. (1979). Hypnotherapy for Reynaud's disease. In G. D. Burroughs, D. R. Collison, & L. Dennerstein, (Eds.), *Hypnosis.* Elsevier/North Holland Biomedical Press.

Brehm, J. W. (1966). *A theory of cognitive reactance.* New York: Academic Press.

Brenman, M. (1942). Experiments in the hypnotic production of antisocial and self-injurious behavior. *Psychiatry, 5,* 49-61.

British Society of Experimental and Clinical Hypnosis. (1984). Use of hypnosis by the police in the investigation of crime (Oct. 1983). *British Journal of Experimental and Clinical Hypnosis, 1,* 57-58.

Brower, D. (1947). The experimental study of imagery: II. The relative predominance of various imagery modalities. *Journal of General Psychology, 37,* 199-200.

Brown, D. P., & Fromm, E. (1986). *Hypnotherapy and hypnoanalysis.* Hillsdale, N.J.: Earlbuaum.

——. (1987). *Hypnosis and behavioral medicine.* Hillsdale, N.J.: Earlbaum.

Brown, G. K., & Nicassio, P. M. (1987). Development of a questionnaire for the assessment of active and passive coping strategies in chronic pain patients. *Pain, 31,* 53-64.

Brown, J., Chaves, J. F., & Leoniff. (1981). Spontaneous hypnotic strategies in two groups of chronic pain patients. Presented at the Annual Meeting of the American Psychological Association, Los Angeles, Calif.

Brown, P. E. (1972). Use of acupuncture in major surgery.. *Lancet, 1,* 1328-1330.

Brown, R. A., Fader, K., & Barber, T. X. (1973). Responsiveness to pain: Stimulus-specificity versus generality. *Psychological Record, 23,* 1-7.

Brown, R., & McNeill, D. (1966). The "tip of the tongue" phenomenon. *Journal of Verbal Learning and Verbal Behavior, 5,* 325-337.

Brown, S. W. (1984). Retrospective duration judgments of a hypnotic time interval. In J. Gibbom & L. Allan (Eds.), Timing and time perception (Vol. 423, pp. 583-584). New York: New York Academy of Sciences.

Buckhout, R., Eugenio, P., Licitra, T., Oliver, L., & Kramer, T. H. (1981). Memory, hypnosis and evidence. *Social Action and the Law, 7,* 67-72.

Buckley, J. P. (1911). The treatment of sensitive dentin. In C. N. Johnson (Ed.), *A textbook of operative dentistry.* Philadelphia: P. Blakistons Sons & Co.

Buckner, L. C., & Coe, W. C. (1972). Imaginative skill, wording of suggestions, and hypnotic susceptibility. *International Journal of Clinical and Experimental Hypnosis, 25,* 27-35.

Buranelli, V. (1975). *The wizard from Vienna.* New York: Coward, McCann and Geoghegen.

Butler, B. (1954). The use of hypnosis in the care of the cancer patient. *Cancer, 7,* 1-14.

Callan, T. D. (1961). Can hypnosis be used routinely in obstetrics? *Rocky Mountain Medical Journal.*

Campbell, D. T. and Stanley, J. C. (1963). *Experimental and quasi-experimental designs for research.* Chicago: Rand-McNally.

Calverley, D. S., & Barber, T. X. (1965). "Hypnosis" and antisocial behavior: An experimental evaluation. Harding, Mass.: Medfield Foundation (Mimeo). Cited by Barber, 1969.

Cangello, V. W. (1961). The use of hypnotic suggestion for pain relief in malignant disease. *International Journal of Clinical and Experimental Hypnosis, 9,* 17-22.

——. (1962). Hypnosis for the patient with cancer. *American Journal of Clinical Hypnosis, 4,* 215-226.

Cantor, N., Mischel, W., & Schwartz, J. C. (1982). A prototype analysis of psychological situations. *Cognitive Psychology, 14,* 45-77.

Capperauld, I. (1972). Acupuncture anesthesia and medicine in China today. *Surgery, Gynecology and Obstetrics, 135,* 440-445.

Caracappa, J. M. (1963). Hypnosis in terminal cancer. *American Journal of Clinical Hypnosis, 5,* 205-206.

Carasso, R. L., Peded, O., Kleinhauz, M., & Yehuda, S. (1985). Treatment of cervical headache with hypnosis, suggestive therapy, and relaxation techniques. *American Journal of Clinical Hypnosis, 27,* 216-218.,

Carlin, S., Ward, W. D., Gershon, A., & Ingraham, R. (1962). Sound stimulation and its effect on dental sensation threshold. *Science, 138,* 1258-1260.

Casey, G. A. (1966). Hypnotic time distortion and learning. *Dissertation Abstracts, 27,* 2116A-2117A.

Cassileth, B. R., Lusk, E. J., Strouse, T. B., & Bodenheimer, B. J. (1984). Contemporary unorthodox treatments in cancer medicine. *Annals of Internal Medicine, 101,* 105-112.

Cedercreutz, C. (1978). Hypnotic treatment of 100 cases of migraine. In F. H. Frankel, & H. S. Zamansky (Eds.), *Hypnosis at its Bicentennial.* New York: Plenum Press, pp. 255-259.

Cedercreutz, C., & Uusitalo, E. (1967). Hypnotic treatment of phantom sensations in 37 amputees. In J. Lassner (Ed.), *Hypnosis and psychosomatic medicine.* New York: Springer-Verlag.

Cedercreutz, C., Lahteenmaki, R., & Tulikoura, J. (1976). Hypnotic treatment of headache and vertigo in skull-injured patients. *International Journal of Clinical and Experimental Hypnosis, 24,* 195-201.

Challis, G. B., & Stam, H. J. (1988a). The development of anticipatory nausea and vomiting in cancer chemotherapy patients: A prospective study. Unpublished manuscript, University of Calgary.

———. (1988b). The relationship between the spontaneous regression of cancer and unorthodox methods of treatment: A review and critique. Unpublished manuscript, University of Calgary.

Chapman, C. R., Benedetti, C., Colpitts, Y. H., & Gerlach, R. (1983). Naloxone fails to reverse pain thresholds elevated by acupuncture: acupuncture analgesia reconsidered. *Pain, 16,* 13-31.

Charcot, J. M. (1882). *Physiologie pathologique: Sur les diver états nerveux détermine pur l'hypnotization chez les hysteriques, CR Academy of Science, 94,* 403-405.

Charles, A. G., Norr, K. L., Block, C. R., Meyering, S., & Meyers, E. (1978). Obstetric and psychological effects of psychoprophylactic preparation for childbirth. *American Journal of Obstetrics and Gynecology, 131,* 44-52.

Chaves, J. F. (1968). Hypnosis reconceptualized: An overview of Barber's theoretical and empirical work. *Psychological Reports, 22,* 587-608.

———. (1975). Acupuncture analgesia for surgery: A six-factor theory reconsidered. *Proceedings of the Third World Symposium on Acupuncture and Chinese Medicine. American Journal of Chinese Medicine, 3,* Suppl. 1, 24.

———. (1985a). Hypnosis in the management of phantom limb pain. In T. Dowd, & J. Healy (Eds.), *Case studies in hypnotherapy.* New York: Guilford.

———. (1985b). Hypnosis in the management of behavioral components of Prader-Willi Syndrome. In T. Dowd, & J. Healy (eds.), *Case studies in hypnotherapy.* New York: Guilford.

———. (1986). Using spontaneous trances. In B. Zilbergeld, M. G. Edelstein, & D. L. Araoz (Eds.), *Hypnosis: questions & answers.* New York: Norton.

———. (1973). Needles and knives: Behind the mystery of acupuncture and Chinese meridians. *Human Behavior, 2,* 19-24.

Chaves, J. F., & Barber, T. X. (1974). Cognitive strategies, experimenter modeling and expectation in the attenuation of pain. Journal of Abnormal Psychology, 83, 356-363.

———. (1974b). Acupuncture analgesia: A six factor theory. *Psychoenergetic Systems, 1,* 11-21.

———. (1976). Hypnotic procedures and surgery. A critical analysis with applications to "acupuncture analgesia." *American Journal of Clinical Hypnosis, 8,* 217-236.

Chaves, J. F., & Brown, J. F. (1978). Self-generated strategies for the control of clinical pain and stress. Presented at the Annual Meeting of the American Psychological Association. Toronto, Canada.

Chaves, J. F., & Brown, J. F. (1987). Spontaneous coping strategies for pain. *Journal of Behavioral Medicine, 10,* 263-276.

Chaves, J. F., & Doney, T. (1976). Cognitive attenuation of pain: The roles of imagery, strategy relevance, absorption and expectation. Presented at the annual meeting of the Association for the Advancement of Behavior Therapy, New York.

Chaves, J. F., & Rosentstiel, A. (1975). Cognitive control of pain: From acupuncture and hypnosis to the blue ray. Presented at the Annual Meeting of the American Psychological Association. Chicago, Ill.

Chaves, J. F., & Scott, D. (1979). Effects of cognitive strategies and suggested criterion alteration on pain threshold. Presented at the Annual Meeting of the Eastern Psychological Association. Philadelphia, Pa.

Chaves, J. F., Whilden, D., & Roller, N. (1979). Hypnosis in the dental behavior sciences: Control of surgical and post-surgical bleeding. In B. D. Ingersoll, & W. R. McCutcheon (Eds.), *Clinical research in behavioral dentistry: Proceedings of the second national conference on behavioral dentistry.* Morgantown, W.V.: West Virginia University.

Cheek, D. B. (1959). Use of rebellion against coercion as mechanism for hypnotic trance deepening. *International Journal of Clinical and Experimental Hypnosis, 7.* 223-228.

——. (1976). Hypnotherapy for secondary frigidity after radical surgery for gynecological cancer: Two case reports. *American Journal of Clinical Hypnosis, 19,* 13-19.

Chen, J. Y. P. (1972). Acupuncture. in J. R. Quinn (Ed.), *Medicine and public health in the People's Republic of China.* Washington, D.C.: U.S. Department of Health, Education and Welfare, National Institutes of Health, 1972, pp. 65-90.

Chertok, L. (1969). *Motherhood and personality: Psychosomatic aspects of childbirth.* Philadelphia: Lippincott.

Chong, T. M. (1968). The use of hypnosis in the management of patients with cancer. *Singapore Medical Journal, 9,* 211-214.

——. (1979). Psychological intervention in patients with cancer. *Singapore Family Physician, 4,* 20-25.

——. (1982). Ericksonian approaches in general practice. In J. K. Zeig (Ed.), *Ericksonian approaches to hypnosis and psychotherapy* (pp. 292-298). New York: Brunner/Mazel.

Christensen, L. (1977). The negative subject effect: Myth, reality or a prior experimental experience effect? *Journal of Personality and Social Psychology, 35,* 392-400.

Clark, W. C. (1974). Pain sensitivity and the report of pain: An introduction to sensory decision theory. *Anesthesiology, 40,* 272-287.

Clark, W. C., & Goodman, J. C. (1974). Effects of suggestion on d' and Cx for pain detection and pain tolerance. *Journal of Abnormal Psychology, 83,* 364-372.

Clark, W. C., & Yang, J. C. (1974). Acupuncture analgesia? Evaluation by signal detection theory. *Science, 184,* 1096-1098.

——. (1976). Experimental pain following analgesic, placebo, and acupuncture: An introduction to signal detection theory. *Acupuncture and Electro-Therapeutics Research, 2,* 87-103.

Clawson, T. A., & Swade, R. H. (1975). The hypnotic control of blood flow and pain: The cure of warts and the potential for the use of hypnosis in the treatment of cancer. *American Journal of Clinical Hypnosis, 17,* 160-169.

Cleeland, C. S. (1984). The impact of pain on the patient with cancer. *Cancer, 54,* 2635-2641.

Cleeland, C. S., & Tearnan, B. H. (1986). Behavioral control of cancer pain. In A. D. Holzman & D. C. Turk (Eds.), *Pain management: A handbook of psychological treatment approaches* (pp. 193-212). New York: Pergamon Press.

Clum, G. A., Luscomb, R. L., & Scott, L. (1982). Relaxation training and cognitive redirection strategies in the treatment of acute pain. *Pain, 12,* 175-183.

Coates, A., Abraham, S., Kay, S. B., Sowerbutts, T., Frewin, C., Fox, R. M., & Tattersall, M. H. N. (1983). On the receiving end—patient perception of the side-effects of cancer chemotherapy. *European Journal of Cancer and Clinical Oncology, 19,* 203-208.

Coe, W. C. (1964). Further norms on the Harvard Group Scale of Hypnotic Susceptibility: Form A. *International Journal of Clinical and Experimental Hypnosis, 12,* 184-190.

Coe, W. C. (1973). The concept of role skills: Hypnotic behavior. Paper presented in the symposium "Role Theory," annual meeting of the American Psychological Association, Montreal.

———. (1978). The credibility of posthypnotic amnesia: A contextualist's view. *International Journal of Clinical and Experimental Hypnosis, 26*, 218-245.

———. (1980). On defining altered states of consciousness. *Bulletin of the British Society of Experimental and Clinical Hypnosis*, April (3), 5-7.

———. (1980). Posthypnotic amnesia. In R. H. Woody (Ed.), *Encyclopedia of Clinical Assessment*. San Francisco: Jossey-Bass.

———. (1983a). Trance: A problematic metaphor for hypnosis. Invited Address, Division 30, Psychological Hypnosis, annual meeting of the American Psychological Association, Los Angeles, August 29.

———. (1983b). Measuring nonvolitional experiences of hypnotic subjects with state and control reports. Paper presented at the meeting of the American Psychological Association, Anaheim, Calif.

———. (1987a). *Hypnosis: Wherefore Art Thou?* Presidential Address, Division 30, American Psychological Association, New York, N.Y.

———. (1987b). *An analysis of sociopolitical factors in viewing hypnosis as a special state.* Manuscript submitted for publication.

Coe, W. C., Allen, J. L., Krug, W. M., & Wurzman, A. G. (1974). Goal-directed fantasy in hypnotic responsiveness: Skill, item wording, or both? *International Journal of Clinical and Experimental Hypnosis, 22*, 157-166.

Coe, W. C., Basden, B. H., Basden, D., Fikes, T., Gargano, G., & Webb, M. (1988). Directed forgetting and posthypnotic amnesia: Information processing in context. Submitted to the *Journal of Personality & Social Psychology*.

Coe, W. C., Basden, B., Basden, D., & Graham, C. (1976). Posthypnotic amnesia: Suggestions of an active process in dissociative phenomena. *Journal of Abnormal Psychology, 85* (5), 455-458.

Coe, W. C., Kobayashi, K., & Howard, M. L. (1972). An approach toward isolating factors that influence antisocial conduct in hypnosis. *International Journal of Clinical and Experimental Hypnosis, 20*, 118-131.

———. (1973). Experimental and ethical problems of evaluating the influence of hypnosis in antisocial conduct. *Journal of Abnormal Psychology, 82*, 476-482.

Coe, W. C., and Ryken, K. (1979). Hypnosis and risks to human subjects. *American Psychologist, 34*, 673-681.

Coe, W. C., & Sarbin, T. R. (1971). An alternative interpretation to the multiple composition of hypnotic scales: A single role-relevant skill. *Journal of Personality and Social Psychology, 18*, 1-8.

Coe, W. C., & Sarbin, T. R. (1977). Hypnosis from the standpoint of a contextualist. In W. E. Edmonston (Ed.), *Conceptual and investigative approaches to hypnosis and hypnotic phenomena* (Vol. 296, pp. 2-13). New York: *Annals of the New York Academy of Sciences*.

Coe, W. C., & Steen, P. (1981). Examining the relationship between believing one will respond to hypnotic suggestions and hypnotic responsiveness. *American Journal of Clinical Hypnosis, 24*, 22-32.

Coe, W. C., Taul, J. H., Basden, D., & Basden, B. (1973). An investigation of the dissociative hypothesis and disorganized retrieval in posthypnotic amnesia with retroactive inhibition in free-recall learning. *Proceedings, 81st Annual Convention*, American Psychological Association.

Coe, W. C., & Tucibat, M. (1988). The effects of two breaching conditions on posthypnotically amnesic subjects. Manuscript in preparation.

Coe, W. C., & Yashinski, E. (1985). Breaching posthypnotic amnesia: Volitional experiences and their correlates. *Journal of Personality and Social Psychology*.

———. (1985). Volitional experiences associated with breaching posthypnotic amnesia. *Journal of Personality & Social Psychology, 48*, 716-722.

Cogan, R. (1975). Comfort during prepared childbirth as a function of parity, reported by four classes of participant observers. *Journal of Psychosomatic Research, 19,* 33-37.

Commins, J., Fullam, F., & Barber, T. X. (1975). Effects of experimenter modeling, demands for honesty, and initial levels of suggestibility on response to hypnotic suggestions. *Journal of Consulting and Clinical Psychology, 43,* 668-675.

Conn, J. H., & Conn, R. N. (1967). Discussion of T. X. Barber's "Hypnosis as a causal variable in present day psychology: A critical analysis." *International Journal of Clinical and Experimental Hypnosis, 15,* 106-110.

Connors, J. R., & Sheehan, P. W. (1976). Analysis of the cue characteristics of task motivational instructions. *International Journal of Clinical and Experimental Hypnosis, 24,* 287-299.

Connors, J. R., & Sheehan, P. W. (1978). The influence of control comparison tasks and between-versus within-subjects effects in hypnotic responsivity. *International Journal of Clinical and Experimental Hypnosis, 26,* 104-122.

Cooper, L. M. (1966). Spontaneous and suggested posthypnotic source amnesia. *International Journal of Clinical and Experimental Hypnosis, 14*(2), 180-193.

———. (1972). Hypnotic amnesia. In E. Fromm & R. E. Shor (Eds.), *Hypnosis: Research developments and perspectives* (pp. 217-252). Chicago: Aldine-Atherton.

Cooper, L. M., Branford, S. A., Schubot, E., & Tart, C. T. (1967). A further attempt to modify hypnotic susceptibility through repeated individualized experience. *International Journal of Clinical and Experimental Hypnosis, 15,* 118-124.

Cooper, L. F., & Erickson, M. H. (1954). *Time-distortion in hypnosis.* Baltimore: Williams & Williams.

Cooper, L. M., & London, P. (1973). Reactivation of memory by hypnosis and suggestions. *International Journal of Clinical and Experimental Hypnosis, 21,* 312-323.

Cooper, S. R., & Powles, W. E. (1945). The psychosomatic approach in practice. *McGill Medical Journal, 14,* 415-438.

Copp, L. A. (1974). The spectrum of suffering. *American Journal of Nursing, 74,* 491-495.

Coppolino, C. A. (1965). *Practice of hypnosis in anesthesiology.* New York: Grune & Stratton.

Corli, O., Grossi, E., Roma, G., & Battagliarin, G. (1986). Correlation between subjective labor pain and uterine contractions: A clinical study. *Pain, 26,* 53-60.

Cotanch, P., Hockenberry, M., & Herman, S. (1985). Self-hypnosis as antiemetic therapy in children receiving chemotherapy. *Oncology Nursing Forum, 12*(4), 41-46.

Council, J. R., & Kirsch, I. (1983). Absorption: Personality correlate or expectancy mediated artifact? Paper presented at 91st Annual Convention of the American Psychological Association, Anaheim, Calif.

Council, J. R., Kirsch, I., & Hafner, L. P. (1986). Expectancy versus absorption in the prediction of hypnotic responding. *Journal of Personality and Social Psychology, 50,* 182-189.

Council, J. R., Kirsch, I., Vickery, A. R., & Carlson, D. (1983). "Trance" versus "skill" hypnotic inductions: The effects of credibility, expectancy, and experimenter modeling. *Journal of Consulting and Clinical Psychology, 51,* 432-440.

Coulton, D. (1966). Natal and post-partum uses of hypnosis. *The American Journal of Clinical Hypnosis, 8,* 192-197.

Craig, K. D. (1980). Ontogenetic and cultural influences on the expression of pain in man. In H. W. Kosterlitz & L. Y. Terenius (Eds.), *Pain and Society* (pp. 37-52). Dahlem Konferenzen. Weinheim: Verlag Chemie.

Crasilneck. H. B. (1979). Hypnosis in the control of chronic low back pain. *American Journal of Clinical Hypnosis, 22,* 71-78.

Crasilneck, H. B., & Fogelman, J. J. (1957). The effects of hypnosis on blood coagulation. *International Journal of Clinical and Experimental Hyponsis, 5,* 132-137.

Crasilneck, H. B., & Hall, J. A. (1962). The use of hypnosis with unconscious patients. *International Journal of Clinical and Experimental Hypnosis, 10,* 141-144.

———. (1973). Clinical hypnosis in problems of pain. *American Journal of Clinical Hypnosis, 15,* 153-161.

Crasilneck, H. B., & Hall, J. A. (1975). *Clinical hypnosis: Principles and applications.* New York: Grune & Stratton.

Crasilneck, H. B., McCranie, E. J., & Jenkins, M. T. (1956). Special indications for hypnosis as a method of anesthesia. *Journal of the American Medical Association, 162,* 1606-1608.

Crasilneck, H. B., Stirman, J. A., Wilson, B. J., McCranie, E. J., & Fogelman, M. J. (1955). Use of hypnosis in the management of burns. *Journal of the American Medical Association, 158,* 103-106.

Crawford, H. J. (1978). Relationship of Hypnotic Susceptibility to Imagery Vividness, Absorption and Daydreaming Styles. Paper presented at the annual meeting of the Western Psychological Association, San Francisco, Calif.

——. (1979). Can Hypnosis Enhance Visual Imagery Processing and Memory? Paper presented at the 31st Annual Meeting of the Society for Clinical and Experimental Hypnosis, Denver, Colo.

——. (1982). Hypnotizability, daydreaming styles, imagery vividness and absorption: A multidimensional study. *Journal of Personality and Social Psychology, 42,* 915-926.

——. (1982). Cognitive processing during hypnosis: Much unfinished business. *Research Communications in Psychology, Psychiatry and Behavior, 7,* 169-179.

Crawford, H. J., & Allen, S. N. (1983). Enhanced visual memory during hypnosis as mediated by hypnotic responsiveness and cognitive strategies. *Journal of Experimental Psychology (General), 112,* 662-685.

Crawford, H. J., Macdonald, H., & Hilgard, E. R. (1979). Hypnotic deafness: A psychophysical study of response to tone intensity as modified by hypnosis. *American Journal of Psychology, 92,* 193-214.

Cross, W., & Spanos, N. P. (in press, 1988). The effects of imagery vividness and receptivity on skill training induced enhancement in hypnotic susceptibility, *Imagination, Cognition and Personality.*

Crouse, E., & Kurtz, R. (1984). Enhancing hypnotic susceptibility: The efficacy of four training procedures. *American Journal of Clinical Hypnosis, 27,* 122-135.

Crowley, R. J. (1980). Effects of indirect hypnosis (rapid induction analgesia) for the relief of acute pain associated with minor podiatric surgical procedures. *Dissertation Abstracts International, 40 (9-B),* 4549.

Crutchfield, R. S. (1955). Conformity and character. *American Psychologist, 10,* 191-198.

Cunningham, P. V., & Blum, G. S. (1982). Further evidence that hypnotically induced color blindness does not mimic congenital defects. *Journal of Abnormal Psychology, 91,* 139-143.

Curton, E. D., & Lordahl, D. S. (1974). Effects of attentional focus and arousal on time estimates. *Journal of Experimental Psychology, 103,* 861-867.

Curzon, L. B. (1980). *Criminal law.* Plymouth: Macdonald and Evans.

Daniels, L. K. (1976a). The effects of automated hypnosis and hand warming on migraine: A pilot study. *American Journal of Clinical Hypnosis, 19,91-94.*

——. (1976b). The treatment of acute anxiety and postoperative gingival pain by hypnosis and covert conditioning: A case report. *American Journal of Clinical Hypnosis, 19, 116-119.*

Darnton, R. (1968). *Mesmerism and the end of the enlightenment in France.* Cambridge, Mass.: Harvard University Press.

Das, J. P. (1958). Factor analysis of a hypnotic scale. *Indian Journal of Psychology, 33,* 97-99.

Daut, R. L., & Cleeland, C. S. (1982). The prevalence and severity of pain in cancer. *Cancer, 50,* 1913-1918.

Davenport-Slack, B. (1975). A comparative evaluation of obstetrical hypnosis and antenatal childbirth training. *The International Journal of Clinical and Experimental Hypnosis, 23,* 266-281.

Davenport-Slack, B., & Boylan, C. H. (1974). Psychological correlates of childbirth pain. *Psychosomatic Medicine, 36,* 215-223.

Davidson, J. A. (1962). An assessment of the value of hypnosis in pregnancy and labor. *British Medical Journal, 2,* 951-953.

Davis, S., Dawson, J. G., & Seay, B. (1978). Prediction of hypnotic susceptibility from imaginative involvement. *The American Journal of Clinical Hypnosis, 20,* 194-198.

de Beer, M., Fourie, D. P., & Niehaus, C. E. (1986). Hypnotic analgesia: Endorphins or situation? *British Journal of Experimental and Clinical Hypnosis, 3,* 139-145.

Deckert, G. H., & West, L. J. (1963). The problem of hypnotizability: A review. *International Journal of Clinical and Experimental Hypnosis, 11,* 205-235.

de Groh, M. (1986). Accessibility of critical material during hypnotic amnesia. Paper presented at the annual meeting of the American Psychological Association, Washington, D.C.

de Groh, M. M., Cross, W. P., & Spanos, N. P. (1986). Attitudes and Imagery in the Prediction of Hypnotic Susceptibility. Unpublished manuscript, Carleton University, Ottawa, Canada.

de Groot, H. P., Gwynn, M. I., & Spanos, N. P. (in press, 1988). The effects of contextual information and gender on the prediction of hypnotic susceptibility. *Journal of Personality and Social Psychology.*

Deikman, A. J. (1963). Experimental meditation. *Journal of Nervous and Mental Disease, 236,* 329-343.

——. (1966). Deautomization and the mystic experience. *Archives of General Psychiatry, 29,* 329-343.

DeLee, S. T. (1955). Hypnotism in pregnancy and labor. *Journal of the American Medical Association, 159,* 750-754.

Dempster, C. R., Balson, P., & Whalen, B. T. (1976). Supportive hypnotherapy during the radical treatment of malignancies. *International Journal of Clinical and Experimental Hypnosis, 24,* 1-9.

D'Eon, J. L., & Perry, C. W. (1983). Response to pressure pain as moderated by susceptibility, type of suggestion strategy, and choice. Presented at the meeting of the Society for Clinical and Experimental Hypnosis, Boston.

Degenaar, J. J. (1979). Some philosophical considerations on pain. *Pain, 7,* 281-304.

Dehenterova, J. (1967(). Some experiences with the use of hypnosis in the treatment of burns. *International Journal of Clinical and Experimental Hyponsis, 15,* 49-53.

De Piano, F. A., & Salzberg, H. C. (1981). Hypnosis as an aid to recall of meaningful information presented under three types of arousal. *International Journal of Clinical and Experimental Hypnosis, 29,* 383-400.

Dermen, D., & London, P. (1965). Correlates of hypnotic susceptibility. *Journal of Consulting Psychology, 29,* 537-545.

DeStefano, R. (1977). The "inoculation" effect in think-with instructions "hypnotic-like" experiences. Doctoral dissertation, Temple University.

Devine, D., & Spanos, N. P. (1988). Expectations and strategy type in the reduction of experimentally induced pain. Unpublished manuscript, Carleton University, Ottawa, Canada.

Deyoub, P. L. (1980). Hypnosis for the relief of hospital-induced stress. *Journal of the American Society of Psychosomatic Dentistry and Medicine, 27*(4), 105-109.

Dhanens, T. P., & Lundy, R. M. (1975). Hypnotic and waking suggestions and recall. *International Journal of Clinical and Experimental Hypnosis, 23,* 68-79.

Diamond, B. L. (1980). Inherent problems in the use of pretrial hypnosis on a prospective witness. *California Law Review, 68,* 313-349.

Diamond, M. J. (1972). The use of observationally-presented information to modify hypnotic susceptibility. *Journal of Abnormal Psychology, 79,* 174-180.

——. (1974). Modification of hypnotizability: A review. *Psychological Bulletin, 81,* 180-198.

——. (1977a). Hypnotizability is modifiable: An alternative approach. *International Journal of Clinical and Experimental Hypnosis, 25,* 147-165.

——. (1977b). Issues and methods for modifying responsivity to hypnosis. In W. E. Edmonston (Ed.), *Conceptual and investigative approaches to hypnosis and hypnotic phenomena* (pp. 119-128). New York: New York Academy of Sciences Press.

——. (1980). The client-as-hypnotist: Furthering hypnotherapeutic change. *International Journal of Clinical and Experimental Hypnosis, 28,* 197-207.

Diamond, M. J. (1982). Modifying hypnotic experience by means of indirect hypnosis and hypnotic skill training: An update (1981). *Research Communications in Psychology, Psychiatry and Behavior, 7,* 233-239.

———. (1983). Therapeutic indications in applying an innovative hypnotherapeutic technique: The client-as-hypnotist. *American Journal of Clinical Hypnosis, 25,* 242-247.

———. (1984). It takes two to tango: Some thoughts on the neglected importance of the hypnotist in an interactive hynotherapeutic relationship. *American Journal of Clinical Hypnosis, 27,* 3-13.

———. (in press, 1988). The interactional basis of hypnotic experience: On the relational dimensions of hypnosis. *International Journal of Clinical and Experimental Hypnosis.*

Diamond, M. J., Gregory, J., Lenney, E., Steadman, C., & Talone, J. M. (1974). An alternative approach to personality correlates of hypnotizability: Hypnosis-specific mediational attitudes. *International Journal of Clinical and Experimental Hypnosis, 12.* 346-353.

Diamond, M. J., & Taft, R. (1975). The role played by ego permissiveness and imagery in hypnotic responsivity. *International Journal of Clinical and Experimental Hypnosis, 23,* 130-138.

Dickason, E. J., Schult, M. O., & Morris, E. M. (1978). *Maternal and infant drugs and nursing intervention.* New York: McGraw-Hill.

Dillon, R. F., & Spanos, N. P. (1983). Proactive interference and the functional ablation hypothesis: More disconformation data. *International Journal of Clinical & Experimental Hypnosis, 31,* 47-56.

Dimond, E. G. (1971). Acupuncture anesthesia: Western medicine and Chinese traditional medicine. *Journal of the American Medical Association, 218,* 1558-1563.

Dingwall, E. J. (Ed.) (1967). *Abnormal hypnotic phenomena, Vols. 1-4.* New York: Barnes & Noble.

Doberneck, R. C., Griffen, W. O. Jr., & Papermaster, A. A. (1950). Hypnosis as an adjunct to surgical therapy. *Surgery, 46,* 229-304.

Doering, S. G., Entwistle, D. R., & Quinlan, D. (1980). Modeling the quality of women's birth experience. *Journal of Health and Social Behavior, 21,* 12-21.

Dolby, R. M., & Sheehan, P. W. (1975). Cognitive processing and expectancy behavior in hypnosis. *Journal of Abnormal Psychology, 86,* 334-345.

Domangue, B. B., & Margolis, C. G. (1983). Hypnosis and a multidisciplinary cancer pain management team. Role and effects. Paper presented at the 35th Annual Meeting of the Society for Clinical and Experimental Hypnosis, Boston, Mass.

Domangue, B. B., Margolis, C. G., Lieberman, D., & Kaji, H. (1985). Biochemical correlates of hypnoanalgesia in arthritic pain patients. *Journal of Clinical Psychiatry, 46,* 235-238.

Doob, L. W. (1971). *Patterning of time.* New Haven: Yale University Press.

Dorcus, R. M. (1937). Modification by suggestion of some vestibular and visual responses. *American Journal of Psychology, 49,* 82-87.

Drake, S. D., & Nash, M. R. (1986). Imaginative Involvement and Hypnotic Susceptibility: A Relationship Mediated by Context? Paper presented at 94th Annual American Psychological Association Convention, Washington, D.C.

Drummond, F. (1981). Hypnosis in the treatment of headache: A review of the last 10 years. *Journal of the American Society for Psychosomatic Dentistry and Medicine, 28,* 87.

Dubin, L. L. (1976). Subjective apperception and the use of color during dental procedures under hypnosis: Report of a case. *American Journal of Clinical Hypnosis, 18,* 282-284.

Dubin, L. L., & Shapiro, S. S. 1974). Use of hypnosis to facilitate dental extraction and hemostatis in a classic hemophiliac with a high antibody titer to factor VIII. *American Journal of Clinical Hypnosis, 17,* 79-83.

Dubreuil, D., Endler, N. S., & Spanos, N. P. (1988). Distraction and redefinition in the reduction of low and high intensity experimentally-induced pain. *Imagination, Cognition and Personality, 7,* 155-164.

Dubreuil, D. L., Spanos, N. P., & Bertrand, L. D. (1983). Does hypnotic amnesia dissipate with time? *Imagination, Cognition and Personality, 2,* 103-113.

Dwyan, J., & Bowers, K. (1983). The use of hypnosis to enhance recall. *Science, 22,* 184-185.

Edmonston, W. E., Jr. (1977). Neutral hypnosis as relaxation. *American Journal of Clinical Hypnosis, 20,* 69-75.

———. (1979). The effects of neutral hypnosis on conditioned responses: Implications for hypnosis as relaxation. In E. Fromm and R. E. Shor (Eds.), *Hypnosis: Developments in research and new perspectives (2nd ed.).* New York: Aldine.

———. (1980). The effects of rapid induction analgesia (RIA), hypnotic susceptibility and the severity of discomfort on reducing dental pain. *American Journal of Clinical Hypnosis, 27,* 81-90.

———. (1980). *Hypnosis and relaxation: Modern verification of an old equation.* New York: John Wiley.

———. (1981). *Hypnosis and relaxation: Modern verification of an old equation.* New York: John Wiley.

———. (1984). Anesis: Correcting a century-old misnomer. In E. E. Levitt (Chair), *Current status of theories of hypnosis.* Symposium conducted at the meeting of the American Psychological Association, Toronto.

———. (1986). *The induction of hypnosis.* New York: John Wiley.

Edmonston, W. E., Jr. & Erbeck, J. R. (1967). Hypnotic time distortion: A note. *American Journal of Clinical Hypnosis, 10,* 79-80.

Egbert, L. D., Battit, G. E., Welch, C. E., & Bartlett, M. K. 1964). Reduction of postoperative pain by encouragement and instruction of patients. *New England Journal of Medicine, 270,* 825-827.

Egbert, L. D., Battit, Turndorf, H., & Beecher, H. K. (1963). The value of the preoperative visit by an anesthetist. *Journal of the American Medical Association, 185,* 553-555.

Eisele, G., & Higgins, J. J. (1962). Hypnosis in educational and moral problems. *American Journal of Clinical Hypnosis, 4,* 259-263.

Ellenberg, L., Kellerman, J., Dash, J., Higgins, G., & Zeltzer, L. (1980). Use of hypnosis for multiple symptoms in an adolescent girl with leukemia. *Journal of Adolescent Health Care, 1,* 132-136.

Ellenberger, H. (1970). T*he discovery of the unconscious.* New York: Basic Books.

Elton, D., Stanley, G., & Burrows, G. (1983). *Psychological control of pain.* New York: Grune & Stratton.

Epstein, S. (1973). The self-concept revisited, or, a theory of a theory. *American Psychologist, 28,* 404-416.

Erdelyi, M. H. (1985). *Psychoanalysis: Freud's cognitive psychology.* New York: Freeman.

Erickson, M. H. (1938a). A study of clinical and experimental findings on hypnotic deafness: I. Clinical experimentation and findings. *Journal of General Psychology, 19,* 127-150.

———. (1938b). A study of clinical and experimental findings on hypnotic deafness: II. Experimental findings with a conditioned response technique. *Journal of General Psychology, 19,* 151-167.

———. (1939). The induction of color blindness by a technique of hypnotic suggestion. *Journal of General Psychology, 20,* 61-89.

———. (1959). Hypnosis in painful terminal illness. *American Journal of Clinical Hypnosis, 1,* 117-121.

———. (1964). Initial experiments investigating the nature of hypnosis. *Journal of Clinical Hypnosis, 7,* 152-162.

———. (1966). The interpersonal hypnotic technique for symptom correction and pain control. *American Journal of Clinical Hypnosis, 8,* 198-209.

———. (1967). Further experimental investigations of hypnosis: Hypnotic and non-hypnotic realities. *American Journal of Clinical Hypnosis, 10,* 87-135.

———. (1980). *The collected papers of Milton H. Erickson on hypnosis.* (4 volumes). Edited by E. L. Rossi. New York: Irvington.

Erickson, M. H., & Erickson, E. M. (1941). Concerning the nature and character of posthypnotic behavior. *Journal of General Psychology, 24,* 95-113.

Erickson, M. H., Hershman, S., & Sector, I. I. (1961). *The practical application of medical and dental hypnosis.* New York: Julian Press.

Erickson, M. H., & Rossi, E. L. (1977). Autohypnotic experiences of Milton H. Erickson. *American Journal of Clinical Hypnosis, 20,* 36-54.

———. (1979). *Hypnotherapy: An exploratory casebook.* New York: Irvington.

Erickson, M. H., Rossi, E. L., & Rossi, S. H. (1976). *Hypnotic realities: The induction of clinical hypnosis and the indirect forms of suggestion.* New York: Irvington.

Erickson, M. H., Rossi, E. L., & Rossi, S. I. (1976). *Hypnotic Realities.* New York: Halsted.

Esdaile, J. (1957). *Hypnosis in medicine and surgery.* New York: Julian Press. (Originally published 1846).

Evans, F. J. (1968). Recent trends in experimental hypnosis. *Behavioral Science, 13,* 477-487.

———. (1979a). Contextual forgetting: Posthypnotic source amnesia. *Journal of Abnormal Psychology, 88,* 556-563.

———. (1979b). Hot amethysts, eleven fingers and the Oriental Express. In G. D. Burrows, D. R. Collison & L. Dennerstein (Eds.), *Hypnosis 1979,* North-Holland, N.Y.: Elsevier.

———. (1985). Expectancy, therapeutic instructions, and the placebo response. In L. White, B. Tursky & G. E. Schwartz (Eds.), *Placebo. Theory, research, and mechanisms* (pp. 215-228). New York: Guilford Press.

Evans, F. J., & Kihlstrom, J. F. (1973). Posthypnotic amnesia as disrupted retrieval. *Journal of Abnormal Psychology, 82*(2), 327-328.

Evans, F. J., & Schmeidler, D. (1966). Relationship between the Harvard Group Scale of Hypnotic Susceptibility and the Stanford Hypnotic Susceptibility Scale: Form C. *International Journal of Clinical and Experimental Hypnosis, 14,* 333-343.

Evans, F. J., & Thorn, W. A. (1966). Two types of posthypnotic amnesia: Recall amnesia and source amnesia. *International Journal of Clinical and Experimental Hypnosis, 14*(2), 162-179.

Evans, M., & Paul, G. L. (1970). Effects of hypnotically suggested analgesia and subjective responses to cold pressor pain. *Journal of Consulting and Clinical Psychology, 35,* 362-371

Everson, T. C., & Cole, W. H. (1966). *Spontaneous regression of cancer.* Philadelphia: Saunders and Company.

Ewin, D. (1983). Emergency room hypnosis for the burned patient. *American Journal of Clinical Hypnosis, 26,* 5-8.

———. (1984). Hypnosis in surgery and anesthesia. In W. C. Wester II, & A. H. Smith, Jr. (Eds.), *Clinical hypnosis: A multidisiplinary approach.* Philadelphia: J. B. Lippincott.

———. (1985). Emergency room hypnosis for the burned patient. *American Journal of Clinical Hypnosis, 29,* 7-12.

———. (1986). The effect of hypnosis and mental set on major surgery and burns. *Psychiatric Annals, 16,* 115-118.

Eyesenck, H. J. (1941). An experimental study of the improvement of mental and physical functions in the hypnotic state. *British Journal of Medical Psychology, 18,* 304-316.

Farthing, G. W., Brown, S. W., & Venturino, M. (1982). Effects of hypnotizability and mental imagery on signal detection sensitivity and response bias. *International Journal of Experimental and Clinical Hypnosis, 30,* 289-305.

Farthing, G. W., Brown, S. & Venturino, M. (1983). Involuntariness of response on the Harvard Group Scale of Hypnotic Susceptibility. *International Journal of Clinical and Experimental Hypnosis, 31,* 170-180.

Farthing, G. W., Venturino, M., & Brown, S. W. (1983). Relationship between two different types of imagery vividness questionnaire items and three hypnotic susceptibility scale factors. A brief communication. *International Journal of Clinical and Experimental Hypnosis, 31,* 8-13.

Farthing, G. W., Venturino, M., & Brown, S. W. (1984). Suggestion and distraction in the control of pain: Test of two hypotheses. *Journal of Abnormal Psychology, 93,* 259-265.

Faulioner, A., & Keys, T. E. (1965). *Foundations of anesthesiology, volume I.* Springfield, Ill.: Charles C. Thomas.

Faw, C., Ballentine, R., Ballentine, L., & van Eys, J. (1977). Unproved cancer remedies. *Journal of the American Medical Association, 238,* 1536-1538.

Fazio, R. H. (1986). How do attitudes guide behavior? In R. M. Sorrentino & E. T. Higgins (Eds.), *The handbook of motivation and cognition: Foundation of social behavior* (pp. 204-243). New York: Guilford Press.

Fellows, B. J. (1986). The concept of trance. In P. L. N. Naish (Ed.), *What is hypnosis: Current theories and research*. Milton Keynes: Open University Press.

Fellows, B. J., & Armstrong, V. (1977). An experimental investigation of the relationship between hypnotic susceptibility and reading involvement, *American Journal of Clinical Hypnosis, 20*, 101-105.

Fellows, B. J., & Creamer, M. (1978). An investigation of the role of "hypnosis," hypnotic suscepti-bility and hypnotic induction in the production of age regression. *British Journal of Social and Clinical Psychology, 17*, 165-171.

Field, P. B. (1965). An inventory scale of hypnotic depth. *International Journal of Clinical and Experimental Hypnosis, 13*, 238-249.

———. (1966). Some self-rating measures related to hypnotizability. *Perceptual and Motor Skills, 23*, 1179-1187.

———. (1974). Effects of tape-recorded hypnotic preparation for surgery. *International Journal of Clinical and Experimental Hypnosis, 22*, 54-61.

———. (1979). Humanistic aspects of hypnotic communication. In E. Fromm & R. Shor (Eds.), *Hypnosis: Developments in research and new perspectives*. New York: Aldine.

Field, P. B., & Palmer, R. D. (1969). Factor analysis: Hypnosis inventory. *International Journal of Clinical and Experimental Hypnosis, 17*, 50-61.

Finer, B. (1966). Experience with hypnosis in clinical anesthesiology. *Sartryck ur Opuscula Medica, 4*, 1-11.

———. (1979). Hypnotherapy in pain of advanced cancer. In J. J. Bonica and V. Ventafridda (Eds.), *Advances in pain research and therapy* (Vol. 2, pp. 223-230). New York: Raven Press.

Finer, B., & Graf, K. (1968). Circulatory changes accompanying hypnotic imagination of hyperalgesia and hypoalgesia in causalgic limbs. *Zeitschrift fur die gesamte experimentelle Medizin, 146*, 97.

Finer, B. L., & Nylen, B. O. (1961). Cardiac arrest in the treatment of burns and report on hypnosis as a substitute for anesthesia. *Plastic and Reconstructive Surgery, 27*, 49-55.

Fingarette, H. (1969). *Self-deception*. London: Routledge & Kegan Paul.

Finke, R. A., & MacDonald, H. (1978). Two personality measures relating hypnotic susceptibility to absorption. *International Journal of Clinical and Experimental Hypnosis, 26*, 178-183.

Finkelstein, S. (1984). Hypnosis in dentistry. In W. C. Wester, II, & A. H. Smith (Eds.), *Clinical hypnosis: A multidisciplinary approach*. Philadelphia: J. B. Lippincott.

Finkelstein, S., & Howard, M. A. (1983). Cancer prevention—A three-year pilot study. *American Journal of Clinical Hypnosis, 25*(2-3), 177-187.

Fishbein, M., & Ajzen, I. (1975). *Belief, attitude, intention, and behavior: An introduction to theory and research*. Reading, Mass.: Addison-Wesley.

Fisher, S. (1954). The role of expectancy in the performance of posthypnotic behavior. *Journal of Abnormal and Social Psychology, 49*, 503-507.

Foley, K. M. (1985). The treatment of cancer pain. *New England Journal of Medicine, 313*, 84-95.

Fordyce, W. E. (1983). The validity of pain behavior measurement. In R. Melzack, (Ed.), *Pain measurement and assessment*. New York: Raven Press.

Fordyce, W. B., Fowler, R. S., Jr., Lehmann, J. F., DeLatur, B. J., Sand, P. L., & Treischmann, R. (1973). Operant conditioning in the treatment of chronic pain. *Archives of Physical Medicine and Rehabilitation, 54*, 399-408.

Fraiberg, S. (1968). *The magic years*. New York: Scribner's.

Fraisse, P. (1984). Perception and estimation of time. *Annual Review of Psychology, 35*, 1-36.

Frank, J. D., Hoehn-Saric, Imber, S. D., Liberman, B. L., & Stone, A. R. (1978). *Effective ingredi-ents of successful psychotherapy*. New York: Brunner/Mazel.

Frankel, F. H. (1976). *Hypnosis: Trance as a coping mechanism.* New York: Plenum Press.

——. (1987). Significant developments in medical hypnosis during the past 25 years. *International Journal of Clinical and Experimental Hypnosis, 35,* 231-247.

Franklin, B., Bory, Lavoisier, Bailly, D'Arcet, De Borie, Guillotin, & Lavoisier (1970). Report on animal magnetism. In M. M. Tinterow (Ed.), *Foundations of hypnosis: From Mesmer to Freud* (pp. 82-128). Springfield, Ill.: Charles C. Thomas. (Original work dated 1785).

Franklin, C. I. (1982). Spontaneous regression in cancer. In B. A. Stoll (Ed.), *Prolonged arrest of cancer.* Toronto: Wiley & Sons.

Fredericks, L. (1980). The value of teaching hypnosis in the practice of anesthesiology. *International Journal of Clinical and Experimental Hypnosis, 28,* 6-15.

Freedman, L. Z. (1963). Childbirth while conscious: Perspectives and communication. *Journal of Nervous and Mental Disease, 137,* 372-379.

Freedman, L. Z., & Ferguson, V. M. (1950). The question of "Painless Childbirth" in primitive cultures. *American Journal of Orthopsychiatry, 20,* 363-372.

Freud, S. (1957). The psychotherapy of hysteria. In J. Breuer & S. Freud, *Studies on hysteria* (pp. 253-305). New York: Basic Books.

Fricton, J. (1981). The effects of direct and indirect hypnotic suggestions. Presented at The Third World Congress of Pain of the International Association for the Study of Pain, Edinburgh, Scotland.

Fricton, J. R., & Roth, P. (1985). The effects of direct and indirect hypnotic suggestions for analgesia in high and low susceptible subjects. *American Journal of Clinical Hypnosis, 27,* 226-231.

Frid, M., & Singer, G. (1979). Hypnotic analgesia in conditions of stress is partially reversed by naloxone. *Psychopharmacology, 63,* 211-215.

Friedlander, J. W., & Sarbin, T. R. (1938). The depth of hypnosis. *Journal of Abnormal and Social Psychology, 33,* 453-475.

Friedman, H., & Taub, H. A. (1982). An evaluation of hypnotic susceptibility and peripheral temperature elevation in migraine treatment. *American Journal of Clinical Hypnosis, 24,* 172-180.

——. (1984). Brief psychological training procedures in migraine treatment. *American Journal of Clinical Hypnosis, 26,* 187-200.

Friedman, H., & Taub, H. (1985). Extended follow-up study of the effects of brief psychological procedures in migraine therapy. *American Journal of Clinical Hypnosis, 28,* 27-33.

Friedman, H., Thompson, R. B., & Rosen, E. F. (1985). Perceived threat as a major factor in tolerance for experimentally induced cold-water pain. *Journal of Abnormal Psychology, 94,* 624-629.

Fromm, E. (1977). An ego-psychological theory of altered states of consciousness. *International Journal of Clinical and Experimental Hypnosis, 25,* 372-387.

Fromm, E., & Shor, R. E. (1979). Underlying theoretical issues: An introduction. In E. Fromm & R. E. Shor (Eds.), *Hypnosis: Developments in research and new perspectives* (revised 2nd ed., pp. 3-13). New York: Aldine.

Fromm, E., Brown, D. P., Hurt, S. W., Oberlander, J. Z., Boxer, A. M., & Pfeifer, G. (1981). The phenomena and characteristics of self-hypnosis. *International Journal of Clinical and Experimental Hypnosis, 29,* 189-246.

Fuchs, K., Marcovici, R., Peretz, A. B., & Paldi, E. (1980). The use of hypnosis in obstetrics. In M. Oajntar, E. Roskar, & M. Lavric (Eds.), *Hypnosis in psychotherapy and psychosomatic medicine.* Ljubljana, Yugoslavia: University Press.

Fuchs, K., Paldi, E., Abramovici, H., and Peretz, B. A. (1980). Treatment of hyperemesis gravidarum by hypnosis. *The International Journal of Clinical and Experimental Hypnosis, 28,* 313-323.

Fülöp-Miller, R. (1938). *Triumph over pain.* New York: The Bobbs-Merrill Co.

Galbraith, G. C., Cooper, L. M., & London, P. (1972). Hypnotic susceptibility and the sensory evoked response. *Journal of Comparative and Physiological Psychology, 80,* 509-514.

Galeano, C., Leung, C. Y., Robitallie, R., & Roy-Chabot. (1979). Acupuncture analgeisa in rabbits. *Pain, 6,* 71-81.

Gandolfo, R. L. (1971). Role of expectancy, amnesia, and hypnotic induction in the performance of posthypnotic behavior. *Journal of Abnormal Psychology, 77,* 324-328.

Gardner, G. G. (1976). Hypnosis and mastery: Clinical contributions and directions for research. *International Journal of Clinical and Experimental Hypnosis, 24,* 202-214.

———. (1976). Childhood, death, and human dignity: Hypnotherapy for David. *International Journal of Clinical and Experimental Hypnosis, 24,* 122-139.

Gardner, G. G., & Lubman, A. (1983). Hypnotherapy for children with cancer: Some current issues. *American Journal of Clinical Hypnosis, 25*(2-3), 135-142.

Gardner, G. G., & Olness, K. (1981). *Hypnosis and hypnotherapy with children.* New York: Grune and Stratton.

Gardner, W. J., & Licklider, J. C. R. (1959). Auditory analgesia in dental operations. *Journal of the American Dental Association, 59,* 1144-1149.

Geertz, C. (1980). Blurred genres: The refiguration of social thought. *American Scholar, 80,* 158-179.

Geiselman, R. E. (1984). Evidence for retrieval inhibition in motivated forgetting. Paper presented at the symposium "Posthypnotic Amnesia: Concepts and Processes," American Psychological Association annual meeting, Toronto.

Geiselman, R. E., Bagheir, B. (1985). Repetition effects in directed forgetting: Evidence for retrieval inhibition. *Memory and Cognition, 13*(1), 57-62.

Geiselman, R. E., Bjork, R. A., & Fishman, D. L. (1983). Disrupted retrieval in directed forgetting: A link with posthypnotic amnesia. *Journal of Experimental Psychology: General, 112*(1), 58-72.

Geiselman, R. E., Fisher, R. P., MacKinnon, D. P., & Holland, H. L. (1985). Eyewitness memory enhancement in the police interview: Cognitive retrieval mnemonics versus hypnosis. *Journal of Allied Psychology, 70,* 401-412.

Geiselman, R. E., MacKinnon, D. P., Fishman, D. L., Jaenick, C., Larner, B. R., Schoenberg, S., & Swartz, S. (1983). Mechanisms of hypnotic and nonhypnotic forgetting. *Journal of Experimental Psychology: Learning, Memory and Cognition, 9*(4), 626-635.

Geiselman, R. E., & Panting, T. M. (1985). Personality correlates of retrieval processes in intentional and unintentional forgetting. *Personality and Individual Differences, 6*(6), 685-691.

Geiselman, R. E., Rabow, V. E., Wachtel, S. L., & McKinnon, D. P. (1985). Strategy control in intentional forgetting. *Human Learning, 4,* 169-178.

Gelfand, S. (1964). The relationship of experimental pain tolerance to pain threshold. *Canadian Journal of Psychology, 18,* 26-42.

Genest, M. (1978). A cognitive-behavioral bibliotherapy to ameliorate pain. Presented at the annual meeting of the American Psychological Association, Toronto.

Genest, M., Meichenbaum, D. H., & Turk, D. C. (1977). A cognitive-behavioral approach to the management of pain. Presented at the 11th Annual Convention of the Association for the Advancement of Behavior Therapy.

Gfeller, J., Lynn, S., Pribble, W., & Kvinge, D. (1985). Enhancing Hypnotic Susceptibility: Interpersonal and Rapport Factors. Paper presented at the Annual Convention of the American Psychological Association, Los Angeles, Calif.

Gheorghiu, V. A., & Orleanu, P. (1982). Dental implant under hypnosis. *American Journal of Clinical Hypnosis, 25,* 68-70.

Gheorgin, V. (1967). Some peculiarities of posthypnotic source amnesia of information. In L. Chertok (Ed.), *Psychological mechanisms of hypnosis.* New York: Springer.

Gibbons, D. E. (1979). *Applied hypnosis and hyperempiria.* New York: Plenum Press.

Gibson, H. B. (1982). *Pain and its conquest.* London: Peter Owen.

Gidro-Frank, L., & Bowersbuch, M. K. (1948). A study of plantar response in hypnotic age regression. *Journal of Nervous and Mental Disease, 107,* 443-458.

Gilbert, J. E., & Barber, T. X. (1972). Effects of hypnotic induction, motivational suggestions, and level of suggestibility on cognitive performance. *International Journal of Clinical and Experimental Hypnosis, 20,* 156-158.

Gillett, P., & Coe, W. (1984). The effects of rapid induction analgesia (RIA), hypnotic susceptibility and the severity of discomfort on reducing dental pain. *American Journal of Clinical Hypnosis, 27,* 81-90.

Gilligan, R. M., Ascher, L. M., Wolper, J., & Bochachevsky, C. (1984). Comparing three cognitive strategies in altering pain behaviors on a cold pressor task. *Perceptual and Motor Skills, 59,* 235-240.

Ginzberg, E. (1986). The destabilization of health care. *New England Journal of Medicine, 315,* 757-761.

Girodo, M., & Wood, D. (1979). Talking yourself out of pain: The importance of believing that you can. *Cognitive Therapy and Research, 3,* 23-33.

Glass, L. B., & Barber, T. X. (1961). A note on hypnotic behavior, the definition of the situation and the placebo effect. *Journal of Nervous and Mental Disease, 132,* 539-541.

Goffman, E. (1959). *The presentation of self in everyday life.* Garden City: Doubleday.

———. (1969). *Strategic interaction.* Philadelphia: University of Pennsylvania Press.

Golan, H. P. (1975). Further case reports from the Boston City Hospital. *American Journal of Clinical Hypnosis, 18,* 55-59.

Goldberger, S. M., & Tursky, B. (1976). Modulation of shock-elicited pain by acupuncture and suggestion. *Pain, 2,* 417-429.

Goldblatt, M., & Munitz, H. (1976). Behavioral treatment of hysterical leg paralysis. *Journal of Behavior Therapy and Experimental Psychiatry, 7,* 259-263.

Golden, W. L., Dowd, E. T., & Friedberg, F. (1987). *Hypnotherapy: A modern approach.* New York: Permagon.

Goldie, L. (1956). Hypnosis in the casualty department. *British Medical Journal, 2,* 1340-1342.

Goldstein, A. (1976). Opioid peptides (endorphins) in pituitary and brain. *Science, 193,* 1081-1086.

Goldstein, A., & Hilgard, E. R. (1975). Failure of opiate antagonist naloxone to modify hypnotic analgesia. *Proceedings of the National Academy of Sciences, 72,* 2041-2043.

Gorassini, D. R. (1983). Hypnotic involuntariness as mere compliance. Unpublished doctoral dissertation. Carleton University, Ottawa, Canada.

Gorassini, D. R., & Spanos, N. P. (1986). A social cognitive skills training program for the successful modification of hypnotic susceptibility. *Journal of Personality and Social Psychology, 50,* 1004-1012.

———. (1986). A social-cognitive skills approach to successful modification of hypnotic susceptibility. *Journal of Consulting and Clinical Psychology,* in press.

Gottfredson, D. (1973). Hypnosis as an anesthetic in dentistry. *Dissertation Abstracts International, 33,* 7-8.

Gracely, R. H. (1980). Pain measurement in man. In L. K. Y. Ng & J. J. Bonica (Eds.), *Pain, discomfort and humanitarian care.* New York: Elsevier/North-Holland.

Gracely, R. H., Dunbar, R., Wolskee, P. J., & Deeter, W. R. (1983). Placebo and naloxone can alter post-surgical pain by different mechanisms. *Nature, 306,* 264-265.

Graham, C., & Leibowitz, H. W. (1972). The effects of suggestions on visual acuity. *International Journal of Clinical and Experimental Hypnosis, 20,* 169-186.

Graham, K. R., & Patton, A. (1968). Retroactive inhibition, hypnosis and hypnotic amnesia. *International Journal of Clinical and Experimental Hypnosis, 16,* 68-74.

Graham, K. R., & Pernicano, K. (1979). Laterality, hypnosis, and the autokinetic effect. *American Journal of Clinical Hypnosis, 22,* 79-84.

Graham, K. R., & Schwartz, L. M. (1973). Suggested deafness and auditory signal detectability. *Proceedings of the 81st Annual Convention of the American Psychological Association, 8,* 1091-1092.

Gravitz, M. A. (1985). An 1846 report of tumor remission associated with hypnosis. *American Journal of Clinical Hypnosis, 28,* 16-19.

Gravitz, M. A. (1988). Early uses of hypnosis as surgical anesthesia. *American Journal of Clinical Hypnosis, 30*, 201-208.

Gravitz, M. A., & Gerton, M. I. (1984). Origin of the term hypnotism prior to Braid. *American Journal of Clinical Hypnosis, 27*, 107-110.

Green, D. M., & Swets, J. A. (1966). *Signal detection theory and psychophysics.* New York: John Wiley.

Greenhill, J. P., & Friedman, S. A. (1974). *Biological principles and modern practice of obstetrics.* Philadelphia: W. B. Saunders Co.

Greenwald, A. G., & Pratkanis, A. R. (1984). The self. In R. Wyer & T. K. Srull (Eds.), *Handbook of social cognition.* Hillsdale, N.J.: Erlbaum.

Gregg, V. H. (1987). Hypnotic pseudomemory: Continuing issues. *British Journal of Experimental and Clinical Hypnosis, 4*, 109-111.

Gregg, V. H., & Mingay, D. J. (1987). Influence of hypnosis on riskiness and discriminability in recognition memory for faces. *British Journal of Experimental and Clinical Hypnosis, 4*, 65-75.

Gregg, V. H., & Whiteley, A. E. (1985). Hypnosis and signal detection theory: Reservations concerning Naish's theory. *British Journal of Experimental and Clinical Hypnosis, 2*, 139-141.

Gregory, J., & Diamond, M. J. (1973). Increasing hypnotic susceptibility by means of positive expectancies and written instructions. *Journal of Abnormal Psychology, 82*, 363-367.

Grevert, P., Albert, L. H., & Goldstein, A. (1983). Partial antagonism of placebo analgesia by naloxone. *Pain, 16*, 143.

Grevert, P., & Goldstein, A. (1985). Placebo analgesia, naloxone, and the role of endogenous opiates. In L. White, B. Tursky & G. E. Schwartz (Eds.), *Placebo. Theory research and mechanisms.* New York: Guilford.

Griffin, G. R. (1980). Hypnosis: Towards a logical approach in using hypnosis in law enforcement agencies. *Journal of Police Science and Administration, 8*, 385-389.

Grimm, L., & Kanfer, F. H. (1976). Tolerance of aversive stimulation. *Behavior Therapy, 7*, 593-601.

Grinder, J., DeLozier, J., & Bandoler, R. (1977). *Patterns of the hypnotic techniques of Milton H. Erickson, M.D.: Vol. 2.* Cupertino, Calif.: Meta Publications.

Gross, H. N., & Posner, N. A. (1963). An evaluation of hypnosis for obstetric delivery. *American Journal of Obstetrics and Gynecology, 76*, 912-920.

Grosz, H. J. (1979). Hypnotherapy in the management of terminally ill cancer patients. *Journal of the Indiana State Medical Association, 72*, 126-129.

Gruen, W. (1972). A successful application of systematic self-relaxation and self-suggestions about postoperative reactions in a case of cardiac surgery. *International Journal of Clinical and Experimental Hypnosis, 20*, 143-151.

Grzesiak, R. C. (1977). Relaxation techniques in treatment of chronic pain. *Archives of Physical and Medical Rehabilitation, 58*, 270-272.

Gur, R. C. (1974). An attention-controlled operant procedure for enhancing hypnotic susceptibility. *Journal of Abnormal Psychology, 8*, 644-650.

——. (1976). Sex differences in personality correlates of hypnotic susceptibility. Paper presented at the 7th International Congress of Hypnosis and Psychosomatic Medicines of the International Society of Hypnosis, Philadelphia.

Gwynn, M. I., de Groot, H. P., & Spanos, N. P. (1988). Hidden observer responding and its relationship to tests of trance logic. Unpublished manuscript, Carleton University, Ottawa, Canada.

Haley, J. (1967). *Advanced techniques of hypnosis and therapy: Selected papers of Milton H. Erickson, M.D.* New York: Grune & Stratton.

——. (1973). *Uncommon therapy: The psychiatric techniques of Milton H. Erickson, M.D.* New York: W. W. Norton & Company.

Hall, H. R. (1983). Hypnosis and the immune system. A review with implications for cancer and the psychology of healing. *American Journal of Clinical Hypnosis, 25*(2-3), 92-102.

Hall, M. D. (1983). Using relaxation imagery with children with malignancies:A developmental perspective. *American Journal of Clinical Hypnosis, 25*(2-3), 143-149.

Halpern, S., & White, L. (1962). Experimental hypnotherapy with a cancer patient. *Journal of the American Society of Psychosomatic Dentistry and Medicine, 9*(1), 7-12.

Ham, M. L., Radtke, L. H., & Spanos, N. P. (1981). The effects of suggestion type and the experience of involuntariness on the breaching of posthypnotic amnesia. Unpublished manuscript, Carleton University, Ottawa, Canada.

Ham, M. W., & Spanos, N. P. (1974). Suggested auditory and visual hallucinations in task-motivated and hypnotic subjects. *American Journal of Clinical Hypnosis, 17*, 94-101.

Hammer, A. G., & Arkins, W. J. (1964). The role of photic stimulation in the induction of hypnotic trance. *International Journal of Clinical and Experimental Hypnosis, 12*, 81-87.

Hammer, E. F. (1954). Post-hypnotic suggestion and test performance. *Journal of Clinical and Experimental Hypnosis, 2*, 178-185.

Hammond, D. C. (1984). Myths about Erickson and Ericksonian hypnosis. *American Journal of Clinical Hypnosis, 26*, 346-245.

Harding, H. C. (1961). Hypnosis and migraine or vice versa. *Northwest Medicine*, February, 168-172.

Harriman. P. L. (1942). Hypnotic induction of color vision anomalies: I. The Isihara and Jensen tests. *Journal of General Psychology, 26*, 289-298.

Hartley, F. B. (1968). Hypnosis for the alleviation of pain in treatment of burns: Case report. *Archives of Physical Medicine, 49*, 39-41.

Hartmann, W., & Rawlins, C. M. (1960). Hypnosis in the management of a case of placenta abruptio. *The International Journal of Clinical and Experimental Hypnosis, 8*, 103-107.

Harvey, M. A., & Sipprelle, C. N. (1978). Color blindness, perceptual interference, and hypnosis. *American Journal of Clinical Hypnosis, 20*, 189-193.

Hastie, R., & Kmar, P. (1979). Person memory: Personality traits as organizing principles in memory for behaviors. *Journal of Personality and Social Psychology, 37*, 25-38.

Hatfield, E. C. (1961). The validity of the LeCron method of evaluating hypnotic depth. *International Journal of Clinical and Experimental Hypnosis, 92*,15-221.

Haward, L., & Ashworth, A. (1980). Some problems of evidence obtained by hypnosis. *Criminal Law Review*, August, 469-485.

He, L. (1987). Involvement of endogenous opioid peptides in acupuncture analgesia. *Pain, 31*, 99-121.

Healy, J. M., & Dowd, J. M. (n.d.). Hypnotherapeutic control of long-term pain. In E. T. Dowd, & J. M. Healy (Eds.), *Case studies in hypnotherapy*. New York: Guilford Press.

Heaton, R. K. (1975). Subject expectancy and environmental factors as determinants of psychedelic flashback experiences. *Journal of Nervous and Mental Disease, 161*, 157-165.

Hedge, A. R. (1960). Hypnosis in cancer. *British Journal of Medical Hypnotism, 12*, 2.

Heide, F. J., Wadlington, W. L., & Lundy, R. M. (1980). Hypnotic responsivity as a predictor of outcome in meditation. *International Journal of Clinical and Experimental Hypnosis, 28*, 358-366.

Helson, H. (1964). *Adaptation-level theory*. New York: Harper & Row.

Hendin, D. (1972). Is acupuncture today's miracle? In *Acupuncture: What can it do for you?* New York: Newspaper Enterprise Association, p. 4-7.

Hendler, C. S., & Redd, W. H. (1986). Fear of hypnosis: The role of labelling in patients' acceptance of behavioral interventions. *Behavior Therapy, 17*, 2-13.

Henry, D. (1985). Subjects' expectancies and subjective experience of hypnosis. Unpublished doctoral dissertation, University of Connecticut.

Higgins, E. T. & King, G. (1981). Accessibility of social constructs: Information-processing consequences of individual and contextual variability. In N. Cantor & J. F. Kihlstrom, *Personality, cognition, and social interaction* (pp. 71-122). Hillsdale, N.J.: Erlbaum.

Hilgard, E. R. (1963). Ability to resist suggestions within the hypnotic state: Responsiveness to conflicting communications. *Psychological Reports, 12*, 3-13.

———. (1965). *Hypnotic susceptibility.* New York: Harcourt, Brace & World.

———. (1969). Pain as a puzzle for psychology and physiology. *American Psychologist, 24*, 103-113.

———. (1974). Toward a neo-dissociation theory: Multiple cognitive controls in human functioning. *Perspectives in Biology and Medicine, 17*, 301-316.

———. (1975a). Hypnosis. *Annual Review of Psychology, 26*, 19-44.

———. (1975b). *Hypnotic susceptibility.* New York: Harcourt, Brace & World.

———. (1975c). The alleviation of pain by hypnosis. *Pain, 1*, 213-231.

———. (1977a). *Divided consciousness. Multiple controls in human thought and action.* New York: John Wiley.

———. (1977b). The problem of divided consciousness: A neodissociation interpretation. *Annals New York Academy of Sciences, 296*, 48-59.

———. (1979). Divided consciousness in hypnosis: The implications of the hidden observer. In E. Fromm & R. E. Shor (Eds.), *Hypnosis: Developments in research and new perspectives* (2nd ed., pp. 45-79). Chicago: Aldine.

———. (1981). Hypnotic susceptibility scales under attack: An examination of Weitzenhoffer's criticisms. *International Journal of Clinical and Experimental Hypnosis, 29*, 24-41.

———. (1982a). Hypnotic susceptibility and implications for measurement. *International Journal of Clinical and Experimental Hypnosis, 30*, 394-403.

———. (1982b). Conscious and unconscious processes in hypnosis. In D. Waxman, P. C. Misra, M. Gibson, & M. A. Basker (Eds.), *Modern trends in hypnosis.* New York: Plenum.

———. (1983). Dissociation theory and hypnosis. Paper presented at the annual meeting of the American Psychological Association, Anaheim.

———. (1986). *Divided consciousness: Multiple controls in human thought and action.* New York: Wiley.

———. (1987). Research advances in hypnosis: Issues and methods. *International Journal of Clinical and Experimental Hypnosis, 35*, 248-264.

Hilgard, E. R., & Hilgard, J. R. (1975). *Hypnosis in the relief of pain.* Los Altos, Calif.: William Kaufmann.

———. (1983). *Hypnosis in the relief of pain* (2nd ed.). Los Altos, Calif.: William Kaufmann.

Hilgard, E. R., Hilgard, J. R., MacDonald, H., Morgan, A. H., & Johnson, L. S. (1978). Covert pain in hypnotic analgesia: Its reality as tested by the real-simulator design. *Journal of Abnormal Psychology, 87*, 655-663.

Hilgard, E. R., & Lauer, L. W. (1962). Lack of correlation between the California Psychological Inventory and hypnotic susceptibility. *Journal of Consulting Psychology, 26*, 331-335.

Hilgard, E. R., & LeBaron, S. (1984). *Hypnotherapy of children with pain.* Los Altos, Calif.: Kaufmann.

Hilgard, E. R., MacDonald, H., Marshall, G. D., & Morgan, A. H. (1974). The anticipation of pain and pain control under hypnosis: Heart rate and blood pressure responses in the cold pressor test. *Journal of Abnormal Psychology, 83*, 561-568.

Hilgard, E. R., MacDonald, H., Morgan, A. H., & Johnson, L. S. (1978). The reality of hypnotic analgesia: A comparison of highly hypnotizables with simulators. *Journal of Abnormal Psychology, 87*, 239-246.

Hilgard, E. R., & Morgan, A. H. (1975). Heart rate and blood pressure in the study of laboratory pain in man under normal conditions and as influenced by hypnosis. *Neurobiologiae Experimentalis, 35*, 741-759.

Hilgard, E. R., Morgan, A. H., & MacDonald, H. (1975). Pain and dissociation in the cold pressor test: A study of hypnotic analgesia with "hidden reports" through automatic key-pressing and automatic talking. *Journal of Abnormal Psychology, 84*, 280-289.

Hilgard, E. R., Ruch, J. C., Lange, A. F., Lenox, J. R., Morgan, A. W., & Sachs, L. B. (1974). The psychophysics of cold pressor pain and its modification through hypnotic suggestion. *American Journal of Psychology, 87,* 17-31.

Hilgard, E. R., Sheehan, P. W., Monteiro, K. P., & MacDonald, H. (1981). Factorial structure of the Creative Imagination Scale as a measure of hypnotic responsiveness. An international comparative study. *International Journal of Clinical and Experimental Hypnosis, 29,* 66-76.

Hilgard, E. R., & Tart, C. T. (1966). Responsiveness to suggestions following waking and imagination instructions and following induction of hypnosis. *Journal of Abnormal Psychology, 71,* 196-208.

Hilgard, J. R. (1970). *Personality and hypnosis: A study of imaginative involvement.* Chicago: University of Chicago Press.

———. (1979). *Personality and hypnosis: A study of imaginative involvement* (2nd ed.). Chicago: University of Chicago Press.

Hilgard, J. R., & LeBaron, S. (1982). Relief of anxiety and pain in children and adolescents with cancer: Quantitative measures and clinical observations. *International Journal of Clinical and Experimental Hypnosis, 30,* 417-442.

———. (1984). Hypnotherapy of pain in children with cancer. Los Altos, Calif.: William Kaufmann.

Hillard, H. (1905). Blue light as an anesthetic. *British Medical Journal,* 1405.

Hiscock, M. (1978). Imagery assessment through self-report: What do imagery questionnaires measure? *Journal of Consulting and Clinical Psychology, 46,* 223-230.

Hockenberry, M. J., & Bologna-Vaughan, S. (1985). Preparation for intrusive procedures using noninvasive techniques in children with cancer: State of the art vs. new trends. *Cancer Nursing, 8,* 97-102.

Hockenberry, M. J., & Cotanch, P. H. (1985). Hypnosis as adjuvant antiemetic therapy in childhood cancer. *Nursing Clinics of North America, 20*(3), 105-107.

Hodson, W. J. (1907). The blue ray in therapeutic dentistry. *Practice Dental Journal,* 845-849.

Hoffmann, E. (1959). Hypnosis in general surgery. *American Surgeon, 25,* 163-169.

Hoffman, M. L. (1983). Hypnotic desensitization for the management of anticipatory emesis in chemotherapy. *American Journal of Clinical Hypnosis, 25*(2-3), 173-176.

Holden, C. (1977). Pain control with hypnosis. *Science, 198,* 808.

Holland, J. (1982). Why patients seek unproven cancer remedies: A psychological perspective. *Ca— A Cancer Journal for Clinicians, 32,* 3-7.

Holmes, J. D., Hekmat, H., & Mozingo, B. S. (1983). Cognitive and behavioral regulation of pain: The facilitative effects of analgesic suggestions. *Psychological Record, 33,* 151-159.

Horan, J. J., Hackett, G., Buchanan, J. S., Stone, C. I., & Demchik-Stone, D. (1977). Coping with pain: A component analysis of stress inoculation. *Cognitive Therapy and Research, 1,* 111-221.

Horan, J. S. (1953). Hypnosis and recorded suggestion in the treatment of migraine: Case report. *Journal of Clinical and Experimental Hypnosis, 1,* 7-10.

Horowitz, M. J. (1978). *Image formation and cognition.* New York: Appleton-Century-Crofts.

Howard, A., Pion, G. M., Gottfredson, G. O., Flattau, P. E., Oskamp, S., Pfafflin, S. M., Bray, D. W., & Burstein, A. G. (1986). The changing face of American psychology: A report from the Committee on Employment and Human Resources. *American Psychologist, 41,* 1311-1327.

Howard, M. L., & Coe, W. C. (1980). The effects of context and subjects' perceived control in breaching posthypnotic amnesia. *Journal of Personality, 48,* 342-359.

Hoyt, I. F. & Kihlstrom, J. F. (1986). Posthypnotic suggestion and waking instruction. Paper presented at the meeting of the American Psychological Association, Washington, D.C.

———. (1987). Posthypnotic suggestion and waking instruction: Allocation of attentional resource in simultaneous tasks. Paper presented at the meeting of the Society for Clinical and Experimental Hypnosis, Los Angeles, Calif.

Huesmann, L. R., Gruder, C. L., & Dorst, G. (1987). A process model of posthypnotic amnesia. *Cognitive Psychology, 19,* 33-62.

Hull, C. L. (1933). *Hypnosis and suggestibility: An experimental approach.* New York: Appleton-Century-Crofts.

Hunt, H. T., & Chefurka, C. M. (1976). A test of the psychedelic model of altered states of consciousness: The role of introspective sensitization in eliciting unusual subjective reports. *Archives of General Psychiatry, 33,* 867-876.

Hyghey, M. J., McElin, T. W., & Young, T. (1978). Maternal and fetal outcome of Lamaze-prepared patients. *Obstetrics and Gynecology, 51,* 643-647.

Ikemi, Y., & Nakagawa, S. (1962). A psychosomatic study of contagious dermatitis. *Kyushu Journal of Medical Science, 13,* 335-350.

Illovsky, J. (1963). An experience with group hypnosis in reading disability in primary behavior disorders. *Journal of Genetic Psychology, 102,* 61-67.

International Society of Hypnosis. (1979). Resolution (adopted August 1979). *International Journal of Clinical and Experimental Hypnosis, 27,* 453.

Israeli, N. (1953). Experimental study of projection in time: 1. Outlook upon the remote future—Extending through the quintillionth year. *Journal of Clinical and Experimental Hypnosis, 1,* 49-60.

Istvan, J. (1986). Stress, anxiety, and birth outcomes: A critical review of the evidence. *Psychological Bulletin, 100,* 331-348.

Jacobson, A. M., Hackett, T. P., Surman, O. S., & Silverberg, E. L. (1973). Reynaud's phenomenon: Treatment with hypnotic and operant techniques. *Journal of the American Medical Association, 225,* 739-740.

Janet, P. (1901). *The mental states of hystericals.* Translated by C. R. Corson. From *L'etat mental des hysteriques,* Vol. 1, 1893; *Les accidents mentaux,* Vol. 2, 1894; Paris: Ruff; New York.: Putnam and Sons.

Janssen, W. F. (1979). Cancer quackery—The past in the present. *Seminars in Oncology, 6,* 526-536.

Jaremko, M. E. (1978). Cognitive strategies in the control of pain tolerance. *Behavior Therapy and Experimental Psychiatry, 9,* 239-244.

Javert, C. T., & Hardy, J. D. (1951). Influence of analgesics on pain intensity during labor (with a note on "Natural Childbirth"). *Anesthesiology, 12,* 189-215.

Jenness, A. J. (1965). *Anxiety, imagery and hypnotizability.* (NIMH Project Report, United States Public Health Service). Washington, D.C.: United States Government Printing Office.

Johnson, R. F. Q. (1974). Suggestions for pain reduction and response to cold induced pain. *Psychological Record, 2,* 138-156.

———. (1976). Hypnotic time-distortion and the enhancement of learning: New data pertinent to the Krauss-Katzell-Krauss experiment. *American Journal of Clinical Hypnosis, 19,* 89-102.

Johnson, R. F. Q., Maher, B. A., & Barber, T. X. (1972). Artifact in the "essence of hypnosis": An evaluation of trance logic. *Journal of Abnormal Psychology, 79,* 212-220.

Jones, B. (1979). Signal detection theory and pain research. *Pain, 7,* 305-312.

———. (1980). Algebraic models for integration of painful and nonpainful electric shock. *Perception and Psychophysics, 28,* 572-576.

Jones, B., & Gwynn, M. I. (1984). Functional measurement scales of painful electric shock. *Perception and Psychophysics, 35,* 193-200.

Jones, B., & Spanos, N. P. (1982). Suggestions for altered auditory sensitivity, the negative subject effect and hypnotic susceptibility: A signal detection analysis. *Journal of Personality and Social Psychology, 43,* 637-647.

———. (1987). Variations in accuracy and response bias following hypnotic and non-hypnotic suggestions in a visual discrimination experiment. Unpublished manuscript, Carleton University, Ottawa, Canada.

Jones, B., Spanos, N. P., & Anuza, T. (1987). Functional measurement analysis of suggestions for hypnotic analgesia. Unpublished manuscript, Carleton University, Ottawa, Canada.

Jones, C. G. (1962). Associated uses of hypnosis in surgery. *American Journal of Clinical Hypnosis,* *4,* 270-271.

Juhasz, J. B. (1972). On the reliability of two measures of imagery. *Perceptual and Motor Skills,* *35,* 874.

———. (1979). Theories of hypnosis and theories of imagining. *Academic Psychology Bulletin, 1,* 119-128.

Juhasz, J. B., & Sarbin, T. R. (1966). On the false alarm metaphor in psychophysics. *Psychological Record, 16,* 323-327.

Kahneman, D. (1973). *Attention and effort.* Englewood Cliffs, N.J.: Prentice-Hall.

Karlin, R. A. (1979). Hypnotizability and attention. *Journal of Abnormal Psychology, 88,* 92-95.

Katcher, A., Segal, H. & Beck. A. (1984). Comparison of contemplation and hypnosis for the reduction of anxiety and discomfort during dental surgery. *American Journal of Clinical Hypnosis, 27,* 14-25.

Katsanis, J., Barnard, J., & Spanos, N. P. (in press, 1988). Self-predictions, interpretational set and imagery vividness as determinants of hypnotic responding. *Imagination, Cognition and Personality.*

Katz, E. R., Kellerman, J., & Ellenberg, L. (1987). Hypnosis in the reduction of acute pain and distress in children with cancer. *Journal of Pediatric Psychology, 12,* 379-394.

Katz, N. (1978). Hypnotic inductions as training in cognitive self-control. *Cognitive Therapy and Research, 2,* 365-369.

———. (1979). Comparative efficacy of behavioral training, training plus relaxation, and a sleep/ trance hypnotic induction in increasing hypnotic susceptibility. *Journal of Consulting and Clinical Psychology, 47,* 536-541.

Katz, N. W. (1979). Comparative efficacy of hypnotic induction and behavior modification procedures in enhancing hypnotic susceptibility. *Journal of Consulting and Clinical Psychology, 47,* 119-127.

———. (1980). Hypnosis and the addictions. A critical review. *Addictive Behaviors, 5,* 41-47.

Katz, N. W., & Crawford, V. L. (1978). A little trance and a little skill: Interaction between models of hypnosis and type of hypnotic induction. Paper presented at the Society for Clinical and Experimental Hypnosis, Asheville, N.C.

Katz, R. L., Kao, C. Y., Speigel, H., & Katz, G. J. (1974). Pain, acupuncture, hypnosis. In J. J. Bonica (Ed.), *Advances in neurology* (Vol. 4). N.Y.: Raven Press.

Kaye, J. M. (1984). Hypnotherapy and family therapy for the cancer patient: A case study. *American Journal of Clinical Hypnosis, 27,* 38-41.

———. (1987). Use of hypnosis in the treatment of cancer patients. *Journal of Psychosocial Oncology, 5,* 11-22.

Kellerman, J., Zeltzer, L., Ellenberg, L., & Dash, J. (1983). Adolescents with cancer: Hypnosis for the reduction of the acute pain and anxiety with medical procedures. *Journal of Adolescent Health Care, 4,* 85-90.

Kelsey, D., & Barron, J. N. (1958). Maintenance of posture by hypnotic suggestion in a patient undergoing plastic surgery. *British Medical Journal, 1,* 756-757.

Kepes, E. R., Chen, M., & Schapira, M. (1976). A critical evaluation of acupuncture in the treatment of chronic pain. In J. J. Bonica (Ed.), *Advances in pain research and therapy* (Vol. 1). New York: Raven Press.

Kidder, L. H. (1972). On becoming hypnotized: How skeptics become convinced. A case study of attitude change. *Journal of Abnormal Psychology, 80,* 317-322.

Kihlstrom, J. F. (1977). Models of posthypnotic amnesia. *Annals New York Academy of Sciences, 296,* 284-301.

———. (1978). Context and cognition in posthypnotic amnesia. *International Journal of Clinical and Experimental Hypnosis, 26*(4), 246-267.

———. (1980). Posthypnotic amnesia for recently learned material: Interactions with "episodic" and "semantic" memory. *Cognitive Psychology, 12,* 227-251.

Kihlstrom, J. F. (1982,). *Self-appraisals of hypnotic "depth."* Paper presented at the 34th Annual Meeting of the Society for Clinical and Experimental Hypnosis, Indianapolis.

————. (1983). Instructed forgetting: Hypnotic and nonhypnotic. *Journal of Experimental Psychology; General, 112,* 73-79.

————. (1984). Conscious, subconscious, unconscious: A cognitive perspective. In K. S. Bowers & D. Meichenbaum (Eds.), *The unconscious reconsidered* (pp. 149-211). New York: John Wiley & Sons.

————. (1985). Hypnosis. *Annual Review of Psychology, 36,* 385-418.

————. (1987). The cognitive unconscious. *Science, 237,* 1445-1452.

Kihlstrom, J. F. & Cantor, N. (1983). Mental representations of the self. In L. Berkowitz (Ed.), *Advances in experimental social psychology* (Vol. 17). New York: Academic Press.

Kihlstrom, J. F., Diaz, W. A., McClellan, G. E., Ruskin, P. M., Pistole, D. D., & Shor, R. E. (1980). Personality correlates of hypnotic susceptibility: Needs for achievement and autonomy, self-monitoring and masculinity-femininity. *The American Journal of Clinical Hypnosis, 22,* 225-229.

Kihlstrom, J. F., Easton, R. D., & Shor, R. E. (1983). Spontaneous recovery of memory during posthypnotic amnesia. *International Journal of Clinical and Experimental Hypnosis, 31,* 309-323.

Kihlstrom, J. F., & Evans, F. J. (1976). Recovery of memory after posthypnotic amnesia. *Journal of Abnormal Psychology, 85*(6), 564-569.

Kihlstrom, J. F., & Evans, F. J. (1979). Memory retrieval processes during posthypnotic amnesia. In J. F. Kihlstrom & F. J. Evans (Eds.), *Functional disorders of memory.* New York: Erlbaum.

Kihlstrom, J. F., Evans, F. J., Orne, E. C., & Orne, M. T. (1980). Attempting to breach posthypnotic amnesia. *Journal of Abnormal Psychology, 89,* 603-616.

Kihlstrom, J. F., & Shor, R. E. (1978). Recall and recognition during posthypnotic amnesia. *International Journal of Clinical and Experimental Hypnosis, 26,* 246-267.

Kihlstrom, J. F., & Wilson, L. (1984). Temporal organization of recall during posthypnotic amnesia. *Journal·of Abnormal Psychology, 93*(2), 200-208.

Kimble, G., & Perlmutter, L. (1970). The problem of volition. *Psychological Review, 77,* 361-384.

Kinney, J. M., & Sachs, L. B. (1974). Increasing hypnotic susceptibility. *Journal of Abnormal Psychology, 83,* 145-150.

Kirsch, I. (1978). The placebo effect and the cognitive-behavioral revolution. *Cognitive Therapy and Research, 2,* 255-274.

————. (1985). Response expectancy as a determinant of experience and behavior. *American Psychologist, 40,*1189-1202.

————. (1986). Role playing versus response expectancy and explanations of hypnotic behavior. *Behavioral and Brain Sciences, 9,* 475-476.

Kirsch, I., Carone, J. E., & Johnston, D. J. (1986). The surreptitious observation design. A new experimental paradigm for distinguishing artifact from essence in hypnosis. Manuscript submitted for publication.

Kirsch, I., Council, J. R., & Vickery, A. R. (1984). The role of expectancy in eliciting hypnotic responses as a function of type of induction. *Journal of Consulting and Clinical Psychology, 52,* 708-709.

Kir-Stimon, W. (1978). Hypnosis as a tool for termination of therapy. *International Journal of Clinical and Experimental Hypnosis, 26,* 134-142.

Kleinhaus, M., Eli, I., & Rubinstein, Z. (1985). Treatment of dental and dental-related behavioral dysfunctions in a consultative outpatient clinic: A preliminary report. *American Journal of Clinical Hypnosis, 28,* 3-9.

Kleinhaus, M., Horowitz, I., & Tobin, T. (1977). The use of hypnosis in police investigation: A preliminary communication. *Journal of the Forensic Science Society, 17,* 77-80.

Klemp, R. H. (1969). The Rotter I-E Scale and hypnotic susceptibility. *Psychological Reports, 24,* 660.

Klepac, R. K., Hauge, G., Dowling, J., & McDonald, M. (1981). Direct and generalized effect of three components of stress inoculation for increased pain tolerance. *Behavior Therapy, 12,* 417-424.

Kline, M. V. (1958). The dynamics of hypnotically induced antisocial behavior. *Journal of Psychology, 45,* 239-245.

———. (1983). *Forensic hypnosis: Clinical tactics in the courtroom.* Springfield, Ill.: C. C. Thomas.

Kline, M. V., & Guze, H. (1955). Self-hypnosis in childbirth: A clinical evaluation of a patient conditioning program. *Journal of Clinical and Experimental Hypnosis, 3,* 142-147.

Klinger, B. (1970). Effect of peer model responsiveness and length of induction procedure on hypnotic responsiveness. *Journal of Abnormal Psychology, 75,* 15-18.

Klinger, E. (1971). *Structure and functions of fantasy.* New York: John Wiley.

Knox, V. J., Gekoski, W. L., Shum, K., & McLaughlin, D. M. (1981). Analgesia for experimentally induced pain: Multiple sessions of acupuncture compared to hypnosis in high-and low-susceptible subjects. *Journal of Abnormal Psychology, 90,* 28-34.

Knox, V. J., Morgan, A. H., & Hilgard, E. R. (1974). Pain and suffering in ischemia: The paradox of hypnotically suggested anesthesia as contradicted by the reports from the "hidden observer." *Archives of General Psychiatry, 30,* 840-847.

Knox, V. J., & Shum, K. (1977). Reduction of cold pressor pain with acupuncture analgesia in high- and low-hypnotic subjects. *Journal of Abnormal Psychology, 86,* 639-643.

Knox, C. J., Shum, K., & McLaughlin, D. M. (1977). Response to cold pressor pain and to acupuncture analgesia in oriental and occidental subjects. *Pain, 4,* 49-57.

Knox, V. J., Shum, K., & McLaughlin, D. M. (1978). Hypnotic analgesia vs. acupuncture analgesia in high- and low-susceptible subjects. In F. H. Frankel and H. S. Zamansky (Eds.), *Hypnosis at its bicentennial: Selected papers.* New York: Plenum.

Kohl, G. C. (1962). Anesthesia in obstetrics. *Medical Times, 90,* 368-378.

Kohut, H. (1977). *The restoration of the self.* New York: International Universities Press.

Kolata, G. B. (1979). Scientists attack report that obstetrical medications endanger children. *Science, 204,* 390-391.

Kolouch, F. T. (1962). Role of suggestion in surgical convalescence. *Archives of Surgery, 85,* 304-315.

———. (1964). Hypnosis and surgical convalescence: A study of subjective factors in postoperative recovery. *American Journal of Clinical Hypnosis, 7,* 120-129.

———. (1968). The frightened surgical patient. *American Journal of Clinical Hypnosis, 10,* 89-98.

Kopel, S. A., & Arkowitz, H. S. (1974). Role playing as a source of self-observation and behavior change. *Journal of Personality and Social Psychology, 29,* 677-686.

Korotkin, I., Pleshkova, T. V., & Suslova, M. M. (1969). Changes in auditory thresholds as a result of hypnotic suggestion. *Soviet Neurology and Psychiatry, 1,* 33-40.

Kotarba, J. A. (1983). *Chronic pain: Its social dimension.* Beverly Hills: Sage.

Kraft, W. A., and Rodolfa, E. R. (1982). The use of hypnosis among psychologists. *American Journal of Hypnosis, 24*(4), 249-257.

Krauss, H. K., Katzell, R., & Krauss, B. J. (1974). Effect of hypnotic time-distortion upon free-recall learning. *Journal of Abnormal Psychology, 83,* 141-144.

Krippner, S. (1963). Hypnosis and reading improvement among university students. *American Journal of Clinical Hypnosis, 5,* 187-193.

Kroger, W. S. (1953). "Natural childbirth": Is Read's method of "natural childbirth" waking hypnotism? *British Journal of Medical Hypnotism, 4,* 29-43.

———. (1957). Introduction and supplemental reports. In J. Esdaile, *Hypnosis in medicine and surgery.* New York: Julian Press.

———. (1972). Hypnotism and acupuncture. *Journal of the American Medical Association, 220,* 1012-1013.

———. (1977a). *Clinical and experimental hypnosis* (2nd ed.). Philadelphia: J. B. Lippincott.

———. (1977b). *Clinical and experimental hypnosis in medicine, dentistry and psychology.* Philadelphia: J. B. Lippincott.

Kroger, W. S., & DeLee, S. T. (1957). Use of hypnoanesthesia for caesarean section and hysterectomy. *Journal of the American Medical Association, 163,* 442-444.

Kroger, W. S., & Fezler, W. D. (1976). *Hypnosis and behavior modification: Imagery conditioning.* Philadelphia: Lippincott.

Kroger, W. S., & Schneider, S. A. (1959). An electronic aid for hypnotic induction: A preliminary report. *International Journal of Clinical and Experimental Hypnosis, 7,* 93-98.

Kruglanski, A. W. (1975). The endogenous-exogenous partition in attribution theory. *Psychological Review, 82,* 387-405.

Kubiak, R. V. (1983). Hypnosis: Anesthetic agent in major surgery: A case report. *Medical Hypnoanalysis, 4,* 46-48.

Kuhn, T. S. (1962). *The structure of scientific revolutions.* Chicago: University of Chicago Press.

———. (1970). *The structure of scientific revolutions, 2nd ed.,* Chicago: University of Chicago Press.

Kuhnmeunch, A. J. (1908). Discussion on the paper of Dr. Raiche on "The value of light energy in dental practice." *Dental Review,* 80-86.

LaBaw, W. C. (1973). Adjunctive trance therapy with severely burned chldren. *International Journal of Child Psychotherapy, 2,* 80-92.

LaBaw, W. L. (1969). Terminal hypnosis in lieu of terminal hospitalization. *Gerontologia Clinica, 11,* 312-320.

LaBaw, W., Holton, C., Tewell, K., & Eccles, D. (1975). The use of self-hypnosis by children with cancer. *American Journal of Clinical Hypnosis, 17,* 233-245.

Lamaze, F. (1958). *Painless childbirth.* London: Burke.

Lana, R. (1959). Pretest-treatment interaction in longitudinal studies. *Psychological Bulletin, 56,* 293-300.

Lang, P. J., & Lazovik, M. (1962). Personality and hypnotic susceptibility. *Journal of Consulting Psychology, 26,* 317-322.

Langer, E. (1978). Rethinking the role of thought in social interaction. In J. Harvey, W. Ickes, & R. Kidd (Eds.), *New directions in attribution research* (Vol. 2, pp. 35-58). Hillsdale, N.J.: Erlbaum.

Langs, R. (1976). *The therapeutic interaction* (2 vols). New York: Jason Aronson.

Lansky, P. (1982). Possibility of hypnosis as an aid in cancer therapy. *Perspectives in Biology and Medicine, 25,* 496-509.

Lanzetta, J. T., Cartwright-Smith, J., & Kleck, R. E. (1976). Effects of nonverbal dissimulation on emotional experience and autonomic arousal. *Journal of Personality and Social Psychology, 33,* 354-370.

Laurence, J.-R., & Nadon, R. (1986). Reports of hypnotic depth: Are they more than mere words? *International Journal of Clinical and Experimental Hypnosis, 34,* 215-233.

Laurence, J.-R., Perry, C., and Kihlstrom, J. F. (1983). "Hidden observer" phenomenon in hynosis: An experimental creation, *Journal of Personality and Social Psychology, 44*(1), 163-169.

Laurence, J.-R., & Perry, C. (1981). The "hidden observer" phenomenon in hypnosis: Some additional findings. *Journal of Abnormal Psychology, 90,* 334-344.

Laurence, J.-R., & Perry, C. (1982). Montreal norms for the Harvard Group Scale of Hypnotic Susceptibility: Form A. *International Journal of Clinical and Experimental Hypnosis, 30,* 167-176.

Laurence, J., & Perry, C. (1983). Hypnotically created memory among highly hypnotizable subjects. *Science, 222,* 523-524.

Lazar, B. S., Tellerman, K., Tylke, L., & Gruenewald, D. (1983). Hypnotic intervention on a pediatric oncology unit. Paper presented at the 35th Annual Meeting of the Society for Clinical and Experimental Hypnosis, Boston.

Lazarus, A. (1971). *Behavior therapy and beyond.* New York: McGraw-Hill.

Lea, P. A., Ware, P. D., & Monroe, R. R. (1960). The hypnotic control of intractable pain. *American Journal of Clinical Hypnosis, 3,* 3-8.

Leckie, F. H. (1964). Hypnotherapy in gynecological disorders. *The International Journal of Clinical and Experimental Hypnosis, 12,* 121-146.

———. (1965). Further gynecological conditions treated by hypnotherapy. *The International Journal of Clinical and Experimental Hypnosis, 13,* 11-25.

LeCron, L. M. (1953). A method of measuring the depth of hypnosis. *Journal of Clinical and Experimental Hypnosis, 1,* 4-7.

Lefebvre, L. and Carli, G. (1985). Parturition in non-human primates: Pain and auditory concealment. *Pain, 21,* 315-327.

Lee-Teng, E. (1965). Trance-susceptibility, induction-susceptibility and acquiescence as factors in hypnotic performance. *Journal of Abnormal Psychology, 70,* 383-389.

Lederman, E. I., Fordyce, C. Y., & Sracy, T. E. (1958). Hypnosis, an adjunct to anesthesiology. *Maryland Medical Journal, 7,* 192-194.

Leibowitz, H. E., Lundy, R. M., & Guez, J. R. (1980). The effect of testing distance on suggestion-induced visual field narrowing. *International Journal of Clinical and Experimental Hypnosis, 28,* 409-420.

Lennander, K. G. (1901). Beobachtungen über die Sensibilität der Bauchhöhle und uber lokale and allgemaine Anästhesia bei Bruch-und Bauchoperationen. *Centralblatt für Chirurgie, 8,* 209-223.

———. (1902). Beobachtungen über die Sensibilität in der Bauchhöhle. *Mitteilungen aus den Grenzgebieten der Medizin und Chirurgie, 10,* 38-104.

———. (1904). Weitere Beobachtungen über Sensibilität in Organ und Gewebe und über lokale Anästhesie. *Deutsche Zeitschrift für Chirurgie, 73,* 297-350.

———. (1906a). Ueber Hofrat Nothnagels zweite Hypothese der Darmkolokschmerzen. *Mitteilungen aus den Grenzgebieten der Medizin und Chirurgie, 16,* 19-28.

———. (1906b). Ueber lokale Anästhesie und über Sensibilität in Organ und Gewebe, weitere Beobachtungen. *Mitteilungen aus den Grenzgebieten der Medizin und Chirurgie, 15,* 465-494.

Lennane, K. J., & Lennane, R. J. (1973). Alleged psychogenic disorders in women—A possible manifestation of sexual prejudice. *New England Journal of Medicine, 288,* 288-292.

Leonard, A. S., Papermaster, A. H., & Wangensteen. (1957). Treatment of postgastrectomy dumping syndrome by hypnotic suggestion. *Journal of the American Medical Association, 165,* 1957-1959.

Leonard, R. F. (1973). Evaluation of selection tendencies of patients preferring prepared childbirth. *Obstetrics and Gynecology, 42,* 371-377.

LeShan, L. (1977). *You can fight for your life.* New York: M. Evans & Company.

Leva, R. A. (1974). Modification of hypnotic susceptibility through audiotape relaxation training: Preliminary report. *Perceptual and Motor Skills, 39,* 872-874.

Levendula, D. (1962). A contemporary view of hypnosis. *Headache, 1,* 15-19.

Levine, J. D., Gordon, N. C., & Fields, H. L. (1978). The mechanism of placebo analgesia. *Lancet, 2,* 654-657.

Levine, J. D., Gormley, J., & Fields, H. L. (1976). Observations on the analgesic effects of needle puncture (acupuncture). *Pain, 2,* 149-159.

Levine, M. (1930). Psychogalvanic reaction to painful stimuli in hypnotic and hysterical anesthesia. *Bulletin of the Johns Hopkins Hospital, 46,* 331-339.

Levitan, A. A., & Jevne, R. (n.d.) Patients fearful of hypnosis. In B. Zilbergeld, M. G. Edelstein, & D. L. Araoz (Eds.), *Hypnosis: Questions and answers.* New York: Norton.

Levitt, E. E. (1986). Compliance, voluntariness, and resistance: Reflections of the essence of hypnosis. Paper presented to the meeting of the American Psychological Association, Washington, D.C.

Levitt, E. E., Arnott, G., Duane, M., Toner, M. O., & Parrish, M. J. (1975). Testing the coercive power of hypnosis: Committing objectionable acts. *International Journal of Clinical and Experimental Hypnosis, 23,* 59-67.

Levitt, E. E., & Baker, E. (1983). The hypnotic relationship—Another look at coercion, compliance, and resistance: A brief communication. *International Journal of Clinical and Experimental Hypnosis, 23,* 59-76.

Levitt, E. E., Brady, J. P., & Lubin, B. (1963). Correlates of hypnotizability in young women: Anxiety and dependency. *Journal of Personality, 31,* 52-57.

Levitt, E. E., Brady, J. P., Ottinger, D., & Hinesley, R. (1962). Effects of sensory restriction on hypnotizability. *Archives of General Psychiatry, 7,* 343-345.

Levitt, E. E., & Henderson, G. H. (1980). Voluntary resistance to neural hypnotic suggestions. Paper presented to the meeting of the Society for Clinical and Experimental Hypnosis, Chicago, Ill.

Lewenstein, L. N., Iwamoto, K., & Schwartz, H. (1981). Hypnosis in high risk surgery. *Ophthalmic Surgery, 12,* 39.

Lewit, K. (1979). The needle effect in the relief of myofascial pain. *Pian, 6,* 83-90.

Li, C. L., Ahlberg, D., Lansdell, H., Gravitz, M. A., Chen, T. C., Ting, C. Y., & Bak, A. F. (1975). Acupuncture and hypnosis: Effects on induced pain. *Experimental Neurology, 49,* 272-280.

Licklider, J. C. R. (1961). On psychophysiological models. In W. A. Rosenblith (Ed.), *Sensory Communication: contributions to the symposium on principles of sensory communication.* Cambridge, Mass.: MIT Press.

Lindauer, M. S. (1969). Subject characteristic in hypnosis research: I. A survey of experience, interest and opinion. *International Journal of Clinical and Experimental Hypnosis, 9,* 151-166.

Locke, S. E., Ransil, B. J., Covino, N. A., Toczydlowski, J., Lohse, C. M., Dvorak, H. F., Arndt, K. A., & Frankel, F. H. (1987). Failure of hypnotic suggestion to alter immune response to delayed-type hypersensitivity antigens. *Annals of the New York Academy of Sciences, 496,* 745-749.

London, P. (1962). Subject characteristic in hypnosis research: I. A survey of experience, interest and opinion. *International Journal of Clinical and Experimental Hypnosis, 9,* 151-166.

London, P., Conant, M., & Davidson, G. C. (1966). More hypnosis in the unhypnotizable: Effects of hypnosis and exhortation on rote learning. *Journal of Personality, 34,* 71-79.

London, P., Cooper, L. M., & Engstrom, D. R. (1974). Increasing hypnotic susceptibility by brain wave feedback. *Journal of Abnormal Psychology, 83,* 554-560.

London, P., Cooper, L. M., & Johnson, H. J. (1962). Subject characteristics in hypnosis research: I. Attitudes towards hypnosis, volunteer status and personality measures: Some correlates of hypnotic susceptibility. *International Journal of Clinical and Experimental Hypnosis, 10,* 13-21.

London, P., Hart, J. T., & Leibovitz, M. P. (1968). EEG alpha rhythms and susceptibility to hypnosis. *Nature, 219,* 71-72.

Longo, D. J., Clum, G. A., & Yaeger, N. J. (1988). Psychosocial treatment for recurrent genital herpes. *Journal of Consulting and Clinical Psychology, 56,* 61-66.

Loomis, E. A. (1951). Space and time perception and distortion in hypnotic states. *Personality, 1,* 283-293.

Lozanov, G. (1967). Anesthetization through suggestion in a state of wakefulness. *Proceedings of the 7th European conference on Psychosomatic Research.* Rome, 399-402.

Luchins, A. S. (1942). Mechanization in problem solving—the effect of Einstellung. *Psychological Monographs, 54*(6).

Lynn, B., & Perl, E. R. (1967). Failure of acupuncture to produce localized analgesia. *Pain, 3,* 339-351.

Lynn, S. J., Jacquith, L. Jothiratnam & Rhue, J. W. (1987). Hypnosis and imagination: A multicultural comparison. Unpublished manuscript, Ohio University.

Lynn, S. J., Nash, M. R., Rhue, J. W., Carlson, V., Sweeney, C., Frauman, D., & Givens, D. (1985). Nonvolition and hypnosis. Reals vs. simulators: Experimental and behavioral differences in response to conflicting suggestions during hypnosis. In D. Waxman, P. C. Misra, M. Gibson, & M. A. Basker (Eds.), *Modern trends in hypnosis.* New York: Plenum.

Lynn, S. J., Nash, M. R., Rhue, J. W., Frauman, D. C., & Stanley, S. (1983). Hypnosis and the experience of nonvolition. *International Journal of Clinical and Experimental Hypnosis, 31,* 293-308.

Lynn, S. J., Nash, M. R., Rhue, J. W., Frauman, D. C., & Sweeney, C. A. (1984). Nonvolition, expectancies, and hypnotic rapport. *Journal of Abnormal Psychology, 93,* 295-303.

Lynn, S. J., Neufeld, V., & Matyi, C. L. (1987). Hypnotic inductions versus suggestions: The effects of direct and indirect wording. *Journal of Abnormal Psychology, 96,* 76-80.

Lynn, S. J., & Rhue, J. W. (1986). The fantasy-prone personality: Hypnosis, imagination and creativity. *Journal of Personality and Social Psychology, 5,* 404-408.

Lynn, S. J., Snodgrass, M., Hardaway, R., & Lenz, J. (1984). Hypnotic susceptibility: Predictions and evaluations of performance and experience. Paper presented at the meeting of the American Psychological Association.

Lynn, S. J., Snodgrass, M., Rhue, J. W., & Hardaway, R. (1987). Goal-directed fantasy, hypnotic susceptibility, and expectancies. *Journal of Personality and Social Psychology, 53,* 933-938.

Lynn, S. J., Snodgrass, M., Rhue, J. W., Nash, M. R., & Frauman, D. C. (1987). Attributions, involuntariness, and hypnotic rapport. *American Journal of Clinical Hypnosis, 30,* 36-43.

Lynn, S. J., Weekes, J. R., Matyi, C. L., & Neufeld, V. (in press, 1988). Direct versus indirect suggestions, archaic involvement, and hypnotic experience. *Journal of Abnormal Psychology.*

Lynn, S. J., Weeks, J., Nuefeld, V., Zivney, O., Brentar, J., & Weiss, F. (1987). Interpersonal climate and hypnotizability level: Effects on hypnotic performance, rapport and archaic involvement. Manuscript submitted for publication.

Lynn, S. J., Weekes, J., Snodgrass, M., Abrams, L., Weiss, F., & Rhue, J. (1986). Control and countercontrol in hypnosis. Meeting of the American Psychological Association.

MacCracken, P. J., Gogel, W. C., and Blum, G. S. (1980). Effects of post-hypnotic suggestion on perceived egocentric distance. *Perception, 9,* 561-568.

Marcel, A. (1983). Conscious and unconscious perception: An approach to the relations between phenomenal experience and perceptual processes. *Cognitive Psychology, 15,* 238-300.

Macfarlane, A. (1977). *The Psychology of childbirth.* Cambridge: Harvard University Press.

MacLeod-Morgan, C., & Lack, L. (1982). Hemispheric specificity: A physiological concomitant of hypnotizability. *Psychophysiology, 19,* 687-690.

Mahoney, M., & Thoresen, C. (1974). *Self-control: Power to the person.* Monterey, Calif.: Brooks/ Cole.

Malyon, A. K., Harris, G. N., Griffin, S., & Pinsky, J. J. (1978). Psychosocial assessment of patients with chronic intractible benign pain syndromes. In B. L. Crue, Jr. (Ed.), *Chronic Pain: Further observations from city of Hope Medical Center.* New York: SP Medical & Scientific Books.

Man, P. L., & Chen, C. H. (1972). Acupuncture "anesthesia"—a new theory and clinical study. *Current Therapeutic Research, 14,* 390-394.

Mandy, A. J., Mandy, T. E., Farkas, R., & Scher, E. (1952). Is natural childbirth natural? *Psychosomatic Medicine, 14,* 431-438.

Mann, F. (1972). The probable neurophysiological mechanisms of acupuncture. In *Transcript of the Acupuncture Symposium.* Los Altos, Calif.: Academy of Parapsychology and Medicine, pp. 24-31.

Marcuse, F. L. (1976). *Hypnosis: Fact and fiction.* Harmondsworth, Middlesex: Penguin Books.

Margolis, C. G. (1983). Hyponotic imagery with cancer patients. *American Journal of Clinical Hypnosis, 25* (2-3), 128-134.

Margolis, R. B., Zimny, G. H., Miller, D., & Taylor, J. M. (1984). Internists and the chronic pain patient. *Pain, 20,* 151-156.

Marino, J. C., Gwynn, M. I., & Spanos, N. P. (1988). Cognitive mediators in the reduction of pain: The role of expectancy, strategy use, and self-presentation. *Journal of Abnormal Psychology.*

Markman, H., & Kadushin, F. S. (1986). Preventive effects of Lamaze training for first-time parents: A short-term longitudinal study. *Journal of Consulting and Clinical Psychology, 54,* 872-874.

Marks, D. F. (1972). Vividness of visual imagery and effect of function. In P. W. Sheehan (Eds.), *The Function and nature of imagery* (pp. 83-108). New York: Academic Press.

———. (1973). Visual imagery differences in recall of pictures. *British Journal of Psychology, 64,* 17-24.

Markus, H. (1986). Possible selves. *American Psychologist.*

Marmer, M. J. (1956). The role of hypnosis in anesthesiology. *Journal of the American Medical Association, 162,* 441-443.

———. (1957). Hypnoanalgesia: The use of hypnosis in conjunction with chemical anesthesia. *Anesthesia and Analgesia, 36,* 27-32.

———. (1959). *Hypnosis in anesthesiology.* Springfield, Ill.: C. C. Thomas.

———. (1964). Discussion in J. Lassner, (Ed.), *Hypnosis in anesthesiology.* Berlin: Springer-Verlag.

Mason, A. A. (1952). A case of congenital ichthyosiform erythrodermia of Brocq threatened by hypnosis. *British Medical Journal, 2,* 422-423.

———. (1955). Surgery under hypnosis. *Anesthesia, 10,* 295-299.

Matthews, W. J., Bennett, H., Bean, W., & Gallagher, M. (1985). Indirect versus direct hypnotic suggestions—An initial investigation: A brief communication. *International Journal of Clinical and Experimental Hypnosis, 3,* 219-223.

Mayer, D. J., Price, D. D., & Rafii, A. (1977). Antagonism of acupuncture analgesia in man by the narcotic antagonist naloxone. *Brain Research, 121,* 368-372.

McCann, T. E., & Sheehan, P. W. (1987). The breaching of pseudomemory under hypnotic instruction: Implications for original memory retrieval. *British Journal of Experimental and Clinical Hypnosis, 4,* 101-108.

McCaul, K. D., & Malott, J. M. (1984). Distraction and coping with pain. *Psychological Bulletin, 95,* 516-633.

McCauley, J. D., Thelan, M. J., Frank, R. G., Willard, R. R., & Callan, K. E. (1983). Hypnosis compared to relaxation in the outpatient management of chronic low back pain. *Archives of Physical Rehabilitation, 64,* 548-552.

McConkey, K. M. (1979). Conflict in hypnosis: Reality versus suggestion. In G. D. Burrows, D. R. Collison, & L. Dennerstein, *Hypnosis.* Amsterdam: Elsevier/North Holland Biomedical Press.

———. (1986). Opinions about hypnosis and self-hypnosis before and after hypnotic testing. *International Journal of Clinical and Experimental Hypnosis, 34,* 311-319.

McConkey, K. M., & Cottee, H. E. (1985). Clinical hypnosis and cognitive skills. *The Cognitive Behaviorist, 7,* 6-8.

McConkey, K. M. & Sheehan, P. W. (1976). Contrasting interpersonal orientations in hypnosis: Collaborative versus contractual modes of response. *Journal of Abnormal Psychology, 85,* 390-397.

McConkey, K. M., Sheehan, P. W., & Cross, D. G. (1980). Posthypnotic amnesia: Seeing is not remembering. *British Journal of Social & Clinical Psychology, 19,* 99-107.

McConkey, K. M., & Sheehan, P. W. (1981). The impact of videotape playback of hypnotic events on posthypnotic amnesia. *Journal of Abnormal Psychology, 90* (1), 46-54.

McCord, H. (1961). The image of the trance. *International Journal of Clinical Hypnosis, 9,* 305-307.

McCord, H., & Sherrill, C. J. (1961). A note on increased ability to do calculus posthypnotically. *American Journal of Clinical Hypnosis, 4,* 124.

McCutcheon, N. (1985). The influence of absorption on time perception in the hypnotic context. Unpublished Master's thesis, California State University, Fresno.

McDonald, R. D., & Smith, J. R. (1975). Trance logic in tranceable and simulating subjects. *International Journal of Clinical and Experimental Hypnosis, 23,* 80-89.

McGlashan, T. H., Evans, F. J., & Orne, M. T. (1969). The nature of hypnotic analgesia and placebo response to experimental pain. *Psychosomatic Medicine, 31,* 227-246.

McKeller, P. (1972). Imagery from the standpoint of introspection. In P. W. Sheehan (Ed.), *The function and nature of imagery* (pp. 35-61). New York: Academic Press.

McKelvie, S. J., & Gingras, P. P. (1974). Reliability of two measures of visual imagery. *Perceptual and Motor Skills, 39,* 417-418.

McKinley, S. J., & Gur, R. C. (1975). Imagery, absorption, meditation and drug use as correlates of hypnotic subjects' descriptions of visual hallucinations. *American Journal of Clinical Hypnosis, 15,* 239-244.

McPeake, J. D., & Spanos, N. P. (1973). The effects of the wording of rating scales on hypnotic subjects' descriptions of visual hallucinations. *American Journal of Clinical Hypnosis, 15,* 239–244.

Meares, M. (1976). Regression of cancer after intensive meditation. *Medical Journal of Australia, 5,* 184.

———. (1977). Atavistic regression as a factor in the remission of cancer. *Medical Journal of Australia, 2,* 132–133.

———. (1979). Regression of cancer of the rectum after intensive meditation. *Medical Journal of Australia, 2,* 539–540.

———. (1980). Remission of massive metastasis from undifferentiated carcinoma of the lung associated with intensive meditation. *Journal of the American Society for Dentistry and Medicine, 27,* 40–41.

———. (1981). Regression of recurrence of carcinoma of the breast at mastectomy site associated with intensive meditation. *Australian Family Physician, 10,* 218–219.

Meeker, W. B., and Barber, T. X. (1971). Toward an explanation of stage hypnosis. *Journal of Abnormal Psychology, 77* (1), 61–70.

Meichenbaum, D. (1977). *Cognitive-behavior modification: An integrative approach.* New York: Plenum Press.

Meichenbaum, D., & Cameron, R. (1984). Issues in cognitive assessment. In T. V. Merluzzi, C. R. Glass, & M. Genest (Eds.), *Cognitive assessment.* New York: Guilford Press.

Meichenbaum, D., & Gilmore, J. B. (1984). The nature of unconscious processes: A cognitive-behavioral perspective. In K. S. Bowers & D. Meichenbaum (Eds.), *The Unconscious Reconsidered.* New York: Wiley.

Melei, J. P., & Hilgard, E. R. (1964). Attitudes toward hypnosis, self-predictions and hypnotic susceptibility. *International Journal of Clinical and Experimental Hypnosis, 12,* 99–108.

Mellers, B. A., & Birnbaum, M. H. (1982). Loci of contextual effects in judgment. *Journal of Experimental Psychology: Human Perception and Performance, 8,* 582–601.

Melzack, R. (1973a). How acupuncture can block pain. *Impact of Science on Society, 23,* 65–75.

———. (1973b). Why acupuncture works. *Psychology Today, 7, 28–37.*

———. (1973c). *The puzzle of pain.* New York: Basic Books.

———. (1974). Central neural mechanisms in phantom limb pain. *Advances in Neurology, 4,* 319–326.

———., (Ed.) (1983). *Pain Measurement and Assessment.* New York: Raven Press.

———. (1984). The myth of painless childbirth. *Pain, 19,* 321–337.

Melzack, R., & Chapman, C. R. (1973). Psychologic aspects of pain. *Postgraduate Medicine, 53,* 69–75.

Melzack, R., Kinch, R. A., Dobkin, P., Lebrun, M., & Taenzer, P. (1984). Severity of labor pain: Influence of physical as well as psychological variables. *Canadian Medical Association Journal, 130,* 579–584.

Melzack, R., & Perry, C. (1975). Self-regulation of pain: The use of alpha-feedback and hypnotic training for the control of chronic pain. *Experimental Neurology, 46,* 452–469.

Melzack, R., Taenzer, P., Feldman, P., & Kinch, R. A. (1981). Labor is still painful after prepared childbirth training. *Canadian Medical Association Journal, 125,* 357–363.

Melzack, R., Terrence, C. Fromm, Ansel, R. (1986). Trigeminal neuralgia and atypical facial pain: Use of the McGill Pain Questionnaire for discrimination and diagnosis. *Pain, 27,* 297–302.

Melzack, R., & Wall, P. (1965). Pain mechanisms: A new theory. *Science, 150,* 971–979.

Melzack, R., & Wall, P. D. (1983). *The challenge of pain.* New York: Basic Books.

Melzack, R., Weisz, A. Z., & Sprague, L. T. (1963). Strategems for controlling pain: Contributions of auditory stimulation and suggestion. *Experimental Neurology,8,* 239–247.

Mersky, H. (1980). Some features of the history of the idea of pain. *Pain, 9,* 3–8,.

Michael, A. M. (1952). Hypnosis in childbirth. *British Medical Journal,* April, 734–737.

Michon, J. A., & Jackson, J. L. (1984). Attentional effort and cognitive strategies in the processing of temporal information. In J. Gibbon & L. Allan (Eds.). *Timing and time perception* (Vol. 423, pp. 298-321). New York: New York Academy of Sciences.

Michotte, A. E. (1946/1963). *The perception of causality.* London: Methuen. (trans.) Miles, T. R., & Miles, E. *La perception de la causalité,* Louvain, France.

Mikail, S. F., Vandeursen, J., & von Baeyer, C. (1986). Rating pain or rating serenity: Effects on cold-pressor pain tolerance. *Canadian Journal of Behavioral Science, 18,* 126-132.

Milgram, S. (1974). *Obedience to authority.* New York: Harper & Row; London: Tavistock.

Miller, A. G. (1986). *The obedience experiments.* New York: Praeger.

Miller, G. A., Galanter, E., & Pribram, K. H. (1960). *Plans and the structure of behavior.* New York: Holt, Rinehart and Winston.

Miller, J. (1973). Ph.D. dissertation, University of Southern California.

Miller, J. A. (1980). Hypnosis in a boy with leukemia. *American Journal of Clinical Hypnosis, 22,* 231-235.

Miller, M. E., & Bowers, K. W. (1986). Hypnotic analgesia and stress inoculation in the reduction of pain. *Journal of Abnormal Psychology, 95,* 6-14.

Miller, R. J., & Leibowitz, H. W. (1976). A signal detection analysis of hypnotically induced narrowing of the visual field. *Journal of Abnormal Psychology, 856,* 446-454.

Milne, G. (1982). Hypnotic treatment of a cancer patient. *Australian Journal of Clinical and Experimental Hypnosis, 10* (2), 123-125.

Mingay, D. J. (1986). Hypnosis and memory for incidentally learned scenes. *British Journal of Experimental and Clinical Hypnosis, 3,* 173-183.

Mischel, W. (1968). *Personality and assessment.* New York: Wiley.

Mixon, P. (1972). Instead of deception. *Journal of the Theory of Social Behavior, 2,* 145-177.

Moir, D.. (1977). Pain relief in labor. *British Journal of Hospital Medicine,* March, 226-234.

Moll, A. (1897). *Hypnotism.* New York: Charles Scribner's Sons.

———. (1958). *The study of hypnosis: Historical, clinical, and experimental research in the techniques of hypnotic induction.* New York: Julian Press. (Original work published 1889).

Moore, M. E., & Berk, S. N. (1976). *Annals of internal medicine, 84,* 381-384.

Moore, R. K. (1964). Susceptibility to hypnosis and susceptibility to social influence. *Journal of Abnormal and Social Psychology, 68,* 282-294.

Morgan, A. H., & Hilgard, J. R. (1978/79). The Stanford Hypnotic Clinical Scale for Children. *American Journal of Clinical Hypnosis, 21,* 148-169.

———. (1979). The Stanford Hypnotic Clinical Scale for Adults. *American Journal of Clinical Hypnosis, 21,* 134-147.

Morgan, A. H., & Lam, D. (1969). The relationship of the Betts vividness of imagery questionnaire and hypnotic susceptibility: Failure to replicate. *Hawthorn House Research Memorandum* (No. 103).

Morrow, G. R. (1986). Effect of the cognitive hierarchy in the systematic desensitization treatment of anticipatory nausea in cancer patients: A component comparison with relaxation only, counselling, and no treatment. *Cognitive Therapy and Research, 10,* 421-446.

Morse, D. R. (1975). Hypnosis in the practice of endodontics. *Journal of the American Society of Psychosomatic Medicine and Dentistry, 22,* 17-22.

Morse, D. R., Martin, J. S., Furst, M. L., & Dubin, L. L. (1977). A physiological and subjective evaluation of meditation, hypnosis, and relaxation. *Psychosomatic Medicine, 39,* 304-324.

Morse, D. R., & Wilcko, J. M. (1979). Nonsurgical endodontic therapy for a vital tooth with meditation-hypnosis as the sole anesthetic: A case report. *American Journal of Clinical Hypnosis, 21,* 258-262.

Morton, J. (1984). Hypnosis: Should we use it? *Police Review,* February 3, p. 228.

Moss, A. A. (1963). Hypnodontics: Hypnosis in dentistry. In W. S. Kroger (Ed.), *Clinical and experimental hypnosis.* Philadelphia: Lippincott.

Mott, T. (1985). Editorial: Are hypotherapy patients hypnotized? *American Journal of Clinical Hypnosis, 27* (3), 151-152.

Mun, C. T. (1966). The use of hypnosis as an adjunct in surgery. *American Journal of Clinical Hypnosis, 8,* 178-180.

Murphy, G. (1935). *A briefer general psychology.* New York: Harper & Brothers.

Murray-Jobsis, J. M. (n.d.) Patients who claim they are not hypnotizable. In B. Zilbergeld, M. G. Edelstein, & D. L. Araoz (Eds.), *Hypnosis: Questions and answers.* New York: Norton.

Naish, P. L. N. (1985). The "trance" described in signal detection terms. *British Journal of Experimental and Clinical Hypnosis, 2,* 133-177.

———. (1986). Hypnosis and signal detection. In P. L. N. Naish (Ed.), *What is hypnosis: Current theories and research.* Milton Keynes: Open University Press.

Nash, M. R. (1984). Preliminary findings on a scale of interpersonal regression during hypnosis: A measure of archaic involvement. Paper presented at the Annual Meeting of the American Psychological Association, Toronto, Canada.

Nash, M. R., Johnson, L. S., & Tipton, R. D. (1979). Hypnotic age regression and the occurrence of transitional object relationships. *Journal of Abnormal Psychology, 88,* 547-555.

Nash, M. R., Lynn, S. J., & Givens, D. L. (1984). Adult hypnotic susceptibility, childhood punishment and child abuse: A brief communication. *International Journal of Clinical and Experimental Hypnosis, 32,* 6-11.

Nettelbaldt, P., Fagerstrom, C. F., & Uddenberg, N. (1976). The significance of reported childbirth pain. *Journal of Psychosomatic Research, 20,* 215-221.

Neufeld, W. J., & Thomas, P. (1977). Effects of perceived efficacy of a prophylactic controlling mechanism on self-control under pain stimulation. *Canadian Journal of Behavioral Science, 9,* 224-232.

Newton, B. W. (1983a). Hypnosis and cancer. *American Journal of Clinical Hypnosis, 25,* 89-91.

———. (1983b). The use of hypnosis in the treatment of cancer patients. *American Journal of Clinical Hypnosis, 25* (2-3), 104-113.

Nisbett, R. E., & Schachter, S. (1966). Cognitive manipulation of pain. *Journal of Experimental Social Psychology, 2,* 227-236.

Nisbett, R. E., & Wilson, T. D. (1977). Telling more than we can know: Verbal reports on mental processes. *Psychological Review, 84,* 231-259.

Nogrady, H., McConkey, K. M., Laurence, J.-R., & Perry, C. (1983). Dissociation, duality, and demand characteristics in hypnosis. *Journal of Abnormal Psychology, 92,* 223-235.

Nogrady, H., McConkey, K. M., & Perry, C. (1985). Enhancing visual memory: Trying hypnosis, trying imagination, and trying again. *Journal of Abnormal Psychology, 2,* 194-204.

Nolan, R. P., & Spanos, N. P. (1987). Hypnotic analgesia and stress inoculation: A critical analysis of Miller and Bowers. *Psychological Reports, 61,* 95-102.

Norr, L. K., Block, C. R., Charles, A., Meyering, S., & Meyers, E. (1977). Explaining pain and enjoyment in childbirth. *Journal of Health and Social Behavior, 18,* 260-275.

Norvell, K. T., Gaston-Johansson, F., & Fridh, G. (1987). Remembrance of labor pain: How valid are retrospective pain measurements? *Pain, 31,* 77-86.

Nowlis, D. P. (1969). The child-rearing antecedents of hypnotic susceptibility and of naturally occurring hypnotic-like experiences. *International Journal of Clinical and Experimental Hypnosis, 17,* 109-120.

Nugent, W. R. (1985). A methodological review of case studies published in the American Journal of Clinical Hypnosis. *American Journal of Clinical Hypnosis, 27,* 191-199.

Nuland, W. (1983). The sexually dysfunctional cancer patient. Paper presented at the 35th Annual Meeting of the Society for Clinical and Experimental Hypnosis, Boston.

Oakley, A. (1983). Social consequences of obstetric technology: The Importance of measuring "soft" outcomes. *Birth, 10,* 99-108

Obstoj, J., & Sheehan, P. W. (1977). Aptitude for trance, task generalizability, and incongruity response in hypnosis. *Journal of Abnormal Psychology, 86,* 543-552.

O'Connell, C. N., Shor, R. E., & Orne, M. T. (1970). Hypnotic age regression: An empirical and methodological analysis. *Journal of Abnormal and Social Psychology*, Monograph supplement, *76* (3), Part 2, pp. 1-32.

O'Connell, D. M. (1964). An experimental comparison of hypnotic depth measured by self-ratings and by an objective scale. *International Journal of Clinical and Experimental Hypnosis, 12*, 34-46.

O'Grady, K. E. (1980). The absorption scale: A factor-analytic assessment. *The International Journal of Clinical and Experimental Hypnosis, 28*, 281-288.

Oliver, G. W. (1983). A cancer patient and her family: A case study. *American Journal of Clinical Hypnosis, 25* (2-3), 156-160.

Olness, K. (1981). Imagery (self-hypnosis) as adjunct therapy in childhood cancer: Clinical experience with 25 patients. *American Journal of Pediatric Hematology/Oncology, 3*, 313-321.

Orne, M. T. (1951). The mechanisms of hypnotic age regression: An expermental study. *Journal of Abnormal and Social Psychology, 16*, 213-225.

————. (1959). The nature of hypnosis: Artifact and essence. *Journal of Abnormal and Social Psychology, 58*, 277-299.

————. (1962a). Hypnotically induced hallucinations. In L. J. West (Ed.), *Hallucinations*. New York: Grune & Stratton.

————. (1962b). On the social psychology of the psychological experiment with particular reference to demand characteristics and their implications. *American Psychologist, 17*, 776-783.

————. (1962c). Antisocial behavior and hypnosis: Problems of control and validation in empirical studies. In G. H. Estabrooks (Ed.), *Hypnosis: Current problems* (pp. 137-192). New York: Harper & Row.

————. (1966). Hypnosis, motivation and compliance. *American Journal of Psychiatry, 122*, 721-726.

————. (1969). Demand characteristics and the concept of quasi-controls. In R. Rosenthal & R. L. Rosnow (Eds.), *Artifact in behavioral research*. New York: Academic Press.

————. (1971). The simulation of hypnosis: Why, how, and what it means. *International Journal of Clinical and Experimental Hypnosis, 19*, 183-210.

————. (1977). On the construct of hypnosis: Implications of the definition for research and practice. *Annals of the New York Academy of Sciences, 296*, 14-33.

————. (1979). The use and misuse of hypnosis in court. *International Journal of Experimental and Clinical Hypnosis, 27*, 311-341.

————. (1979). On the simulating subject as a quasi-control group in hypnosis research: What, why, and how. In E. Fromm & R. E. Shor (Eds.), *Hypnosis: Developments in research and new perspectives* (2nd ed.). New York: Aldine.

————. (1980a). Nonpharmacological approaches to pain relief: Hypnosis, biofeedback, placebo effects. In L. K. Y. Ng & J. J. Bonica (Eds.), *Pain, discomfort and humanitarian care*. New York: Elsevier/North Holland.

————. (1980b). Hypnotic control of pain: Toward a clarification of the different psychological processes involved. In J. J. Bonica (Ed.), *Pain* (pp. 155-172). New York: Raven Press.

Orne, M. T., Dinges, D. F., & Orne, E. C. (1984). On the differential diagnosis of multiple personality in the forensic context. *International Journal of Clinical and Experimental Hypnosis, 32*, 118-169.

————. (1986). Hypnotic experience: A cognitive social psychological reality. *Behavioral and Brain Sciences, 9*, 477-478.

Orne, M. T., & Evans, F. J. (1965). Social control in the psychological experiment: Antisocial behavior and hypnosis. *Journal of Personality and Social Psychology, 1*, 189-200.

Orne, M. T., & Hammer, A. G. (1974). Hypnosis. *Encyclopedia Britannica* (pp. 133-140). Chicago: William Benton.

Orne, M. T., & Holland, C. C. (1968). On the ecological validity of laboratory deceptions. *International Journal of Psychiatry, 6*, 282-293.

Orne, M. T., & O'Connell, D. N. (1967). Diagnostic ratings of hypnotizability. *International Journal of Clinical and Experimental Hypnosis, 15,* 125-133.

Orne, M. T., Sheehan, P. W., & Evans, F. J. (1968). The occurrence of posthypnotic behavior outside the experimental setting. *Journal of Personality and Social Psychology, 26,* 217-221.

Orne, M. T., Soskis, D. A., Dinges, D. F., & Orne, E. C. (1984). Hypnotically induced testimony. In G. L. Wells and E. F. Loftus (Eds.), *Eyewitness testimony: Psychological perspectives* (pp. 171-213). Cambridge University Press.

Ornstein, R. F. (1969). *On the experience of time.* Harmondsworth, England: Penguin Books.

Overstad, B. (1981). *Bibliotherapy: Books to help young children.* St. Paul, Minn.: Toys 'n Things Press.

Palmer, R. O., & Field, P. B. (1968). Visual imagery and susceptibility to hypnosis. *Journal of Consulting and Clinical Psychology, 32,* 456-461.

Papermaster, A. A., Doberneck, R. C., & Bonello, F. J. (1960). Hypnosis in surgery. II Pain. *American Journal of Clinical Hypnosis, 2,* 200-224.

Parducci, A. (1974). Contextual effects: A range theory analysis. In E. C. Carterette & M. P. Friedman (Eds.), *Handbook of Perception* (Vol. 2). New York: Academic Press.

Parfitt, R. R. (1980). *The Birth primer.* New York: Signet.

Parker, P. D., & Barber, T. X. (1964). Hypnosis, task-motivating instructions and learning performance. *Journal of Abnormal and Social Psychology, 69,* 499-504.

Parrish, M. J. (1974). Moral predisposition and hypnotic influence on "immoral" behavior: An exploratory study. *American Journal of Clinical Hypnosis, 17,* 115-124.

Parrish, M., Lundy, R. M., & Leibowitz, H. W. (1969). Effect of hypnotic age regression on the magnitude of the Ponzo and Poggendorff Illusions. *Journal of Abnormal Psychology, 74,* 693-698.

Pattie, F. A. (1935). A report of attempts to produce uniocular blindness by hypnotic suggestion. *British Journal of Medical Psychology, 15,* 230-241.

———. (1941). The production of blisters by hypnotic suggestions: A review. *Journal of Abnormal and Social Psychology, 36,* 62-72.

———. (1950). The genuineness of bilateral deafness produced in hypnosis. *American Journal of Psychology, 63,* 84-86.

———. (1967). A brief history of hypnotism. In J. E. Gordon (Ed.), *Handbook of clinical and experimental hypnosis.* New York: Macmillan.

Pennebaker, J. W. (1982). *The psychology of physical symptoms.* New York: Springer-Verlag.

Pepper, S. C. (1942). *World hypotheses.* Berkeley: University of California Press.

Perchard, S. D. (1960). Hypnosis in obstetrics. *Proceedings of the Royal Society of Medicine, 53,* 458-460.

Perky, C. W. (1910). An experimental study of imagination. *American Journal of Psychology, 21,* 422-452.

Pernick, M. S. (1985). *A calculus of suffering: Pain, Professionalism, and anesthesia in nineteenth-century America.* New York: Columbia University Press.

Perry, C. (1973). Imagery, fantasy and hypnotic susceptibility: A multidimensional approach. *Journal of Personality and Social Psychology, 26,* 217-221.

———. (1977). Is hypnotizability modifiable? *International Journal of Clinical and Experimental Hypnosis, 25,* 125-146.

———. (1979). Hypnotic coercion and compliance to it: A review of evidence presented in a legal case. *International Journal of Clinical and Experimental Hypnosis, 27,* 187-218.

Perry, C. W., Gelfand, R., & Marcovitch, P. (1979). The relevance of hypnotic susceptibility in the clinical context. *Journal of Abnormal Psychology, 88,* 592-603.

Perry, C. W., & Laurence, J.-R. (1980). Hypnotic depth and hypnotic susceptibility: A replicated finding. *International Journal of Clinical and Experimental Hypnosis, 28,* 272-280.

———. (1983). The enhancement of memory by hypnosis in the legal investigative situation. *Canadian Psychology, 24,* 155-167.

Perry, C., & Nogrady, H. (1985). Use of hypnosis by the police in the investigation of crime: Is guided memory a safe substitute? *British Journal of Experimental and Clinical Hypnosis, 2,* 25-31.

Perry, C., & Walsh, B. (1978). Inconsistencies and anomalies of response as a defining characteristic of hypnosis. *Journal of Abnormal Psychology, 87,* 575-577.

Pesce, G. (1987). Measurement of reported pain of childbirth: A comparison between Australian and Italian subjects. *Pain, 31,* 87-98.

Peters, J. E. (1973). Trance logic: Artifact or essence in hypnosis? Unpublished doctoral dissertation, Pennsylvania State University.

Peters, R. S. (1958). *The concept of motivation.* New York: Humanities Press.

Pettitt, G. A. (1979). Adjunctive trance and family therapy for terminal cancer. *New Zealand Medical Journal, 89* (627), 18-21.

Pistole, D. D. (1979). A multivariate study of hypnotic susceptibility as a function of locus of control, method of induction and sex of subject. *Dissertation Abstracts International, 40,* 1403B.

Plotkin, W. B. (1976). On the self-regulation of the occipital alpha rhythm: Control strategies, states of consciousness, and the role of physiological feedback. *Journal of Experimental Psychology: General, 105,* 66-69.

———. (1979). The alpha experience revisited: Biofeedback in the transformation of psychological state. *Psychological Bulletin, 85,* 1132-1148.

Plunkett, R. J. (1958). Medical use of hypnosis. *Journal of the American Medical Association, 168,* 186.

Poore, M., and Foster, J. C. (1985). Epidural and nonepidural anesthesia: Differences between mothers and their experiences of birth. *Birth, 12,* 205-214.

Popper, K. (1963). *Conjectures and Refutations.* New York: Harper & Row.

Potash, M., & Jones, B. (1977). Aging and decision criteria for the detection of tones in noise. *Journal of Gerontology, 32,* 436-440.

Poulton, E. C. (1973). Unwanted range effects from using within-subject experimental designs. *Psychological Bulletin, 80,* 113-121.

———. (1975). Range effects in experiments on people. *American Journal of Psychology, 88,* 3-32.

———. (1979). Models for biases in judging sensory magnitude. *Psychological Bulletin, 86,* 777-803.

———. (1982). Influential companions: Effects of one strategy on another in the within-subject design of cognitive psychology. *Psychological Bulletin, 91,* 673-690.

Poulton, E. C., & Freeman, P. R. (1966). Unwanted asymmetrical transfer effects with balanced experimental designs. *Psychological Bulletin, 66,* 1-8.

Price, D. D., & Barber, J. (1987). An analysis of factors that contribute to the efficacy of hypnotic analgesia. *Journal of Abnormal Psychology, 96,* 45-61.

Price, D. D., Rafii, A., Watkins, L. R., & Buckingham, B. (1984). A psychophysical analysis of acupuncture analgesia. *Pain, 19,* 27-42.

Priebe, F. A., & Wallace, B. (1986). Hypnotizability, imaging ability and the detection of embedded objects. *International Journal of Clinical and Experimental Hypnosis, 35,* 320-329.

Pritchard, J. A., & MacDonald, P. C. (1980). *Williams obstetrics: Sixteenth edition.* New York: Appleton-Century-Crofts.

Prkachin, K. M., & Craig, K. D. (1985). Influencing non-verbal expressions of pain: Signal detection analysis. *Pain, 21,* 399-409.

Putnam, W. H. (1979). Hypnosis and distortions in eyewitness memory. *International Journal of Clinical and Experimental Hypnosis, 27,* 437-448.

Radtke, H. L., & Spanos, N. P. (1981a). Temporal sequencing during posthypnotic amnesia: A methodological critique. *Journal of Abnormal Psychology, 90,* 476-485.

———. (1981b). Was I hypnotized? A social-psychological analysis of hypnotic depth reports. *Psychiatry, 44,* 359-376.

Radtke,H. L., & Spanos, N. P. (1982). The effect of rating scale descriptors on hypnotic depth reports. *Journal of Psychology, 3,* 235-245.

Radtke, H. L., Spanos, N. P., Armstrong, L. A., Dillman, N., & Boisvenue, M. E. (1983). Effects of electromyographic feedback and progressive relaxation on hypnotic susceptibility: Disconfirming results. *International Journal of Clinical and Experimental Hypnosis, 31,* 98-106.

Radtke, H. L., Spanos, N. P., & Bertrand, L. D. (1983). Serial organization during posthypnotic amnesia. Unpublished manuscript, University of Calgary.

Radtke, H. L., Spanos, N. P., Della Malva, C. L., & Stam, H. J. (1986). Temporal organization and hypnotic amnesia using a modification of the Harvard Group Scale of Hypnotic Susceptibility. *International Journal of Clinical and Experimental Hypnosis, 34,* 41-45.

Radtke, H. L., Thompson, V. A., & Egger, L. A. (1987). Use of retrieval cues in breaching hypnotic amnesia. *Journal of Abnormal Psychology, 96* (4), 335-340.

Radtke-Bodorik, H. L., Planas, M., & Spanos, N. P. (1980). Suggested amnesia, verbal inhibition, and disorganized recall for a long word list. *Canadian Journal of Behavioral Science, 12,* 87-97.

Radtke-Bodorik, H. L., Spanos, N. P., & Haddad, M. G. (1979). The effects of spoken versus written recall on suggested amnesia in hypnotic and task-motivated subjects. *American Journal of Clinical Hypnosis, 22,* 8-16.

Raginsky, B. B. (1951). Use of hypnosis in anesthesiology. *Personality, 1,* 340-348.

Raiche, F. E. (1908). The value of light energy in dental practice. *Dental Review,* 42-50.

Raikov, V. L. (1982). Hypnotic age regression to the neonatal period: Comparisons with role-play. *International Journal of Clinical and Experimental Hypnosis, 30,* 108-116.

Rausch, V. (1980). Cholecystectomy with self-hypnosis. *American Journal of Clinical Hypnosis, 22,* 121-129.

Read, G. D. (1933). *Natural childbirth.* London: Heinemann.

Reading, A. E., & Cox, D. N. (1985). Psychosocial predictors of labor pain. *Pain, 22,* 309-315.

Redd, W. H. (1986). Use of behavioral methods to control the aversive effects of chemotherapy. *Journal of Psychosocial Oncology, 3,* 17-22.

Redd, W. H., & Andresen, G. V. (1981). Conditioned aversion in cancer patients. *Behavior Therapist, 4* (2), 3-4.

Redd, W. H., Andresen, G. V., & Minagawa, R. Y. (1982). Hypnotic control of anticipatory emesis in patients receiving cancer chemotherapy. *Journal of Consulting and Clinical Psychology, 50,* 14-19.

Redd, W. H., & Andrykowski, M. A. (1982). Behavioral intervention in cancer treatment: Controlling aversion reactions to chemotherapy. *Journal of Consulting and Clinical Psychology, 50,* 1018-1029.

Redd, W. H., Rosenberger, P. H., & Hendler, C. S. (1983). Controlling chemotherapy side effects. *American Journal of Clinical Hypnosis, 25* (2-3), 161-172.

Reese, L. (1983). Coping with pain. The role of perceived self-efficacy. Unpublished doctoral dissertation. Stanford University.

Reeves, J. L., Redd, W. H., Storm, F. K., & Minagawa, R. Y. (1983). Hypnosis in the control of pain during hyperthermia treatment of cancer. In J. J. Bonica, U. Lindblom, & A. Iggo (Eds.), *Advances in pain research and therapy* (Vol. 5, pp. 857-861). New York: Raven Press.

Reiff, R., & Scheerer, M. (1959). *Memory and hypnotic age regression.* New York: International Universities Press.

Register, P. A., & Kihlstrom, J. F. (1986). Finding the hypnotic virtuoso. *International Journal of Clinical and Experimental Hypnosis, 34,* 84-97.

Reilley, R. R., Parisher, D. W., Carona, A., & Dobrovolosky, N. W. (1980). Modifying hypnotic susceptibility by practice and instruction. *International Journal of Clinical and Experimental Hypnosis, 28,* 29-45.

Reis, M. (1966). Subjective reactions of a patient having surgery without chemical anesthetic. *American Journal of Clinical Hypnosis, 9,* 122-124.

Reiser, M. (1980). *Handbook of investigative hypnosis.* Los Angeles: Lehi.

Relman, A. S. (1987). Practicing medicine in the new business climate. *New England Journal of Medicine, 316,* 1150-1151.

Reyher, J. (1977). Clinical and experimental hypnosis: Implications for theory and methodology. In W. E. Edmonston (Ed.), *Conceptual and investigative approaches to hypnosis and hypnotic phenomena* (pp. 69-85). New York: New York Academy of Sciences.

Reston, J. (1972). Now, about my operation. In *Acupuncture: What can it do for you?* New York: Newspaper Enterprise Association, pp. 8-11.

Rhee, J. L. (1972). Introductory remarks: Acupuncture: The need for an in-depth appraisal. In *Transcript of the Acupuncture Symposium.* Los Altos, Calif.: Academy of Parapsychology and Medicine, pp. 8-10.

Rhue, J. W., & Lynn, S. J. (1987). Fantasy proneness: The ability to hallucinate "as real as real." *British Journal of Experimental and Clinical Hypnosis, 4,* 173-180.

——. (1988). Fantasy proneness: Developmental antecedents. *Journal of Personality.*

Richards, M. P. M. (1982). The trouble with "choice" in childbirth. *Birth, 9,* 253-260.

Richardson, P. H. & Vincent, C. A. (1986). Acupuncture for the treatment of pain: A review of evaluative research. *Pain, 24,* 15-40.

Roberts, A. H., & Tellegen, A. (1973). Ratings of "trust" and hypnotic susceptibility. *The International Journal of Clinical and Experimental Hypnosis, 21,* 289-297.

Rock, N. L., Shipley, T. E., & Campbell, C. (1969). Hypnosis with untrained, nonvolunteer patients in labor. *The International Journal of Clinical and Experimental Hypnosis, 17,* 25-36.

Rollman, G. B. (1977). Signal detection theory assessment of pain: A review and critique. *Pain, 4,* 187-211.

——. (1983). Measurement of experimental pain in chronic pain patients: Methodological and individual factors. In R. Melzack (Ed.), *Pain Measurement and Assessment.* New York: Raven Press.

Ronnestad, M. H. (1985). Hypnosis and autonomy: An empirical investigation. Unpublished manuscript.

Rosberger, Z., Perry, C., Thirlwell, M. P., & Hollingworth, L. (1983). Hypnosis in the relief of anxiety, nausea, and vomiting associated with cancer chemotherapy. Paper presented at the 35th Annual Meeting of the Society for Clinical and Experimental Hypnosis, Boston.

Rosenberg, S. W. (1983). Hypnosis in cancer care: Imagery to enhance the control of the physiological and psychological "side-effects" of cancer therapy. *American Journal of Clinical Hypnosis, 25* (2-3), 122-127.

Rosenhan, D., & London, P. (1963). Expectation, susceptibility, and performance. *Journal of Abnormal and Social Psychology, 66,* 71-81.

Rosenhan, D. L., & Tomkins, S. S. (1964). On preference for hypnosis and hypnotizability. *International Journal of Clinical and Experimental Hypnosis, 12,* 109-114.

Rosenthal, R., & Rosnow, R. L. (1975). *The Volunteer subject.* New York: Wiley.

Rosnow, R. L., & Suls, J. L. (1970). Reactive effects of pretesting in attitude research. *Journal of Personality and Social Psychology, 15,* 338-343.

Rossi, E. L. (1986). *The psychobiology of mind-body healing.* New York: W. W. Norton.

Rowland, L. W. (1939). Will hypnotized persons try to harm themselves or others? *Journal of Abnormal and Social Psychology, 34,* 114-117.

Ruch, J. C. (1975). Self-hypnosis: The result of heterohypnosis or vice versa? *International Journal of Clinical and Experimental Hypnosis, 4,* 282-304.

Ruch, J. C., Morgan, A. H., & Hilgard, E. R. (1974). Measuring hypnotic responsiveness: A comparison of the Barber Suggestibility Scale and the Stanford Hypnotic Susceptibility Scale: Form A. *International Journal of Clinical and Experimental Hypnosis, 22,* 365-376.

Ryle, G. (1949). *The concept of mind.* New York: Barnes and Noble.

Saavedra, R. L., & Miller, R. J. (1983). The influence of experimentally induced expectations on responses to the Harvard Group Scale of Hypnotic Susceptibility, Form A. *International Journal of Clinical and Experimental Hypnosis, 31,* 37-46.

Sacerdote, P. (1962). The place of hypnosis in the relief of severe protracted pain. *American Journal of Clinical Hypnosis, 4,* 150-157.

———. (1965). Additional contributions to the hypnotherapy of the advanced cancer patient. *American Journal of Clinical Hypnosis, 7,* 308-319.

———. (1966). Hypnosis in cancer patients. *American Journal of Clinical Hypnosis, 9,* 100-108.

———. (1968a). Psychophysiology of hypnosis as it relates to pain and pain problems. *American Journal of Clinical Hypnosis, 10,* 236-243.

———. (1968b). Involvement and communication with the terminally ill patient. *American Journal of Clinical Hypnosis, 10,* 244-248.

———. (1970). Theory and practice of pain control in malignancy and other protracted or recurring painful illnesses. *International Journal of Clinical and Experimental Hypnosis, 18,* 160-180.

———. (1977). Applications of hypnotically elicited mystical states to the treatment of physical and emotional pain. *International Journal of Clinical and Experimental Hypnosis, 25,* 309-324.

———. (1982a). Erickson's contribution to pain control in cancer. In J. K. Zeig (Ed.), *Ericksonian approaches to hypnosis and psychotherapy* (pp. 336-345). New York: Brunner/Mazel.

———. (1982b). Techniques of hypnotic intervention with pain patients. In J. Barber & C. Adrian (Eds.), *Psychological approaches to the management of pain* (pp. 60-83). New York: Brunner/Mazel.

Sachs, L. B. (1971). Construing hypnosis as modifiable behavior. In A. Jacobs & L. B. Sachs (Eds.), *Psychology of private events* (pp. 61-75). New York: Academic Press.

Sachs, L. B., & Anderson, W. L. (1967). Modification of hypnotic susceptibility. *International Journal of Clinical and Experimental Hypnosis, 15,* 172-180.

St. Jean, R. (1978). Posthypnotic behavior as a function of experimental surveillance. *American Journal of Clinical Hypnosis, 20,* 250-255.

———. (1980). Hypnotic time distortion and learning: Another look. *Journal of Abnormal Psychology, 89,* 20-24.

St. Jean, R., & MacLeod, C. (1983). Hypnosis, absorption, and time perception. *Journal of Abnormal Psychology, 92,* 81-86.

St. Jean, R., & Coe, W. C. (1981). Recall and recognition memory during posthypnotic amnesia: A failure to confirm the disrupted retrieval hypothesis and memory disorganization hypothesis. *Journal of Abnormal Psychology, 90,* 231-241.

St. Jean, R., MacLeod, C., Coe, W. C., & Howard, M. L. (1982). Amnesia and hypnotic time estimation. *International Journal of Clinical and Experimental Hypnosis, 30,* 127-137.

St. Jean, R., & Robertson, L. (1986). Attentional versus absorptive processing in hypnotic time estimation. *Journal of Abnormal Psychology, 95.*

Salancik, G. R., & Conway, M. (1970). Attitude inferences from salient and relevant content about behavior. *Journal of Personality and Social Psychology, 32,* 829-840.

Sampimon, R. L. H., & Woodruff, M. F. A. (1946). Some observations concerning the use of hypnosis as a substitute for anesthesia. *Medical Journal of Australia, 1,* 393-395.

Samuelly, I. (1972). Lamaze method of childbirth, conditioning or hypnosis. *The American Journal of Clinical Hypnosis, 5,* 136-139.

Sanders, G. S., & Simmons, W. L. (1983). Use of hypnosis to enhance eyewitness accuracy: Does it work? *Journal of Applied Psychology, 68* (1), 70.

Sanders, R. S., & Reyher, J. (1969). Sensory deprivation and the enhancement of hypnotic susceptibility. *Journal of Abnormal Psychology, 74,* 375-381.

Sarbin, T. R. (1943). The concept of role-taking. *Sociometry, 6,* 273-284.

———. (1950). Contributions to role-taking theory: I. Hypnotic behavior. *Psychological Review, 57,* 255-270.

Sarbin, T. R. (1962). A historical sketch of theories of hypnosis. In L. Postman (Ed.), *Psychology in the making.* New York: Knopf.

———. (1962). Attempts to understand hypnotic phenomena. In L. Postman (Ed.), *Psychology in the making: Histories of selected research problems* (pp. 745-785). New York: Alfred A. Knopf.

Sarbin, T. R. (1968). Ontology recapitulates philology: The mythic nature of anxiety. *American Psychologist, 26* (6), 411-418.

——. (1973). On the recently-reported physiological and pharmacological reality of the hypnotic state. *Psychological Record, 23,* 501-510.

——. (1977). Contextualism: A world view for modern psychology. In A. Landfield (Ed.)., (1976) *Nebraska Symposium on Motivation.* Lincoln: University of Nebraska Press.

——. (1980). Hypnosis: Metaphorical encounters of the fourth kind. *Semiotica. 30,* 195-209.

——. (1981). On self-deception. In T. Sebeok & R. Rosenthal (Eds.), *The clever Hans phenomenon: Communication with horses, whales, apes, and people.* New York: Annals of the New York Academy of Sciences, *364,* 22-35.

——. (1984). Nonvolition in hypnosis: A semiotic analysis. *Psychological Record, 34,* 537-549.

——. (Ed.) (1986). *Narrative psychology: The storied nature of human conduct.* New York: Praeger.

Sarbin, T. R., & Adler, N. (1971). Self-reconstitutive processes: A preliminary report. *Psychoanalytic Review, 57,* 599-616.

Sarbin, T. R., & Allen, V. L. (1968). Role theory. In G. Lindzey & E. Aronson (Eds.), *Handbook of Social Psychology,* Vol. II, Reading, Mass. Addison-Wesley.

Sarbin, T. R., & Coe, W. C. (1972). *Hypnosis: A social psychological analysis of influence communication.* New York: Holt, Rinehart & Winston.

Sarbin, T. R., & Coe, W. C. (1979). Hypnosis and psychopathology: Replacing old myths with fresh metaphors. *Journal of Abnormal Psychology, 88,* 506-526.

——. (1979). Hypnosis and psychopathology: Replacing old myths with fresh metaphors. *Journal of Abnormal Psychology, 88,* 506-526.

Sarbin, T. R., & Juhasz, J. B. (1970). Toward a theory of imagination. *Journal of Personality, 38,* 52-76.

——. (1975). The social context of hallucinations. In R. K. Siegel & L. J. West (Eds.), *Hallucinations: Behavior, experience, and theory.* New York: Wiley Biomedical.

Sarbin, T. R., & Lim, D. T. (1963). Contributions to role-taking theory X: Some evidence in support of the role-taking hypothesis in hypnosis. *Journal of Clinical and Experimental Hypnosis, 11,* 98-103.

Sarbin, T. R., & Mancuso, J. C. (1980). *Schizophrenia: Medical diagnosis or verdict?* Elmsford, N.Y.: Pergamon.

Sarbin, T. R., & Slagle, R. W. (1972). Hypnosis and psychophysiological outcomes. In E. Fromm & R. E. Shor (Eds.), *Hypnosis: Research developments and perspectives.* Chicago: Aldine.

——. (1979). Hypnosis and psychophysiological outcomes. In E. Fromm & R. E. Shor (Eds.), *Hypnosis: Developments in research and new perspectives* (2nd ed.). New York: Aldine.

Schafer, D. W. (1975). Hypnosis use on a burn unit. *International Journal of Clinical and Experimental Hypnosis, 23,* 1-14.

Schank, R., & Abelson, R. P. (1979). *Scripts, plans, goals and understanding.* Hillsdale, N.J.: Erlbaum.

Scheibe, K. E. (1979). *Mirrors, masks, lies, and secrets.* New York: Praeger.

Schibley, W. J., & Aanonsen, G. A. (1966). Hypnosis—Practical in obstetrics? *Medical Times, 94,* 340-343.

Schlutter, L. C., Golden, C., & Blume, H. G. (1980). A comparison of treatments for prefrontal muscle contraction headache. *British Journal of Medical Psychology, 53,* 47-52.

Schon, R. C. (1960). Addendum to "hypnosis in painful terminal illness." *American Journal of Clinical Hypnosis, 3,* 61-62.

Schreiber, Y. L. (1961). The method of indirect suggestion as used in hysteria. In R. B. Winn (Trans. & Ed.), *Psychotherapy in the Soviet Union.* New York: Philosophical Library.

Schubot, E. D. (1964). Trance and waking performance in the perception of time. Unpublished masters thesis, Stanford University, Stanford, Calif..

Schuyler, B. A., & Coe, W. C. (1981). A physiological investigation of volitional and nonvolitional experience during posthypnotic amnesia. *Journal of Personality and Social Psychology, 40,* 1160-1169.

Schuyler, B. A., & Coe, W. C. (1987). Volitional and nonvolitional experiences during posthypnotic amnesia. Manuscript submitted for publication.

Schwarcz, B. E. (1965). Hypnoanalgesia and hypnoanesthesia in urology. *Surgical Clinics of North America, 45,* 7547-7555.

Schwartz, W. S. (1978). Time and context during hypnotic involvement. *International Journal of Clinical and Experimental Hypnosis, 26,* 307-316.

———. (1980). Hypnosis and episodic memory. *International Journal of Clinical & Experimental Hypnosis, 28,* 375-385.

Scott, D. L. (1975). Hypnosis in plastic surgery. *American Journal of Clinical Hypnosis, 18,* 98-104.

Scott, D. S. (1980). Pain endurance induced by a subtle social variable (demand) and the "reverse Milgram effect." *British Journal of Social and Clinical Psychology. 19,* 137-139.

Scott, D. S., & Barber, T. X. (1977). Cognitive control of pain: Effects of multiple cognitive strategies. *Psychological Record, 27,* 373-383.

Scott, D. S., & Leonard, C. E. Jr. (1978). Modification of pain threshold by the covert reinforcement procedure and a cognitive stategy. *Psychological Record, 28,* 49-57.

Scott, J. R., & Rose, N. B. (1976). Effects of psychoprophylaxis (Lamaze preparation) on labor and delivery in primiparas. *New England Journal of Medicine, 294,* 1205-1207.

Sears, A. B. (1955). A comparison of hypnotic and waking recall. *Journal of Clinical and Experimental Hypnosis, 3,* 215-221.

———. (1956). Hypnosis and recall. *Journal of Clinical and Experimental Hypnosis, 4,* 165-171.

Serafetinides, E. A. (1986). Electrophysiological responses to sensory stimulation under hypnosis. *American Journal of Psychiatry, 125,* 150-151.

Serly, A. (1987). A trance to remember. *The Law Magazine, June, 12.*

Shapiro, A. (1983). Psychotherapy as adjunct treatment for cancer patients. *American Journal of Clinical Hypnosis, 25* (2-3), 150-155.

Shapiro, D. H. (1978). *Precision nirvana.* Englewood Cliffs, N.J.: Prentice-Hall.

Sheehan, E. P., Smith, H. V., & Forrest, D. W. (1982). A signal detection study of the effects of suggested improvement on the monocular visual acuity of myopes. *International Journal of Clinical and Experimental Hypnosis, 30,* 138-146.

Sheehan, P. J. (1971). Countering preconceptions about hypnosis: An objective index of involvement with the hypnotist [monograph]. *Journal of Abnormal Psychology, 78,* 299-322.

Sheehan, P. J., & Perry, C. W. (1976). *Methodologies of hypnosis.* Hillsdale, N.J.: Erlbaum.

Sheehan, P. W. (1967a). A shortened form of Bett's questionnaire upon mental imagery. *Journal of Clinical Psychology, 23,* 386-389.

———. (1967b). Reliability of a short test of imagery. *Perceptual and Motor Skills, 25,* 744.

———. (1970). Analysis of the treatment effects of simulation instructions in the application of the real-simulating model of hypnosis. *Journal of Abnormal Psychology, 75,* 98-103.

———. (1971a). A methodological analysis of the simulating technique. *International Journal of Clinical and Experimental Hypnosis, 19,* 83-99.

———. (1971b). Countering preconceptions about hypnosis: An objective index of involvement with the hypnotist. *Journal of Abnormal Psychology, 78,* 299-322.

———. (1971c). Task structure as a limiting condition of the occurrence of the treatment effects of simulating instruction in application of the real-simulating model of hypnosis. *International Journal of Clinical and Experimental Hypnosis, 19,* 260-276.

———. (1973a). Escape from the ambiguous: Artifact and methodologies of hypnosis. *American Psychologist, 28,* 983-993.

———. (1973b). Analysis of the heterogeneity of "faking" and "simulating" performance in the hypnotic setting. *International Journal of Clinical and Experimental Hypnosis, 21,* 213-225.

———. (1977). Incongruity in trance behavior: A defining property of hypnosis? *Annals of the New York Academy of Sciences, 296,* 194-207.

———. (1979). Hypnosis and the process of imagination. In E. Fromm & R. E. Shor (Eds.), *Hypnosis: Developments in research, and new perspectives.* New York: Aldine.

Sheehan, P. W. (1980). Factors influencing rapport in hypnosis. *Journal of Abnormal Psychology, 89* (2), 263-281.

Sheehan, P. W., & Dolby, R. M. (1974). Artifact and Barber's model of hypnosis: A logical-empirical analysis. *Journal of Experimental Social Psychology, 10,* 171-187.

Sheehan, P. W., Griff, L., & McCann, T. (1984). Memory distortion following exposure to false information in hypnosis. *Journal of Abnormal Psychology, 93,* 259-265.

Sheehan, P. W., McConkey, K. M., & Cross, D. (1978). Experimental analysis of hypnosis: Some new observations on hypnotic phenomena. *Journal of Abnormal Psychology, 87,* 570-573.

Sheehan, P. W., & McConkey, K. M. (1979). Australian norms for the Harvard Group Scale of Hypnotic Susceptibility: Form A. *International Journal of Clinical and Experimental Hypnosis, 27,* 294-304.

Sheehan, P. W., & McConkey, K. (1982). *Hypnosis and experience: The exploration of phenomena and processes.* Hillsdale, N.J.: Erlbaum.

Sheehan, P. W., Obstoj, I., & McConkey, K. M. (1976). Trance logic and cue structure as supplied by the hypnotist. *Journal of Abnormal Psychology, 85,* 459-472.

Sheehan, P. W., & Perry, C. W. (1976). *Methodologies of hypnosis: A critical appraisal of contemporary paradigms of hypnosis.* Hillsdale, N.J.: Erlbaum.

——. (1980). Research in hypnosis: An overview of current methods. In G. D. Burrows & L. Dennerstein (Eds.), *Handbook of hypnosis and psychosomatic medicine.* Amsterdam: Elsevier/ North Holland Biomedical Press.

Sheehan, P. W., & Tilden, J. (1983). Effects of suggestibility and hypnosis on accurate and distorted retrieval from memory. *Journal of Experimental Psychology: Learning, Memory and Cognition, 9,* 283-293.

——. (1984). Real and simulated occurrences of memory distortion in hypnosis. *Journal of Abnormal Psychology, 93,* 47-57.

——. (1986). The consistency of occurrences of memory distortion following hypnotic induction. *International Journal of Clinical and Experimental Hypnosis, 2,* 122-137.

Sherman, R. A., Sherman, C. J., & Parker, L. (1984). Chronic phantom in stump pain among American veterans: Results of a survey. *Pain, 18,* 83-96.

Sherman, R. A., Gall, N., & Gormaly, J. (1979). Treatment of phantom limb pain with muscular relaxation training to disrupt the pain-anxiety-tension cycle. *Pain, 6,* 47-56.

Sherman, R. A., Sherman, C. J., & Gall, N. G. (1980). A survey of current phantom limb pain treatments in the United States. *Pain, 8,* 85-100.

Sherman, S. J. (1988). Ericksonian psychotherapy and social psychology. In S. Lankton (Ed.), *Advances in Ericksonian hypnosis, Monograph series, No. 2.*

Sherman, S. J., Zehner, K. S., Johnson, J., & Hirt, E. R. (1983). Social explanation: The role of timing, set, and recall on subjective likelihood estimates. *Journal of Personality and Social Psychology, 44,* 1127-1143.

Shevrin, H., & Dickman, S. (1980). The psychological unconscious: A necessary assumption for all psychological theory? *American Psychologist, 35,* 421-434.

Shor, R. E. (1959). Hypnosis and the concept of the generalized reality-orientation. *American Journal of Psychotherapy, 13,* 582-602.

——. (1960). The frequency of naturally occurring "hypnotic-like" experiences in the normal college population. *International Journal of Clinical and Experimental Hypnosis, 8,* 151-163.

——. (1962a). Three dimensions of hypnotic depth. *International Journal of Clinical and Experimental Hypnosis, 10,* 23-28.

——. (1962b). Physiological effects of painful stimulation during hypnotic analgesia under conditions designed to minimize anxiety. *International Journal of Clinical and Experimental Hypnosis, 10,* 183-202.

——. (1967). Physiological effects of painful stimulation during hypnotic analgesia. In J. E. Gordon (Ed.), *Handbook of clinical and experimental hypnosis* (pp. 511-547). New York: Macmillan.

Shor, R. E. (1970). The three-factor theory of hypnosis as applied to the book-reading fantasy and to the concept of suggestion. *International Journal of Clinical and Experimental Hypnosis, 18,* 89-98.

——. (1971). Expectancies of being influenced and hypnotic performance. *International Journal of Clinical and Experimental Hypnosis, 19,* 154-166.

——. (1979). A phenomenological method for the measurement of variables important to an understanding of the nature of hypnosis. In E. Fromm & R. E. Shor (Eds.), *Hypnosis: Developments in research and new perspectives* (revised 2nd ed., pp. 105-135). New York: Aldine.

Shor, R. E., & Cobb, J. C. (1968). An exploratory study of hypnotic training using the concept of plateau responsiveness as a referent. *American Journal of Clinical Hypnosis, 10,* 178-197.

Shor, R. E., & Easton, E. D. (1973). Preliminary report on research comparing self- and hetero-hypnosis. *American Journal of Clinical Hypnosis, 1,* 37-44.

Shor, R. E., & Orne, E. C. (1962). *Harvard Group Scale of Hypnotic Susceptibility, Form A.* Palo Alto, Calif.: Consulting Psychologists Press.

——. (1963). Norms on the Harvard Group Scale of Hypnotic Susceptibility: Form A. *International Journal of Clinical and Experimental Hypnosis, 11,* 39-48.

Shor, R. E., Orne, M. T., & O'Connell, D. N. (1962). Validation and cross-validation of a scale of self-reported personal experiences which predict hypnotizability. *Journal of Psychology, 53,* 55-75.

——. (1966). Psychological correlates of plateau hypnotizability in a special volunteer sample. *Journal of Personality and Social Psychology, 3,* 80-95.

Shor, R. E., Pistole, D. D., Easton, R. D., & Kihlstrom, J. F. (1984). Relation of predicted to actual hypnotic responsiveness, with special reference to posthypnotic amnesia. *International Journal of Clinical and Experimental Hypnosis, 32* (4), 376-387.

Siegel, E. F. (1979). Control of phantom limb pain by hypnosis. *American Journal of Clinical Hypnosis, 21,* 285-286.

Silva, C. E., & Kirsch, I. (1987). Breaching hypnotic amnesia by manipulating expectancy. *Journal of Abnormal Psychology, 96* (4), 325-329.

Silverberg, E., & Lubera, J. A. (1988). Cancer statistics, 1988. *Ca—A Cancer Journal for Clinicians, 38,* 5-22.

Simon, J. M., & Salzberg, H. (1981). Electromyographic feedback and taped relaxation instructions to modify hypnotic susceptibility and amnesia. *American Journal of Clinical Hypnosis, 24,* 14-21.

Simonton, D. C., Matthews-Simonton, S., & Creighton, J. L. (1978). *Getting well again.* New York: Bantam Books.

Sims, S. E. R. (1987). Relaxation training as a technique for helping patients cope with the experience of cancer: A selective review of the literature. *Journal of Advanced Nursing, 12,* 583-591.

Sinclair-Gieben, A. H. C., & Chalmers, D. (1959). Evaluation of treatment of warts by hypnosis. *Lancet, 2,* 480-482.

Singer, J. L. (1974). *Imagery and daydream methods in psychotherapy and behavior modification.* New York: Academic Press.

Sjolund, B., & Ericksson, M. (1976). Electro-acupuncture and endogenous morphines. *Lancet, 2,* 1085.

Sluis, A., & Coe, W. C. (1987). Posthypnotic amnesia. Findings on breaching, volition and the dissipation hypothesis. Manuscript submitted for publication.

Smilkstein, G., Helsper-Lucas, A., Ashworth, C., Montano, D., & Pagel, M. (1984). Prediction of pregnancy complications: An application of the biopsychosocial model. *Social Science and Medicine, 18,* 315-321.

Smith, M. C. (1983). Hypnotic memory enhancement of witnesses: Does it work? *Psychological Bulletin, 94,* 387-407.

Smith, M. S., & Kamitsuka, M. (1984). Self-hypnosis misinterpreted as CNS deterioration in an adolescent with leukemia and vincristine toxicity. *American Journal of Clinical Hypnosis, 26*, 280-282.

Smith, S. J., & Balaban, A. B. (1983). A multidimensional approach to pain relief: Case report of a patient with systemic lupus erythematosus. *International Journal of Clinical and Experimental Hypnosis, 31*, 72-81.

Smyth, L. D. (1981). Toward a social learning theory of hypnosis. I. Hypnotic suggestibility. *American Journal of Clinical Hypnosis, 23*, 147-168.

Snow, L. (1979). The relationship between "rapid induction" and placebo analgesia, hypnotic susceptibility and chronic pain intensity. *Dissertation Abstracts International, 40*, 937.

Snyder, C. R., & Higgins, R. L. (1988). Excuses: Their effective role in the negotiation of reality. *Psychological Bulletin, 104*, 23-35.

Society for Clinical and Experimental Hypnosis. (1979). Resolution (adopted October 1978). *International Journal of Clinical and Experimental Hypnosis, 27*, 452.

Spanos, N. P. (1971). Goal-directed fantasy and the performance of hypnotic test suggestions. *Psychiatry, 34*, 86-96.

———. (1981). Hypnotic responding: Automatic dissociation or situation-relevant cognizing? In E. Klinger (Ed.), *Imagery: Concepts, results and applications*. New York: Plenum.

———. (1982a). A social psychological approach to hypnotic behavior. In G. Weary & H. L. Mirels (Eds.), *Integrations of clinical and social psychology* (pp. 231-271). New York: Oxford University Press.

———. (1982b). Hypnotic behavior: A cognitive social psychological perspective. *Research Communications in Psychology, Psychiatry, and Behavior, 7*, 199-213.

———. (1983). The hidden observer as an experimental creation. *Journal of Personality and Social Psychology, 44*, 170-176.

———. (1986a). Hypnosis and the modification of hypnotic susceptibility: A social psychological perspective. In P. L. N. Naish (Ed.), *What is hypnosis?* (pp. 85-120). Philadelphia: Open University Press.

———. (1986b). Hypnotic behavior: A social psychological interpretation of amnesia, analgesia and trance logic. *Behavioral and Brain Sciences, 9*, 449-467.

———. (1986b). More on the social psychology of hypnotic behavior. *Behavioral and Brain Sciences, 9*, 489-497.

———. (1986c). Hypnosis, nonvolitional responding and multiple personality: A social psychological perspective. In B. Maher & W. Maher (Eds.), *Progress in experimental personality research* (Vol. 14, pp. 1-62). New York: Academic Press.

Spanos, N. P., & Barber, T. X. (1968). "Hypnotic" experiences as inferred from subjective reports: Auditory and visual hallucinations. *Journal of Experimental Research in Personality, 3*, 136-150.

———. (1972). Cognitive activity during "hypnotic" suggestibility: Goal-directed fantasy and the experience of nonvolition. *Journal of Personality, 40*, 510-524.

Spanos, N. P., & Barber, T. X. (1974). Toward a convergence in hypnosis research. *American Psychologist, July*, pp. 500-511.

Spanos, N. P., Barber, T. X., & Lang, G. (1974). Cognition and self-control: Cognitive control of painful sensory input. In H. London & R. E. Nisbit (Eds.), *Thought and feeling: Cognitive alteration of feeling states* (pp. 144-158). Chicago: Aldine.

Spanos, N. P., & Bertrand, L. D. (1985). EMG biofeedback, attained relaxation, and hypnotic susceptibility: Is there a relationship? *American Journal of Clinical Hypnosis, 27*, 219-225.

Spanos, N. P., Bertrand, L. D., & Perlini, A. H. (1988). Reduced clustering during hypnotic amnesia for a long word list: A reply to Wilson and Kihlstrom. *Journal of Abnormal Psychology*.

Spanos, N. P., & Bodorik, H. L. (1977). Suggested amnesia and disorganized recall in hypnotic and task-motivated subjects. *Journal of Abnormal Psychology, 86* (3), 295-305.

Spanos, N. P., Bodorik-Radtke, H. L., & Shabinsky, M. A. (1980). Amnesia, subjective organization and learning a list of unrelated words in hypnotic and task-motivated subjects. *International Journal of Clinical and Experimental Hypnosis, 28,* 126-139.

Spanos, N. P., Brett, P. J., Menary, E. P., & Cross, W. P. (1987). A measure of attitudes toward hypnosis: Relationships with absorption and hypnotic susceptibility. *American Journal of Clinical Hypnosis, 30,* 139-150.

Spanos, N. P., Bridgeman, M., Stam, H. J., Gwynn, M. I., & Saad, C. I. (1983). When seeing is not believing: The effects of contextual variables on the reports of hypnotic hallucinations. *Imagination, Cognition and Personality, 2,* 195-209.

Spanos, N. P., Brown, J. M., Jones, B., & Horner, D. (1981). The effects of cognitive activity and suggestions for analgesia in the reduction of reported pain. *Journal of Abnormal Psychology, 90,* 554-561.

Spanos, N. P., & Chaves, J. F. (1970). Hypnotic research: A methodological critique of experiments generated by two alternative paradigms. *American Journal of Clinical Hypnosis, 13*(2), 108-127.

Spanos, N. P., Cobb, P. C., & Gorassini, D. R. (1985). Failing to resist hypnotic test suggestions: A strategy for self-presenting as deeply hypnotized. *Psychiatry, 48,* 282-292.

Spanos, N. P., Cross, W. P., Menary, E. P., Brett, P. J., & de Groh, M. (1987). Attitudinal and imaginal ability predictors of social cognitive skill-training enhancements in hypnotic susceptibility. *Personality and Social Psychology Bulletin, 13,* 379-398.

Spanos, N. P., Cross, W. P., Menary, E. P., & Smith, J. (1986). Long-term effects of cognitive skill-training for the enhancement of hypnotic susceptibility. Unpublished Manuscript, Carleton University, Ottawa, Canada.

Spanos, N. P., & D'Eon, J. L. (1980). Hypnotic amnesia, disorganized recall and inattention. *Journal of Abnormal Psychology, 89,* 744-750.

Spanos, N. P., D'Eon, J. L., Pawlak, A. E., Mah, C. D., & Ritchie, G. (1988). A multivariate study of hypnotizability. *Imagination, Cognition and Personality.* Robertson, L.A.

Spanos, N. P., & de Groh, M. (1983). Structure of communication and reports of involuntariness by hypnotic and nonhypnotic subjects. *Perceptual and Motor Skills, 57,* 1179-1186.

———. (1984). Effects of active and passive wording of inattention strategies on response to suggestions for complete and selective amnesia. Unpublished manuscript, Carleton University, Ottawa, Canada.

Spanos, N. P., de Groh, M., & de Groot, H. P. (1987). Skill training for enhancing hypnotic susceptibility and word list amnesia. *British Journal of Experimental and Clinical Hypnosis, 4* (1), 15-23.

Spanos, N. P., de Groot, H. P., & Gwynn, M. I. (1987). Trance logic as incomplete responding. *Journal of Personality and Social Psychology, 53,* 911-921.

Spanos, N. P., de Groot, H. P., Tiller, D. K., Weekes, J. R., & Bertrand, L. D. (1985). "Trance logic" duality and hidden observer responding in hypnotic, imagination control, and simulating subjects. *Journal of Abnormal Psychology, 94,* 611-623.

Spanos, N. P., Flynn, D. M., & Gwynn, M. I. (1988). Contextual demands, negative hallucinations, and hidden observer responding: Three hidden observers observed. *British Journal of Experimental and Clinical Hypnosis, 5,* 5-10.

Spanos, N. P., Gabora, N. J., Jarrett, L. E., & Gwynn, M. I. (1988). Contextual determinants of hypnotizability and of relationships between hypnotizability scales. Unpublished manuscript, Carleton University, Ottawa, Canada.

Spanos, N. P., & Gorassini, D. R. (1984). Structure of hypnotic test suggestions and attributions of responding involuntarily. *Journal of Personality and Social Psychology, 46,* 688-696.

Spanos, N. P., & Gottlieb, J. (1979). Demonic possession, mesmerism, and hysteria: A social psychological perspective on their historical interrelationships. *Journal of Abnormal Psychology, 88,* 527-546.

Spanos, N. P., Gottlieb, J., & Rivers, S. M. (1980). The effects of short-term meditation training on hypnotic responsivity. *Psychological Record, 30,* 343-348.

Spanos, N. P., Gwynn, M. I., Gabora, N. J., & Jarrett, L. E. (1988). Response expectancies and interpretational sets as determinants of hypnotic responding. Unpublished manuscript, Carleton University, Ottawa, Canada.

Spanos, N. P., Gwynn, M. I., Malva, L. D., & Bertrand, L. D. (1988). Social psychological factors in the genesis of posthypnotic source amnesia. *Journal of Abnormal Psychology, 97*, 322-329.

Spanos, N. P., Gwynn, M. I., & Stam, H. J. (1983). Instructional demands and ratings of overt and hidden pain during hypnotic analgesia. *Journal of Abnormal Psychology, 92*, 479-488.

Spanos, N. P., Ham, M. W., & Barber, T. X. (1973). Suggested ('hypnotic') visual hallucinations: Experimental and phenomenological data. *Journal of Abnormal Psychology, 81*, 96-106.

Spanos, N. P., & Ham, M. L. (1973). Cognitive activity in response to hypnotic suggestion: Goal-directed fantasy and selective amnesia. *American Journal of Clinical Hypnosis, 15* (3), 191-198.

Spanos, N. P., & Ham, M. W. (1975). Involvement in suggestion-related imaginings and the "hypnotic dream." *American Journal of Clinical Hypnosis, 18*, 43-51.

Spanos, N. P., & Hewitt, E. C. (1980). The hidden observer in hypnotic analgesia: Discovery or experimental creation? *Journal of Personality and Social Psychology, 39*, 1201-1214.

Spanos, N. P., Hodgins, D. C., Stam, J. H., & Gwynn, M. I. (1984). Suffering for science: The effects of implicit social demands on response to experimentally induced pain. *Journal of Personality and Social Psychology, 46*, 1162-1172.

Spanos, N. P., Horton, C., & Chaves, J. F. (1975). The effects of two cognitive strategies on pain threshold. *Journal of Abnormal Psychology, 84*, 677-681.

Spanos, N. P., Jones, B., Brown, J. M., & Horner, D. (1983). Magnitude estimates of cold pressor pain: Effects of suggestions, cognitive strategy, and tolerance. *Perception, 12*, 355-362.

Spanos, N. P., Jones, B., & Malfara, A. (1982). Hypnotic deafness: Now you hear it—Now you still hear it. *Journal of Abnormal Psychology, 90*, 75-77.

Spanos, N. P., & Katsanis, J. (1988). Effects of instructional set on attributions of nonvolition during hypnotic and nonhypnotic analgesia. *Journal of Personality and Social Psychology.*

Spanos, N. P., Kennedy, S. K. & Gwynn, M. I. (1984). The moderating effect of contextual variables on the relationship between hypnotic susceptibility and suggested analgesia. *Journal of Abnormal Psychology, 93*, 285-294.

Spanos, N. P., Lush, N., & Gwynn, M. I. (1987). Cognitive skill training enhancement of hypnotizability: Generalization effects and trance logic responding. Unpublished manuscript, Carleton University, Ottawa, Canada.

Spanos, N. P., Lush, N. I., Smith, J. E., & de Groh, M. (1986). Effects of two hypnotic induction procedures on overt and subjective response to two measures of hypnotic susceptibility. *Psychological Reports, 59*, 1227-1230.

Spanos, N. P., MacDonald, D. K., & Gwynn, M. I. (1988). Instructional set and the relative efficacy of hypnotic and waking analgesia. *Canadian Journal of Behavioral Science, 26*, 64-72.

Spanos, N. P., McLean, J. M., & Bertrand, L. D. (1986). Serial organization during hypnotic amnesia under two conditions of item presentation. *Journal of Research in Personalty, 21*, 361-374.

Spanos, N. P., McNeil, C., Gwynn, M. I., & Stam, J. J. (1984). The effects of suggestions and distraction on reported pain in subjects high and low on hypnotic susceptibility. *Journal of Abnormal Psychology, 93*, 277-284.

Spanos, N. P., & McPeake, J. D. (1974). Involvement in suggestion-related imaginings, experienced involuntariness, and credibility assigned to imaginings in hypnotic subjects. *Journal of Abnormal Psychology, 83* (6), 687-690.

——. (1975a). Involvement in everyday imaginative activities, attitudes toward hypnosis, and hypnotic susceptibility. *Journal of Personality and Social Psychology, 31*, 594-598.

Spanos, N. P., & McPeake, J. D. (1975b). The interaction of attitudes toward hypnosis and involvement in everyday imaginative activities on hypnotic susceptibility. *The American Journal of Clinical Hypnosis, 17*, 247-252.

Spanos, N. P., & McPeake, J. D. (1977). Cognitive strategies, goal-directed fantasy, and response to suggestions in hypnotic subjects. *American Journal of Clinical Hypnosis, 20*, 114-123.

Spanos, N. P., McPeake, J. D., & Churchill, N. (1976). Relationships between imaginative ability variables and the Barber Suggestibility Scale. *International Journal of Clinical and Experimental Hypnosis, 19,* 39-46.

Spanos, N. P., Menary, E., Brett, P. J., Cross, W., & Ahmed, Q. (1987). Failure of posthypnotic responding to occur outside the experimental setting. *Journal of Abnormal Psychology, 96,* 52-57.

Spanos, N. P., & Moretti, P. (1988). Mysticism, absorption and hypnotic responding. *Journal for the Scientific Study of Religion, 27,* 105-116.

Spanos, N. P., Mullens, D., & Rivers, S. M. (1979). The effects of suggestion structure and hypnotic vs. task motivation.instructions on response to hallucination suggestions. *Journal of Research in Personality, 13,* 59-70.

Spanos, N. P., & O'Hara, P. (1988). Effects of hypnotizability, strategy type, strategy use and expectations on reported reductions in experimentally induced pain. Unpublished manuscript, Carleton University, Ottawa, Canada.

Spanos, N. P., Ollerhead, V. G., & Gwynn, M. I. (1986). The effects of three instructional treatments on pain magnitude and pain tolerance. *Imagination, Cognition and Personality, 5,* 321-337.

Spanos, N. P., & Perlini, A. (1988). Placebo analgesia and hypnotic and nonhypnotic suqqested analgesia in high and low hypnotizable subjects. Unpublished manuscript, Carleton University, Ottawa, Canada.

Spanos, N. P., & Radtke, H. L. (1981). Hypnotic amnesia, optional responding, and compliance. *Bulletin of the British Society of Experimental and Clinical Hypnosis, 4,* 18-19.

Spanos, N. P., & Radtke, H. L. (1981). Hypnotic visual hallucinations as imaginings: A cognitive social psychological perspective. *Imagination, Cognition and Personality, 1,* 147-170.

———. (1982). Hypnotic amnesia as strategic enactment: A cognitive, social-psychological perspective. *Research Communications in Psychology, Psychiatry, and Behavior, 7,* 215-231.

Spanos, N. P., Radtke, H. L., & Bertrand, L. D. (1985). Hypnotic amnesia as a strategic enactment: Breaching amnesia in highly susceptible subjects. *Journal of Personality and Social Psychology, 47,* 1155-1169.

Spanos, N. P., Radtke, H. L., Dubreuil, D. L. (1982). Episodic and semantic memory in posthypnotic amnesia: A reevaluation. *Journal of Personality and Social Psychology, 43,* 565-573.

Spanos, N. P., Radtke, H. L., Hodgins, D. C., Bertrand, L. D., Stam, H. J., & Dubreuil, D. L. (1983a). The Carleton University Responsiveness to Suggestion Scale: Stability, reliability, and relationships with expectancy and hypnotic experiences. *Psychological Reports, 53,* 555-563.

Spanos, N. P., Radtke, H. L., Hodgins, D. C., Bertrand, L. D., Stam, H. J., & Moretti, P. (1983b). The Carleton University Responsiveness to Suggestion Scale: Relationship with other measures of hypnotic susceptibility, expectancies, and absorption. *Psychological Reports, 53,* 723-734.

Spanos, N. P., Radtke, H. L., Hodgins, D. C., Stam, H. J., & Bertrand, L. D. (1983c). The Carleton University Responsiveness to Suggestion Scale: Normative data and psychometric properties. *Psychological Reports, 53,* 523-535.

———. (1983d). Scoring manual for the Carleton University Responsiveness to Suggestion Scale. Unpublished manuscript, Carleton University, Ottawa, Canada.

Spanos, N. P., Radtke-Bodorik, H. L. (1980). Integrating hypnotic phenomena with cognitive psychology: An illustration using suggested amnesia. *Bulletin of the Society of Experimental and Clinical Psychology, 3,* 4-7.

Spanos, N. P., Radtke-Bodorik, H. L., Ferguson, J. D., & Jones, B. (1979). The effects of hypnotic susceptibility, suggestions for analgesia and the utilization of cognitive strategies on the reduction of pain. *Journal of Abnormal Psychology, 88,* 282-292.

Spanos, N. P., Radtke-Bodorik, H. L., & Shabinsky, M. A. (1980). Amnesia, subjective organization, and learning of a list of unrelated words in hypnotic and task-motivated subjects. *International Journal of Clinical and Experimental Hypnosis, 28* (2), 126-139.

Spanos, N. P., Radtke-Bodorik, H. L., & Stam, H. J. (1980). Disorganized recall during suggested amnesia: Fact not artifact. *Journal of Abnormal Psychology, 89,* 1-19.

Spanos, N. P., Rivers, S. M., & Gottlieb, J. (1978). Hypnotic responsivity, meditation an laterality of eye-movements. *Journal of Abnormal Psychology, 87,* 566-569.

Spanos, N. P., Rivers, S. M., & Ross, S. (1977). Experienced involuntariness and response to hypnotic suggestions. In W. E. Edmonston (Ed.), *Conceptual and investigative approaches to hypnosis and hypnotic phenomena* (Vol. 296, pp. 208-221). New York: New York Academy of Sciences.

Spanos, N. P., Robertson, L. A., Menary, E. P., & Brett, P. J. (1986). Component analysis of cognitive skill training for the enhancement of hypnotic susceptibility. *Journal of Abnormal Psychology, 95,* 350-357.

Spanos, N. P., Salas, J., Bertrand, L. D., & Johnston, J. C. (1987). Occurrence schemes, context ambiguity and hypnotic responding. *Imagination, Cognition and Personality.*

Spanos, N. P., Salas, J. A., Menary, E. P., & Brett, P. J. (1986). A comparison of overt and subjective responses to the Carleton University Responsiveness to Suggestion Scale and the Stanford Hypnotic Susceptibility Scale under conditions of group administration. *Psychological Reports, 58,* 847-856.

Spanos, N. P., Spillane, J., & McPeake, J. C. (1976). Suggestion elaborateness, goal-directed fantasy, and response to suggestion in hypnotic and task-motivated subjects. *American Journal of Clinical Hypnosis, 18,* 254-262.

Spanos, N. P., Stam, H. J., & Brazil, K. (1981). The effects of suggestion and distraction on coping ideation and reported pain. *Journal of Mental Imagery, 5,* 75-89.

Spanos, N. P., Stam, H. J., D'Eon, J. L., Pawlak, A. E., & Radtke-Bodorik, H. L. (1980). The effects of social psychological variables on posthypnotic amnesia. *Journal of Personality and Social Psychology, 39,* 737-750.

Spanos, N. P., Stam, H. J., Rivers, S. M., & Radtke, H. L. (1980). Meditation, expectation, and performance on indices of nonanalytic attending. *International Journal of Clinical and Experimental Hypnosis, 28,* 244-251.

Spanos, N. P., Stenstrom, R. J., & Johnston, J. C. (1988). Hypnosis, placebo and suggestion in the treatment of warts. *Psychosomatic Medicine, 50,* 245-260.

Spanos, N. P., Tkachyk, M., Bertrand, L. D., & Weekes, J. R. (1984). The dissipation hypothesis of amnesia: More disconfirming evidence. *Psychological Reports, 55,* 191-196.

Spanos, N. P., Voorneveld, P. W., & Gwynn, M. I. (1987). The mediating effects of expectation on hypnotic and nonhypnotic pain reduction. *Imagination, Cognition, and Personality. 6,* 231-246.

Spanos, N. P., Weekes, J. R., & Bertrand, L. D. (1985). Multiple personality: A social psychological perspective. *Journal of Abnormal Psychology, 9,* 362-376.

Spanos, N. P., Weekes, J. R., & de Groh, M. (1984). The "involuntary" countering of suggested requests: A test of the ideomotor hypothesis of hypnotic responsiveness. *British Journal of Experimental and Clinical Hypnosis, 1,* 3-11.

Spanos, N. P., Williams, V., & Gwynn, M. I. (1988). A comparison of hypnotic, salicylic acid, and placebo treatments for the remission of warts. Unpublished manuscript, Carleton University, Ottawa, Canada.

Spiegel, D. (1985). The use of hypnosis in controlling cancer pain. Ca—*A Cancer Journal for Clinicians, 35,* 221-231.

Spiegel, D., & Albert, L. H. (1983). Naloxone fails to reverse hypnotic alleviation of chronic pain. *Psychopharmacology, 81,* 140-143.

Spiegel, D., & Bloom, J. R. (1983). Group therapy and hypnosis reduce metastatic breast carcinoma pain. *Psychosomatic Medicine, 45,* 333-339.

Spiegel, D., Cutcomb, S., Ren, C., & Pribram, K. (1985). Hypnotic hallucination alters evoked potentials. *Journal of Abnormal Psychology. 94,* 249-255.

Spiegel, H., & Spiegel, D. (1978). *Trance and treatment: Clinical uses of hypnosis.* New York: Basic Books.

Spinhoven, P. (1987). Hypnosis and behavior therapy: A review. *International Journal of Clinical and Experimental Hypnosis, 35*(1), 8-31.

Spinhoven, P. (1988). Similarities and dissimilarities in hypnotic and nonhypnotic procedures for headache control: A review. *American Journal of Clinical Hypnosis, 30,* 183-194.

Spinhoven, P., Van Dyck, R., Zitman, F. G., & Linssen, A. C. G. (1985). Treating tension headache: Autogenic training and hypnotic imagery. Presented at the 10th International Congress of Hypnosis and Psychosomatic Medicine, Toronto, Canada.

Springer, C. J., Sachs, L. B., & Morrow, J. E. (1977). Group methods of increasing hypnotic susceptibility. *International Journal of Clinical and Experimental Hypnosis, 25,* 184-191.

Stacher, G., Schuster, P., Bauer, P., Lahoda, R., & Schulze, D. (1975). Effects of relaxation or analgesia on pain threshold and pain tolerance in the waking and in the hypnotic state. *Journal of Psychosomatic Research, 19,* 259-265.

Stalnaker, J. M., & Richardson, M. W. (1930). Time estimation in the hypnotic trance. *Journal of General Psychology, 4,* 362-366.

Stalnaker, J. M., & Riddle, E. E. (1932). The effect of hypnosis on long-delayed recall. *Journal of General Psychology, 6,* 429-440.

Stam, H. J. (1984). Hypnotic analgesia and the placebo effect: Controlling ischemic pain. Dissertation Abstracts International, 44, 2286B.

——. (1989). The practice of Health Psychology and Behavioral Medicine: Whither theory? In W. J. Baker, H. Rappard, L. Mos, & H. J. Stam (Eds.), *Recent trends in theoretical psychology.* New York: Springer.

Stam, H. J., Bultz, B. D., & Pitman, C. A. (1986). Psychosocial problems and interventions in a referred sample of cancer patients. *Psychosomatic Medicine, 48,* 539-548.

Stam, H. J., & Challis, C. B. (in press). Oncologists', nurses' and pharmacists' ratings of cancer chemotherapy toxicity. *Journal of Pain and Symptom Management.*

Stam, H. J., & Fraser, L. C. (1986). Inducing hypnosis: Toward a social constructionist perspective. Paper presented at the annual meeting of the American Psychological Association, Washington, D.C.

Stam, H. J., Goss, C., Rosenal, L., Ewens, S., & Urton, B. (1985). Aspects of psychological distress and pain in cancer patients undergoing radiotherapy. In H. L. Fields et al. (Eds.), *Advances in pain research and therapy* (Vol. 9, pp. 569-573). New York: Raven Press.

Stam, H. J., McGrath, P. A., & Brooke, R. I. (1984). The effects of a cognitive-behavioral treatment program on temporo-mandibular pain and dysfunction syndrome. *Psychosomatic Medicine, 46,* 534-545.

Stam, H. J., Petrusic, W. M. P., & Spanos, N. P. (1981). Magnitude scales for cold pressor pain. *Perception and Psychophysics, 29,* 612-617.

Stam, H. J., & Scott, C. (1988). Knowledge and attitudes about cancer: Canadian Cancer Society surveys, 1954-1986. Unpublished manuscript, University of Calgary.

Stam, H. J., & Spanos, N. P. (1980). Experimental designs, expectancy effects, and hypnotic analgesia. *Journal of Abnormal Psychology, 89,* 551-559.

——. (1987). Hynotic analgesia, placebo analgesia and ischemic pain: The effects of contextual variables. *Journal of Abnormal Psychology, 96,* 313-320.

Stam, H. J., & Steggles, S. (1987). Predicting the onset of progression of cancer from psychological characteristics: Psychometric and theoretical issues. *Journal of Psychosocial Oncology, 5*(2), 35-46.

Stambaugh, E. E., & House, A. E. (1977). Multimodality treatment of migraine headache: A case study utilizing biofeedback, relaxation, autogentic and hypnotic treatments. *American Journal of Clinical Hypnosis, 19,* 235-240.

Standley, K., & Nicholson, J. (1980). Childbirth events and changes in maternal health locus of control beliefs. Paper presented at the annual meeting of the American Psychological Association, Montreal, Canada.

Stanley, S. M., Lynn, S. J., & Nash, M. R. (1986). Trance logic, susceptibility screening, and the transparency response. *Journal of Personality and Social Psychology, 50,* 447-454.

Stenoff, D. N. (1961). Maxillofacial surgery and hypnosis in the emergency and operating room. *Journal of the American Association of Nurses Anesthetists.* February.

Steggles, S., Stam, H. J., Fehr, R., & Aucoin, P. (1987). Hypnosis and cancer: An annotated bibliography 1960-1985. *American Journal of Clinical Hypnosis, 29,* 281-290.

Steinberg, S., & Pennell, E. L., Jr. (1965). Hypnoanesthesia—A case report on a 90-year-old patient. *American Journal of Clinical Hypnosis, 7,* 355-356.

Sterling, K., & Miller, J. G. (1940). The effect of hypnosis upon visual and auditory acuity. *American Journal of Psychology, 53,* 269-276.

Stern, J. A., Brown, M., Ulett, A., & Sletten, I. (1977). A comparison of hypnosis, acupuncture, morphine, Valium, aspirin, and placebo in the management of experimentally induced pain. *Annals of the New York Academy of Sciences, 296,* 175-193.

Sternbach, R. A., & Tursky, B. (1965). Ethnic differences among housewives in psychophysical and skin potential responses to electric shock. *Psychophysiology, 1,* 241-246.

Stevens, R. J. (1976). Psychological strategies for management of pain in prepared childbirth. 1: A review of the research. *Birth and the Family Journal, 3,* 157-164.

Stevens, S. S. (1971). Issues in psychophysical measurement. *Psychological Review, 78,* 426-450.

Stolar, D. (1979). The effect of contingent praise upon hypnotic susceptibility and insusceptibility. Paper presented at the annual meeting of the Society of Clinical and Experimental Hypnosis, Denver.

Stolzenberg, J., & Droger, W. S. (1961). *Dental hypnosis.* Hollywood: Wilshire Book Co.

Stone, C. I., Demchik-Stone, D. A., & Horan, J. (1977). Coping with pain: A component analysis of Lamaze and cognitive-behavioral procedures. *Journal of Psychosomatic Research, 21,* 451-456.

Stone, G. C., Weiss, S. M., Matarazzo, J. D., Miller, N. E., Rodin, J., Belar, C. D., Follick, M. J., & Singer, J. E. (1987). *Health psychology: A discipline and a profession.* Chicago: University of Chicago Press.

Stone, H. (1977). Pain, fear and stress phenomena in dental patients. In A. R. Guerra (Ed.), *Modern anesthesia in dentistry.* Philadelphia: Franklin Institute Press.

Stone, J. A., & Lundy, R. M. (1985). Behavioral compliance with direct and indirect body movement suggestions. *Journal of Abnormal Psychology, 94,* 256-263.

Stone, P., & Burrows, D. (1980). Hypnosis and obstetrics. In G. D. Burrows & L. Dennerstein (Eds.), *Handbook of hypnosis and psychosomatic medicine.* New York: Elsevier/North Holland.

Strack, F., Schwartz, N. & Gschneidinger, E. (1985). Happiness and reminiscing: The role of time perspective, affect, and mode of thinking. *Journal of Personality and Social Psychology, 49,* 1460-1469.

Straus, R. A. (1982). *Strategic self-hypnosis.* Englewood Cliffs, N.J.: Prentice Hall.

———. (1983). Cooperative hypnosis: A less manipulative alternative based upon "non-state theory." *The Annual Review of Hypnosis,* May, pp. 21-33.

Stricherz, M. E. (1982). Social influence, Ericksonian strategies and hypnotic phenomena in the treatment of sexual dysfunction. *American Journal of Clinical Hypnosis, 24* (3), 211-218.

Strosberg, I. M. (1982). Notes on treatment of cancer by hypnosis. *Journal of the American Society of Psychosomatic Dentistry and Medicine. 29* (3), 74-76.

Surman, O. S., Gottlieb, S. K., Hackett, T. P., & Silverberg, E. L. (1973). Hypnosis in the treatment of warts. *Archives of General Psychiatry, 28,* 439-441.

Surman, O. S., Hackett, T. P., Silverberg, E. L., & Behrendt, D. M. (1974). Usefulness of psychiatric interventions in patients undergoing carcdiac surgery. *Archives of General Psychiatry, 30,* 830-835.

Sutcliffe, J. P. (1960). "Credulous" and "skeptical" views of hypnotic phenomena: A review of certain evidence and methodology. *International Journal of Clinical and Experimental Hypnosis, 8,* 73-101.

———. (1961). "Credulous" and "skeptical" views of hypnotic phenomena: Experiments on esthesia, hallucination and delusion. *Journal of Abnormal and Social Psychology, 62,* 189-200.

Sutcliffe, J. P., Perry, C. W., & Sheehan, P. W. (1970). Relation of some aspects of imagery and fantasy to hypnotic susceptibility. *Journal of Abnormal Psychology, 76,* 279-287.

Swedlow, M., & Stjernswärd, J. (1982). Cancer pain relief—an urgent problem. *World Health Forum, 3,* 325-330.

Sweet, W. H. (1981). Some current problems in pain research and therapy (including needle puncture, "acupuncture"). *Pain, 10,* 297-309.

Swirsky-Sacchetti, T., & Margolis, C. G. (1986). The effects of a comprehensive self-hypnosis training program on the use of factor VIII in severe hemophilia. *International Journal of Clinical and Experimental Hypnosis, 34,* 71-83.

Syrjala, K. L., Cummings, C., Donaldson, G., & Chapman, C. R. (1987). Hypnosis for oral pain following chemotherapy and irradiation. Paper presented at the fifth World Conference on Pain, Hamburg, West Germany, August.

Talone, J. M., Diamond, M. J., & Steadman, C. (1975). Modifying hypnotic performance by means of brief sensory experiences. *International Journal of Clinical and Experimental Hypnosis, 25,* 184-191.

Tan, S. Y. (1982). Cognitive and cognitive-behavioral methods for pain control: A Selective Review. *Pain,* 201-208.

Tart, C. T. (1963). Hypnotic depth and basal skin resistance. *International Journal of Clinical and Experimental Hypnosis, 11,* 81-92.

———. (1966). Types of hypnotic dreams and their relation to hypnotic depth. *Journal of Abnormal Psychology, 71,* 377-382.

———. (1970a). Self-report scales of hypnotic depth. *International Journal of Clinical and Experimental Hypnosis, 18,* 105-125.

———. (1970b). Increases in hypnotizability resulting from a prolonged program for enhancing personal growth. *Journal of Abnormal Psychology, 75,* 260-266.

———. (1979a). Quick and convenient assessment of hypnotic depth: Self-report scales. *American Journal of Clinical Hypnosis, 21,* 186-207.

Tart, C. T. (1979b). Measuring the depth of an altered state of consciousness with particular reference to self-report scales of hypnotic depth. In E. Fromm & R. E. Shor (Eds.), *Hypnosis: Developments in research and new perspectives (2nd ed.).* New York: Aldine.

Tart, C. T., & Hilgard, E. R. (1966). Responsiveness to suggestions under "hypnosis" and "waking-imagination" conditions: A methodological observation. *International Journal of Clinical and Experimental Hypnosis, 14,* 247-256.

Taugher, V. J. (1958). Hypno-anesthesia. *Wisconsin Medical Journal, 57,* 95-96.

Tebecis, A. K., & Provins, K. A. (1974). Accuracy of time estimation during hypnosis. *Perceptual and Motor Skills, 39,* 1123-1126.

Tellegen, A. (1976). *Differential personality questionnaire.* University of Minnesota.

———. (1979). On measures and conceptions of hypnosis. *American Journal of Clinical Hypnosis, 21,* 219-237.

———. (1981). Practicing the two disciplines for relaxation and enlightenment: Comment on "Role of the feedback signal in electromyograph biofeedback: The relevance of attention" by Qualls and Sheehan. *Journal of Experimental Psychology: General, 110,* 217-226.

Tellegen, A., & Atkinson, G. (1974). Openness to absorbing and self-altering experiences ("absorption"), a trait related to hypnotic susceptibility. *Journal of Abnormal Psychology, 83,* 268-277.

———. (1976). Complexity and measurement of hypnotic susceptibility: A comment on Coe's and Carbin's alternative interpretation. *Journal of Personality and Social Psychology, 33,* 142-148.

Thelen, M. H., & Fry, R. A. (1981). The effects of modeling and selective attention on pain tolerance. *Journal of Behavior Therapy and Experimental Psychiatry, 12,* 225-229.

Theodor, L. H., & Mandelcorn, M. S. (1973) Hysterical blindness: A case report and study using modern psychophysical technique. *Journal of Abnormal Psychology, 82,* 552-553.

t'Hoen, P. (1978). Effects of hypnotizability and visualizing ability on imagery mediated learning. *International Journal of Clinical and Experimental Hypnosis, 26,* 45-54.

Thomas, H., & Karlovsky, E. D. (1954). Two thousand deliveries under a training for childbirth program: A statistical survey and commentary. *American Journal of Obstetrics and Gynecology, 68,* 279-284.

Tiba, J., Balogh, I., Meszaros, I., Banyai, E., Greguss, A. C., & Jakubecz, S. (1980). Hypnotherapy during pregnancy, delivery and child-bed: First steps in Hungary. In M. Panjntar, E. Roskar, & M. Lavric (Eds.), *Hypnosis in Psychotherapy and Psychosomatic Medicine.* Ljubljana, Yugoslavia: University Press.

Timm, H. W. (1981). The effects of forensic hypnosis techniques on eyewitness recall and recognition. *Journal of Police Science and Administration, 9,* 188-194.

———. (1985). An examination of the effects of forensic hypnosis. In D. Waxman et al., *Modern Trends in Hypnosis.* New York: Plenum.

Tinterow, M. M. (1960). The use of hypnotic anesthesia for major surgical procedures. *American Surgeon, 26,* 732-737.

Titchener, E. B. (1909). *Lectures on the experimental psychology of the thought-processes.* New York: The Macmillan Company.

Tkach, W. (1972). A firsthand report from China: "I have seen acupuncture work," says Nixon's doctor. *Today's Health, 50,* 50-56.

Tkachyk, M., Spanos, N. P., & Bertrand, L. D. (1985). Variables affecting subjective organization during posthypnotic amnesia. *Journal of Research in Personality, 19,* 95-108.

Todorovic, D. D. (1959). Hypnosis in military medical practice. *Military Medicine, 34,* 121-125.

Tomkins, S. S. (1979). Script theory: Differential magnification of affects. In H. E. Howe, Jr., & R. A. Diensbier (Eds.), *Nebraska Symposium on Motivation,* (Vol. 26). Lincoln: University of Nebraska Press.

Tower, R. B. (1982). Imagery: Its role in development. In A. A. Sheikh (Ed.), *Imagery, current theory, research and application.* New York: John Wiley & Sons.

True, R. M. (1949). Experimental control in hypnotic age regression states. *Science, 110,* 583-584.

Trzebinski, J. (1985). Action-oriented representations of implicit personality theories. *Journal of Personality and Social Psychology, 48,* 1266-1278.

Tsao, Y., Wittlieb, E., Miller, B., & Wang, T. (1983). Time estimation of a secondary event. *Perceptual and Motor Skills, 57,* 1051-1055.

Tuckey, C. L. (1889). Psychotherapeutics; or treatment by hypnotism. *Woods Medical and Surgical Monographs, 3,* 721-795.

Tulving, E. (1972). Episodic and semantic memory. In E. Tulving & W. Donaldson (Eds.), *Organization of memory.* New York: Academic Press.

Tulving, E., & Perlstone, Z. (1966). Availability vs. accessibility of information in memory for words. *Journal of Verbal Learning and Verbal Behavior, 5,* 381-391.

Turk, D. C. (1977). A coping skills-training approach for the control of experimentally produced pain. Unpublished doctoral dissertation, University of Waterloo.

Turk, D., & Salovey, P. (1985). Cognitive structures, cognitive processes, and cognitive behavior modification: II. Judgments and inferences of the clinician. *Cognitive Therapy and Research, 9,* 19-33.

Turk, D. C., Meichenbaum, D., & Genest, M. (1983). *Pain and behavioral medicine: A cognitive behavioral perspective.* New York: Guilford.

Turner, P. S. (1906). Some results withblue rays in the relief of pain. *Practical Dental Journal,* 653-656.

Udolf, R. (1983). *Forensic hypnosis: Psychological and legal aspects.* Lexington, Mass.: Lexington Books.

Udolf, R. (1987). *Handbook of hypnosis for professionals, 2nd edition.* New York: Van Nostrand Reinhold.

Ulett, G. A., Akpinar, S., & Itil, T. M. (1972). Hypnosis: Physiological, pharmacological reality. *American Journal of Psychiatry, 138,* 799-805.

Ullman, M. (1947). Herpes simplex and second degree burn induced under hypnosis. *American Journal of Psychiatry, 103,* 828-830.

Underwood, B. J., & Shaughnessy, J. J. (1975). *Experimentation in psychology.* New York: Wiley.

Vallacher, R. R., & Wegner, D. M. (1987). What do people think they are doing? Action identification and human behavior. *Psychological Review, 94,* 3-5.

Van Dyke, P. B. (1965). Hypnosis in surgery. *Journal of Abdominal Surgery, 7,* 1-5.

Van Gorp, W. G., Meyer, R. G. & Dunbar, K. (1985). The efficacy of direct versus indirect hypnotic induction techniques on reduction of experimental pain. *International Journal of Clinical and Experimental Hypnosis, 33,* 329-328.

Van Nuys, D. (1973). Meditation, attention and hypnotic susceptibility: A correlational study. *International Journal of Clinical and Experimental Hypnosis, 21.*

———. (1977). Successful treatment of sacroiliac pain by telephone. *Journal of the American Society of Psychosomatic Dentistry and Medicine, 24,* 73-75.

Venn, J. (1987). Hypnosis and Lamaze Method—an exploratory study: A brief communication. *The International Journal of Clinical and Experimental Hypnosis, 35,* 79-82.

Vickery, A. R., & Kirsch, I. (1985). Expectancy and skill training in the modification of hypnotizability. Paper presented at the meeting of the American Psychological Association, Los Angeles.

Vickery, A. R., Kirsch, I., Council, J. R., & Sirkin, M. I. (1985). Cognitive skill and traditional trance hypnotic inductions: A within-subject comparison. *Journal of Consulting and Clinical Psychology, 53,* 131-133.

Vincent, C. AS., & Richardson, P. H. (1986). The evaluation of therapeutic acupuncture. *Pain, 24,* 1-13.

Wachtel, P. (1984). Foreword to *The Unconscious reconsidered.* K. S. Bowers & D. Meichenbaum, (Eds.) New York: Wiley.

Wack, J. T., & Turk, D. C. (1984). Latent structure of strategies used to cope with nociceptive stimulation. *Health Psychology, 3,* 27-43.

Wadden, T. A., & Anderton, C. H. (1982). The clinical uses of hypnosis. *Psychological Bulletin, 91,* 215-243.

Wagman, R., & Stewart, C. G. (1975). Visual imagery and hypnotic susceptibility. *Perceptual and Motor Skills, 38,* 815-822.

Wagstaff, G. F. (1977). Posthypnotic amnesia as disrupted retrieval: A role playing paradigm. *Quarterly Journal of Experimental Psychology, 29,* 499-500.

———. (1981). *Hypnosis as compliance and belief.* New York: St. Martin's.

———. (1981). Hypnotic amnesia and compliance. *Bulletin of the British Society for Experimental and Clinical Hypnosis, 4,* 17-18.

———. (1981). Source amnesia and trance logic: Artifacts in the essence of hypnosis? *Bulletin of the British Society of Experimental and Clinical Hypnosis, 4,* 3-5.

———. (1981). Suggested amnesia: Compliance or inattention-encoding specificity? *Bulletin of the British Journal of Experimental and Clinical Hypnosis, 4,* 3-5.

———. (1981). The use of hypnosis in police investigation. *Journal of the Forensic Science Society, 21,* 3-7.

———. (1981). The validity of posthypnotic amnesia. Paper presented to the Experimental Psychology Society, Liverpool.

———. (1982a). Amnesia, compliance and men of straw: A tailpiece. *Bulletin of the British Society of Experimental and Clinical Hypnosis, 5,* 42-45.

———. (1982b). Hypnosis and recognition of a face. *Perceptual and Motor Skills, 55,* 816-818.

———. (1982c). Hypnosis and witness recall: A discussion paper. *Journal of the Royal Society of Medicine, 75,* 793-797.

———. (1983a). A comment on McConkey's "Challenging hypnotic effects: The impact of conflicting influences on response to hypnotic suggestions." *British Journal of Experimental and Clinical Hypnosis, 1,* 11-15.

Wagstaff, G. F. (1983b). Suggested improvement of visual acuity: A statistical reevaluation. *International Journal of Clinical and Experimental Hypnosis, 31,* 239-240.

———. (1984). The enhancement of witness memory by "hypnosis": A review and methodological critique of the experimental literature. *British Journal of Experimental and Clinical Hypnosis, 2,* 3-12.

———. (1985). A reply to Perry and Nogrady's "Use of hypnosis by the police in the investigation of crime: Is guided memory a safe substitute?" *British Journal of Experimental and Clinical Hypnosis, 3,* 39-42.

———. (1986). Hypnosis as compliance and belief: A sociocognitive view. In P. Naish (Ed.), *What is hypnosis?* (pp. 59-84). Philadelphia: Open University Press.

———. (1987). Is hypnotherapy a placebo? *British Journal of Experimental and Clinical Hypnosis, 4,* 135-140.

———. (in press, 1989). Public conceptions of forensic hypnosis: Implications for education and practice. In M. Heap (Ed.), *Experimental and clinical hypnosis: Current practices.* Croom Helm.

Wagstaff, G. E., & Carroll, R. (1987). The cognitive-simulation of hypnotic amnesia and disorganized recall. *Medical Science Research, 15,* 85-86.

Wagstaff, G. F., & Maguire, C. (1983). An experimental study of hypnosis, guided memory and witness memory. *Journal of the Forensic Science Society, 23,* 73-78.

Wagstaff, G. F., & Ovenden, M. (1979). Hypnotic time distortion and free-recall learning—An attempted replication. *Psychological Research, 40,* 291-298.

Wagstaff, G. F., & Sykes, C. T. (1984). Hypnosis and the recall of emotionally toned material. *IRCS Medical Science, 12,* 137-138.

Wagstaff, G. F., Traverse, J., & Milner, S. (1982). Hypnosis and eyewitness memory: Two experimental analogues. *IRCS Medical Science, 10,* 894-895.

Wahl, C. W. (1962). Contraindications and limitations of hypnosis in obstetric analgesia. *American Journal of Obstetrics and Gynecology, 84.*

Wain, H. (1980). Pain control through the use of hypnosis. *American Journal of Clinical Hypnosis, 23,* 41-46.

Wakeman, R. J., & Kaplan, J. Z. (1978). An experimental study of hypnosis in painful burns. *American Journal of Clinical Hypnosis, 21,* 3-12.

Walker, N. S., Garratt, J. B., & Wallace, B. (1976). Restoration of eidetic imagery via hypnotic age regression: A preliminary report. *Journal of Abnormal Psychology, 85,* 335-337.

Wallace, B. (1979). Hypnotic susceptibility and the perception of after-images and dot stimuli. *American Journal of Psychology, 92,* 681-691.

———. (1984). Apparent equivalence between perception and imagery in the production of various visual illusions. *Memory and Cognition, 12,* 156-162.

Wallace, B., & Patterson, S. L. (1984). Hypnotic susceptibility and performance on various attention specific cognitive tasks. *Journal of Personality and Social Psychology, 47,* 175-181.

Wallace, G. (1959). Hypnosis in anesthesiology. *International Journal of Clinical and Experimental Hypnosis, 7,* 129-137.

Wallace, G., & Coppolino, C. A. (1960). Hypnosis in anesthesiology. *New York Journal of Medicine, 60,* 3258-3273.

Warren, F. D. (1972). Panel discussion. *Transcripts of the Acupuncture Symposium.* Los Altos, Calif.: Academy of Parapsychology and Medicine, pp. 86-92.

Watkins, J. (1978). *The therapeutic self.* New York: Human Sciences Press.

Watkins, J. G. (1984). The Bianchi (L. A. Hillside Strangler) case: Sociopath or multiple personality? *International Journal of Clinical and Experimental Hypnosis, 32,* 67-101.

Watkins, J. G., & Watkins, H. H. (1979). The theory and practice of ego-state therapy. In H. Grayson (Ed.), *Short-term approaches to psychotherapy* (pp. 176-226). New York: Human Sciences Press.

Watson, C. S., & Clopton, D. M. (1969). Motivated changes of auditory sensitivity in a simple detection task. *Perception and Psychophysics, 5,* 281-287.

Watzlawick, P. (1978). *The language of change.* New York: Basic Books.

Waxman, D. (1983). Use of hypnosis in criminology: Discussion paper. *Journal of the Royal Society of Medicine, 76,* 480-484.

Weber, S. J., & Cook, T. D. (1972). Subject effects in laboratory research: An examination of subject roles, demand characteristics, and valid inferences. *Psychological Bulletin, 77,* 273-295.

Wedemeyer, C., & Coe, W. C. (1981). Hypnotic state reports: Contextual variation and phenomenological criteria. *Journal of Mental Imagery, 5,* 107-118.

Weinstock, C. (1983). Psychosomatic elements in 18 consecutive cancer regressions positively not due to somatic therapy. *Journal of the American Society for Dentistry and Medicine, 30,* 151-155.

Weisenberg, M. (1977). Pain and pain control. *Psychological Bulletin, 84,* 1008-1044.

Weishaar, B. B. (1986). A comparison of Lamaze and hypnosis in the management of labor. *American Journal of Clinical Hypnosis, 24,* 149-171.

Weitz, R. D. (1983). Psychological factors in the prevention and treatment of cancer. *Psychotherapy in Private Practice, 1* (4), 69-76.

Weitzenhoffer, A. M. (1953). *Hypnotism: An objective study in suggestibility.* New York: Wiley.

————. (1957). *General techniques of hypnotism.* New York: Grune and Stratton.

————. (1963). The nature of hypnosis, Part 1. *American Journal of Clinical Hypnosis, 5,* 295-321.

————. (1964). Explorations in hypnotic time distortion I: Acquisition of temporal reference frames under conditions of time distortion. *Journal of Nervous and Mental Disease, 138,* 354-366.

————. (1974). When is an "instruction" an "instruction"? *American Journal of Clinical Hypnosis, 22,* 258-269.

————. (1978). What did he (Bernheim) say? In F. H. Frankel & H. S. Zamansky (Eds.), *Hypnosis at its bicentennial.* New York: Plenum.

————. (1980). Hypnotic susceptibility revisited. *American Journal of Clinical Hypnosis, 22,* 130-146.

————. (1982). In search of hypnosis. In D. Waxman, P. C. Misra, M. Gibson, & M. A. Basker (Eds.), *Modern Trends in Hypnosis.* New York: Plenum.

————. (1986). Scientific support for hypnosis and its effects. In B. Zilbergeld, M. G. Edelstein & D. Araoz (Eds.), *Hypnosis: Questions and answers.* New York: W. W. Norton.

Weitzenhoffer, A. M., & Hilgard, E. R. (1959). *The Stanford Scale of Hypnotic Susceptibility, Forms A and B.* Palo Alto, Calif.: Consulting Psychologists Press.

————. (1962). *Stanford Scale of Hypnotic Susceptibility, Form C.* Palo Alto, Calif.: Consulting Psychologists Press.

Weitzenhoffer, A. M., & Weitzenhoffer, G. R. (1958). Personality and hypnotic susceptibility. *American Journal of Clinical Hypnosis, 1,* 79-82.

Wellisch, D. K., & Yager, J. (1981). Is there a cancer-prone personality? In M. B. VanScoy-Mosher (Ed.), *Medical oncology: Controversies in cancer treatment.* Boston: G. K. Hall.

Wells, W. R. (1940). Ability to resist artificially induced dissociation. *Journal of Abnormal and Social Psychology, 35,* 261-272.

Welwood, J. (1980). *The meeting of the ways: Explorations in East/West psychology.* New York: Schocken Books.

Werbel, E. W. (1965). *One surgeon's experience with hypnosis.* New York: Pagent Press.

————. (1967). Hypnosis in serious surgical problems. *American Journal of Clinical Hypnosis, 10,* 44-47.

Werner, W. E. F., Schauble, P. G., & Knudson, M. S. (1982). An argument for the revival of hypnosis in obstetrics. *The American Journal of Clinical Hypnosis, 24,* 149-171.

Weyandt, J. A. (1976). Hypnosis in a dental patient with allergies. *American Journal of Clinical Hypnosis, 19,* 123-125.

White, K. D., Ashton, R., & Brown, R. M. D. (1977). The measurement of imagery vividness: Normative data and their relationship to sex, age, and modality differences. *British Journal of Psychology, 68,* 203-211.

White, K. D., Ashton, R., & Law, H. (1974). Factor analyses of the shortened form of Betts' questionnaire upon mental imagery. *Australian Journal of Psychology, 26,* 183-190.

White, P. A. (1988). Casual processing: Origins and development. *Psychological Bulletin, 104,* 36-52.

White, R. W. (1941a). A preface to the theory of hypnotism. *Journal of Abnormal and Social Psychology, 36,* 477-505.

——. (1941b). An analysis of motivation in hypnosis. *Journal of General Psychology, 24,* 145-162.

White, R. W., Fox, G. F., & Harris, W. W. (1940). Hypnotic hyperamnesia for recently learned material. *Journal of Abnormal and Social Psychology, 35,* 88-103.

Wick, E. (1982). Foreword to D. L. Araoz. *Hypnosis and sex therapy.* New York: Brunner/Mazel.

Wickless, C. & Kirsch, I. (1988). The effects of verbal and experimental expectancy manipulation on hypnotic susceptibility. *Journal of Personality and Social Psychology.*

Wickramasekera, I. (1972). Effects of EMG feedback training on susceptibility to hypnosis: Preliminary observations. In J. Stoyva, T. X. Barber, L. V. DiCara, J. Kamiya, N. E. Miller, & D. Shapiro (Eds.), *Biofeedback and self-control: 1971.* Chicago, Ill.: Aldine-Atherton.

——. (1973). Effects of electromyographic feedback on hypnotic susceptibility: More preliminary data. *Journal of Abnormal Psychology, 82,* 74-77.

Wideman, M. V., & Singer, J. E. (1984). The role of psychological mechanisms in preparation for childbirth. *American Psychologist, 39,* 1357-1371.

Wiggins, J. S. (1973). *Personality and prediction: Principles of personality assessment.* Mass.: Addison-Wesley Publishing.

Wilber, K. (1980). *The human project.* Wheaton, Ill.: Theosophical Publishing House.

Willard, R. D. (1974). Perpetual trance as a means of controlling pain in the treatment of terminal cancer with hypnosis. *Journal of the American Institute of Hypnosis, 15* (3), 111-131.

Williamsen, J. A., Johnson, H. J., & Eriksen, C. W. (1965). Some characteristics of posthypnotic amnesia. *Journal of Abnormal Psychology, 70,* 123-131.

Wilson, D. L. (1967). The role of confirmation of expectancies in hypnotic induction. *Dissertation Abstracts, 28,* 4787-B.

Wilson, L., Greene, E., & Loftus, E. F. (1986). Beliefs about forensic hypnosis. *International Journal of Clinical and Experimental Hypnosis, 34,* 110-121.

Wilson, L., and Kihlstrom, J. F. (1986). Subjective and categorical organization of recall during posthypnotic amnesia. *Journal of Abnormal Psychology, 95* (3), 264-273

Wilson, N. J. (1968). Neurophysiologic alternations with hypnosis. *Diseases of the Nervous System, 29,* 618-629.

Wilson, S. C., & Barber, T. X. (1978). The creative imagination scale as a measure of hypnotic responsiveness. *American Journal of Clinical Hypnosis, 20,* 235-249.

——. (1981). Vivid fantasy and hallucinatory abilities in the life histories of excellent hypnotic subjects ("somnambules"): Preliminary report with female subjects. In E. Klinger (Ed.), *Imagery Volume 2: Concepts, results and applications* (pp. 133-152). New York: Plenum Press.

——. (1983). The fantasy-prone personality: Implications for understanding imagery, hypnosis, and parapsychological phenomena. In A. A. Sheikh (Ed.), *Imagery: Current theory, research, and application* (pp. 340-387). New York: John Wiley & Sons.

Wilson, T. (1985). Self-deception without repression. In M. W. Martin (Ed.), *Self-deception and self-understanding.* University of Kansas Press.

Winkelstein, L. B., & Levinson, J. (1959). Fulminating pre-eclampsia with caesarean section performed under hypnosis. *American Journal of Obstetrics and Gynecology, 78,* 420-423.

Winsberg, B., & Greenlick, M. (1976). Pain response in Negro and White obstetrical patients. *Journal of Health and Social Behavior, 8,* 222-228.

Winnicott, D. W. (1965). The theory of the parent-infant relationship. In D. W. Winnicott's (Ed.), *The maturational processes and the facilitating environment* (pp. 37-55). New York: International Universities Press.

Wittgenstein, L. (1953). *Philosophical investigations* (2nd ed.). Oxford: Blackwell.

——. (1980). *Remarks on the philosophy of psychology* (Vol. 1). Oxford: Blackwell.

Wolberg, (1972). *Hypnosis: Is it for you?* New York: Harcourt Brace Jovanovich.

Wolff, B. B. (1971). Factor analysis of human pain response: Pain endurance as a specific pain factor. *Journal of Abnormal Psychology, 78,* 292-298.

Wolff, B. B., & **Langley, S.** (1968). Cultural factors and the response to pain: A review. *American Anthropologist, 70,* 494-501.

Wolff, B. B., & **Horland, A. A.** (1967). Effects of suggestion upon experimental pain: A validation study. *Journal of Abnormal Psychology, 72,* 402-407.

Wollman, L. (1964). Hypnosis for the surgical patient. *American Journal of Clinical Hypnosis, 7,* 83-85.

Woodforde, L. M., & **Fielding, J. R.** (1975). Pain and cancer. In M. Weisenburg (Ed.), *Pain: Clinical and experimental perspectives* (pp. 332-336). St. Louis: Mosby.

Wooley-Hart, ʾA. (1979). Slowing down the inevitable. *Nursing Mirror, 149,* 36-39.

World Health Organization. (1986). *Cancer pain relief.* Geneva: Author.

Worthington, E. L. (1978). The effects of imagery content, choice of imagery context and self-verbalization on the self-control of pain. *Cognitive Theory and Research, 2,* 225-240.

Wyer, R. S., Jr., & **Srull, T. K.** (1981). Category accessibility. Some theoretical and empirical issues concerning the processing of social stimulus information. In J. H. Flavell & L. Ross (Eds.), *Social cognitive development: Frontiers and possible futures.* New York: Cambridge University Press.

Yanchar, R. J., & **Johnson, H.** (1981). Absorption and attitudes toward hypnosis: A moderator analysis. *International Journal of Clinical and Experimental Hypnosis, 29,* 375-382.

Yanovski, A., & **Briklin, B.** (1967). Spontaneous abreaction during major surgery under hypnosis. *Psychiatry Quarterly, 41,* 496-5124.

Yates, A. J. (1961). Hypnotic age regression. *Psychological Bulletin, 58,* 429-440.

Young, J., & **Cooper, L. M.** (1972). Hypnotic recall amnesia as a function of manipulated expectancy. *Proceedings of the 80th Annual Convention of the American Psychological Association, 7,* 857-858.

Young, P. C. (1927). Is rapport an essential characteristic of hypnosis? *Journal of Abnormal and Social Psychology, 22,* 130-139.

——. (1928). The nature of hypnosis: As indicated by the presence or absence of posthypnotic amnesia and rapport. *Journal of Abnormal and Social Psychology, 22,* 372-382.

——. (1948). Antisocial uses of hypnosis. In L. M. LeCron (ed.), *Experimental hypnosis* (pp. 376-409). New York: Macmillan.

——. (1952). Antisocial uses of hypnosis. In L. M. Le Cron (Ed.), *Experimental hypnosis, 2nd ed.* (pp. 376-409). New York: Macmillan.

Yuille, J. C., & **McEwan, N. J.** (1985). Use of hypnosis as an aid to eyewitness memory. *Journal of Applied Psychology, 70,* 389-400.

Zamansky, H. S. (1977). Suggestion and countersuggestion in hypnotic behavior. *Journal of Abnormal Psychology, 86,* 346-351.

Zamansky, H. S., & **Bartis, S. P.** (1985). The dissociation of an experience: The hidden observer observed. *Journal of Abnormal Psychology, 94,* 243-248.

Zamansky, H. S., & **Clark, L. R.** (1986). Cognitive competition and hypnotic behavior: Whither absorption. *International Journal of Clinical and Experimental Hypnosis, 34,* 20-214.

Zelig, M., & **Beidleman, W. B.** (1981). The investigative use of hypnosis: A word of caution. *International Journal of Clinical and Experimental Hypnosis, 29* (4), 401-412.

Zeltzer, L., Kellerman, J., Ellenberg, L., & **Dash, J.** (1983). Hypnosis for reduction of vomiting associated with chemotherapy and disease in adolescents with cancer. *Journal of Adolescent Health Care 4,* 77-84.

Zeltzer, L., & LeBaron, S. (1982). Hypnosis and nonhypnotic techniques for reduction of pain and anxiety during painful procedures in children and adolescents with cancer. *Journal of Pediatrics, 101,* 1032-1035.

——. (1983). Behavioral intervention for children and adolescents with cancer. *Behavioral Medicine Update, 5* (2-3), 17-22.

Zeltzer, L., LeBaron, S., & Zeltzer, P. M. (1984). The effectiveness of behavioral intervention for reduction of nausea and vomiting in children and adolescents receiving chemotherapy. *Journal of Clinical Oncology, 2,* 683-689.

Zilberfeld, B. (1978). *Male sexuality: A guide to sexual fulfillment.* Boston: Little, Brown and Company.

Zimbardo, P. G., Marshall, G., & Maslach, C. (1971). Liberating behavior from time-bound control: Expanding the present through hypnosis. *Journal of Applied Social Psychology, 1,* 305-323.

Zimbardo, P. G., Marshall, G., White, G., & Maslach, C. (1973). Objective assessment of hypnotically induced time distortion. *Science, 181,* 282-284.

Contributors

LORNE D. BERTRAND, PH.D., is a Postgraduate Fellow in the Department of Psychology at the University of Calgary. His research interests are in human memory, hypnotizability, and hypnotic amnesia.

JOHN F. CHAVES, PH.D., is Professor and Head of the Section of Behavioral Science in the Department of Community Dentistry at the School of Dental Medicine, Southern Illinois University. His research interests are psychological aspects of anxiety and pain management, as well as behavioral medicine and dentistry.

WILLIAM C. COE, PH.D., is Professor of Psychology at California State University at Fresno. His research interests are hypnosis, hypnotic amnesia, social influence processes, and psychopathology.

JAMES R. COUNCIL, PH.D., is Assistant Professor of Psychology at the University of North Dakota. His research interests are hypnosis, expectancy effects, and fantasy and imaginal processes.

MARGARET DE GROH is a doctoral candidate in the Department of Psychology at Carleton University, Ottawa. Her research interests are hypnosis and issues of psychological measurement.

HANS P. DE GROOT is a doctoral candidate in the Department of Psychology at Carleton University, Ottawa. His research interests are hypnosis and the psychology of occult beliefs.

JOYCE L. D'EON, PH.D., manages the Center for Chronic Pain at the Rehabilitation Center, Ottawa. Her research interests are hypnosis, chronic pain and its management, the psychology of childbirth, and behavioral medicine.

MICHAEL JAY DIAMOND, Ph.D., is an Adjunct Professor of Psychology at the University of California in Los Angeles and a clinical psychologist in private practice. His research interests are hypnosis, hypnotherapy, and the modification of hypnotizability.

DEBORA M. FLYNN is a doctoral candidate in the Department of Psychology at Carleton University, Ottawa. Her research interests are perception, social psychology, and hypnosis.

MAXWELL I. GWYNN is a doctoral candidate in the Department of Psychology at Carleton University, Ottawa. His research interests are hypnosis, pain, eyewitness testimony, and suggestibility.

RICHARD F. Q. JOHNSON, PH.D., is a research psychologist for the U.S. Army. His research interests include hypnosis and suggestion-induced dermatological changes.

WILLIAM J. JONES, PH.D., is Professor and Chairman of the Department of Psychology at Carleton University, Ottawa. His research interests are perception and psychophysics, cerebral laterality, pain, and hypnosis. He also has scholarly interests in the philosophy of science and the history of psychoanalysis.

IRVING KIRSCH, PH.D., is Professor of Psychology at the University of Connecticut. His research interests are hypnosis, behavior modification, expectancy effects, and the history of psychology and psychiatry.

STEVEN J. LYNN, PH.D., is Professor of Psychology at Ohio University. His research interests are hypnosis, hypnotherapy, and imaginal and fantasy processes.

H. LORRAINE RADTKE, PH.D., is Associate Professor of Psychology at the University of Calgary. Her research interests are in hypnosis and in the psychology of women.

JUDITH W. RHUE, PH.D., is Assistant Professor of Psychology at the University of Toledo. Her research interests are hypnosis and the assessment and correlates of fantasy.

RICHARD ST. JEAN, PH.D., is Professor of Psychology at the University of Prince Edward Island, Canada. He has research interests in cognitive psychology, the psychology of time perception, and hypnosis.

THEODORE R. SARBIN, PH.D., is Professor Emeritus at the University of California at Santa Cruz. He is a distinguished pioneer in the areas of hypnosis research and social role theory. He maintains research interests in these areas as well as in psychopathology, criminality, and the history of psychology and psychopathology.

NICHOLAS P. SPANOS, PH.D., is Professor of Psychology and Director of the Laboratory for Experimental Hypnosis at Carleton University, Ottawa. His research interests include hypnosis, pain control, psychopathology, the social psychology of the courtroom, and the history of psychology and psychopathology.

HENDERIKUS J. STAM, PH.D., is Associate Professor of Psychology at the University of Calgary. His research interests are hypnosis, the history of psychology, and psychological aspects of cancer and its treatment.

GRAHAM F. WAGSTAFF, PH.D., is in the Psychology Department at the University of Liverpool, England. His research interests are the social psychology of hypnosis, forensic aspects of hypnosis, compliance, and the psychology of belief.

JOHN R. WEEKES is a doctoral candidate in the Department of Psychology at Ohio University. His research interests are hypnosis, imagination, and the forensic aspects of hypnosis.